Sally MILIAN
Phmy 7T7
731511439.

BACTERIOLOGY AND IMMUNOLOGY
FOR STUDENTS OF MEDICINE

F. S. STEWART
M.D., F.R.C.P.I., F.C.Path., M.R.I.A.

Fellow of Trinity College, Dublin
Professor of Bacteriology and Preventive Medicine, University of Dublin
Consultant Bacteriologist, Sir Patrick Dun's, Adelaide, Meath
and Royal City of Dublin Hospitals
Consultant Serologist, Rotunda Hospital

Bacteriology and Immunology for Students of Medicine

FORMERLY BIGGER'S HANDBOOK OF BACTERIOLOGY

Ninth Edition

F. S. Stewart

Baillière Tindall & Cassell
LONDON

First Edition	January 1925
Second Edition	February 1929
Reprinted	October 1930
Third Edition	March 1932
Reprinted	August 1933
Fourth Edition	September 1935
Reprinted	February 1938
Fifth Edition	May 1939
Reprinted	September 1945
Reprinted	September 1946
Reprinted	March 1948
Sixth Edition	October 1949
Seventh Edition	February 1959
Reprinted	October 1961
Eighth Edition	July 1962
Reprinted	December 1963
Ninth Edition	August 1968
Reprinted	July 1970
Reprinted	February 1971
Reprinted	November 1972

© 1968 Baillière, Tindall and Cassell Ltd
7–8 Henrietta Street, London, WC2 E 8QE

I.S.B.N. 0–7020–0265–8

Published in the United States by
The Williams & Wilkins Company, Baltimore

Made and printed in Great Britain by
William Clowes and Sons, Limited, London, Beccles and Colchester

CONTENTS

COLOUR PLATES

PREFACE TO THE NINTH EDITION

With this edition *Bigger's Handbook of Bacteriology* appears under a new title. The change in title was made for two reasons. Firstly, it had for some time been clear that the designation 'Handbook', suggesting as it does a practical laboratory manual, was no longer appropriate to its content. Secondly, as compared with the last of Bigger's own editions—the 6th in 1949—it has become, to all intents and purposes, a new book. Nevertheless the scaffolding of the book and its primary objective—that is to present within a reasonable compass the fundamental principles of medical microbiology and immunology—are still the same.

In the five years since the appearance of the last edition the explosive growth of microbiology and immunology has continued—a growth which necessarily involved a substantial rewriting of the text. The major changes have been in the sections on immunology, virology and chemotherapy. In addition the introductory chapter on bacterial cytology, physiology and genetics has been considerably expanded. No part of the book however has escaped major revision and about half the text is new. As well as the new textual material there are a considerable number of new photographs, diagrams and tables, prepared or selected primarily on the basis of their informational or explanatory content. At the same time there has been a further rigorous pruning of descriptions and data of purely technical or taxonomic interest. The progress of recent years not only has required the substitution of new material for old but has also involved a change in orientation. Progress has been most conspicuous at fundamental levels and has led to a great increase in our understanding, still far from complete, of basic biological mechanisms. This has been particularly the case in respect of microbial genetics, the mode of action of antimicrobial drugs, the structure and intracellular replication of viruses, the composition and production of antibodies and the nature and consequences of immune and allergic reactions. As a result the book is more clearly based on general biological and biochemical principles than its predecessors. Nevertheless like the latter it has been designed specifically to meet the requirements of students of medicine, and microbiology and immunology are presented in the first instance as providing a scientific basis for the practice of medicine.

In the preface to *The Concise Oxford Dictionary*, H. W. Fowler says 'A dictionary maker, unless he is a monster of omniscience, must deal with a great many matters of which he has no firsthand knowledge'. This can certainly be taken to apply *a fortiori* to the author of a scientific work attempting to present an up to date and authoritative account of an area as extensive as that covered in this book. It has, of course, only been possible to do so by drawing extensively on the works of other authors, and in the bibliography I have listed those sources which I have found most valuable. In addition I am indebted to Dr J. D. McKeever for his careful and critical reading of the proofs and for valuable suggestions, to Mrs Mary McLoughlin for assistance in the compilation of abstracts and references, to Mr T. Harvey and Miss Doreen Miggin for photographic and technical assistance respectively, to Miss Doreen O'Driscoll for her painstaking typing of the text, to my daughter Caroline and my son Bruce for their help in the preparation of the index, to my wife for a further diagram, to Dr June D. Almeida, Dr E. M. Brieger, Professor J. P. Duguid, Dr R. W. Horne, Professor M. A. Epstein and Dr T. H. Flewett for new photographs, and, for permission to reproduce photographic material first published elsewhere, to the Academic Press (*Virology*, *Journal of Molecular Biology*, 'Structure and Ultrastructure of Micro-organisms' by E. M. Brieger), Messrs Oliver and Boyd (*Journal of Pathology and Bacteriology*) and the Editor, the *British Medical Journal*.

Dublin   F. S. Stewart
April 1968

CHAPTER 1

THE GENERAL PROPERTIES OF BACTERIA

The term bacteria is applied in a general sense to a somewhat heterogeneous collection of minute unicellular organisms of relatively simple structure. As a group bacteria are closely related both to the simpler plants—the microscopic algae and fungi—and to the simpler animals—the protozoa—but may be regarded as even simpler and more primitive. On the whole their resemblance to the algae and fungi is greater than to the protozoa and they are therefore usually classified in the plant kingdom in which they are assigned to the class *Schizomycetes* or fission fungi.

In certain respects, however, bacteria obviously possess properties normally associated with the animal kingdom, many being actively motile and owing their motility to the possession of organelles-flagella similar to those found in motile protozoa. In fact van Lewenhoek, the discoverer of bacteria, referred to them because of their frequent motility as little animals or 'animalcules'. In order to deal with this dilemma some microbiologists, following the proposal of Haeckel, a nineteenth-century biologist, assigned bacteria and unicellular micro-organisms in general to a kingdom distinct from both the animal and plant kingdoms—the protista. The protista have in turn been divided into higher and lower protists differentiated by the presence or absence of a nuclear membrane. Protozoa and fungi which possess this membrane are classified as higher protists, while others, such as bacteria and blue-green algae are classed as lower protists. This classification is on the whole acceptable since it more explicitly allows us to recognize in bacteria a spectrum of micro-organisms forming a natural bridge between the plant and animal kingdoms. It also has the advantage of making it easier to regard bacteria as being more primitive, in an evolutionary sense, than either plants or animals, and to envisage the common progenitor of both these kingdoms as having been an organism resembling a simpler bacterium.

The number of types of bacteria is enormous, but we are concerned mainly with the small number which is associated with disease in man and other animals. It may be said, however, that the popular conception of bacteria as harmful and unnecessary parasites is very far from the truth. It is almost certain that human life on the earth would be impossible were it not for the innumerable activities of bacteria. They form the link between the animal and vegetable kingdoms and render the dead and useless material of the former available for the growth of plants, on which the life of all animals depends. Further, they fix atmospheric nitrogen and render it available for plant life, which explains the fact that the soil of the earth, suitably tended, is always capable of sustaining vegetation. They are the active agents in many phenomena which are taken so much for granted that the role of the bacteria is often scarcely suspected. The souring of milk, the ripening of cheese, the curing of tobacco, the preparation of leather and a number of other industrial processes depend on the action of bacteria.

The classification of the various types of bacteria presents considerable difficulties and will be more fully considered in a later chapter (Chapter 7). For the moment, however, we may note that on purely morphological grounds they may be subdivided into six main groups.

1. *Bacteria proper or true bacteria.* These are rigid unbranched free-living organisms. To the medical bacteriologist they are the most important of the

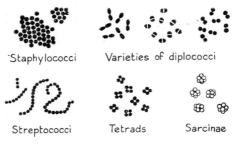

Staphylococci   Varieties of diplococci

Streptococci   Tetrads   Sarcinae

FIG. 1. TYPES OF COCCI

Schizomycetes. They may be further subdivided according to their shape into *cocci, bacilli, vibrios* and *spirilla.*

Cocci are more or less spherical organisms. They are given descriptive names depending on the ways in which the individual organisms are arranged. *Diplococci* are cocci arranged in pairs. *Streptococci* are cocci arranged in chains.

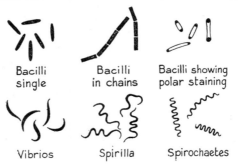

Bacilli
single   Bacilli
in chains   Bacilli showing
polar staining

Vibrios   Spirilla   Spirochaetes

FIG. 2. BACILLI, VIBRIOS, SPIRILLA AND SPIROCHAETES

Staphylococci are cocci arranged in clusters like bunches of grapes. *Tetrads* are cocci arranged in groups of four cells. *Sarcinae* are cocci arranged in cubical packets of eight cells.

Bacilli are rod-shaped bacteria whose length is at least twice their width. Some of the smaller bacilli may, however, assume an almost coccal appearance. *Vibrios* are curved rods the curve of which forms less than one complete spiral. Longer rigid curved organisms usually with several spirals are known as *spirilla*.

2. *Actinomycetes*. These, like the bacteria proper, are rigid organisms but resemble the fungi in that they may show true branching, and in tending to form filaments.

3. *Spirochaetes*. These are flexuous non-branched organisms of spiral shape.

4. *Mycoplasmas*. These are highly pleomorphic organisms of indefinite shape. In general they resemble bacteria which have been deprived of their rigid cell walls (p. 5).

5. *Rickettsiae and chlamydiae*. These are very small organisms which were at one time regarded as being intermediate between viruses and bacteria. The chlamydiae have frequently been described as large viruses, but are now recognized as bacteria, though differing from the true bacteria in being so highly parasitic that they can multiply only within other living cells. This obligatory parasitism is due to a deficiency in the full complement of metabolic enzymes necessary for the maintenance of a free-living existence. Nevertheless, though highly parasitic, these organisms have some independent metabolic capability, and can be regarded as living organisms, in a sense in which viruses (p. 413) manifestly cannot. It seems likely that both rickettsiae and chlamydiae have developed from true bacteria by a process of retrograde evolution.

6. *Miscellaneous higher bacteria*. These have been very inadequately studied and are of doubtful status. They are free-living organisms of unusual morphology, comprising stalked, sheathed, budding and slime forms. Though of great intrinsic interest, they are of no importance in medical microbiology.

Structure of Bacteria

Bacteria are the smallest free-living organisms; their size is measured in microns, one micron (μ) being 1/1000 millimetre, i.e. 1/25,000 inch. Because of this a microscope affording a considerable degree of magnification is necessary for their demonstration. Most of the cocci have a diameter of about 1μ and most of the bacilli measure from 2 to 5μ in length and from 0·5 to 1μ in width. Different species of bacteria tend to have characteristic average dimensions but individual strains may show appreciable deviation from these.

When examined in the living condition bacteria are seen to be transparent, colourless and homogeneous or finely granular. Their presence in liquid, when examined microscopically, can be detected only on account of their refractivity which is close to that of water. Consequently in unstained wet preparations the contrast between bacteria and background is poor. They are therefore usually examined in stained preparations. Staining not only increases contrast and therefore facilitates the visualization of bacteria but also, when stains specific for these are employed, permits the recognition of certain structural features.

For general purposes the stain most frequently employed is Gram's stain (p. 35). On the basis of their reactions in this stain bacteria may be classified into two large groups—the Gram positive and the Gram negative. This classification is of great importance in relation to bacterial identification.

In spite of their small size bacteria have a well organized cellular structure. Like the cells of higher organisms the bacterial cell possesses a *nucleus*, a *cytoplasm* and a *cytoplasmic membrane*. The true bacteria and the actinomycetes resemble plant cells in possessing, in addition, a *cell wall* which is distinct from the cytoplasm and cytoplasmic membrane.

The cell wall is a complex rigid structure which gives bacteria their definite shape. It must possess considerable strength so as to enable it to withstand the osmotic pressure—in some cases this is as much as 20 atmospheres—of the intracellular constituents. Were it not in fact for the cell wall, bacteria would burst since the delicate cytoplasmic membrane would by itself be unable to withstand this high internal pressure. The relationship of the cell wall to the underlying cytoplasmic membrane may be thought of as being like that of a bicycle tyre to its inner tube. The thickness of most bacterial cell walls under normal conditions of growth is in the range of from 10 to 20 mμ—the cell walls of Gram positive bacteria being in general somewhat thicker than those of Gram negative bacteria.

The rigidity of the bacterial cell wall is due to the presence of a basal three-dimensional enveloping structure known as *mucopeptide* or *murein*. The cell wall mucopeptides so far examined have been found to be composed chemically of a backbone consisting of the amino sugars N-acetyl glucosamine and N-acetyl muramic acid, to the muramic acid residues of which are attached peptide side-chains comprising a limited number of amino acids, D- and L-alanine, D-glutamic acid and either L-lysine, diaminopimelic acid, diaminobutyric acid or ornithine. The latter two dibasic amino acids have only recently been

RIBITOL TEICHOIC ACID FROM A STRAIN OF *Staphylococcus aureus*

Gl·N·Ac = N-acetyl glucosamine. $n = 12–16$
Molecule contains one alanine residue for every two ribitol residues

recognized in cell walls. In some species either glycine or aspartic acid is also present. In the intact cell the three-dimensional structure of the mucopeptide is completed by extensive cross linking between neighbouring peptide chains. In *Staphylococcus aureus* this appears to occur through a glycine pentapeptide, linking lysine and terminal D-alanine residues.

The cell wall is the first defence of bacteria against a hostile environment. It is not surprising therefore, that the natural biological destruction of bacteria often starts with an attack on the cell wall. Some hostile micro-organisms, e.g. certain fungi and bacteriophages, produce lysozyme-like enzymes which attack cell walls by hydrolysing the glycosidic linkages between the amino sugars of the mucopeptide backbone. Other micro-organisms appear to secrete enzymes which are capable of splitting off the peptide chains of the mucopeptide. Lysozyme-like enzymes are also found in animal tissues and cells, and there is some evidence that the bactericidal and bacteriolytic action of complement (p. 137) against Gram negative bacteria may require an initial stage of lysozyme activity.

In the case of certain bacteria, notably *Bacillus* species, *Micrococcus lysodeikticus* and *Streptococcus faecalis*, the wall mucopeptide of the intact cell is susceptible to the action of lysozyme. As a result of this action the wall is broken down leaving a structure known as a *protoplast*, which is bounded only by the cytoplasmic membrane. Protoplasts are osmotically sensitive and undergo rapid lysis in isotonic or hypotonic solutions. Because of this they can only be maintained in intact form in hypertonic solutions. Protoplasts may also be obtained from certain bacteria by growing them in the presence of penicillin or other antibiotics which are capable of inhibiting cell wall synthesis. Protoplasts are much more readily prepared from Gram positive than from Gram negative bacteria. This is not surprising, as the mucopeptide is a relatively minor component of the Gram negative cell wall. In fact, protoplasts obtained from Gram negative organisms appear to retain a good deal of the cell wall lipopolysaccharide and lipoprotein.

Mucopeptide is the major constituent of the cell walls of Gram positive bacteria constituting from 50 to as much as 90 per cent of the wall. In Gram negative species, however, mucopeptide constitutes only from 5 to 10 per cent of the wall, but even under these circumstances it is responsible for the osmotic stability of the cell. This is because the osmotic pressure of the Gram negative cell appears to be considerably less than that of the Gram positive cell. In addition to mucopeptide, Gram positive cell walls contain polysaccharides and teichoic acids. The latter are polymeric complexes of ribitol phosphate or glycerol phosphate with simple sugar or amino sugar residues, together with alanine in the unnatural D-configuration. It now seems possible that some at least of these additional components are bound to the mucopeptide by covalent bonds. Their precise significance in cell wall structure is at present unknown. Gram positive cell walls do not appear to contain protein as an integral component of the wall but in some cases protein may be present in a microcapsular or capsular layer, e.g. the M proteins of the streptococci (p. 254), and the glutamyl polypeptides of *Bacillus* species (p. 277).

Gram negative cell walls are biochemically considerably more complex than Gram positive cell walls, and unlike the latter contain a high concentration of lipid and protein. The precise anatomical arrangement of the various components in the Gram negative cell wall is not fully understood. It would appear, however, that the cell wall mucopeptide occurs as an inner layer, outside which is the lipoprotein and lipopolysaccharide, each possibly occurring as further distinct layers.

From the marked difference in cell wall composition shown between the Gram positive and Gram negative bacteria it might be expected that the chemical composition of the cell wall could be useful as a taxonomic criterion. That this is the case was first shown by Cummins and Harris who found that the sugar composition of the cell walls of various Gram positive bacteria was of particular value for differentiation at both generic and species level. Thus the cell walls of *Staphylococcus aureus* contain hexosamine but no simple sugars. Rhamnose is found in the cell walls of many streptococci but is absent from the pneumococcus cell wall, and arabinose is apparently a universal component of the cell walls of the corynebacteria. Recent evidence suggests that the presence of diaminobutyric acid may be associated significantly with plant pathogenicity in the corynebacteria.

Beneath the cell wall, as an anatomically distinct structure, is the cytoplasmic membrane. The membrane is semipermeable, allowing the passage of water but impermeable to large molecular weight compounds and also to many small molecular weight compounds, e.g. simple sugars and amino acids. Because of this it constitutes the osmotic barrier of the cell, controlling the passage of nutrients into the cytoplasm and of end products of metabolism out of it.

Compared with the cell wall the cytoplasmic membrane is very thin, from 60 to 100 Å in cross-section. In many bacteria it has been found possible to achieve some separation of the membrane from the wall—a phenomenon known as plasmolysis—by suspension of the bacteria in a medium of high osmotic tension. This has been much easier to achieve with Gram negative than with Gram positive cells, possibly indicating a closer association of the membrane of the Gram positive cell with the cell wall. This closer association appears also to be borne out by electron micrographs. Chemically the membrane consists of lipoprotein but with up to 20 per cent of carbohydrate. The membranes are thought to have a bimolecular leaflet structure consisting of a double layer of lipid sandwiched between two outer layers of protein. The major portion of the lipid appears to be diphospatidyl glycerol containing long-chain— C-15 and C-17—branched fatty acids. It is possible that the cell membrane may be the main location of the glycerol teichoic acids.

There is considerable evidence that the cytoplasmic membrane, together with its cytoplasmic extensions (see below), may be the functional equivalent of the mitochondria of higher cells. Thus in *Staphylococcus aureus* and *Micrococcus lysodeikticus* it has been found to be the main location of Krebs cycle enzymes (p. 22), of the electron transport chain and of oxidative phosphorylation. It also contains *permeases* which are necessary for the active transport of many small molecular weight organic compounds across the membrane. In addition, recent evidence indicates that, at least in Gram positive cells, the membrane participates in the synthesis of the cell wall.

Morphologically, the bacterial cytoplasm is much simpler than the cytoplasm of higher organisms. Electron micrographs of bacteria have failed to reveal structures analogous to mitochondria, and the complex membranous system of higher organisms known as endoplasmic reticulum and the Golgi apparatus are notably absent. However, recent work has shown the presence, particularly in Gram positive bacteria, of a coiled tubular membranous structure morphologically distinct from a mitochondrium, and occurring in juxtaposition to and apparently continuous with the cytoplasmic membrane of dividing cells. These organelles have been variously designated as *mesosomes* or, because of possible analogy to mitochondria, as chondriods. In function, they are probably similar to the cytoplasmic membrane of which, in the present state of our knowledge, they appear to be intracytoplasmic extensions. Additionally, recent evidence would indicate an important regulatory role in cell division. Evidence that the bacterial chromosome may be physically attached to a mesosome, and the association of mesosomes with the septa of dividing cells suggests an important role for the mesosome in co-ordinating chromosomal replication with cell division.

The main structural components of the bacterial cytoplasm would appear to be the ribonucleoprotein granules, known as *ribosomes*. These measure from 100 to 200 Å units in diameter, and are the sites of protein synthesis. It has been estimated that a single bacterium may contain upwards of 10,000 ribosomes. The ribosomes have been shown to occur in groups, known as *polysomes*, linked together like beads on a chain by messenger RNA (p. 22). The individual ribosomes have a sedimentation coefficient of 70 Svedberg units. Each 70S ribosome is a complex of two smaller units with sedimentation coefficient of 50S and 30S. In the presence of magnesium these form stable complexes to yield a 70S ribosome. In low magnesium concentrations, however, they dissociate and in the absence of magnesium further degradation occurs. Ribosomes appear to be the points of attack of certain antibiotics which act on bacteria by interfering with protein synthesis (Chapter 10).

Although it was for a long time disputed, bacteria are now accepted to possess a structure which is the morphological and functional equivalent of the nucleus of higher organisms. Like the latter it carries the genetic blueprint of the cell coded in the nucleotide sequence of its desoxyribonucleic acid (DNA).

DNA AND PROTEIN COMPOSITION OF AN AVERAGE BACTERIAL CELL

Volume 10^{-12} ml. Dry weight 1.5×10^{11} daltons

DNA	Protein
Single molecule 2000μ long	2×10^6 molecules
Weight 5×10^9 daltons	Weight 9×10^{10} daltons
1.6×10^7 nucleotides	8×10^8 amino acids
2500 nucleotides/gene	400 amino acids/molecule
6400 genes	Possibly 1000 molecular species

Data from K. McQuillen in *Function and Structure in Micro-organisms*. 15th Symposium of the Society for General Microbiology.

The bacterial nucleus can be demonstrated in two ways.

1. It can be stained with basic stains, e.g. Giemsa, following breakdown of

ribosomal RNA by acid hydrolysis or by the action of ribonuclease. As demonstrated by staining procedures nuclei are usually referred to as *chromatin bodies*. Resting cells contain only one chromatin body per cell but dividing cells may contain two or even four. This is due to an asynchrony of nuclear and cellular division.

2. Nuclei may also be seen in electron micrographs of very thin sections of bacteria, where they appear as central areas of lower electron density than the rest of the cell. These areas consist of interlacing bundles of very thin fibrils, about 20 to 60 Å in diameter, in a clear structureless matrix. The nuclear area defined by electron microscopy is usually referred to as the *nucleoplasm*. There is convincing autoradiographic evidence that, in the case of *E. coli* and probably other organisms as well, the nuclear DNA occurs in the form of a single chromosomal thread of about 2000μ in length. Except when mobilized for transfer (p. 27), it exists in the cell as a circular closed loop. One can imagine the coiling necessary to fit this long thread into the nuclear area of a cell which is in itself only 2 to 3μ in length. It is this folding which gives the appearance of bundles of fibrils seen in electron micrographs. This concept of a single chromosomal thread is in agreement with the genetic evidence indicating the determinants of transmissible characters on a single linkage group. The bacterial cell thus differs genetically from the cells of other organisms in being genetically haploid, and in possessing only a single chromosome. There is, therefore, no necessity for the occurrence in bacteria of the complicated series of changes associated with mitosis and meiosis in higher organisms.

The bacterial nucleus differs from the nucleus of higher cells in two further respects.

1. It does not possess a nuclear membrane, and is therefore in direct contact with the cytoplasm of the cell. This may well facilitate rapid transfer of messenger RNA from the nucleus to the ribosomes. Cells lacking a nuclear membrane are sometimes referred to as *procaryotic* in contrast to *eucaryotic* cells which possess a nuclear membrane.

2. The bacterial DNA does not appear to be associated with a basic protein, though the presence of some protein in the nucleus has not been excluded.

Many bacteria possess in addition to the above structures *flagella*, *fimbriae* or *pili*, *capsules*, *spores* and various types of *granules*. Since these structures are found only in certain species their demonstration is of importance in bacterial identification.

Flagella are the locomotor organs of bacteria. They are long, contractile hair-like filaments measuring from 120 to 190 Å in diameter, and usually several microns in length. In some bacterial species, e.g. the enterobacteriaceae, they are arranged along the sides of the organism. This is known as *peritrichous* flagellation. In others, such as *Pseudomonas*, flagella occur singly or in tufts at one or both ends—*polar* flagellation. Individually, flagella are too thin to be seen by ordinary light microscopy but they can be stained by silver impregnation methods. They are best demonstrated by electron microscopy when they appear, particularly those from peritrichously flagellated bacteria, as helical or wave-like structures. In electron micrographs the flagella can be seen to pass through the cell wall and to originate either from the cytoplasm or the cytoplasmic membrane. Though they are not attached to the cell wall, flagella apparently can only initiate movement when the cell wall is present. Thus protoplasts prepared from *Bacillus* species by lysozyme treatment, and possessing apparently normal flagella are non-motile.

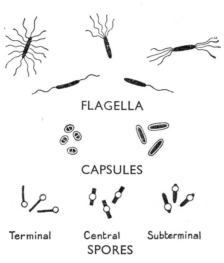

FLAGELLA

CAPSULES

Terminal   Central   Subterminal

SPORES

FIG. 3. FLAGELLA, CAPSULES AND SPORES

From studies with a variety of peritrichously flagellated species it would appear that the standard method of attachment is through a hook at the proximal end of the flagellum. The hook appears to be attached to a disc-like or spherical basal structure the whole complex being closely associated with, and probably directly attached to, the cytoplasmic membrane. The basal structure may have some analogy with the blepharoplasts of the flagellates.

Chemically flagella are composed mainly, if not entirely, of protein. The flagellar protein, known as *flagellin*, appears to have many of the properties of the fibrous proteins, keratin and myosin. In general, flagellar proteins appear to lack a full complement of amino acids, being deficient particularly in tryptophane, histidine, proline and cysteine. The flagellar protein of *Salmonella typhimurium* is of interest in that it contains an unusual amino acid, ε-N-methyllysine.

The flagella of *Salmonella typhimurium* are built up from globular subunits of flagellin apparently disposed helically around a hollow core, five subunits forming one complete turn of the helix. Under acid conditions the subunits dissociate but on reversal of these conditions they reaggregate spontaneously to reform intact flagella. This process is analogous to the self-assembly of virus capsids (p. 418), and suggests that under in vivo conditions flagella may be spontaneously assembled from prefabricated flagellin subunits. Some support for this concept has been obtained from the observation that the regeneration of flagella by organisms that have been deflagellated by mechanical means is insensitive to chloramphenicol—an active inhibitor of protein synthesis. In this case it was found that if the organisms prior to exposure to chloramphenicol had been labelled with C[14] the resynthesized flagella were radioactive. These findings are consistent with the concept of spontaneous assembly of the flagella from a pool of flagellin subunits. Serological evidence for the existence of an intracellular pool of flagellin has also been obtained. However the discovery of a bacterial mutant capable of synthesizing flagellin at 45° C, but incapable of synthesizing intact flagella at this temperature, indicates the possibility that some biological assembly process over and above spontaneous self-assembly may be involved. There is also some evidence that a primer consisting of a short flagellar fragment is a necessary prerequisite for the assembly process, in which the fragment might act as a nucleus for crystallization.

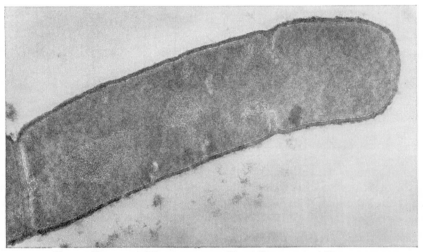

FIG. 4. ELECTRON MICROGRAPH OF THIN SECTION OF A BACILLUS
Note cell wall, transverse septum and nucleoids
(From Glauert, Brieger and Allen (1961) *Exp. Cell Res.*, 22, 73: Academic Press)

The most conclusive evidence that flagella are the organs of bacterial motility, is the fact that bacteria from which the flagella have been removed by violent agitation are non-motile, though still viable. Motility appears to be due to the passage of helical waves of contraction down the flagellum, the waves tending to propel the bacterium forward. How the contraction wave is generated, and the mechanism by which it obtains its energy, are not known. The presence of adenosine triphophatase, which by breaking down ATP might release the necessary energy, has not so far been demonstrated in bacterial flagella. The speed with which flagella can propel bacteria is considerable, actively motile species being capable of travelling at speeds of up to 50μ per second. For a typical Gram negative bacillus of approximately 5μ in length this would mean moving at the rate of ten times its own length per second—equivalent for an adult man of a 100 yard dash in 5 seconds.

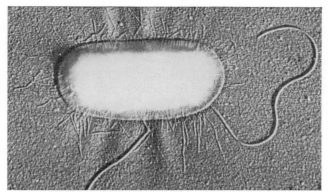

FIG. 5. ELECTRON MICROGRAPH OF *E. coli* SHOWING FIMBRIAE
AND TWO LONG WAVY FLAGELLA (From Duguid, *J. Path. Bact.*
1955, *70*, 335)

Fimbriae or *pili* are hair-like processes attached to the cell wall and are only found in certain bacteria, particularly in the Gram negative bacilli. They differ from flagella in being shorter and thinner, straight, and play no part in the motility of the organism. Fimbriae cannot be demonstrated with the light microscope but can be seen in suitably prepared electron micrographs. They are best developed when the bacteria are grown in fluid media. They are probably structures by which bacteria can attach themselves to cells and to other particulate material. Fimbriated bacteria readily adsorb to and agglutinate the red cells of certain animal species. Fimbriae possess antigens different from those of the body of the organism and of the flagella. Recent evidence indicates that, at least in the enterobacteriaceae, highly specialized pili constitute the conjugation tubes through which genetic material is transferred from one cell to another in bacterial conjugation (p. 26).

Bacteria of the genera *Bacillus* and *Clostridium* produce highly resistant dormant forms known as *spores*. These appear first as round or oval bodies which form within the cytoplasm of the organism. They are highly refractile but stain with great difficulty. In simple Gram stained preparations they appear as clear unstained areas. When stained, however, e.g. by Möller's method, they hold the stain firmly and are not readily decolorized. The spore may be situated in the centre of the bacillus-equatorial, near one end-subterminal, or protruding from one end-terminal, the precise location being constant within a single species. In the *Bacillus* genus the diameter of the spore is normally less than that of the bacterium but in the genus *Clostridium* the spore is usually wider than the bacterium.

The first stage in the formation of the spore is a condensation of chromatin, apparently representing half the cellular DNA, in an area at one end of the bacterium known as the *spore field* which is destined to be the site of formation of the new spore. At the same time a transverse septum derived from the cytoplasmic membrane forms by a process of invagination, and divides the developing spore, now known as the *forespore*, from the rest of the bacillus, known as the *sporangium*. From this stage on, the two areas of the cell are functionally distinct, the sporangium continuing to produce components characteristic of the vegetative form, and the forespore producing components characteristic of the spore. The dividing septum eventually completely encircles the fore-spore as a double-layered membrane, the inner layer of which becomes the spore wall. The spore *cortex* is then laid down between the inner and outer layers, and the process completed by transformation of the outer layer into the spore coats and *exosporium*.

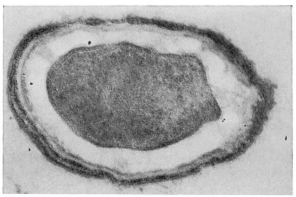

FIG. 6. ELECTRON MICROGRAPH OF THIN SECTION OF SPORE SHOWING SPORE CYTOPLASM AND WALL, CORTEX AND SPORE COATS (From Brieger, *Structure and Ultrastructure of Micro-organisms*: Academic Press)

Finally, when the spore is fully formed, the body of the organism degenerates and the spore is set free, the entire process culminating in the release of the mature spore taking from 4 to 8 hours to complete. Although sporulation is initiated by nutrient deprivation, it is nevertheless a phase of high metabolic activity in the developing spore. There is an active synthesis of new proteins—both of new enzymes and new structural proteins. If this synthesis is inhibited by suspension of the vegetative cells in media containing amino acid analogues, or by exposure to protein inhibitors such as chloramphenicol or actinomycin D, sporulation will not occur. During sporulation major changes are observed in energy metabolism. Thus in *Bacillus* species there is an activation of the enzymes of the tricarboxylic and glyoxylic acid cycles which are present, though dormant, in the vegetative cells. The primary function of this activation appears to be the provision of Krebs cycle intermediates for the synthesis of the characteristic spore component, *dipicolinic acid*. In this process poly β-hydroxy butyrate, which is synthesized during the early stages of sporulation and which disappears during the later stages, appears to play an important intermediary role.

Spores are dormant bacterial forms; they are non-metabolizing and non-reproducing. Spore DNA is not replicated, messenger RNA is not produced, and the spore protein synthesizing system is defective as judged by in vitro incorporation experiments. Their biological importance derives from their high resistance to a variety of agencies to which the vegetative form is susceptible—

heat, ultra-violet irradiation, mechanical disruption and most chemical disinfectants. They can, as a result, survive for much longer periods than the vegetative form in environments which would be completely inimical to the latter. Spores have, in fact, been recovered from dried plants which have been preserved for some 300 years. It has been estimated that spores may show a death rate under natural conditions of about 90 per cent each 100 years. Because of their superior viability they may therefore be regarded as specialized forms which certain bacteria have evolved to survive under otherwise adverse conditions. Of particular importance to medicine is their high resistance to heat; some will resist boiling for several hours. This necessitates the employment, as in the autoclave, of temperatures of over 100° C for the sterilization of sporulating species.

Spores show marked differences from vegetative organisms in morphology, chemical composition and antigenic structure. The structure of the spore shows up well in electron micrographs of very thin sections. In the centre is the cytoplasm of the spore which appears to be much more homogeneous than the cytoplasm of the vegetative form. The cytoplasm is bounded by a delicate membrane or spore wall; outside the spore wall is a thick *cortex* of low density and low affinity for dyes. The cortex appears to contain most of the mucopeptide of the spore. This is surrounded by the coats of the spore of which up to three may be present. Finally, outside the spore coats there is in many cases a loosely attached outer layer or *exosporium*. Recent electron micrographic evidence indicates a nap of numerous, very thin filaments on the exosporia of certain spores.

The most striking chemical differences between spores and vegetative cells are their lower free-water content, and the presence of a large amount—on average about 10 per cent of the mass of the spore—of an unusual compound, dipicolinic acid (DPA), occurring as its calcium salt. Spores have been shown to possess a number of spore-specific antigens, and to produce a variety of enzymes differing both in antigenic and physical properties from the corresponding enzymes of the vegetative form. The spores are unusually rich in sulphur-containing amino acids, notably cysteine, which appears to be located mainly in the spore coat. The disulphide linkages derived from these are thought to be responsible for the increased radiation resistance of the spore. Most workers believe that the heat resistance of the spore is in some way related to the presence of a calcium dipicolinic acid chelate. This view is supported by the findings that during sporulation the accumulation of DPA is associated with the development of heat resistance, and that spores formed in the presence of low calcium concentration possess a low heat resistance. This compound might act by binding to the peptide chains of spore proteins, and in some way as yet unknown, rendering these less liable to heat denaturation.

In general, sporulation is initiated in conditions where, as a result of nutrient limitation, rapid growth is terminated; the precise mechanism by which this occurs is not known. It would appear, however, that sporing bacteria possess in effect two genomes, one for the vegetative cell and one for the spore. During vegetative growth transcription of the spore genome is inhibited, and as sporulation proceeds the transcription of the vegetative genome is inhibited.

Evidence has been obtained by Halvorson for the presence during sporulation in *Bacillus* of a *sporulation factor* which he believes may have the effect of derepressing the transcription of the spore genome. In addition he has postulated the production by the spore genome of a substance which inhibits the transcription of the vegetative genome. This latter substance may be identical for the *Bacillus* genus with an antibiotic compound shown by Balassa to be produced during sporulation.

Under suitable conditions the spore regenerates the vegetative form. This process, known as *germination* is initiated apparently by the stimulation of certain so-called trigger nutrients, usually simple sugars, amino acids and ribosides present in the environment. It can also be induced in some cases by unnatural means, e.g. by mechanical abrasion or by exposure to certain surface active compounds. For the *Bacillus* genus, germination has been found to be produced maximally by a mixture of L-alanine and inosine, as organic trigger nutrients acting in relatively high salt concentrations. In general, the readiness with which sporulation may be induced under such conditions is greatly increased by prior mild heat treatment.

At the physiological level, germination involves a dissolution, presumably as a result of an enzymic process of the cortex and coats of the spore. In the case of *Bacillus cereus*, evidence has recently been obtained that the spores contain a lysozyme-like enzyme which has been found capable, under experimental conditions, of inducing germination of spores treated with reagents capable of reducing disulphide linkages. This treatment might initiate a breakdown of the spore coats, sufficiently to allow the enzyme to gain access to the mucopeptide of the spore cortex. Under similar conditions spore germination has also been induced by exposure to lysozyme. In natural germination the hypothetical germination enzyme must, of course, act from within the spore. In this case it is possible that the enzyme might be activated by contact of the spore with the various trigger nutrients which have been found capable of inducing germination. It would presumably be necessary for the trigger nutrient to gain access to the spore cytoplasm, and its efficiency as a trigger might therefore well depend on its capacity to do so.

The *capsule* is an outer covering of jelly-like material surrounding the cell wall. It is not essential to the life of the cell since it may be lost spontaneously by mutation, and in some cases, removed enzymically without loss of viability. Occasionally, the outer limit of the capsule may be poorly defined; it is then usually referred to as a *slime layer*. The capsules of most of the pathogenic bacteria are viscous polysaccharide gums which give the colony of the organism a mucoid appearance. Capsules have a low affinity for aniline dyes, and are most reliably demonstrated by the so-called 'negative staining' procedures. Polysaccharide capsules are readily washed off the cell with water, and water must therefore be avoided in capsule stains. Organisms of the *Bacillus* genus are unusual in that their capsules are composed largely of polypeptide. In pathogenic species the capsules inhibit the engulfment of the bacteria by the phagocytes, and play an important part in determining virulence; if the capsule is lost either by mutation or enzymic degradation the organism becomes avirulent.

Certain bacteria are known to possess surface antigens, which exist in a distinct layer external to the cell wall, though insufficiently thick to be seen by ordinary microscopic methods. This layer is sometimes referred to as a *micro-capsule*. Important examples of microcapsular antigens are the M antigens of the streptococci and the Vi antigens of *Salmonella typhi*. Of these, the M antigens of the streptococci have probably most claim to be described as microcapsular, since they can be removed enzymically without affecting the viability of the organism or the integrity of the cell wall. In the intact cell they are normally covered by a true capsule. The O antigens of the enterobacteriaceae are sometimes described as being microcapsular. However, they occur naturally as integral cell wall components, and to apply the term microcapsular to them is confusing, except in so far as it indicates their surface location.

Intracellular *granules* may be observed in many species of bacteria. The most important of these are the *metachromatic* or *volutin* granules which are highly characteristic of the corynebacteria and which are of practical importance in the identification of these organisms. Metachromatic granules stain very intensely with basic dyes; because of this it was at one time thought that they consisted largely of ribonucleic acid. It is now known, however, that they are in fact granules of highly polymerized metaphosphate. Metachromatic granules accumulate in the bacterial cell only when the latter is grown on relatively rich media. Certain bacterial species show the presence of granules of glycogen like polysaccharide and of lipid. Their demonstration is not of any diagnostic importance.

Many bacteria when grown under unsuitable environmental conditions assume an unusual and frequently bizarre morphology; this may take the form of spherical, lemon-shaped, boat-shaped or irregular coarse spiral structures usually known as *involution forms*. Most involution forms appear to be non-viable under ordinary conditions of cultivation. They are probably forms in which the synthesis of the bacterial cell wall is defective and therefore analogous to sphaeroplasts and L forms (p. 377).

Growth of Bacteria

Bacteria multiply by simple division or *fission*. Fission occurs when the cell reaches a critical size, but the immediate stimulus of the division process is unknown. The first stage in fission consists of a division of the nucleus, followed by division of the cell. Nuclear division generally occurs in phase with cell division but when cells are growing rapidly it tends to outpace cell division. Consequently during rapid growth the cells usually show two or more nuclei, and one or more transverse septa prior to division. The rate at which fission occurs varies with different species. Many species, e.g. *E. coli*, and many Gram negative bacilli, multiply very rapidly, dividing, in their most rapid growth phase and under optimal conditions, once in every 20 to 30 minutes. Some organisms, however, e.g. tubercle bacilli, grow very slowly, dividing only once or twice in 24 hours.

Two main types of cell division have been described. During the first, characteristic of the Gram negative bacteria, the cell appears to divide by a constrictive or pinching process. In the second, there is an ingrowth of the cytoplasmic membrane to form a transverse septum, the new transverse cell wall being laid down between adjacent layers of membrane.

The growth of individual cells has recently been studied by the fluorescent antibody technique. This has shown two main types of growth mechanism.

1. The cell wall may grow by intercalation, i.e. by the insertion at several foci throughout the wall of segments of new material. There is some evidence that this involves a preliminary autolysis at the sites of fresh synthesis. This type of growth appears to be common in Gram negative bacteria.

2. The new material is laid down largely at the point at which cell division is going to occur. This seems to occur particularly in Gram positive organisms.

Bacteria may be cultivated in the laboratory by providing them with suitable nutrient material. This may be supplied either in fluid or in solid media. When inoculated into fluid media most species grow diffusely throughout the medium but some, particularly those which prefer a high oxygen tension, grow mainly on the surface of the medium while others grow mainly at the bottom. A fluid culture of a rapidly growing organism such as *E. coli* may contain after overnight incubation as many as 10^9 to 10^{10} organisms per ml. On solid media bacteria grow in the form of colonies each colony consisting of the descendants of a single cell deposited on the surface of the medium. If a large number of organisms is seeded onto the medium the colonies will fuse together and produce a confluent sheet of growth.

When bacteria are inoculated into a fluid medium there is a delay of some hours before they begin to multiply. This period of delay is known as the *lag phase*. Although there is no obvious multiplication during the lag phase, bacteria are nevertheless highly active in it. From the beginning they increase in size and synthesize cellular material. This synthetic activity is clearly shown if the nitrogen concentration of a culture, which is a measure of the amount of bacterial protein present, is plotted against time.

The lag phase is followed by the *logarithmic phase*, during which the bacteria are multiplying at their maximum rate. The time required for one bacterial division during the logarithmic phase is known as the *generation time*. In the log phase the number of organisms present in each generation period is virtually twice that in the previous period. Consequently if the logarithm of the number of organisms is plotted against time the result is a straight line. The phase is of relatively short duration, lasting at most for some hours. In its termination three factors are of importance. (1) Exhaustion of nutrients. This factor is probably of much greater importance to bacteria growing naturally than under the usual conditions of a laboratory culture. (2) The accumulation of toxic metabolic end products which inhibit bacterial growth. (3) The achievement of a maximum population density. It would appear that even under conditions of optimal nutrition, and in the absence of significant inhibition by metabolic and products, there is a minimal amount of living space in which a bacterium will grow.

Following the log phase there is a *stationary phase*, during which the bacterial population remains roughly constant. In this phase a balance is apparently struck between bacterial multiplication and bacterial death. The stationary phase is followed by the *phase of decline*, during which the number of organisms progressively decreases, the culture eventually becoming sterile. Complete sterility may not be achieved, however, for a considerable time.

Nutritional Requirements

During the growth of bacteria there occurs an active synthesis of the complex constituents of the cell. In order that this synthesis may take place, the elements, which are ultimately incorporated in the cell protoplasm, must be present in an assimilable form in the medium in which the organism is growing. Phosphorus, sulphur, sodium, potassium, iron and other elements required in small amounts are readily assimilated from simple salts present in the environment of the organism. Different types of bacteria, however, show considerable differences in the nature of the food material which they can accept as sources of the elements carbon and nitrogen. These differences correspond in general with differences in the synthetic power of the bacteria. Some organisms—*autotrophs* —are endowed with considerable synthetic power and can utilize very simple inorganic compounds, such as carbon dioxide and nitrates or ammonium salts, as sources of carbon and nitrogen respectively. From these they can build up their complex carbohydrates, proteins, fats and other essential constituents.

The bacteria in which we are mainly interested are classed as *heterotrophs*. These differ from the autotrophs in requiring organic sources of carbon such as are found in carbohydrates, proteins, amino acids and fatty acids, for growth. There is in fact virtually no type of organic compound which cannot be utilized by some species of bacteria. These compounds serve not only as sources of energy but also as sources of the carbon required for the synthesis of cell material. Among the heterotrophic bacteria, however, there are marked differences in nutritional requirements. Some, such as *E. coli*, are relatively non-exacting in their demands, being capable of growing on fairly simple media containing glucose or other carbohydrate as a source of energy, and common inorganic salts as a source of nitrogen, phosphorus, sulphur and other mineral requirements. Many of the parasitic bacteria, however, are much more fastidious than *E. coli*, and will not grow on a simple glucose salt medium such as described above, but require the addition of complex organic compounds, which they are unable to synthesize for themselves. Such compounds are known as *growth factors*. In general, the nutritional demands of bacteria—that is, the range of growth factors they require—can be correlated with their degree of parasitism. As a result of long habituation, the more highly parasitic bacteria have become adapted to the well-stocked nutritional environment of the animal body, and finding many of their complex organic requirements preformed, do not need the elaborate synthetic powers of the less exacting free-living bacteria. This development of nutritional needs and the loss of synthetic power may therefore be considered as a sort of retrograde evolution during which bacteria have lost more and more of their synthetic capacity and have in consequence become increasingly dependent on an adequate supply of preformed growth factors.

Bacterial growth factors can be conveniently classified in three large groups: (1) amino acids; (2) bacterial vitamins; (3) a miscellaneous group of compounds of unrelated chemical composition.

Amino acid requirement may vary from that of comparatively non-exacting organisms, such as *Salmonella typhi*, which needs only a single amino acid—tryptophane—to that of highly exacting organisms such as *Leuconostoc mesenteroides*, which require 17 amino acids, none of which it can synthesize. In general, the requirement for amino acids is most frequently for the aromatic type, since these are the most difficult to synthesize. Gram positive bacteria are much more exacting in their demands for amino acids than are Gram negative bacteria. On the other hand, since they must obtain their amino acid requirements preformed from the environment, Gram positive bacteria have had to develop the capacity to maintain a high intracellular concentration of amino acid against a concentration gradient. Even where considerable amino acid requirement exists, bacteria are nevertheless able to meet some of their needs by synthesis from ammonium salts. Nitrate can be utilized as an alternative source of nitrogen by some of the heterotrophic bacteria. The organism must, however, first reduce it to ammonia through the action of the enzyme nitratase. In some cases amino acid requirement depends on the vitamin composition of the medium. If the medium is deficient in a vitamin required for amino acid synthesis, the vitamin being one that the organism cannot synthesize, the appropriate corresponding amino acid must be supplied preformed.

Bacterial vitamins play a catalytic role in bacterial metabolism, generally as constituents of coenzymes, which—in contrast to the amino acids—are required by bacteria in very low concentrations. The most important of the bacterial vitamins are those belonging to the B group of animal vitamins—biotin, nicotinic acid, pantothenic acid, pyridoxine, paraminobenzoic acid, riboflavine, thiamine and folic acid. Their role in bacterial metabolism is essentially similar to their role in tissue metabolism. Other important bacterial vitamins are lipoic acid, which is required in the oxidative decarboxylation of pyruvic acid, and haematin which is a component of bacterial cytochromes and of the enzymes peroxidase and catalase. The need for purines and pyrimidines is related to the growth factor composition of the medium. Oleic acid is required by the corynebacteria and *Erysipelothrix*, and the polyamines putrescine and spermidine by *Haemophilus influenzae* and *H. parainfluenzae*.

It is probable, however, that most bacteria require all or practically all these factors and that they can synthesize the majority of those they require from simpler substances. Those they cannot synthesize must be supplied preformed in the medium. The power of bacteria to synthesize growth factors is of great importance in connexion with animal nutrition, since animals can utilize vitamins produced by bacteria in the intestine.

Bacteria in the body have an ample supply of their required growth materials. In the laboratory, however, it is essential, when attempting to grow a particular organism, to ensure that the medium satisfies all its nutritional requirements.

Blood or other body fluids can usually be relied on to supply a considerable variety of food materials such as amino acids and growth factors lacking in the simpler laboratory media. When the needs of an organism are exactly known, it is possible to prepare a *synthetic medium* satisfying these and containing only known constituents. Such defined media have been particularly valuable in the production of pure bacterial toxins where it is desirable to reduce unwanted material to a minimum. They have little, if any, application in routine bacteriological work.

All bacteria require for the initiation of growth a low concentration of carbon dioxide (CO_2); this is essential to heterotrophic organisms as a means of replenishing the dicarboxylic acids of the Krebs cycle. Sufficient CO_2 both to initiate and to maintain growth is usually obtained from endogenous metabolism. Large amounts of CO_2 are, however, indispensable to gonococci and meningococci, and to the bovine variety of *Brucella abortus*.

Bacteria show considerable differences in their requirement for and tolerance of molecular oxygen. Some—the *obligatory aerobes*—grow only in its presence. Organisms of this type, e.g. gonococci, meningococci and *Vibrio cholerae*, grow poorly in the depths of fluid media where the oxygen tension is insufficiently high for significant growth. Others, the *obligatory anaerobes*, grow only when all traces of oxygen are absent from the medium. The majority of pathogenic bacteria are *facultative anaerobes*, i.e. organisms which will grow in both aerobic and anaerobic conditions. Why oxygen inhibits the growth of some organisms is not fully understood. It has been suggested that it is due to the production of hydrogen peroxide, a substance highly toxic to bacteria, coupled with a lack of the detoxicating enzyme—*catalase*—of aerobic organisms. An alternative possibility is that the obligatory anaerobes possess enzymes which, for activity, must be in the reduced state. Most, if not all, bacteria appear to require carbon dioxide in small amounts and some, such as *Brucella abortus*, in relatively large amounts. As carbon dioxide is produced by the metabolism of bacteria, enough is usually present in a normal inoculum to initiate growth.

Each type of bacterium multiplies best within a restricted temperature range. For most of the pathogenic bacteria the optimum growth temperature (i.e. the temperature at which the organism multiplies at a maximum rate but which is not necessarily the temperature of maximum yield) is 37° C with upper and lower growth limits of 40 to 45° C and 15 to 20° C respectively. In general, the more highly parasitic a bacterium the closer does its temperature range of growth approximate to 37° C, the temperature to which it has become accustomed by association with the animal body. Organisms with an optimal temperature of about 37° C are known as *mesophiles*.

Some bacteria, notably certain free-living members of the *Pseudomonas* genus, have an optimum temperature of around 20° C, and are capable of significant growth in temperatures below 10° C a temperature at which mesophiles will not grow. Organisms of this type, which are known as *psychrophiles*, are widely distributed in nature; they are not of pathogenic importance though they may be responsible for food decomposition. The precise reason for the low growth range of the psychrophiles is unknown. In some cases it has been suggested that this is due to the inactivity of certain permease mechanisms at low temperatures but in other cases no such correlation has been established.

At the other extreme are the *thermophiles*—bacteria many of which have optimum temperatures in the range of 50 to 60° C, some being capable of growing up to 75° C. It is probable that the unusual behaviour of the thermophilic bacteria is due to the high heat resistance of their enzyme proteins. Thermophilic bacteria, though not pathogenic, are of importance since they may be responsible for spoilage in food that has been processed by heat.

Bacterial Metabolism

The mechanisms involved in the breakdown and utilization of foodstuffs by bacteria are basically similar to those occurring in higher organisms. The similarity is in fact so great that bacteria are frequently the material of choice for the investigation of general biochemical mechanisms. Bacteria nevertheless show certain important metabolic differences. First, they are metabolically much more active. In general the metabolic activity of an organism depends on the ratio of its surface area to its volume, a ratio which in the case of bacteria is extremely high. Thus the surface area: volume ratio for man is 0·024; for bacteria it is in the region of 5000. Bacteria therefore possess, relatively, a very large surface through which nutrients may be absorbed and through which metabolic end products may be released into the environment and this in turn results in a high metabolic rate. Second, bacteria differ from other organisms in the types of substrate that they can utilize for the production of energy and for the synthesis of cell material; amongst different bacteria there are in addition important species differences in the types of substrates that can be metabolized—differences which are of considerable importance in diagnostic bacteriology. Thus the capacity to utilize and break down lactose is of importance in the differentiation of the enterobacteriaceae. Third, bacteria differ in the types of end product which they produce. Here again differences of diagnostic importance are encountered amongst various bacterial species.

In order that a molecule can be metabolized it must first gain access to the cell. The cell wall and cytoplasmic membrane of bacteria appears to be normally completely impermeable to large molecular weight compounds such as proteins, polysaccharides and lipids. Such molecules must therefore be broken down in the extracellular environment to smaller units before they can be assimilated; this the cell achieves by the secretion of various hydrolytic enzymes—proteases, polysaccharidases and lipases. The component parts into which large molecules are thus broken down, namely the amino acids, fatty acids and simple sugars constitute the fundamental building blocks of the cell.

Nutrient material which is absorbed into the cell is utilized by the organism for two purposes. First, for the production of energy which is required for the synthesis of cell material and in the case of motile organisms for motility. A considerable amount of energy is of course lost to the cells as heat through the large surface of the organism. Second, the nutrient materials are utilized for the synthesis of the various structural components of the cell and of the enzymes and coenzymes required in bacterial metabolism.

The energy required for bacterial growth is supplied mainly by oxidation. As in other organisms bacterial oxidation consists in the removal of hydrogen from an oxidizable substrate; essentially the process is one of removing electrons which is followed by hydrogen transfer. This is effected by the agency of various dehydrogenases which are specific for the substrate attacked. The hydrogen is then transferred to an appropriate hydrogen acceptor, the process therefore being one of a coupled oxidation and reduction. Most oxidations involve the transfer of hydrogen through a series of such acceptors. The energy released by oxidation is used in the first place to effect the synthesis of high energy bonds. These are the readily hydrolysable phosphate anhydride bonds of adenosine diphosphate (ADP) and adenosine triphosphate (ATP). The energy stored in such compounds is released by rupture of the phosphate bond, and in this way can be used to drive endergonic synthetic reactions. Energy is also transferred by the high energy C—S bonds of acetyl coenzyme A and acetyl lipoic acid.

Two main types of oxidation may be distinguished; first, oxidation occurring under aerobic conditions and involving the uptake of molecular oxygen. In this process which is known as *respiration* the hydrogen is transferred through a series of hydrogen acceptors and ultimately to molecular oxygen. Most pathogenic bacteria can effect this change and as in mammalian tissues it is dependent on the presence of the respiratory pigment *cytochrome*. Respiration is a highly efficient energy yielding mechanism since by it the substrate can be completely metabolized; in the case of glucose this results in the complete breakdown of the glucose molecule to yield carbon dioxide and water.

Certain bacteria, however, notably the streptococci and the clostridia, do not possess any cytochrome components. As a result such organisms cannot obtain energy by aerobic oxidation. In the presence of oxygen the streptococci can however effect some aerobic oxidation through the agency of flavoprotein. The energy released by this process is however apparently not utilizable for growth. Oxidation by flavoprotein per se results in the production of hydrogen peroxide, a substance which is highly toxic to many species of bacteria. Some streptococci appear to break down the hydrogen peroxide thus formed by the action of peroxidase. As a general rule, however, aerobic bacteria which produce hydrogen peroxide during aerobic growth break it down by the action of catalase (p. 227).

The second main type of oxidation—that which is not associated with the uptake of molecular oxygen—is known as *fermentation*. In this case hydrogen is transferred to some other organic compound which is correspondingly reduced. Thus in the bacterial breakdown of glucose by the Embden–Meyerhof–Parnas route, the oxidation of 3-phosphoglyceraldehyde to 1,3-diphosphoglyceric acid is associated with a concomitant reduction of pyruvic to lactic acid. The breakdown of the substrate is not as complete in fermentation as it is in respiration; fermentation is therefore a much less efficient energy yielding process.

The most important group of substrates used for the production of energy by the pathogenic bacteria are the carbohydrates. The carbohydrate most usually available is glucose, and this can be utilized by most of the heterotrophic bacteria. The main mechanism involved in the bacterial breakdown of glucose is by the Embden–Meyerhoff–Parnas route identical with that occurring in yeast and muscle. Other mechanisms by which glucose may be broken down are by the Entner–Doudoroff pathway, and the pentose pathway or hexose monophosphate shunt. The latter is of importance in supplying the intermediate erythrose-4-phosphate required for the synthesis of the aromatic amino acids. All three of these pathways involve the initial phosphorylation of glucose to glucose-6-phosphate, and the production of pyruvic acid—a key intermediary in bacterial metabolism—as a principal end product. The fate of pyruvate is varied. It can be completely oxidized via the Krebs citric acid cycle, coenzyme and cytochrome to carbon dioxide and water or it can be broken down by changes of fermentative type to give a variety of end products—formic, acetic, propionic, lactic, butyric and succinic acids, ethyl, propyl and butyl alcohols, acetyl methyl carbinol and 2,3-butylene glycol, hydrogen and carbon dioxide. The precise end products formed by the fermentative breakdown of pyruvate differ with different organisms and in certain cases these differences are of diagnostic importance.

It would be beyond the scope of this chapter to attempt to review the multiplicity of mechanisms involved in bacterial syntheses. It is sufficient to say that bacteria can build up complex molecules from simple precursors by a series of elaborate and sequential biosynthetic pathways. These are mediated by enzymes the synthesis of which is controlled directly by the bacterial genome, the energy for synthesis being derived by breakdown of the high energy phosphate bonds generated from bacterial oxidation. The enzymes involved in metabolism and on which the life of the cell depends, are themselves synthesized from their constituent amino acids under the direct control of chromosomal DNA; this carries in the sequence of its nucleotide bases the genetic code indicating the sequence of incorporation of amino acids into protein. There is now conclusive evidence for a triplet code, each amino acid being denoted by a nucleotide sequence or word of three bases. Different amino acids are represented by different triplets produced by various combinations of the four DNA bases—adenine, guanine, cytosine and thymine. The triplet code corresponding to all the commonly occurring amino acids has now been determined.

In the translation of the genetic code into protein, three phases may be distinguished.

1. The base sequence of one of the strands of the chromosomal DNA is transcribed into a complementary sequence of bases in a high molecular weight RNA known as messenger RNA (m-RNA). Its composition is determined as in the case of the DNA double helix by hydrogen bonding properties. Thus guanine pairs with cytosine, RNA uracil pairs with DNA adenine and DNA thymine with RNA adenine.

Messenger RNA is synthesized on a template of chromosomal DNA through the activity of the enzyme RNA polymerase. On completion, the messenger RNA becomes detached from the template and migrates to the cytoplasm where it becomes associated with a group of ribosomes to form a polysome (p. 7).

As a component of the polysome it serves as a template for the assembly of the amino acids into proteins.

2. Each amino acid activated by reaction with ATP combines with a low molecular weight RNA known as transfer RNA (t-RNA) to form an amino acyl RNA complex. These reactions are catalysed by enzymes—amino acyl RNA synthetases—specific for each amino acid. Each amino acid has a specific transfer RNA, characterized by a specific site for the corresponding amino acyl t-RNA synthetase, and also by a specific triplet of nucleotide bases through which it pairs with messenger RNA.

3. The final stage is initiated by the alignment of transfer RNA molecules with their associated amino acids, along the messenger RNA in a sequence determined by the complementarity of their bases with those of messenger RNA. As a result of this alignment the amino acids are arranged in a sequence determined by the base sequence of chromosomal DNA. The process appears to involve first the attachment of an amino acyl t-RNA molecule to a ribosome located at the 5′hydroxyl end of the messenger RNA chain. The t-RNA appears to attach to a 50S ribosome, and the messenger RNA to lie in a groove between the 50S and 30S ribosomes. The entire 70S ribosome then moves along the m-RNA strand, and as it does, combines successively with the molecules of amino acyl t-RNA, as dictated by the associated m-RNA codon. As this occurs each amino acyl t-RNA molecule attaches in turn to the ribosome, displacing from it the amino acyl RNA molecule previously combined. At the same time a peptide bond forms between the amino group of the incoming amino acyl t-RNA and the carboxyl of the amino acid previously in situ. Finally, when the ribosome has traversed the entire length of the messenger RNA chain it becomes detached from the latter, and the completed peptide chain is released.

Bacterial Genetics

As we have seen, bacteria possess a single circular chromosome. In the case of E. coli and Salmonella typhimurium the location of many of the genes on the chromosome has been determined, and detailed chromosome maps prepared. The chromosome nucleic acid, which has a molecular weight of approximately 5×10^9, contains about 6000 genes, each containing an average of 1200 nucleotide pairs and capable of coding at three base pairs per amino acid, for proteins with an average composition of 400 amino acids and corresponding to a molecular weight of about 100,000. Although our knowledge of the details of chromosome replication are incomplete it is clear that the first stage must be a separation of the two DNA strands, new complementary strands being laid down on each of the original strands acting as an initiator by a process of base pairing. The new DNA strand is synthesized from nucleotide triphosphates through the action of a DNA polymerase. There is, in addition, evidence that the DNA double helix is attached at some point to the cytoplasmic membrane, possibly to a mesosome. It seems likely that this attachment constitutes a firm base for the uncoiling process, and is at the same time involved in the co-ordination of chromosomal replication and cell division. There are two principal models for this process:

1. Growth of the cell membrane or its incipient division may serve as a stimulus initiating the unwinding process.

2. The initial event may be a replication of the DNA, and only when this is completed can the cell divide. An hypothesis on these lines has been put forward by Lark. This proposes that one strand of the double helix is attached to the cytoplasmic membrane via a protein *replicator*. The second strand is detached and broken at this point by interaction with a protein *initiator*, and the double helix opens by a swivelling action at the replicator. Complementary polynucleotide chains are then laid down on the separating strands. Meanwhile, the initiator attaches to another site on the cell membrane via another protein designated a *proreplicator*. When the entire duplex has been replicated the free end joins up at the proreplicator, converting the latter into a replicator. It is suggested that, when this transformation has occurred, cell division can be initiated.

Extrachromosomal Genetic Determinants

Recent work has shown that a variety of bacterial properties are determined by extrachromosomal genetic determinants. The following have so far been described.

1. F or fertility factors (sex factors). F factors were first identified by their role in bacterial conjugation (p. 26). They have an independent genetic role, however, in that they can determine the occurrence of a surface antigen necessary for conjugation and for synthesis of the specialized pilus or fimbria capable of adsorbing F plus bacteriophage (see p. 28). In addition F factors may occasionally incorporate chromosomal genes.

2. C or colicinogeny factors. These are the determinants of colicine production in *E. coli* (p. 566).

3. Resistance transfer factors—RTFs (p. 198). These factors have been found to carry genetic determinants for drug resistance, a single factor being capable of carrying genes controlling resistance to a variety of drugs. So far, they have not been shown to be capable of determining bacterial properties other than drug resistance but it is probable that other similar factors capable of doing so will be discovered.

4. Factors usually referred to as *plasmids*, determining the capacity to produce penicillinase in *Staphylococcus aureus* (p. 249).

All of the above extrachromosomal determinants occur in the cytoplasm of the cell, where they undergo a replication normally co-ordinated with cell division. It seems likely, as shown for the F factor, that only one copy of the determinant exists per cell. This restriction on autonomous replication is probably due, as in the case of prophages, to the production by the determinant of a cytoplasmic repressor which prevents the spontaneous transcription of its genetic information. Presumably, at cell division some signal is transmitted to the cytoplasmic factor initiating its replication. F factors, some C factors and resistance transfer factors are spontaneously transferred from one cell to another in a conjugation-like act requiring cell to cell contact. It is likely that some change resulting from cell to cell contact initiates replication. Staphylococcal plasmids differ from the other extrachromosomal genetic determinants mentioned, in being incapable of spontaneous transfer from one cell to another. They may, however, be passively transferred by bacterial viruses, i.e. by transduction (p. 558). Extrachromosomal determinants which are spontaneously transferable, are usually referred to as *episomes*, though when this term was first introduced by Jacob and Monod, it also implied a capacity for chromosomal integration.

Bacterial Variation

When maintained in the same environment bacteria, like other organisms, exhibit a high degree of stability in their properties. This stability is due to the fact that their properties are controlled by genes which are replicated at cell division—an identical set of genes being transmitted to each daughter cell. When, however, the environmental conditions are altered bacteria exhibit a marked capacity to change their properties in such a way as to ensure their survival in the altered environment. This change in properties is known as *variation*. Variation may occur in two ways: (*a*) As a result of a genotypic change. Changes of this type are heritable, i.e. are transmitted to daughter cells. (*b*) As a result of a phenotypic change. This is a change in the behaviour of the cell which is not associated with a change in genotype. Phenotypic changes are therefore non-heritable.

Genotypic Variation

There are two main varieties of genotypic variation: (1) by mutation; and (2) by various forms of genetic transfer or exchange, in which genetic material is transferred from one bacterial cell to another.

Mutation

This, as in other organisms, is the occurrence of a change in the structure of a single gene leading to an alteration or loss in its function, and as a result an alteration of the properties of the cell. The chemical basis for this change, as has recently been shown by Brenner, is an alteration in the base sequence of the chromosomal DNA. Such a change may occur spontaneously or as a result of the action of mutagenic agents, the most important of which are base analogues, alkylating agents and ultra-violet irradiation. Spontaneous mutations are rare events usually occurring with a frequency of about 1 in 10^7 to 10^{10} cell divisions. The change in base sequence may be due to the substitution of one base pair in the DNA double helix for another, the deletion of a base pair or the insertion of a new base pair. Under natural conditions mutation is by far the most important source of genotypic variation in bacteria. Since bacteria are haploid, a mutated gene has considerable freedom of expression as no complementary gene exists—as in diploid organisms—to which it may be recessive. Moreover, bacteria are relatively simple in structure, and a mutated gene may be able to express itself without necessity for alteration in the other properties of the organism. As a result of these factors, bacteria show much greater potential for variation than do higher organisms. They are consequently less dependent than diploid organisms on genetic exchanges for the degree of variation which will permit successful environmental adaptation.

Mutations may occur in relation to most, if not all, of the observable properties of bacteria, viz. morphology, colonial appearance, biochemical activity, antigenic structure, drug sensitivity and pathogenicity. As a general rule provided the environmental conditions remain unchanged mutants do not replace the parent strain. The environment may, however, be such as to select certain mutants. In such circumstances the mutant will tend to replace the parent strain. Its success in doing so will depend on its relative superiority in the selective environment. Thus mutants to drug resistance, for example, rapidly replace their drug-sensitive parents in the presence of the drug. In this case the mutant has an absolute superiority over the parent in an environment in which the drug is present. As in other organisms, the environmental selection of chance mutations form the basis of bacterial evolution.

Genetic Exchange

This denotes the change in the properties of a cell by transfer to it of genetic material from another cell. Four types of genetic exchange can be distinguished —*transformation, conjugation, phage-mediated transfer* and *episomal transfer*. Transformation and conjugation are processes involving the transfer of chromosomal genes while episomal transfer is the spontaneous transfer of extrachromosomal genes. In phage-mediated transfer, bacteriophages act as carriers of genetic material from one cell to another; this is considered in more detail in Chapter 42.

Conjugation

This phenomenon was first described by Lederberg and Tatum in 1946, as occurring among certain nutritionally exacting or auxotrophic mutants of a strain of *E. coli* K12, and is the nearest equivalent to sexuality amongst bacteria. It differs from other types of exchange involving chromosomal genes: (1) in requiring physical contact between the conjugating pair; and (2) in that the participants exhibit sexual polarization. Lederberg and Tatum showed that when two auxotrophic K12 mutants with complementary nutritional deficiencies were mixed together a small number of hybrids without nutritional defect, known as prototrophs, were produced. These would grow on an unsupplemented minimal medium on which the parental strains would not grow. It was subsequently shown by Hayes that in the parental strains participating in conjugation, one of the parents functioned as a male or donor cell and the other as a female or recipient cell. The capacity of a strain to act as donor depends on the sex or fertility factor (F) in the cytoplasm. Strains possessing this factor are known as F plus (F+) and behave as males. Strains lacking this factor are known as F minus (F−) and behave only as females. Several functions can be ascribed to the F factor.

CONJUGATION OF AUXOTROPHIC MUTANTS OF *Escherichia coli* K12 TO YIELD PROTOTROPHS

Mutant	can synthesize	cannot synthesize
58.161 F+	threonine, leucine, B_1	methionine
W.677 F−	methionine	threonine, leucine, B_1

Neither mutant will grow on 'minimal' ammonium salt–glucose medium, lacking threonine, leucine, methionine and B_1. When conjugation occurs however and W.677 receives a section of the 58.161 chromosome which carries genes for the synthesis of threonine, leucine and B_1 the resultant hybrid will grow on minimal medium.

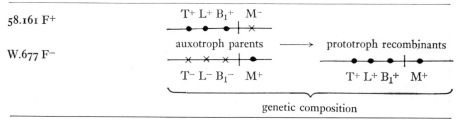

58.161 F+

$T^+ L^+ B_1^+ \ M^-$

W.677 F−

auxotroph parents   ⟶   prototroph recombinants

$T^- L^- B_1^- \ M^+$ $T^+ L^+ B_1^+ \ M^+$

genetic composition

1. It determines the production of a specific antigen on the surface of F+ strains. This antigen diminishes the charge on the surface of the F+ cells, so that on random collision they tend to adhere to F− cells.

2. It controls the synthesis of specialized pili through which a chromosome fragment can be injected from the male into the female cell. These pili have been

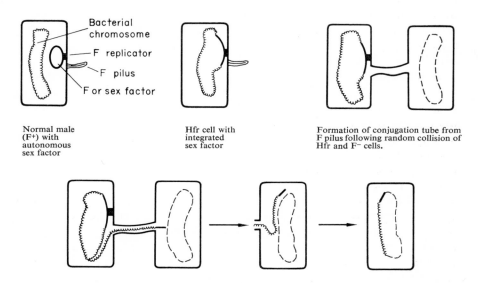

Bacterial chromosome
F replicator
F pilus
F or sex factor

Normal male (F+) with autonomous sex factor

Hfr cell with integrated sex factor

Formation of conjugation tube from F pilus following random collision of Hfr and F− cells.

Replication of the integrated sex factor with its associated chromosome, starting from the F replicator, is triggered by conjugation. One of the daughter double strands becomes detached from the replicator and is propelled, presumably by the energy of replication, through the conjugation tube into the F− cell. A chromosomal fragment is formed by random breakage and is ultimately incorporated into the recipient's chromosome

FIG. 7. POSSIBLE MODEL OF CONJUGATION IN *Escherichia coli* K12

found to carry receptors for certain bacteriophages which are specific for F+ cells.

3. It mobilizes the F+ chromosome for transfer. In the normal F+ *E. coli*, the chromosomal DNA exists as a closed, circular loop and the F agent occurs free in the cytoplasm. Before conjugation can occur, the F agent must migrate from its normal cytoplasmic location to the chromosome into which it becomes inserted. Cells with F factors integrated in this way are known as Hfr (high frequency) cells. In the absence of conjugation the chromosome replicates normally. If contact with an F− cell is established, however, replication is initiated at the site of F insertion but one of the new chromosomes fails to undergo ring closure, remaining straight and passing in this form through the conjugation tube into the female cell. In this process the proximal end of the chromosome, known as the origin, carries only a small moiety of the replicated F factor, the major portion of which is at the distal end of the now linear chromosome. The size of the chromosomal fragment transferred depends on random breakage of the chromosome during transfer. Consequently, the closer to the origin a particular gene is situated, the more frequently will the marker property controlled by that gene be transferred in conjugation. Frequency of transfer in conjugation can therefore be used as a basis for the preparation of a chromosome map. The position of a marker can also be determined by inter-rupted mating experiments in which mating cells are separated mechanically in a Waring blendor. The earlier the entry of a marker the closer it is to the origin. The transferred fragment is then incorporated into the homologous portion of the recipient's chromosome. The process appears to have some analogy with the crossing over mechanism in diploid cells, but the eliminated chromosomal fragment does not form a reciprocal recombinant with the complementary section of the donor chromosome. The bacterial male, therefore, is rather like the male of the praying mantis which dies in the act of copulation.

There is considerable evidence, necessarily of an indirect character, that the F factor is a large molecule of DNA apparently containing about 2×10^5 base pairs. On this estimate it is about the size of a bacteriophage chromosome. In the cytoplasm of F+ cells, the F agent is capable of autonomous replication. This replication is nevertheless under the control of the cell genome, and does not proceed uncontrolledly, as in bacteriophage replication (p. 550), with resulting damage to the structure of the cell.

F− cells readily become infected with the F agent when grown with F+ cells; this is a form of spontaneous episomal transfer. Unlike bacteriophage infection, F infection cannot be produced by exposing the F− cell to culture filtrates of F+ cells, the F agent being transferred only by an act analogous to conjugation. Spontaneous F transfer requires the replication of the F agent, to ensure its presence in both the donor and recipient cell. Its replication is presumably stimulated by the act of conjugation involved. Since the F agent is free in the cytoplasm, its transfer does not involve the transfer of chromosomal genes. Occasionally however, integrated F agents are ejected from the Hfr chromo-some and are found to have incorporated some chromosomal genes through recombination with an area contiguous to the F locus. Such modified F factors are known as F prime factors or *F genotes*, and their transfer coupled with the transfer of the associated chromosomal marker is known as F-duction or sexduction.

In *E. coli*, conjugation in the sense of chromosomal transfer can also be promoted by certain C factors and by RTF's, but with much less efficiency than by F.

Conjugation has been demonstrated in organisms other than *E. coli* K12. It can be shown to occur between various wild type *E. coli* strains, which act as both gene donors and acceptors, and between various strains of shigellae as recipients and *E. coli* K12 as donor; between strains of *Pseudomonas aeruginosa* and between strains of *Vibrio cholerae*. In wild type *E. coli* and *Pseudomonas* the donor state appears to depend on the occurrence of a sex factor similar to, but not apparently identical with, that of *E. coli* K12. In *Vibrio cholerae*, conjugation seems to depend on a bacteriocinogeny determinant known as P. In none of these cases has the Hfr transformation been observed.

Transformation

This phenomenon, discovered in the pneumococcus by Griffith in 1928, was the first demonstration that genetic material could be transferred from one bacterium to another. Griffith observed that mice which had been injected with live, non-capsulated variants of capsulated type 2 pneumococci, and heat-killed pneumococci of capsular type 1, died of a septicaemia due to capsulated type 1 strains. It was apparent that the non-capsulated type 2 organisms had in some way been transformed into capsulated type 1 organisms. This transformation was subsequently demonstrated under in vitro conditions, and the general principle established that non-capsulated pneumococci derived from one type could be transformed into capsulated pneumococci of another, by exposure to a transforming agent present in cell-free filtrates or extracts of the capsulated strain. The transforming agent was later identified by Avery, McLeod and McCarty as DNA.

Intraspecific transformation has been recognized in strains of *Haemophilus influenzae*, *Bacillus subtilis*, *Neisseria meningitidis* and in various streptococci, as well as in the pneumococcus. It has been studied mostly in the pneumococcus, a species in which a wide range of readily recognizable characteristics may be transferred. Transforming agents appear to consist of large fragments of DNA equivalent to about one per cent of the total bacterial genome. Under optimal conditions each cell is capable of taking up about ten such molecules. Consequently, in the presence of an excess of transforming agent, about 10 per cent of the cells of a transformable culture can be shown to be transformed in respect of a specific marker characteristic. There is clear evidence that transformation is due to the incorporation of the DNA fragment, or more probably a single strand of the DNA double helix, into the chromosome of the recipient where it exchanges for the corresponding segment of the latter, and becomes thenceforth an integral part of the recipient's genome. In the pneumococcus the capacity to be transformed, known as *competence*, only appears transitorily in a culture, being found only for about 40 minutes towards the end of the logarithmic phase of growth. This is presumably the only time during growth when the cells are permeable to the large DNA molecule. There is some reason to believe that this permeability may arise from a physical breakdown of the cell membrane. Another possibility is that competence may require the synthesis of appropriate receptor sites on the bacterial surface, and that this may only occur at a particular stage in growth.

Phenotypic Variation

This defines a change in the behaviour of the cell produced in response to some environmental stimulus. Such changes do not involve the genome, and are temporary in character—reversal to the normal pattern occurring when the environmental stimulus producing them has been withdrawn. In contrast to mutational changes they are acquired by the bacterial population as a whole rather than by a few mutant cells. Changes of this type may be broadly described as adaptive. They may be divided into two main categories.

I. Environmental control of the rate of enzyme synthesis. Many bacterial enzymes are *inducible*, the synthesis of the enzyme only occurring to a significant extent in the presence of the enzyme substrate or a substrate analogue. Inducible enzymes are usually, though not invariably, enzymes involved in the breakdown of exogenous substrates. Non-inducible enzymes, whose rate of synthesis is independent of the presence of substrates, are referred to as *constitutive*. Notable examples of inducible enzymes are: (*a*) those involved in the transport and breakdown of lactose by *E. coli*, namely β-*galactosidase, galactoside permease* and *thiogalactoside transacetylase*, all of which are inducible by lactose; and (*b*) the extracellular *penicillinases* produced by various *Bacillus* species and by *Staphylococcus aureus* which are inducible by penicillin.

The model currently invoked to explain enzyme induction is the one proposed by Jacob and Monod. It postulates the participation in enzyme production of three distinct genetic components:

1. A structural gene, or genes, which code for the synthesis of the enzyme protein and of any other protein which forms a functional unit with the enzyme. Thus in *E. coli* the synthesis of β-galactosidase is co-ordinated with the synthesis of β-galactoside permease and thiogalactoside transacetylase.

2. The transcription of the structural genes into messenger RNA is controlled by an operator gene, which when active, as it were, switches on the transcription mechanism.

3. A *regulator* gene which is responsible for the production of a cytoplasmic *repressor* whose function is to inhibit the action of the *operator*. When the operator is inhibited the messenger RNA providing the information for the synthesis of the enzyme is not transcribed, and the enzyme is not produced.

If, however, the substrate, i.e. lactose or certain substrate analogues such as thiogalactosides, are present they combine with the repressor and prevent it from inhibiting the activity of the operator. There is now considerable evidence that where, as in lactose fermentation, a number of enzymes are involved in the metabolism of a compound, the genes responsible for determining their synthesis are arranged sequentially on the chromosome, and are under the

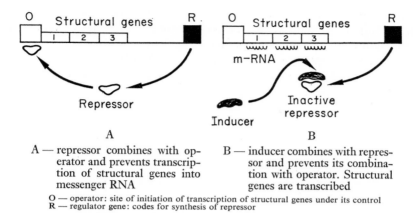

A — repressor combines with operator and prevents transcription of structural genes into messenger RNA

B — inducer combines with repressor and prevents its combination with operator. Structural genes are transcribed

O — operator: site of initiation of transcription of structural genes under its control
R — regulator gene: codes for synthesis of repressor

FIG. 8. JACOB-MONOD MODEL FOR ENZYME INDUCTION

control of a single operator. Such a co-ordinated genetic unit is referred to as an *operon*. Mutations may occur at various sites in such a system. The regulator gene may fail to produce a repressor or the operon may become insensitive to the repressor; under these circumstances the production of the enzyme becomes constitutive rather than inducible. On the other hand, the regulator gene may produce repressor incapable of being inhibited by inducer or the structural genes may become insensitive to the operon. In these cases no enzyme is produced, and the presence of the corresponding structural genes can only be demonstrated in recombination experiments. The lactose repressor has recently been demonstrated directly; in general it would appear to possess the properties of an allosteric protein (see below), capable of combining specifically both with the operator and with the inducer. However, the production of repressor is not inhibited by exposure of the cell to agents which inhibit protein synthesis. This suggests the possibility that the repressor might not be a protein. Nevertheless, inhibition could fail to occur because only a few molecules of repressor per cell may be required for effective repression.

The process of enzyme induction obviously gives bacteria great flexibility in their capacity to respond to changes in the nutritional composition of an environment. Enzymes involved in biosynthetic pathways, e.g. in the synthesis of amino acids, are non-inducible, unlike the enzymes considered above. Their production may, however, be inhibited by the biosynthetic end product. This was first shown by Cohn and Monod in 1953. They found that the production of tryptophane synthetase and methionine synthetase were repressed if the organisms were supplied with tryptophane and methionine respectively. Where a number of enzymes are involved in a synthesis the end product appears to be capable of repressing the production of most, if not all, of the enzymes involved simultaneously. This mechanism is easily explained on the basis of a model similar to that devised by Jacob and Monod for inducible enzymes. The enzymes involved in the synthetic sequence are arranged sequentially in an operon under the control of an operator gene. In this case, however, the regulator gene is postulated to produce an inactive *apo-repressor* which is incapable of combining with the operator gene. It is transformed into a fully active repressor by combination with the end product of the biosynthetic pathway. This mechanism permits a great economy for the cell in the synthesis of enzyme protein since it allows the production of a particular biosynthetic enzyme to be switched off when the enzyme is no longer required.

II. A second major way in which bacteria may respond to environmental changes is the process known as *feedback inhibition*, in which the activity, but not the production, of a biosynthetic enzyme is damped down by the biosynthetic end product. In this case the end product appears to combine with the first enzyme of the metabolic pathway so as to inhibit its activity. The end product responsible for feedback inhibition shows no structural resemblance to the substrate of the inhibited enzyme. Thus threonine, which is synthesized from aspartic acid will inhibit the formation of an aspartokinase which is involved in the formation of aspartyl phosphate from aspartate. The inhibited enzyme must therefore have two distinct combining specificities: (1) for its normal substrate; and (2) for the biosynthetic end product. For proteins of this type Jacob and Monod have proposed the name of *allosteric* proteins. Feedback inhibition may be thought of primarily as a fine control of metabolism, in contrast to co-ordinated enzyme repression which may be regarded as a coarse control.

CHAPTER 2

MICROSCOPIC EXAMINATION OF BACTERIA

Because of the extremely small size of bacteria a high degree of magnification is necessary for their demonstration. This degree of magnification is achieved by the use of the $\frac{1}{12}$-in. and $\frac{1}{6}$-in. objectives which give magnifications of $95\times$ and $45\times$ respectively. These are usually employed, when a monocular microscope is used, with oculars giving a magnification of $10\times$; with binocular instruments $6\times$ or $8\times$ oculars are used. The $\frac{1}{12}$-in. objective is an oil-immersion lens and is used in the examination of stained preparations; when it is used a drop of oil is placed on the slide and the lens immersed in the oil. Since the refractive index of the oil is approximately the same as that of glass the loss of light which would otherwise occur at the air–glass interface is reduced and more light passes into the objective. This permits a closer working distance between the lens and the film and consequently a lens of shorter focal length and greater magnification can be employed. The $\frac{1}{6}$-in. lens commonly known as the 'dry high power' is used for the examination of wet unstained preparations. In addition the bacteriologist also requires a $\frac{2}{3}$-in. lens (magnification $10\times$); this lens is used mainly for the preliminary examination of infected tissues.

The magnification with sharp definition attainable by the ordinary microscope is limited partly by the wave-length of light and partly by the physical properties of glass used as a refracting medium in lenses. As a result, it is not possible to obtain satisfactory definition of objects less than 0.25μ in diameter. Theoretically, greater magnification with clear definition should be possible, but the degree of magnification attained is limited by the quality of the lenses obtainable.

When, instead of light, a beam of electrons is used, as in the *electron microscope*, the limitation imposed in optical microscopes by the wave-length of light is eliminated and a magnification of up to 200,000 can be obtained. The electron microscope is so costly and complicated that it is unlikely to replace the normal microscope except where very high magnifications are required. It has, however, been of great value in the investigation of the finer details of cellular structure and in the demonstration of viruses and rickettsiae (Chapter 31).

The Use of the Microscope

Bacteria may be examined microscopically either in unstained wet preparations or in stained preparations.

WET PREPARATIONS

Unstained preparations have a restricted application in bacteriology. They are mainly used for the demonstration of bacterial motility and for the demonstration of spirochaetes.

Motility is best demonstrated microscopically in hanging drop preparations in which a drop of culture or other bacteria-containing fluid is deposited on the centre of a coverslip which is then inverted over the concavity of a specially prepared glass slide, or over a metal ring attached by petroleum jelly to the surface of an ordinary slide. Alternatively, the fluid may be placed on the surface of a slide and a coverslip dropped over it.

True motility must be distinguished both from Brownian movement, which is due to molecular bombardment, and is also seen in minute, lifeless particles, and from the flowing of the bacteria owing to currents set up by uneven heating. The best test is to observe carefully two bacteria lying close together and sharply in focus at the same time. If these move in different directions, they exhibit true motility.

Motility may also be demonstrated by stab inoculation down the centre of a tube of nutrient agar containing a low concentration of agar. On incubation non-motile organisms remain confined to the line of the stab while motile organisms produce a diffuse growth spreading out towards the sides and bottom of the tube.

For the demonstration of spirochaetes, which are not visible under direct illumination, dark ground illumination is employed. This requires the use of a special condenser which reflects the light on the object obliquely so that only the rays refracted by the object enter the objective. With this technique the organisms are seen brightly outlined against a dark background.

STAINED PREPARATIONS

Preparation of Films

A film of the preparation to be examined is first made on a glass slide by spreading with a wire loop. If the material to be examined is from a solid culture it is first emulsified in a drop of water on the slide, and the film is then spread. The technique requires practice, and only with experience can films be prepared, which are not too thick or too thin.

Before staining, films must be dried and fixed. Drying is best carried out by holding the slide between fingers and thumb and moving gently to and fro above a Bunsen flame. The film is then fixed by passing it three times through the flame. It is of the greatest importance that during drying and fixation the film should not be overheated.

The stains most commonly used in bacteriology are solutions of basic aniline dyes in water. Many types of bacteria can be satisfactorily stained by flooding the fixed film with the stain, which is allowed to act for a period ranging from a few seconds to several hours, depending on the intensity of action of the particular stain used and the type of bacteria. After staining, the slide is thoroughly washed with tap water and dried by blotting.

Gram's Method

This is the staining method most frequently used in diagnostic bacteriology. The organisms are first stained with an aniline dye of the violet series—usually crystal violet—and are then treated with an iodine solution which acts as a mordant. Next they are washed in alcohol and finally counterstained with a dye of contrasting colour, e.g. fuchsin. On the basis of their reaction to the Gram stain bacteria can be divided into two great groups—the Gram positive and Gram negative. Gram positive organisms retain the violet stain after decolorization with alcohol; with Gram negative organisms, on the other hand, the violet stain is removed by alcohol treatment and the organisms are seen to be stained with the counterstain employed. Gram positive organisms are, therefore, purple in colour, and when fuchsin is used as counterstain Gram negative organisms are pink.

The determination of the Gram character of an organism is of great importance in identification. The pathogenic cocci, with the exception of the neisseriae, are Gram positive. The pathogenic bacilli are Gram negative, except the following genera: *Corynebacterium, Bacillus, Clostridium, Actinomyces, Listeria* and *Erysipelothrix* which are Gram positive. Mycobacteria stain with difficulty by Gram's method but when stained are also Gram positive.

In the past, numerous attempts have been made to attribute the Gram positive character to particular chemical compounds, notably nucleoproteins, nucleic acids and polyglycerophosphate in the Gram positive cell. In none of these cases, however, has a satisfactory correlation between staining properties and chemical composition been established. On the whole it seems more likely that the difference between Gram positive and Gram negative cells is due to a difference in the permeability of their cell membranes, in particular, that the membranes of Gram positive organisms are less permeable to the dye iodine complex in alcoholic solution.

The distinction between Gram positive and Gram negative shows a high degree of correlation with certain biological properties. (1) As previously mentioned the cell walls of Gram positive bacteria differ considerably in chemical composition from those of Gram negative bacteria (p. 5). (2) Gram positive organisms are much less susceptible to mechanical damage than are Gram negative but show on the whole a greater susceptibility to inimical chemical agencies. (3) Gram positive organisms are on the whole more nutritionally exacting than Gram negative. (4) The production of potent exotoxins (Chapter 5) is almost exclusively a property of Gram positive organisms.

There are many modifications of the original Gram's method, but the one here described, that of Jensen, is probably the simplest and most reliable.

1. Stain with crystal violet for $\frac{1}{2}$ minute.

2. Pour off excess stain and wash off residual stain with Lugol's iodine. Cover with fresh iodine and allow to act for 1 minute.

3. Pour the iodine solution off the slide and shake it so as to free it as completely as possible of the solution.

4. Flood with alcohol, rock and pour off. Repeat until alcohol removes no further stain from the film.

5. Wash with water.

6. The film is then counterstained. The object of this is to render visible Gram negative bacteria and cells from which the alcohol has removed the violet colour. The counterstain must contrast in colour with the violet of Gram positive bacteria and should not be too intense. Dilute carbol fuchsin is the counterstain most commonly used. For the demonstration of intracellular Gram negative organisms, e.g. gonococci and meningococci, neutral red is better since it gives sharper differentiation between the bacteria and the cell nucleus.

7. Wash with water. Blot. Dry.

Ziehl–Neelsen Method

Next to the Gram stain this is the method most frequently used in diagnostic bacteriology. It is the method routinely employed for the demonstration of tubercle bacilli—organisms which are not normally stainable by Gram's method.

1. The fixed film is covered with strong carbol fuchsin which should be filtered onto the slide through a filter paper funnel. Heat is then applied below the slide either with a small flame of the Bunsen, a spirit lamp or spirit torch. The heating should be sufficient to cause steam to rise, but boiling the stain must be avoided. Staining should last for at least 10 minutes, heat being applied occasionally. Care must be taken to prevent the stain drying on the slide, fresh stain being added if necessary.

2. Wash well in water.

3. Flood the slide with 20 per cent sulphuric acid in water and leave on for 1 or 2 minutes. In the acid the pink colour changes to yellow or brown.

4. Wash in water. The pink colour may return. If so, steps 3 and 4 are repeated as many times as necessary, until the film has not more than a faint pink tinge.

5. Wash in 95 per cent alcohol for 1 minute.

6. Wash in water.

7. Counterstain. Löffler's methylene blue applied for ½ minute is commonly used.

8. Wash with water. Blot. Dry.

Steps 3 and 5 may be replaced by treatment with acid alcohol. After treatment for 5 minutes, the film is rinsed with water and, if the pink colour returns, the acid alcohol is replaced. It may be necessary to alternate acid alcohol and water several times before the film has been sufficiently decolorized.

Tubercle bacilli resist decolorization with acid and appear bright red because of which they are referred to as acid-fast; other bacteria and cells take the colour of the counterstain used.

After films have been examined microscopically the objective should be wiped free of oil. If this is not done, tubercle bacilli may be transferred in the oil to the films subsequently to be examined. For the same reason it is important that when the oil is placed on the slide prior to examination, the glass rod used should not be allowed to touch the slide.

PLATE I

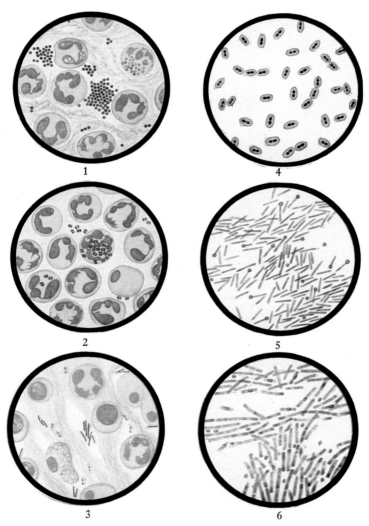

1

4

2

5

3

6

BACTERIA AS SEEN WITH THE OIL-IMMERSION LENS

1. Staphylococci in pus
2. Gonococci in pus
3. Tubercle bacilli in sputum

4. Pneumococci stained to show capsules
5. *Cl. tetani* stained to show spores
6. *B. anthracis* stained to show spores

[*To face p.* 36

Stains for *Corynebacterium diphtheriae*

For routine use Neisser's stain gives excellent results, demonstrating both the morphology of the organisms and the characteristic metachromatic granules.

Neisser's Stain

1. Neisser's methylene blue—3 minutes.
2. Wash rapidly with water.
3. Counterstain with either Bismarck brown, Löffler's methylene blue or neutral red for 3 minutes.

Methods of Demonstrating Spirochaetes

With the exception of the borreliae, spirochaetes cannot be stained with aniline dyes and must therefore be stained by special methods.

Fontana's Method

This is probably the most satisfactory method of demonstrating spirochaetes in films. It is a silver impregnation method, the spirochaetes being rendered visible by the deposition of metallic silver on their surfaces, which makes them appear much coarser than they really are.

1. Dry film without heat.
2. Fix in acid formalin solution for about 1 minute, the reagent being renewed three times during this period.
3. Wash well with water.
4. Treat with mordant for $\frac{1}{2}$ minute, gentle heat being applied.
5. Wash well with water.
6. Treat with silver solution for $\frac{1}{2}$ minute, gentle heat being applied.
7. Wash well with water.

The spirochaetes are stained dark brown or black.

The silver solution should not be kept for more than a few hours as, if kept for a longer time, a brown precipitate may form and this is a most violent explosive.

Giemsa's Stain

For the demonstration of spirochaetes in blood, e.g. in relapsing fever, Giemsa's method, as used for the demonstration of malaria parasites, is of value.

Levaditi's Method

This is a silver impregnation method which is used for the demonstration of spirochaetes in tissues.

Capsule Stains

In the tissues capsules are usually visible in Gram stained preparations but the Gram stain is not satisfactory for their demonstration in cultures.

India Ink Method

In cultures capsules are probably best demonstrated by the wet India ink technique. This is not strictly a staining method since the ink is used merely to provide a dark background against which bacteria and their capsules stand out in sharp relief.

1. Place a loopful of India ink on the slide.
2. Emulsify a small amount of the culture in the ink and cover with a coverslip.
3. Press the coverslip down applying pressure through a sheet of blotting paper so as to flatten out the ink into a thin pale film.

On examination the capsule may be seen as a clear area between the highly refractile outline of the cell wall and the greyish background formed by the India ink.

Hiss's Method

This method is most successful when applied to films freshly made from infected body fluids. If a film is to be made from a culture, the growth should be emulsified in serum instead of in water and only the slightest degree of heat necessary for fixation should be used.

1. Crystal violet with heat—$\frac{1}{2}$ minute.
2. Wash off with a 20 per cent solution of copper sulphate: do not use water.
3. Blot and dry.

The body of the bacterium is stained a deep purple and the capsule a lilac colour.

Spore Stains

Spores are usually visible in Gram stained films. Their positive identification however requires the use of special spore stains.

Moller's Method

1. Carbol fuchsin with heat—10 minutes.
2. Wash with water.
3. Decolorize with 5 per cent solution of sodium sulphite—$\frac{1}{2}$ minute.
4. Wash with water.
5. Counterstain with Löffler's methylene blue—1 minute.
6. Wash with water. Blot. Dry.

Spores are stained bright red, and the vegetative cells blue. The optimum time for step 3 must be determined by trial as spores of some bacteria are more easily decolorized than those of others.

Demonstration of Fungi

In tissues fungi are most readily demonstrated by the periodic acid Schiff (PAS) technique. This method is specific for glycogen-like polysaccharide which is a characteristic component of the cytoplasm of fungi.

For the demonstration of fungi in cultures the lactophenol blue method is normally used. A drop of lactophenol blue is placed on a slide and a small portion of the culture is gently teased out in it with needles. The preparation is covered with a coverslip which is pressed down firmly. Excess stain is then removed from the edges of the preparation with blotting paper. For optimum staining some hours' contact should be allowed. The characteristic morphology of the filamentous fungi is best seen in cultures grown on slides or coverslips. For microscopic examination these should be mounted directly in lactophenol blue.

Fluorescence Microscopy

This technique depends on the capacity of bacteria which have been stained with a fluorescent dye—auramine being generally used—to fluoresce in ultraviolet light. Its only application in medical bacteriology is in the demonstration of tubercle bacilli, the staining technique employed for this purpose being similar in principle to that of the Ziehl-Neelsen. The advantage of the method over the Ziehl-Neelsen technique is that it will permit the use of the 1/6 or 2/3 objective thus allowing the rapid scrutiny of a large area of film. The method is mainly used in laboratories examining large numbers of specimens for tubercle bacilli. For the ordinary diagnostic laboratory the Ziehl-Neelsen method is usually preferred.

Fluorescent Antibody Technique

This technique, devised by Coons, has been extensively used for the microscopic demonstration of viral antigens in infected tissues. It has also been employed on a limited scale for bacterial identification.

Two procedures are employed—direct and indirect. In the direct technique the material to be examined is exposed to an antiserum specific for the antigen under investigation and coupled chemically with a fluorochrome or compound which fluoresces in ultra-violet light. The fluorochromes most frequently used for this purpose are fluorescein isothiocyanate and Lissamine-Rhodamine. After washing, the 'stained' preparations are examined in a dark field under UV illumination, when the sites at which antibody has combined with antigen show up with a bright fluorescence. In the indirect procedure the material to be examined is treated with an uncoupled antiserum and, after washing, the preparation is exposed to a coupled antiserum containing antibody specific for the γ globulin of the species from which the serum used in the first stage of the technique was obtained.

CHAPTER 3

THE CULTIVATION OF BACTERIA

As we have seen, the nutritional requirements of the pathogenic bacteria may be very complex, these being capable of growing only when supplied with a variety of complex growth factors. Their needs can be met by preparing completely defined or *synthetic* media made from the particular compounds, e.g. amino acids, etc., required by the organisms. Such media are used considerably in research and in the preparation of bacterial end products as free as possible from unnecessary foreign material. The requirements of the pathogenic bacteria for complex substances are, however, more easily met from naturally occurring material such as blood, serum, yeast, meat extract and egg. Such substances are therefore used as the basis of the media most frequently employed in diagnostic bacteriology.

Both solid and fluid media are used. Solid media are essential for the isolation of bacteria in pure culture. A single organism deposited on the surface of a solid medium will multiply to form a *colony*. This colony, which is invisible to the naked eye, is composed of millions of daughter cells of the original organism. It is, however, a pure culture and can be picked off and seeded into or onto other media for further investigation. In a fluid medium, on the other hand, the bacteria grow diffusely; consequently, if it has been inoculated with material containing more than one species, these will grow as a mixed culture.

Fluid media, although of great importance in pure culture study of bacteria, are not by themselves suitable for the isolation of organisms from mixtures. They may, however, be used as *enrichment* media prior to plating. Thus, if material containing a small number of organisms is inoculated into a fluid medium and the latter, after incubation, is subcultured onto a solid medium, the chances of isolation will be much greater, since the organisms will have multiplied in the fluid medium.

Many media incorporate substances which render them *differential* or *selective*. A differential medium is one which contains some substance on which a particular organism or group of organisms has a characteristic action. The alteration in the medium resulting from this action enables one to recognize the presence, in the material cultured, of this organism or group of organisms. Thus by adding lactose and an indicator, broth is rendered a differential medium for lactose fermenting bacteria. If these are present they ferment the lactose, producing acid which changes the colour of the indicator; if absent, the indicator does not change.

40

A selective medium is one which inhibits the growth of all bacteria except those of a particular type or group. A medium is usually made selective by adding to it some substance which tends to prevent the growth of unwanted types while having little or no effect on those which are desired. Selective media are of particular importance in the isolation of bacteria from some site in the body, such as the throat or intestinal tract, which has an extensive normal flora.

Most of the pathogenic bacteria will grow only in the range of pH 6 to pH 8. Optimum growth is usually restricted to the range pH 7 to pH 7·4, which corresponds to the pH of the body fluids in which these organisms are accustomed to live. The media used for their cultivation are therefore usually adjusted to a pH within this range. During their growth, however, bacteria produce various end products which tend to alter the pH of the medium. This effect is counteracted by the use of buffers. Most of the media used in diagnostic bacteriology have considerable intrinsic buffering power due to the presence of peptone or animal protein. When, however, media deficient in such natural buffers are used salts with a buffering action must be incorporated in the medium. The salts most generally used for this purpose are NaH_2PO_4, Na_2HPO_4 and $NaHCO_3$.

The media must be sterile, i.e. they must contain no living organisms. Sterilization of media is usually carried out in the *autoclave*. Certain media, however, deteriorate at the high temperature of the autoclave and for these the *steamer* is used. Some of the substances used in the preparation of media may be adversely affected by any form of heat sterilization. These ingredients can be sterilized by *filtration*.

Types of Media Employed in the Cultivation of the Pathogenic Bacteria

Nutrient Broth

Nutrient broth is the basis of many of the media used in the cultivation of the pathogenic bacteria. By itself it is a valuable subculture medium for bulk preparation of organisms for a variety of purposes, e.g. to provide antigens for serological examination, as inocula for sensitivity testing and in vaccine production. Three types of broth are used: *infusion* broth, *extract* broth and *digest* broth. Infusion broth and extract broth contain as their main ingredients peptone and meat extract. Fresh extracts of meat, usually of ox heart, are used in infusion broth, and commercial extracts, e.g. Lab Lemco, in extract broth.

Digest broth is a special type which is made from an enzymatic digest of meat. Peptone is not required since the digest contains a considerable amount of protein breakdown products. Digest broth is a much richer medium than nutrient broth and is of particular value in the cultivation of pneumococci and streptococci.

Nutrient Agar

By the addition of agar to nutrient broth, a solid medium, nutrient agar, is obtained. Agar is an extract of certain seaweeds and consists mainly of polysaccharide. By itself it has virtually no nutrient properties.

Nutrient agar is a gel which can be melted by heating to 100° C and becomes solid at about 45° C. It is not liquefied by the action of any of the pathogenic bacteria. Nutrient agar is usually used in Petri dishes in quantities of 15 to 20 ml of agar. For subcultures and for the preparation of suspensions for slide agglutination tests, agar slopes or slants containing about 5 ml of agar, solidified in a sloped position, are commonly employed.

Blood Agar

By itself nutrient agar is not a rich medium. Its nutrient properties are, however, greatly improved by the addition of blood, and the resulting medium which is known as blood agar, is the standard medium for the isolation of many pathogens. In addition to supporting their growth it will indicate whether they are haemolytic or not—an important diagnostic criterion. Citrated or defibrinated human and horse blood are most frequently employed, usually in a concentration of from 5 to 10 per cent.

Media for the Culture of *Corynebacterium diphtheriae*

Coagulated Serum Medium

Serum media, prepared from coagulated bovine, sheep, or horse serum are particularly valuable for the growth of diphtheria bacilli. On these media, the diphtheria bacilli grow very rapidly and produce their most typical morphology.

Löffler's serum medium, the type commonly used, consists of 3 parts of serum and 1 part of broth containing 1 per cent of glucose.

Selective Media for *Corynebacterium diphtheriae*

For the isolation of diphtheria bacilli tellurite media, which are inhibitory for the majority of organisms other than corynebacteria likely to be found in the nose and throat, are commonly employed. In addition to being selective for the diphtheria bacillus tellurite media are also differential—diphtheria bacilli producing black colonies on them due to the reduction of the tellurite to metallic tellurium. In the preparation of the older types of tellurite media the media were heated and because of the resultant change in the blood were brown in colour. One of these heated blood tellurite media, McLeod's medium, is of special value for the differentiation of the cultural types of diphtheria bacilli (p. 282). For diagnostic purposes, however, media prepared with unheated blood, e.g. Hoyle's, are more satisfactory than those prepared with heated blood; this is because the growth of some strains of diphtheria bacilli are inhibited by heated blood and in general most strains produce an atypical morphology on such media. Hoyle's medium contains horse blood, lysed by freezing and thawing or by incubation with saponin, and potassium tellurite in a concentration of 0·04 per cent. Downie's medium, containing unlysed unheated blood, which is easier to prepare, may also be used.

Media for the Isolation of Pathogenic Intestinal Bacteria

Very many media are used to facilitate the isolation of intestinal pathogens from materials, such as faeces, which contain coliform bacilli and other bacteria. They rely for their selective properties either on a dye, e.g. brilliant green as in Wilson and Blair's medium, or on one of the bile salts. Of the solid media used for this purpose only MacConkey's medium, Leifson's desoxycholate citrate medium and Wilson and Blair's medium, which are the most generally useful, will be described.

MacConkey's Agar

MacConkey's medium contains peptone, sodium taurocholate, lactose, neutral red and agar. All enterobacteriaceae grow well on MacConkey's agar; for the isolation of enteric pathogens the medium has therefore low selectivity. Because of the presence of lactose and indicator, lactose fermenting organisms, e.g. the coliform group, produce pink or red colonies while non-lactose fermenting bacteria, such as the salmonellae and shigellae, produce transparent or colourless colonies.

Desoxycholate Citrate Agar

This is similar to but more selective than MacConkey's medium. Since it contains lactose and indicator, lactose fermenting bacteria produce pink colonies; they are usually surrounded by an area of opacity due to the precipitation of the desoxycholate by the acid produced in fermentation. Desoxycholate citrate agar is the most generally useful medium for the isolation of intestinal pathogens.

Wilson and Blair's Medium

In addition to nutrient agar, this medium contains bismuth-ammonium-citrate, sodium sulphite, sodium phosphate, glucose, ferric citrate and brilliant green, all of which appear to be essential. It is the most highly selective of the three media described here, inhibiting the growth of coliforms and shigellae but allowing the growth of salmonellae and, unfortunately, *Proteus*. It is of particular value for the isolation of *Salmonella typhi* and *Salmonella paratyphi B* which, when well dispersed, produce characteristic black colonies surrounded by a black metallic sheen. Other salmonellae may produce either similar colonies or colonies which are green in colour.

Selenite F Medium and Tetrathionate Broth

These are fluid enrichment media which are of considerable value in the isolation of salmonellae, but are of no value for dysentery bacilli. They are to an appreciable extent selective, permitting a much greater initial growth of salmonellae than of coliforms or other organisms normally found in the intestinal tract. This disparity is most marked after 18 to 24 hours' incubation which is therefore the best time for subculture. Either MacConkey's or Leifson's medium is suitable for this purpose.

Media for *Mycobacterium tuberculosis*

Lowenstein–Jensen Medium

This is the medium most frequently used for the isolation of tubercle bacilli from human sources. Its essential ingredients are coagulated egg, potato starch, asparagin, glycerol and malachite green. The concentration of glycerol incorporated in the medium is sufficient to have considerable stimulatory effect on human type tubercle bacilli but not so great as to have more than a relatively slight inhibitory effect on bovine type strains (Chapter 27). To avoid the drying which would otherwise occur during the prolonged period of incubation required for the culture of the tubercle bacillus both of the above media are dispensed in screw capped bottles. A somewhat similar medium, *Stonebrink's medium*, lacks glycerol and has been recommended for the isolation of bovine type tubercle bacilli.

Dorset Egg Medium

This medium which consists simply of coagulated egg and broth may also be used for the isolation of tubercle bacilli, particularly of bovine type strains, but is not as sensitive as the two media previously described. It is an excellent medium for the maintenance of stock cultures of most bacterial species.

Culture of Anaerobic Bacteria

Anaerobic bacteria are usually isolated by inoculation onto an appropriate solid medium, e.g. blood agar, which is then incubated in a McIntosh and Fildes anaerobic jar. This is a jar from which the air may be exhausted and replaced with hydrogen or nitrogen. Anaerobic bacteria may also be grown under aerobic conditions in fluid media containing reducing substances. Two important media of this type are *Robertson's meat medium*, and *Brewer's medium*.

Robertson's Minced Meat Medium

This medium consists of minced meat (which contains reducing substances) covered with a layer of broth. The addition of 0·2 to 0·5 per cent glucose improves the anaerobic conditions in the medium. The top of the broth may be covered with a layer of liquid paraffin or melted petroleum jelly. Capillary pipettes must be used to inoculate and to withdraw samples from the medium when an oil or petroleum jelly seal is used. Robertson's medium is very useful for preserving cultures of certain organisms, such as *Str. pyogenes*, which are facultative but not obligatory anaerobes and which die in a short time under aerobic conditions.

Brewer's Medium

The addition of 0·1 per cent sodium thioglycollate to broth renders it capable of supporting the growth of strict anaerobes. The medium is improved by the further addition of glucose. Very commonly 0·05 per cent of powdered agar and 1 in 500,000 of methylene blue are added to the medium. The incorporation of agar minimizes convection currents and increases the degree of anaerobiosis in the depths of the medium.

Willis and Hobb's Medium

This medium is of considerable value for the isolation of clostridia and especially for the isolation of *Clostridium perfringens* from infected food, in cases of bacterial food poisoning. It contains lactose, egg yolk, milk, and is made selective for clostridia by the incorporation of neomycin to which clostridia are highly resistant. The colonies of organisms which produce lecithinase, e.g. *Clostridium perfringens*, are surrounded by opalescent zones on this medium.

Other Media

Many other media have been recommended and used successfully for the isolation of different species. Some of these are mentioned in the sections on individual organisms.

Media for Biochemical Tests

A great variety of media is used in connexion with the various biochemical tests employed in bacterial identification. The most widely applicable of these are the so-called 'sugar' media which are used to determine the capacity of bacteria to ferment carbohydrates or other fermentable substrates of differential importance.

'Sugar' Media

The most commonly used sugar media are fluid media containing the particular substance under test, together with peptone as a source of nitrogen.

The medium must also contain a pH indicator for which either neutral red, phenol red or more commonly Andrade's indicator is generally employed. The medium is distributed in test tubes on the bottom of which rest, in an inverted position, very small inner tubes known as Durham tubes. Fermentation of the carbohydrate may result in the formation of acid alone or of acid accompanied by the evolution of gas. The production of acid is shown by a change in the colour of the medium—this is to a reddish pink if Andrade's indicator is used, if gas is also produced it collects at the top of the Durham tube.

Peptone water sugars are not satisfactory for certain organisms, e.g. streptococci, pneumococci and neisseriae, with exacting nutritional requirements. For streptococci and pneumococci Hiss's serum water sugars are usually employed; these contain serum in a concentration of 25 per cent sugar and an indicator. Fermentation of the sugar is shown by a change in the colour of the indicator and by coagulation of the serum. The fermentation reactions of the gonococci and meningococci, which are highly aerobic and therefore do not grow well in liquid media, are best determined on agar media containing the appropriate carbohydrate and 5 per cent of rabbit serum.

Dehydrated Media

Many media can now be obtained commercially in dehydrated form. These are particularly valuable for small laboratories which do not have the facilities, or in fact the need, for media preparation on a large scale.

Cultural Technique

In most cases media are inoculated with a wire loop which is sterilized in the Bunsen flame before and after use. Inoculation of plates is usually by the parallel streak method (Fig. 9). The first series of streaks is charged from the material

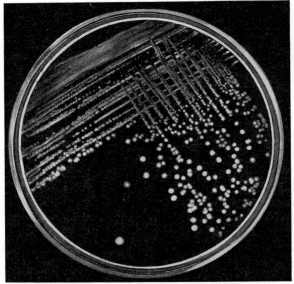

FIG. 9. THE COLONIES ON A PLATE SPREAD BY THE METHOD OF PARALLEL STREAKS ($\times \frac{2}{3}$)

under examination. The second and third series, each at right angles to the previous series, are made without recharging but after sterilization of the loop. In this way the inoculum becomes successively diluted and, provided it has not been too large initially, well isolated colonies are usually found in one quadrant of the plate. Large quantities of material are usually inoculated with a Pasteur pipette as in the isolation of tubercle bacilli.

For the great majority of the pathogenic bacteria the optimum temperature of cultivation is 37° C, the customary period of incubation being from 18 to 48 hours, except for particularly slow-growing organisms such as tubercle bacilli. Plates are incubated in the inverted position, i.e. with the lid downwards so that the water of condensation does not flow over the surface of the medium.

When bacteria from an originally mixed inoculum have been grown in plate culture, pure cultures of individual species may be obtained by picking off single colonies with a wire loop and inoculating them onto an appropriate subculture medium. However, where there has initially been a considerable mixture of organisms, as in the isolation of enteric pathogens from faeces, single colonies from the primary plate should be subcultured to a further plate; single colonies from the latter can usually be assumed to be free from contaminants.

CHAPTER 4

DISINFECTION AND STERILIZATION

The terms *disinfection* and *sterilization* are generally used—rather imprecisely—to indicate the treatment of material so as to destroy or otherwise eliminate any living organisms present. There is, however, a tendency to prefer the term sterilization for physical methods of treatment and the term disinfection for chemical methods. Thus chemicals which will kill bacteria are known as *disinfectants*. Material that has been treated in such a way that it contains no living organisms is said to be *sterile*.

Disinfectant and sterilizing procedures are of great practical importance. Their main applications are as follows:

1. For disinfection in the literal sense of rendering material non-infective. The treatment of material so as to kill any pathogenic organisms present, e.g. in the sterilization of surgical instruments or the disinfection of clothing, is of the greatest value in our efforts to prevent the spread of infection.

2. In the treatment of food so as to kill, or inhibit, the growth of the organisms responsible for food decomposition. Some of the methods used for this purpose, e.g. drying, salting and pickling, are of great antiquity and date as traditional and empirical procedures from the beginnings of civilized society.

3. In the bacteriological laboratory, for the sterilization of media and glassware which are to be used in the cultivation of bacteria.

Natural Disinfection

Although the deliberate application of disinfectant techniques is of great importance in medicine, appreciable disinfection occurs spontaneously under natural conditions—pathogenic organisms which have become adapted to a parasitic role in the animal body, as a rule surviving poorly outside it. The more important factors operating under such conditions and leading to the death of bacteria are deprivation of nutriment and the disinfectant action of light and desiccation. In certain natural environments other special factors come into play; thus in water bacteria are ingested by algae and protozoa, while in the soil they are exposed to the action of antibiotic substances produced by various soil organisms.

PHYSICAL METHODS OF STERILIZATION
Mechanical Trauma

Bacteria can be killed by simple mechanical trauma, e.g. by grinding, by shaking with small particles, by ultrasonic irradiation and by repeated freezing and thawing. Mechanical methods, however, have no practical application in disinfection—although they are of considerable value as research procedures for the rupture of bacteria, so as to release various intracellular constituents.

Heat

The application of heat is the most important of all the methods of disinfection, and provided the heat used is adequate it is the most certain and rapid; it is also easily controlled and unlike chemical disinfection leaves no potentially harmful residue.

As with all other types of disinfection the sterilization of a bacterial population by heat is a gradual process. Throughout most of the process the rate of disinfection is approximately a logarithmic one, i.e. if the logarithm of the number of survivors is plotted against time the resultant curve is a straight line.

The time required for sterilization is inversely related to the temperature of exposure—the higher the temperature the shorter the time required. Thus a culture which requires one hour for sterilization at 60° C will be sterilized in only a few minutes at 80° C; at 100° C sterilization will be virtually instantaneous.

Different types of bacteria show considerable differences in heat susceptibility. In general most vegetative bacteria are killed by exposure, under moist conditions, to temperatures of 60 to 65° C for half an hour. A few species have, however, an unusually high degree of heat susceptibility. Spirochaetes, for example, are killed in a very short time at 40° C and many of the streptococci, with the notable exception of *Streptococcus faecalis*, are killed rapidly in the range of 50 to 55° C. Sporing organisms have on the other hand a very high resistance to heat—most spores being capable of withstanding a temperature of 100° C for very long periods. This is why high temperature sterilization—i.e. by the use of temperatures over 100° C—is obligatory for hospital sterilization and for the sterilization of many types of preserved foods.

Dry Heat

Dry heat is the preferred method of sterilization for glassware, e.g. of glass syringes, and of materials such as oils, jellies and powders which are impervious to steam. It is unsuitable for material, e.g. fabrics, which may be damaged by heat. As compared with steam sterilization it has the disadvantages that a longer time and a higher temperature are required. The most widely used type of dry heat sterilizer is the hot air oven. Hot air ovens are usually electrically heated. In the simpler gravity convection ovens the air circulates by convection. This form of oven is unsatisfactory since it is difficult to ensure that there has been adequate air circulation. The mechanical convection type of oven in which the air is circulated by a fan is much more efficient. Suitable sterilizing times in the hot air oven are 3 hours at 140° C, 1 hour at 160° C and 20 to 30 minutes at 180° C.

Moist Heat

As previously mentioned most vegetative bacteria can be fairly rapidly killed by temperatures in the range of 60 to 65° C. The most important applications of temperatures in this range are in the pasteurization of milk and in the preparation of bacterial vaccines.

Boiling is frequently used for the sterilization of glass syringes, surgical instruments and small pieces of apparatus. Since, however, many spores will withstand boiling for a considerable time, boiling must be regarded as inadequate for the sterilization of such materials.

Steam Sterilization

Exposure to steam is the most widely used and the most effective technique of moist heat sterilization. Steam is a much more efficient sterilizing agent than hot air at the same temperature, for the following reasons. First, bacteria are intrinsically more susceptible to moist than to dry heat. Second, steam is a more rapid sterilizing agent than hot air because on condensation it gives up its latent heat of vaporization thereby rapidly heating the objects on which it condenses. Third, steam has a much greater power of penetrating porous material. This is due to the fact that on condensation a partial vacuum is created which has the effect of sucking in more steam from outside until the material becomes thoroughly permeated.

Steam may be employed in three ways.

Steam at 100° C

This is achieved in a steamer in which the steam is generated at atmospheric pressure by electricity or gas from water in the bottom of the chamber. The materials to be sterilized are placed on perforated shelves through which the steam passes to escape through an opening at the top. The method is mainly used for the sterilization of bacteriological media which would be damaged at the high temperature of the autoclave. The procedure of 'intermittent' or 'fractional' sterilization is usually employed; this ensures the destruction of spores which might not be killed by a single steaming. The procedure involves steaming for short periods on each of three successive days. It should be noted that the method can be applied only to nutrient media in which spores can germinate in the intervals between steaming.

Low Temperature Steam

This method has recently been advocated for the sterilization of materials such as blankets and polythene tubing, which would be damaged by steam at high temperatures. Saturated steam at temperatures of from 70 to 90° C may be generated in sterilizers operating at pressures of 20 to 10 in. of mercury. Under these conditions steam has been found to be a much more effective sporicidal agent than water at the same temperature. The efficiency of the process can be significantly increased by the injection of a small amount of formalin along with the steam.

Steam at Temperatures Greater than 100° C

This is achieved by the use of the autoclave. The use of such high temperatures is necessitated by the high thermal resistance of bacterial spores (p. 13).

Essentially an autoclave is a very strong boiler or cylinder with a door which can be hermetically sealed and constructed sufficiently strongly to withstand the high pressures required. The pressure is maintained at the appropriate level during sterilization by means of a safety valve set to blow off at a predetermined pressure. In construction, autoclaves vary enormously from the simpler laboratory types—in which the steam is generated in the autoclave itself, and which are essentially little more than glorified pressure cookers—to the highly sophisticated hospital sterilizers with virtually automatic control of the sterilizing cycle. Whatever the type of instrument however the same fundamental principles must be borne in mind in its operation.

The steam must be saturated. This in effect means that it should have a temperature appropriate to its pressure, i.e. the temperature it would have as generated from water at the same pressure. Saturated steam condenses readily and has good penetrating power. Steam which is supersaturated or wet has poor penetrating power since the water present causes clogging of porous materials. Supersaturation is only likely to occur when the steam has been piped for long distances during which it has become cool, some of it condensing into water in the process. Superheated steam, i.e. steam with a temperature above that appropriate for its pressure is also a poor sterilizing agent, its loss in sterilizing efficiency being proportional to its degree of superheat. It has a low capacity for condensation and, therefore, as a sterilizing agent behaves essentially like hot air. There are three main causes of superheating, all three arising only where, as in hospital sterilizers, the steam is led into the sterilizing chamber from an outside source—either a central steam supply or an independent boiler.

(*a*) Steam led from an external source is usually generated at a high pressure —of the order of 50 to 60 lb/in². Before admission to the sterilizer its pressure must be brought down by reducing valves to the working pressure of the autoclave, i.e. in the region of 15 to 30 lb/in². Unless prior to this stage, the steam has had an excess water content, the reduction of pressure will automatically create a state of superheating.

(*b*) In jacketed autoclaves, if the air has not been completely exhausted from the sterilizing chamber, the temperature of the latter will be maintained by the heat of the jacket while the partial pressure of the steam will be reduced by the presence of the air. The temperature of the steam will therefore be higher than that corresponding to its pressure.

(*c*) Fabrics which have been rendered excessively dry, perhaps as a result of prolonged evacuation of the cylinder prior to sterilization, will absorb moisture from the steam, thereby reducing its pressure without reducing its temperature.

There must be complete discharge of air from the sterilizing chamber. This is necessary for a number of reasons: If there is appreciable residual air the steam will mix with the air and its temperature will be reduced in proportion to the amount of air originally present.

Pockets of air will collect around the materials and packs to be sterilized and will prevent steam penetration. Hot air being heavier than steam will tend to gravitate to the bottom of the sterilizing chamber. In this part of the chamber sterilization will therefore be much less efficient than at the top.

In the simpler laboratory autoclaves the air is expelled by the flow of steam through a discharge tap sited at the top of the autoclave. This method of air discharge requires skilled supervision and though reasonably satisfactory in the laboratory, is quite unsuitable for hospital sterilizers. In hospital sterilizers the air may be removed in one of two ways: (a) by downward displacement; (b) by evacuation prior to admission of the steam.

(a) Air is heavier than steam and though on first admission the steam mixes freely with it, the air eventually gravitates towards the bottom of the chamber. From here it escapes through an air discharge trap incorporating a thermostatically controlled valve which remains open at temperatures below that of the steam thereby permitting the discharge of air and/or condensate and when the air has been discharged, closing at the temperature of the steam. In this type of instrument the chamber discharge line incorporates a thermometer for recording the lowest temperature reached in the sterilizer; if the temperature recorded is the correct one for saturated steam at the pressure employed, then it can be assumed that all the air has been removed from the cylinder.

(b) In recent years there has been increasing development of high prevacuum sterilizers in which the air is removed by exhaustion with powerful pumps prior to admission of the steam. In order to ensure complete removal of the air, and therefore complete steam penetration of fabric packs, a vacuum must be drawn to a residual absolute pressure of not more than 20 mm of mercury. It has been found, however, that even under these conditions a single cycle of evacuation may not prove completely effective in the sterilization of a small package in a large chamber—the so-called 'small package' effect. This appears to be due to the fact that the residual air in the chamber is for some reason concentrated in the materials in the package. This effect can be overcome either by two or more periods of evacuation with admission of steam between each evacuation, or by a continuous pulsed injection of steam during the pumping-down process.

The autoclave must be loaded in such a way that all the materials to be sterilized can be adequately penetrated by the steam. Hospital packs should therefore not be covered by impervious wrappings. In downward displacement instruments, packs should be disposed in such a way that layers of fabrics are arranged vertically and not horizontally. This arrangement facilitates expulsion of air and condensate. For the same reason jars and cans used as containers, should be laid on their sides.

The duration of the sterilizing period will depend on the steam temperature. For routine disinfection with downward displacement instruments a pressure of 15 lb/in^2 which is equivalent at sea level to a steam temperature of 121° C, is commonly employed. Under these conditions recommended exposures range from 15 to 45 minutes depending on the penetrability of the load. With high prevacuum sterilizers, because of the more rapid penetration of the steam, shorter sterilizing times and therefore higher temperatures can be employed. Exposure at 135° C for 3 minutes is commonly used. This short cycle has the great advantage of permitting a much more rapid turnover than with the downward displacement procedure.

Control of Sterilization

Physical Methods

Ultimately the most satisfactory method of control is by use of thermocouples inserted into test packs which can be appropriately sited in the load. Thermocouples, however, are not generally available on hospital sterilizers.

Chemical Methods

A number of chemical indicators have been used of which the most satisfactory are Brown's tubes. These are sealed glass tubes containing a fluid which undergoes a colour change from red through amber to green when the appropriate sterilizing temperature has been maintained for certain minimal times. Four types of tube are available, two for use with steam sterilizers, and two for use with hot air sterilizers and conveyor ovens. The Bowie Dick autoclave tape is a heat sensitive tape which is widely used for monitoring conditions in the centre of packs in high prevacuum sterilizers. If the centre of the tape fails to undergo a colour change there is incomplete heat penetration into the centre of the pack.

Bacteriological Methods

Suspensions of spores—particularly the highly heat-resistant spores of *Bacillus stearothermophilus*—dried on paper strips or discs are sited in a pack and subsequently tested for sterility. The number of spores present in the strip should be sufficiently large to make a sterility test significant. A recommended minimum is 10^5 spores per test strip. Clostridial spores mixed with sand or soil may also be used. Bacteriological indicator tests have the disadvantages that they do not give an immediate result, and that they require expert supervision.

The crucial test for the efficacy of sterilization is the sterility of the product. Sterility tests cannot be applied readily to hospital materials but in industry they are frequently used for materials which can be readily sampled, e.g. foods. Under these conditions, tests can be seriously misleading, however, since some organisms may remain viable even though sufficiently damaged by heat that they fail to grow under ordinary conditions of cultivation. Because of this, indicator tests designed to reveal the efficiency of the sterilization process are to be preferred.

Cold

Bacteria may also be killed by exposure to cold. Two different circumstances must be distinguished.

Cold Shock

This is a sudden reduction in temperature without actual freezing. Some species are highly susceptible to cold shock. Thus a 95 per cent drop in the number of viable *E. coli* has been reported to occur following sudden chilling from 45 to 15° C. The mechanism of this effect is unknown but it is possibly due to a difference in the rate of contraction on cooling of different intracellular constituents, with a resultant disorganization of cellular structure.

Freezing

It was at one time thought that the lethal effect of freezing was due to physical damage to the cell membrane and/or cell wall by ice crystals. It is now generally accepted that such a mechanism can play only a minor role, if any, in the death of frozen organisms. There are probably two major factors involved. (1) The formation of ice crystals outside the cell by the withdrawal of water from the cell interior increases the intracellular salt concentration. This would in turn be capable of causing considerable damage by protein denaturation, and is probably a major cause of death when bacteria are frozen to temperatures of not lower than − 30 to − 35° C. (2) Formation of ice inside the cell. There is evidence that this can only occur if the bacteria are frozen to temperatures lower than − 35° C, and even then, only under conditions of rapid cooling. The lethal effect of intracellular ice does not appear to be due to a direct action of the ice on the cytoplasm but only occurs during defreezing. It appears to be maximal when the bacteria are heated slowly, and minimal when they are heated rapidly. The formation of intracellular ice therefore appears in some way to condition the cells to damage on slow warming. The precise nature of this damage is unknown.

Ultra-violet Radiation

Light has considerable disinfectant properties and plays a very important part in the spontaneous sterilization which occurs under natural conditions. Its disinfectant action is due mainly to the ultra-violet rays, most of which are screened out by glass and also to a considerable extent by smoky and foggy atmospheres.

The most active of the ultra-violet rays are those with wave-lengths in the region 2400 to 2800 Ångstrom units. Radiation in this region is, however, present to only a small extent in the solar radiation which succeeds in penetrating the earth's atmosphere, the latter containing little radiation with wave-length below 2900 Ångstrom units.

Ultra-violet radiation can be produced artificially by special UV lamps. Those most commonly employed are of the low pressure mercury vapour type. With these, over 95 per cent of the radiation emitted is of wave-length 2537 Ångstrom units. Germicidal UV lamps must be used with care since the radiation has a damaging effect on the eyes; they must consequently be sited in such a way that the eyes are not exposed directly to the radiation.

Most vegetative bacteria appear to exhibit much the same order of susceptibility to ultra-violet irradiation—Gram positive species, however, appearing to show a slightly greater resistance than Gram negatives. Spores are highly

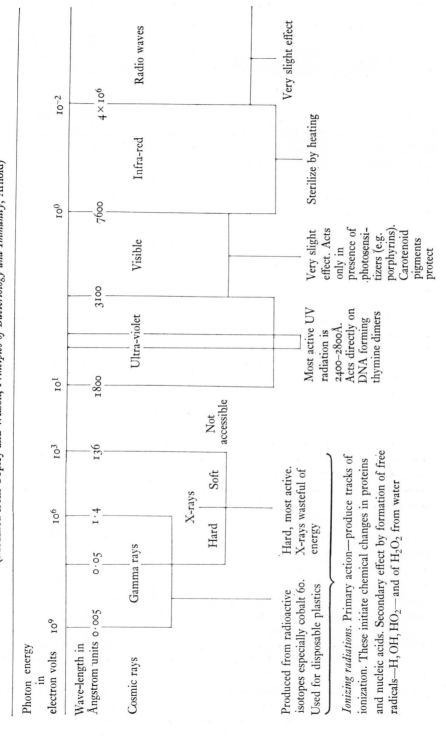

BACTERICIDAL ACTIVITY OF ELECTROMAGNETIC RADIATIONS

(Modified from Topley and Wilson, *Principles of Bacteriology and Immunity*, Arnold)

Photon energy in electron volts: 10^9 10^6 10^3 10^1 10^0 10^{-2}

Wave-length in Ångstrom units: 0·005   0·05   1·4   136   1800   3100   7600 4×10^6

Cosmic rays   Gamma rays   X-rays   Ultra-violet   Visible   Infra-red   Radio waves

Hard   Soft   Not accessible

Produced from radioactive isotopes especially cobalt 60. Used for disposable plastics

Hard, most active. X-rays wasteful of energy

Ionizing radiations. Primary action—produce tracks of ionization. These initiate chemical changes in proteins and nucleic acids. Secondary effect by formation of free radicals—H, OH, HO_2— and of H_2O_2 from water

Most active UV radiation is 2400–2800Å. Acts directly on DNA forming thymine dimers

Very slight effect. Acts only in presence of photosensitizers (e.g. porphyrins). Carotenoid pigments protect

Sterilize by heating

Very slight effect

resistant and the susceptibility of the viruses is variable. As a practical method of disinfection, however, ultra-violet irradiation has the serious disadvantage that its penetrating power is very slight. It is therefore only of value for the sterilization of surfaces, of very thin fluid films, and of the air.

There seems little doubt that the lethal effect of ultra-violet irradiation in the most actively bactericidal range is due to its strong absorption by, and resultant damage to, the nuclear DNA. The most important effect of its action on DNA is the production of *thymine dimers*. Dimer formation occurs in the first place between adjacent thymines of the same DNA strand, and later between thymines on opposite strands. The former leads to a copying error when the DNA is replicated, as a result of interference with hydrogen-bonding relationships. Dimer formation between thymines on opposite strands might be expected to result in an inhibition of the capacity of the nucleic acid to replicate.

In addition to its direct action on DNA ultra-violet irradiation may cause denaturation of bacterial proteins or have an indirectly lethal action through the formation in the presence of oxygen, of hydrogen peroxide and organic peroxides in culture media. The latter effects are probably of greater importance than a direct action on nucleic acid in determining the bactericidal activity of the ultra-violet component of sunlight.

Recovery of damaged, but still viable organisms is considerably enhanced if after irradiation the organisms are washed or mildly heated, or grown on semi-solid media or on media which are slightly deficient nutritionally. Recovery is also enhanced by the presence of pyruvate and dicarboxy and tricarboxy acids of the Krebs cycle and of catalase in the medium. The mechanism by which many of these various manipulations result in enhanced recoveries is not known precisely but they presumably act either by removal or destruction of toxic substances—thus catalase presumably acts by decomposition of hydrogen peroxide—or by permitting repair of the damage effected by the irradiation. The latter is probably the mechanism involved in the enhancement of recovery by growth on suboptimal media. Under normal growth conditions replication of the nucleic acid is attempted and becomes a lethal process. If, however, the onset of growth is delayed some repair of the damage can occur and a viable DNA which can replicate safely, is produced.

The most studied technique for enhancing recovery is that of *photoreactivation*. Considerable repair of irradiation damage can be effected by exposing the organisms to visible light within a few hours of irradiation. The most effective radiation appears to be in the wave-length 3400 to 4000 Å. Photoreactivation will reverse both the bactericidal and mutagenic effects of irradiation. It is due to the activity of a bacterial enzyme which combines with the damaged DNA in the dark but which becomes activated in light, and is released with repair to the ultra-violet lesion. The enzyme is specific for irradiated DNA. It does not combine with unirradiated DNA nor with DNA in which thymine has been substituted by 5-bromouracil. The latter observation makes it very probable that it acts by uncoupling the thymine dimers formed by irradiation. Photoreactivation has so far been described only in strains of *E. coli* and yeast but is possibly of appreciably wider distribution. The existence of 'dark' non-photoreactivable repair enzymes which can repair a variety of types of damage to bacterial DNA has also been demonstrated.

In addition to its bactericidal and mutagenic effect, ultra-violet irradiation can induce vegetative phage production in certain lysogenic bacteria, and colicine production in certain colicinogenic bacteria (p. 567). In both these cases induction is believed to be due to the destruction of a cytoplasmic repressor.

It has been shown by Howarth that certain colicinogeny determinants will increase the ultra-violet resistance of strains of *Salm. typhimurium*. In addition they have been found to depress inducibility of other colicines and of prophage lambda (p. 559). These findings suggest the possibility that some part of the lethal effect of irradiation may be due to the induction of defective prophages, i.e. prophages which are incapable of undergoing vegetative transformation in non-irradiated cultures (p. 558).

Under experimental conditions artifically produced ultra-violet irradiation can cause a considerable reduction in the bacterial content of the air. It does not, however, appear to have been of much practical value in the control of respiratory infection. Probably its most useful application is in the control of contamination and in reducing staff infection, in sterile rooms and cabinets in microbiological laboratories.

Effect of Visible Light

Although most of the disinfectant action of sunlight is due to radiation in the near ultra-violet range, radiation in the visible range has some disinfectant properties. For this, however, the presence of a photodynamic sensitizing substance is required. The phenomenon of photodynamic sensitization can be demonstrated with dyes, e.g. eosin, which fluoresce on exposure to visible light. The phenomen was first demonstrated at the beginning of the century with *Paramecium*. Oxygen is essential and the mechanism involved appears to be a photo-oxidation. Under natural conditions bacterial porphyrins and flavins are believed to be of importance as photodynamic sensitizers. Evidence has been presented by Stanier that bacteria may be protected from photo-oxidation by naturally occurring carotenoid pigments. Non-pigmented mutants of naturally pigmented species show a great increase in susceptibility to visible light. The bacterial chlorophylls of the photosynthetic bacteria appear to be particularly potent in inducing photosensitization, and it is significant that these bacteria invariably possess carotenoid pigments. Stanier suggests that the protective effect of the carotenoid against photo-oxidation is due to some structural change produced by the pigment in the natural sensitizer, so that photo-oxidation cannot occur.

Ionizing Radiations

Ionizing radiations have considerable disinfectant action. They have a much higher energy content than ultra-violet radiation and have consequently a much greater capacity to induce lethal chemical changes. These changes are primarily the result of the production by the radiation of tracks of ionization in the cells. In the killing of bacteria the changes induced in the nucleic acids—particularly in DNA—are probably of greatest importance. Ionizing radiations also affect the cell through the production from water molecules both extracellularly and intracellularly of hydrogen peroxide and of oxidizing free radicals.

Of the various types of ionizing radiation only cathode rays and gamma rays would appear to have any reasonable prospect of practical application. Both these types of radiation have received considerable attention in recent years as possible disinfecting agents. Generators and accelerators are now available which can produce cathode rays on a commercial scale and radioactive isotopes —in particular, cobalt-60 which produces gamma radiation—are now available in substantial quantities as by-products of atomic energy installations.

Cathode rays, being particulate—they are accelerated electrons—have poor penetrating power. This, however, can be compensated for by the fact that they can be given high energies. Gamma rays have relatively greater penetrating power but their potential energy content is much less than that of cathode rays. Ionizing radiations have been used to a limited extent for the sterilization of food and pharmaceutical products. Their main disadvantage is that they can produce chemical changes in the material irradiated. These may result in abnormal odours and colours in food and loss of activity in pharmaceutical compounds. Current research in this field is concerned mainly with the efforts to minimize these effects which appear to be due mainly to free radical formation.

Ionizing radiations are being used on an increasing scale for the sterilization of surgical materials, particularly of disposable items made of rubber or plastic. They are of particular importance in the sterilization of disposable syringes. Other materials which may be sterilized in this way are surgical catgut, bone and tissue grafts and adhesive dressings.

Desiccation

Although lethal to bacteria, drying is not applicable as a practical method of sterilization. Bacterial species differ considerably in their susceptibility to drying. Some, such as gonococci and the cholera vibrio, are rapidly killed. Tubercle bacilli and streptococci on the other hand are resistant and may persist in the dried state, e.g. in dust or in books, for long periods. The effect of drying depends on a number of factors—a low temperature, a protein medium and the absence of oxygen affording bacteria considerable protection. Bacteria that survive the drying process are in a state of suspended animation, and in this condition may remain viable for years. Consequently, drying is widely used as a method of preserving bacterial cultures. The initial mortality is considerably diminished if the cultures are dried in vacuo from the frozen state. This process is known as *lyophilization* or *freeze drying*.

Filtration

Filtration has a number of bacteriological applications. It may be used for the preparation from cultures of cell-free bacterial products, e.g. toxins and enzymes, to free virus-containing fluids from bacteria and for the sterilization of media or media ingredients which would be damaged by heating. For these purposes filters with pores sufficiently small to hold back bacteria must be employed. Many filters are also available in porosities which will retain large particles but which will not effect sterilization. These coarser filters are frequently used in the clarification of culture media which are subsequently to be sterilized by heat.

Filtration is usually carried out under negative pressure, the fluid being sucked through the filter into a receiving flask, which is connected to an exhaust pump. On exhaustion of the flask by the pump the fluid is sucked through the filter. The use of excessive pressure is to be avoided because this might force some bacteria through the filter. On the other hand, filtration should not be allowed to take a long time, since some small organisms might then be able to grow through the filter pores.

During filtration there may be appreciable adsorption of material from the fluid being filtered onto the surface of the filter. This adsorption occurs because filters are not merely mechanical sieves but carry electrical charges by virtue of which they attract material carrying an opposite charge. Adsorption may result in the clogging of the filter or, more serious still, in the retention of substances, e.g. enzymes, which it is desired to obtain in the filtrate.

The most commonly used bacteriological filter is the *Seitz* filter. In this the filtering agent is a pad of asbestos which is discarded after a single filtration. The Seitz filter is easy to use but unfortunately asbestos has considerable adsorptive capacity and also contributes certain ions, particularly magnesium, to the filtrate.

Collodion or *Gradocol* membranes are virtually free from adsorptive capacity and have to a considerable extent replaced Seitz filters for many routine laboratory applications. They can be made with a specific and uniform pore size and have consequently been of great value in the estimation of the size of small particles such as viruses. Gradocol membranes are discarded after a single filtration.

For the filtration of small quantities of fluid, asbestos pads and collodion membranes, which can be fitted between the mouths of two 5 ml bijou bottles with a special collar, are available. The fluid is forced through the filter from one bottle to the other by centrifugation.

Filters of diatomaceous earth (*Berkefeld* and *Mandler*) of unglazed porcelain (*Chamberland* and *Doulton*) and of sintered glass are also used. The diatomaceous earth and porcelain filters are commonly made in the form of thick-walled tubes called candles. In the sintered glass filters the filtering agent is a diaphragm made from small particles of glass which have been fused sufficiently to make the particles adhere. Sintered glass filters and the modern porcelain filters have relatively little adsorptive effect.

Filtration is of considerable importance in the purification of water supplies destined for human consumption. For this purpose two methods are employed.

1. Slow sand filtration. This method employs large filter beds made, from the bottom up, of clinker, gravel and sand. The essential filtering agent, however, is the vital or zoogloeal layer, consisting mainly of algae and protozoa, which forms on the surface of the sand when the water has been allowed to flow through the filter for some time. Until this layer forms the filter cannot be used. Eventually, after prolonged use, the surface of the filter becomes too thick and must be scraped off and allowed to reform.

2. *Rapid sand filtration.* In this method alum is added to the water. The alum precipitates, carrying with it many of the bacteria present. The water is then passed through a sand filter on the surface of which the alum accumulates and acts like the vital layer of a slow sand filter.

Of the two methods the slow sand filter is considerably more efficient but neither can be relied on to render water completely sterile. To reduce its bacterial content still further water after filtration is treated with chlorine. For the filtration of small household supplies unglazed porcelain filters are frequently employed. To maintain their efficiency these must be cleaned at regular intervals.

Another application of filtration of practical importance is for the removal of micro-organisms from the air. Air filtration is of value in industries utilizing fermentation processes, e.g. those concerned with the manufacture of antibiotics in which the control of extraneous contamination is essential. Air filtration is also being employed on an increasing scale in hospital operating theatres and dressing rooms as a means of controlling hospital cross infection. Filters of slag wool, glass wool and spun glass fibres have been mainly used. Cotton wool is also an extremely efficient air filter but is only effective as long as it can be kept dry. It is not used in air filtration on a large scale but is of course of the greatest value to the bacteriologist as a method of preserving the sterility of culture media.

CHEMICAL DISINFECTION

Chemical agents exhibit two distinct types of antibacterial effect—(a) a *bactericidal* or killing effect and (b) a *bacteriostatic* or growth inhibiting effect. Bactericidal activity may be demonstrated by mixing a suspension of bacteria with the disinfectant and then after a period of contact under defined conditions the mixture is subcultured to a nutrient medium. If the compound has a bactericidal action no growth of the organism will occur on subculture. To demonstrate bacteriostatic activity the disinfectant is incorporated in a suitable nutrient medium, e.g. broth which is then inoculated with the organism and incubated. A bacteriostatic effect is shown by the absence of growth after incubation.

Most of the chemical compounds which can kill bacteria exhibit a bacteriostatic effect in concentrations lower than those required to kill. The relationship between bactericidal and bacteriostatic concentrations is not, however, the same for all disinfectants. Some compounds, e.g. the mercurials and the quaternary ammonium compounds, have very marked bacteriostatic properties inhibiting bacterial growth in dilutions very much higher than those required to kill.

Others, e.g. the halogens, which of the commonly used disinfectants are unique in this respect, appear to be exclusively or almost exclusively bactericidal.

On the whole we know relatively little of the precise way in which disinfectants kill bacteria; it is probable that in most cases killing occurs through some form of enzyme inactivation either by protein denaturation, oxidation or by a combination of the antibacterial agent with specific groups of enzyme proteins. Some of the compounds used as disinfectants, e.g. the quaternary ammonium compounds, are capable of damaging the bacterial cell membrane and thus permitting leakage of essential intracellular compounds from the cell into its environment. This type of effect is believed to be of primary importance in the killing action of such compounds.

Kinetics of Disinfection

When a bacterial population is exposed to a disinfectant there is a progressive reduction with time in the number of surviving organisms. Disinfection is therefore a gradual process. In this connection it is important to remember that when we study the killing of bacteria by a disinfectant the observable effect is the effect on a bacterial population not the effect on a single bacterial cell. It follows therefore that the larger the bacterial population exposed the longer is the time required for its sterilization.

It is generally accepted as a working hypothesis that the rate at which disinfection occurs is uniform in the sense that during each unit of time a constant proportion of the organisms present at the beginning of that time is killed. In this event if the logarithm of the number of survivors after exposure to a disinfectant is plotted against the time of exposure the resultant curve is a straight line. This relationship is expressed mathematically in the following formula:

$$K = 1/t \log B/b,$$

where B = the initial number of organisms and b = the number after time t. There is, however, considerable doubt as to whether the logarithmic curve though mathematically convenient is in fact a correct general expression of the process of disinfection. It appears to be approximately correct when relatively high concentrations of disinfectant are used. With lower concentrations, however, many bacteriologists claim that the disinfection curve has a sigmoid character the rate being slow in the early stages then proceeding rapidly for most of the disinfection process and finally slowing down at the end.

As might be expected the rate of disinfection varies with the concentration of disinfectant employed. The effect of concentration on rate however is not constant and varies considerably with different disinfectants. With phenolic compounds, for example, a change in the concentration of the disinfectant has a marked effect on the disinfection rate. Thus with phenol, halving the concentration of disinfectant increases approximately 64-fold the time required for sterilization. With most other disinfectants changes in concentration have a very much less dramatic effect on sterilizing time than in the case of phenol.

For example with the mercurials halving the concentration of disinfectant only doubles the time required for sterilization.

Factors Affecting Disinfectant Action

The efficiency of a disinfectant is affected by a variety of factors.

1. Since disinfection is a chemical process its rate is considerably affected by temperature. In most cases the higher the temperature the more rapid the rate and consequently the shorter the time required for sterilization. The effect of temperature on rate is, however, not the same for different compounds and even with the same compound varies over different parts of the temperature range.

2. Different organisms show considerable differences in their susceptibility to disinfection. Spores in particular are highly resistant, possibly because the relatively impermeable spore coverings form an effective barrier to the passage of the disinfectant into the cell. Of the commonly used disinfectants only the halogens and formaldehyde possess any useful sporicidal activity. Tubercle bacilli also exhibit a high resistance to chemical disinfection, particularly to disinfectants in aqueous solution. This lack of susceptibility is usually attributed to the high lipid content of the tubercle bacillus. On the whole Gram positive organisms appear to be more susceptible to the action of disinfectants than Gram negatives. Of the latter the *Pseudomonas* genus appears to be one of the most resistant.

3. The activity of disinfectants may be markedly affected by substances present in the environment. Most disinfectants are to a greater or lesser extent inhibited by organic material with a high protein content, e.g. serum, blood and pus. This inhibition is most marked in the case of the aniline dyes, the mercurials and the cationic detergents. Certain disinfectants, depending on their nature, are inhibited by specific compounds. The quaternary ammonium compounds, for example, are markedly inhibited by soaps and lipids and the mercurials by compounds containing sulphydryl (SH) groups. The pH of the environment may also have considerable effect. Some compounds, e.g. the cationic detergents and aniline dyes, are most active under alkaline conditions while others, notably the phenols and chlorine, are most active at an acid pH.

Acids and Alkalis

Most bacteria will grow only in a pH range of 5 to 9, and the growth of many is fairly sharply restricted to the neighbourhood of pH 7. The inhibitory action of acid on the growth of bacteria is utilized in the occasional incorporation of benzoic acid and sulphurous acid (as sulphur dioxide) as preservatives in certain foods and of acetic acid as vinegar in pickling.

The disinfectant activity of strong acids and alkalis depends in general on their acid or basic strength. Many weak organic acids have, however, a higher activity than would be expected from their dissociation constants. This activity is due to the toxicity of the organic anion.

The tubercle bacillus is appreciably more resistant than other organisms to disinfection by acid and alkali. Consequently material from which it is proposed to culture tubercle bacilli may be treated with acid or alkali to free it from other bacteria present.

Salts

All salts have some degree of toxicity for bacteria. The most toxic are those of the heavy metals, mercury and silver, and the least toxic the salts of sodium and potassium.

Of the heavy metals the most frequently used is mercury. Two types of compound are employed—the *inorganic salts* and the *organic mercurials* in which mercury is combined with an organic radical. Both types of compound have very marked bacteriostatic properties but cannot be regarded as good disinfectants since their bactericidal activity is relatively slight. Mercury compounds appear to act on bacteria by combining with sulphydryl (SH) groups of bacterial proteins and other essential intracellular compounds. With these they form a relatively loose combination from which they can be dissociated by the addition of SH containing compounds. Since pus and exudates contain a variety of such compounds they antagonize the action of the mercurials. This constitutes a further serious limitation to their medical utility.

The anti-infective properties of silver, as reflected in the use of silver urns as domestic utensils, have been known from antiquity. Metallic silver is itself bacteriostatic in a very high dilution. This effect is known as the *oligodynamic* effect and is probably due to free silver ions released in low concentrations from the metal. The bactericidal effect of silver is made use of in the Katadyn process of water disinfection—a method which is sometimes used for domestic installations. Of the salts of silver—silver nitrate has been most used. Its main medical application is in the prophylaxis of ophthalmia neonatorum and is highly effective for this purpose if instilled into a new-born infant's eyes immediately after delivery. Colloidal silver compounds in which silver is combined with protein and from which silver ions are slowly released have been widely used as antiseptics, particularly in ophthalmology. They have mainly a bacteriostatic action and are relatively poor disinfectants.

Halogens

Chlorine and *iodine* are the only halogens which have any practical application as disinfectants. For certain purposes—chlorine as a water disinfectant and iodine as a skin disinfectant—they are unequalled. Their great value as disinfectants is due to the following:

1. They are bactericidal in a very high dilution. They are in fact unique amongst the disinfectants in that their activity is practically exclusively bactericidal.

2. Their action is very rapid.

3. They possess considerable activity against sporing organisms.

In addition to chlorine itself three types of chlorine compound—the hypochlorites, the inorganic chloramines and the organic chloramines—are available. The disinfectant action of all chlorine compounds is due to their capacity to liberate free chlorine. In solution the liberated chlorine forms hypochlorous acid which in its non-ionized form is believed to be the active disinfectant agent. Since hypochlorous acid is least dissociated at acid pH values chlorine disinfectants are in general most active under acid conditions.

For large scale water disinfection chlorine is usually employed in the form of the compressed gas but for the small scale purification of domestic supplies it is usually employed in the form of chlorinated lime (calcium hypochlorite). When water is treated with chlorine it is first necessary to determine its 'chlorine demand'. This is due to a variety of substances which may be present in the water which are capable of combining with chlorine. Although some of the compounds thus formed, in particular the organic chloramines, may have appreciable disinfectant action—their action is much slower than that of free chlorine. Consequently it is usual to add sufficient chlorine to satisfy the chlorine demand of the water and at the same time to provide enough residual chlorine for active disinfection. A residual chlorine concentration of from 0·2 to 0·4 parts per million is quite adequate for this purpose. In the case of waters which contain a large amount of organic material a considerable amount of chlorine may have to be added initially to leave this amount of residual chlorine.

Hypochlorites have a wide application in the dairy industry for the disinfection of equipment for which they are possibly the best compounds at present available. Calcium hypochlorite is frequently employed for the disinfection of faeces, urine and sanitary utensils, and is highly effective for this purpose. It has however little, if any, activity against tubercle bacilli. Sodium hypochlorite in the form of an aerosol disseminated by spraying has been used extensively as an air disinfectant but its value for this purpose is doubtful.

Inorganic chloramines, which are compounds of chlorine with ammonia, of varying chlorine composition, have appreciable disinfectant action. In solution they are more stable than the hypochlorites releasing their available chlorine more slowly. Consequently they have a much more sustained action but, as might be expected, are active in lower dilution. Because of their persistent action they are of special value for the sterilization of water when there is a delay in its distribution. In some water purification plants, particularly in the United States, chloramines are relied on entirely for disinfection—the water being treated with calculated amounts of ammonium sulphate and chlorine. Organic chloramines were at one time widely used as wound antiseptics but are now rarely employed.

Iodine is used almost exclusively as a skin disinfectant and is the only disinfectant commonly used for this purpose which is active against sporing organisms. It is usually employed as a tincture. This is an alcoholic solution containing 2·5 per cent iodine and 2·5 per cent potassium iodide in 90 per cent alcohol. Lugol's solution—a watery solution containing 5 per cent iodine and 10 per cent potassium iodide may also be employed for skin disinfection and has the advantage that it is less irritant to the tissues than the tincture. In the concentrations in which it is normally used iodine is not appreciably affected by organic matter. Like chlorine it is most active at an acid pH. The active agent in disinfection is the iodine molecule. An occasional disadvantage encountered in the use of iodine as a skin disinfectant is that it can produce skin rashes in individuals who are unduly susceptible to it. In the form of a 2 per cent aqueous solution iodine is probably the best agent available for the sterilization of clinical thermometers.

Mixtures of iodine with various surface active agents, which act as carriers for the iodine, are known as iodophors; they have been widely used in the United States especially for the sterilization of dairy equipment. Compounds of this type, particularly those formed with non-ionic detergents, are claimed to be more active than the alcoholic and aqueous solutions.

Phenols

Phenolic compounds are probably the most widely used of all disinfectants. The disinfectant activity of phenol itself was first discovered by Lister whose use of it to control hospital infections laid the foundation of modern surgical asepsis. Phenol is, however, no longer used as a general disinfectant. It is expensive and compared with its modern derivatives has a relatively low degree of activity. It is in addition not suitable for application to the skin or mucous membranes since it is readily absorbed with the production of severe toxic symptoms. Its main importance is as a standard with which other disinfectants may be compared and as a bacteriostatic agent in materials to be used for injection.

The antibacterial activity of phenol is greatly increased by various forms of substitution in the phenol nucleus—the compounds which are of most importance being the *alkyl-* and *chloro-* derivatives and the *diphenyls*. Many of these derivatives have a very high antibacterial activity some having phenol coefficients of 100 or more. In addition the more active compounds are appreciably less toxic than phenol being much less readily absorbed from the skin and mucous membranes. High activity is, however, associated with certain disadvantages. Whereas the simpler compounds—phenol itself and the cresols—are not significantly affected by the presence of organic matter and have much the same degree of activity against Gram positive and Gram negative organisms, the activity of the more active high molecular weight compounds is appreciably diminished by the presence of organic material and is considerably more marked against Gram positives than against Gram negatives. Most phenolic disinfectants have a low solubility in water; consequently they must be formulated with solubilizing or emulsifying agents. For this purpose various soaps are used—various proprietary preparations differing in the type of soap employed. Soaps not only act as solubilizing or emulsifying agents for phenols, but also, provided an excessive amount of soap is not present, increase their antibacterial action.

The simplest of the alkyl phenols are the cresols—the three isomers of which, o-, m- and p-, show no significant differences in disinfectant activity. Cresols are obtained industrially by the distillation of coal tar and are the principal ingredients of the lower boiling point fractions. The cresols resemble phenol closely in their antibacterial effects but are appreciably more active. Lysol, one of the most commonly used general purpose disinfectants, consists of 50 per cent cresol in soap. Unfortunately Lysol produces a severe brown staining and is consequently unsuitable for the sterilization of fabrics. Like phenol it is too toxic for application to the skin, but is widely used in laboratories for the preliminary sterilization of infected glassware and in hospitals for the disinfection of excreta. It is probably the most suitable disinfectant for disinfecting the floors and furniture of infected rooms.

The xylenols or methyl cresols have provided two extremely important disinfectants—p-chloro-sym-m-xylenol (PCMX) and 2,4-dichloro-sym-m-xylenol (DCMX). Of these PCMX has been more used; it is the main component of a number of commercial preparations of which the best known and most widely used is probably Dettol. PCMX has considerable activity against both Gram positive and Gram negative organisms. Its capacity to retain its activity for a considerable time on the skin and other surfaces is of special value in medicine. It is of low toxicity and is not markedly inhibited by organic matter. It is probably the most widely used domestic disinfectant and mainly as a result of the work of Colebrook and Maxted has become virtually the standard disinfectant in obstetrical practice. It is usually formulated with α terpineol, which is the active agent of pine oil, and with various soaps.

The most important of the diphenyl compounds are the chloro substituted diphenylmethanes—dichlorophane, tetrachlorophane and hexachlorophane. The bactericidal activity of these compounds is somewhat less than that of the chloroxylenols but they are bacteriostatic in very high dilutions. In fact because of their marked bacteriostatic potency they were at first considerably over-rated as bactericidal agents. Hexachlorophane is probably the best known. Unlike other phenols it retains its activity in the presence of large amounts of soap and germicidal soaps containing low concentrations of hexachlorophane have achieved a considerable popularity. Hexachlorophane soaps when frequently used cause a marked reduction of the bacterial flora of the skin and for this reason have been strongly recommended for habitual use by surgeons. Hexachlorophane is appreciably more active against Gram positive than against Gram negative organisms.

Chlorhexidine (1,6-di-4'-chlorphenyldiguanidohexane). This compound has come into extensive use in recent years as a skin disinfectant. It is actively bactericidal for a wide range of Gram positive and Gram negative species and because of its rapid action and low toxicity is of special value for clinical use. A 0·5 per cent solution of the digluconate in 70 per cent ethyl alcohol is reported to be as effective for skin disinfection as tincture of iodine and has the advantage that it lacks the irritative properties of the latter. In addition to its application as a skin disinfectant chlorhexidine applied in a cream base has been favourably reported on for the treatment of nasal carriers of *Staphylococcus aureus*.

Soaps

Though soaps possess disinfectant properties their activity is of a comparatively low order; it is consequently unlikely that much disinfectant action occurs during the short time taken in washing the hands. Nevertheless the process of cleaning with soap and water mechanically removes organisms from the skin and has in effect a disinfectant action.

Soaps are somewhat selective in action being appreciably more active against Gram positive than against Gram negative organisms. Of the pathogenic bacteria the pneumococci appear to be the most susceptible to their action. Staphylococci are highly resistant. Of the fatty acid soaps the most active are those derived from the unsaturated fatty acids.

A variety of so-called 'germicidal' soaps in which low concentrations of various disinfectants, e.g. mercurials, formaldehyde and phenols, are incorporated in soap are available commercially. The majority of these have little germicidal activity apart from that of the soap itself and are quite wrongly described as germicidal. Soaps incorporating diphenyls, however, particularly those containing hexachlorophane seem to be an exception in this respect and appear to have a high degree of germicidal activity.

Alcohols

Ethyl alcohol is the only alcohol which is in general use as a disinfectant. It is extensively used for the sterilization of the skin prior to operation and inoculation. Ethyl alcohol is also widely used for the disinfection of clinical thermometers and provided a sufficient period of contact is allowed is very effective for this purpose.

Ethyl alcohol is non-specific in action being active against both Gram positive and Gram negative organisms. It possesses in addition appreciable activity against tubercle bacilli a property of considerable importance in the sterilization of thermometers. It has no significant sporicidal activity; in fact the recovery of anthrax spores after 20 years exposure to ethyl alcohol has been recorded.

Ethyl alcohol almost certainly acts by protein denaturation and exhibits a bactericidal effect only in the presence of water. Appreciable disinfectant activity only occurs in concentrations of from 40 to 95 per cent—the optimum range being from 50 to 70 per cent. In suitable concentration it is rapidly bactericidal. Because of its lack of sporicidal activity ethyl alcohol should not be used by itself for the sterilization of instruments.

In general the disinfectant activity of the alcohols increases with increase in chain length. Above 10 carbon atoms, however, the solubility of the compound becomes too low for practical use. Apart from ethyl alcohol the only alcohols which have so far had any significant application have been isopropyl alcohol and the dihydric alcohols ethylene and propylene glycol. Iso-propyl alcohol which is appreciably more active and less volatile than ethyl alcohol has been recommended for the sterilization of clinical thermometers. It is claimed to be more effective than ethyl alcohol as a skin disinfectant; its high cost, however, prohibits its general use for this purpose. Ethylene and propylene glycol have been used as aerosols for air disinfection but their value for this purpose is doubtful.

Dyes

Two groups of dyes (*a*) the *aniline* dyes and (*b*) the *acridines* have been considerably used as skin and wound antiseptics. Both groups are bacteriostatic in high dilution but are of low bactericidal activity. Of the aniline dyes brilliant green, malachite green and crystal violet (an impure form of the latter is known as gentian violet) have been mainly used. All are amino derivatives of triphenyl-methane. The aniline dyes are highly selective being much more active against Gram positive than against Gram negative organisms. Staphylococci are particularly susceptible to the dyes of the violet series. The aniline dyes are without activity against tubercle bacilli; in fact because of this malachite green is used as a selective agent in Löwenstein's medium for growth of tubercle bacilli. The use of gentian violet and of brilliant green as selective agents in the isolation of haemolytic streptococci and of salmonellae respectively are considered elsewhere (Chapter 3). The aniline dyes are more active at an alkaline than at an acid pH. They are non-irritant to the tissues and are virtually non-toxic, but have the disadvantage that they are considerably inhibited by organic material; their activity is consequently considerably reduced in the presence of pus.

The acridines have, for clinical purposes, two important advantages over the aniline dyes: (1) Though somewhat more active against Gram positives than against Gram negatives they are not as selective as the aniline dyes. (2) They are little if at all affected by the presence of organic matter. The following compounds all of which are amino substituted acridines are of clinical importance: proflavine, acriflavine, euflavine and aminacrine. These compounds show no significant differences in potency. Proflavine has been the most used since it appears to have the lowest tissue toxicity of the group. A property of the acridines which is of special value for wound antisepsis is the fact that they can be used to impregnate gauze from which they are slowly released in a moist environment.

Quaternary Ammonium Compounds

This group of compounds has the general formula NR_4X where R stands for an alkyl or phenyl radical and X an inorganic radical. They may therefore be regarded as substituted ammonium salts. In solution they ionize to yield an organic cation and an inorganic anion. The organic cation of the quaternaries has lipophilic properties and confers on the compounds marked surface activity.

The antibacterial properties of the group were first systematically investigated by Domagk in 1935 who found that for optimum activity one of the substituent radicals should be a carbon chain of from 8 to 18 carbon atoms. Literally hundreds of such compounds have now been synthesized but the majority of these have, for one reason or another, been unsuitable as disinfectants. The more important compounds now in use are cetrimide, benzalkonium chloride and domiphen bromide.

The quaternary ammonium compounds have very marked antibacterial properties and are bactericidal for a wide range of organisms. Although active against both Gram positive and Gram negative species they are appreciably more active against the Gram positives. They are virtually without activity against tubercle bacilli and spores. A special feature of the group and one in which they resemble the mercurials is that they are bacteriostatic in very high dilution. This can be attributed to the fact that because of their high surface activity they are readily adsorbed to the bacterial surface even when present in very low concentration. Their antibacterial activity, like that of the aniline dyes, is much more marked at alkaline than at acid pH values. Although strongly haemolytic for red cells under in vitro conditions they appear to possess little in vivo toxicity. Unfortunately they are markedly inhibited by organic matter particularly by proteins, phospholipids and fats. In this connexion it has been suggested that the relatively low susceptibility of the Gram negatives is due to their high lipid content. The quaternary ammonium compounds are also antagonized by soaps and other anionic compounds. The possibility of antagonism by soap should be borne in mind when any member of this group is being used for the disinfection of the skin.

The readiness with which quaternaries are adsorbed to surfaces is of practical importance in disinfection for the following reasons: (1) When applied to the skin they form an antibacterial surface film which persists for a considerable time. There is some doubt, however, as to their value as skin disinfectants since the residual detergent may not be actively bactericidal. (2) They are readily adsorbed to glassware and to fabrics. Consequently they are widely used for the sterilization of food utensils in restaurants and hotels, for the sterilization of milk containers in the dairy industry and for the disinfection of blankets in hospitals.

Oxidizing Agents

Potassium permanganate has been considerably used in the tropics for the disinfection of water and vegetables. Although highly active against the cholera vibrio it is not a satisfactory water disinfectant, since when present in effective antibacterial concentration it has an unpleasant taste and in addition leaves a residue of toxic manganese compounds in the water. The intense staining it produces makes it unsuitable as a general disinfectant.

Hydrogen peroxide is used for skin disinfection but undoubtedly owes much of its reputation to the vigorous bubbling which occurs when it is brought into contact with tissue catalase in open wounds.

Formaldehyde

When dispersed in gaseous form formaldehyde has considerable bactericidal activity and is one of the very limited number of disinfectants active against spores. The sterilizing efficiency of formaldehyde is very low under dry conditions but increases with increase in moisture content of the air up to a level of around 50 per cent relative humidity. Sterilization is not strictly gaseous but is as a result of condensation of the gas on exposed surfaces. Consequently formaldehyde has relatively poor penetrating power and this constitutes a considerable limitation to its practical use. Its penetration into clothes and fabrics can, however, be considerably increased by using it in a sterilizing chamber, like a hospital sterilizer, which can be exhausted of air prior to introduction of the gas. Under these conditions sterilization is usually carried out around 60° C. Formaldehyde is frequently used for the sterilization of hospital bedding and fabrics, e.g. woollen materials, which might be damaged by heating to the high temperature of the autoclave. It may, however, take a considerable time to remove all traces of formaldehyde from fabrics which have been exposed to it. Formaldehyde is undoubtedly the most effective of the gaseous disinfectants for room sterilization and though rarely used now for terminal disinfection is occasionally employed for the disinfection of rooms in laboratories and in industries where contamination must be kept to a minimum. In liquid form (Formalin) formaldehyde is used to sterilize materials such as wool and hides which may harbour anthrax spores. It is also employed for the disinfection of the shoes and footwear of persons suffering from athlete's foot since it is very active against the fungi responsible for this condition.

Glutaraldehyde

This relatively new disinfectant has a wide range of action including a marked lethal effect on spores and tubercle bacilli. Its sporicidal action is said to be considerably greater than that of formaldehyde. Like the latter, it probably acts as an alkylating agent. It shows a maximum activity at pH of 7·5 to 8·5 and polymerizes rapidly above pH 9. It is usually employed as a 2 per cent buffered solution (Cidex) which is claimed to be stable for 2 weeks at 20° C. It has been recommended for the sterilization of cystoscopes and other endoscopic instruments which cannot be subjected to heat sterilization.

Ethylene Oxide

Although it has been used in Germany for many years as an insecticide it is only in comparatively recent years that ethylene oxide has received any serious attention as a disinfectant. It is a cyclic ether $(CH_2)_2O$ which boils at 10·8° C and which therefore is a gas at ordinary room temperatures. By itself it is highly inflammable but forms safe non-inflammable mixtures with CO_2 and fluorinated hydrocarbons. It is toxic to man by inhalation, and on contact with the skin has a vesicant action. It cannot be used, therefore, for sterilizing the air of occupied rooms. Ethylene oxide is active against all types of bacteria including spores and tubercle bacilli but its action is slow. It is active at room temperature and is most effective at a relative humidity of about 30 per cent. In the dry state bacteria appear to be highly resistant. Effective bactericidal concentrations are in the region of 400 to 100 mg per litre. It can be used for sterilizing a wide range of materials but is of particular value for the sterilization of materials which would be damaged by heat, e.g. polythene tubing. It has been of special value in the sterilization of heart lung machines. In contrast to formaldehyde, ethylene oxide has marked penetrating power. An important corollary of this property is the readiness with which all traces of the gas disappear from materials which have been exposed to it. It has, however, considerable solubility in certain plastics and in rubber and leather. The most serious objections to its general use are its high cost and the necessity for complex equipment. In addition, it requires highly skilled supervision. Because of these limitations ethylene oxide is unlikely to come into routine use in hospital sterilization.

CHAPTER 5

BACTERIA IN HEALTH AND DISEASE

Most bacteria are free-living organisms deriving their nourishment from inert organic or inorganic materials. Although often of great importance in the economy of nature, these free-living bacteria are of little interest to the medical bacteriologist, who is concerned primarily with the limited numbers of species which are parasitic for man.

In respect of their capacity to produce disease the parasitic bacteria form a continuous series, ranging from those with little or no power of producing disease to those that when present in the body almost invariably produce disease. From the evolutionary point of view the non-pathogenic or occasionally pathogenic bacteria must be regarded as being more successful than the more highly pathogenic varieties. They are able to establish a harmless parasitic relationship with their hosts, sometimes to the advantage of the latter, which ensures their own chances of survival. Highly pathogenic bacteria can rarely if ever establish such a relationship and, by frequently killing the host, diminish their own chances of survival.

The Normal Body Flora

At birth the skin and mucous membranes are, as might be expected, sterile. It is in fact possible by the adoption of stringent isolation procedures to maintain laboratory animals in a germ-free state. Such animals have been of considerable value for research, particularly in connexion with the development of immunity mechanisms.

In the normal animal, however, the surfaces of the body which are in contact with the environment, namely the skin and mucous membranes rapidly become colonized by organisms present in the environment. The organisms that can establish themselves in this way differ in the various parts of the body, which consequently show variations in their normal flora. Such differences are due to the operation of local and environmental factors which favour and tend to select certain species. We know relatively little of the precise nature of these environmental factors and of the way in which they tend to favour particular bacteria. We do know, however, that changes in environmental conditions may result in marked changes in local flora.

The organisms of this normal flora are known as *commensals* and obtain their nutriment from the secretions and waste products of the body. Occasionally species of relatively high pathogenicity may appear in the normal flora without causing disease. When this happens the individual in whose body the pathogen is found is known as a *carrier*. The carrier state is, however, unusual—the highly pathogenic organisms either initiating an infection or being rapidly eliminated from the body.

A knowledge of the types of bacteria found in different areas is of great importance in diagnostic bacteriology and these will be briefly considered.

The skin is constantly receiving bacteria from the air or from objects with which it has come in contact, but the majority of these do not grow on it because of the absence of suitable growth conditions. Few are capable even of surviving on the skin for more than a very short time because of substances which are bactericidal for them. The skin is also highly acid in reaction, pH values of 3 to 5 having been recorded. Another factor of importance in limiting the bacterial population of the skin is the drying that occurs on the skin surface, which can itself cause the rapid death of many pathogenic species. Within a few hours of being contaminated with *E. coli, Salm. typhi* or *Str. pyogenes*, the skin can free itself completely of these foreign bacteria. The most constant of the normal flora of the skin are anaerobic diphtheroids—which belong to the genus *Propioni- bacterium*—and non-pathogenic staphylococci. These organisms are found mostly in the sebaceous glands; their numbers are little affected by washing.

The organisms most frequently and most constantly found in the nose are non-pathogenic corynebacteria. The nose is also the natural home of *Staph. aureus*, and this organism can be isolated from about 50 per cent of nasal swabs taken from normal persons. The occasional *Staph. aureus* on the skin is usually secondary to nasal carriage. About the throat, viridans streptococci, *N. catarrhalis* and staphylococci very commonly occur, while pneumococci and Friedländer's bacillus are not infrequent. The deeper portions of the respiratory tract, the finer bronchioles and the alveoli of the lung, are normally sterile.

The mouth has a very mixed bacterial flora—the abundant moisture and the constant presence of small food particles providing an ideal environment for bacterial growth. Both aerobic and anaerobic types are found. The most important of the aerobic organisms are non-haemolytic streptococci and neisseriae but miscellaneous fungi and actinomycetes are frequently present. Some of the last are believed to be of importance in the formation of dental tartar. Prior to the eruption of the teeth and in the edentulous adult, the flora of the mouth consists almost exclusively of aerobic organisms. Following the eruption of the teeth a number of anaerobic types—spirochaetes, anaerobic vibrios, various anaerobic cocci, and not infrequently *Actinomyces israelii*—are able to establish themselves. These organisms find ideal sites for anaerobic multiplication in the pockets between the gums and the teeth.

The contents of the healthy stomach are practically sterile, as are also those of the duodenum, owing to the presence of hydrochloric acid in the gastric secretion, but the intestine contains an enormous number and variety of bacteria. It has been calculated that an adult excretes in the faeces about 3×10^{13} bacteria daily, the majority of which are dead.

The intestinal flora of the breast-fed infant is almost exclusively lactobacillary in type. With the introduction of bottle feeding the lactobacilli became less numerous, and finally, on substitution of solid food and adult diet the normal mixed but predominantly Gram negative bacillary intestinal flora becomes established. The most numerous of these are the bacteroids—a miscellaneous group of anaerobic Gram negative bacilli—and the coliform bacilli, particularly *E. coli*. A variety of other organisms is also found although to a lesser extent, viz.: *Str. faecalis*, clostridia notably *Cl. perfringens*, paracolon bacilli, and *Bacillus*, *Lactobacillus*, *Proteus* and *Pseudomonas* species. *Staph. aureus* can also usually be isolated from faeces.

In diarrhoea as a result of the rapid movements of the intestinal contents the flora usually undergoes considerable change. Organisms such as *Proteus*, *Pseudomonas* and certain coliforms which are normally found in small numbers may become very numerous. The composition of the intestinal flora may be considerably altered in persons receiving wide-spectrum antibiotics; the normal sensitive organisms are inhibited and may be replaced by resistant organisms.

It was at one time believed that toxic bacterial products absorbed from the intestinal tract might have some deleterious effects on the body—a hypothetical condition known as autointoxication. This view has no scientific foundation but is still maintained with considerable fervour by many 'nature cure' enthusiasts.

About the external genitals, in both sexes, various Gram positive cocci, *E. coli*, smegma bacilli and spirochaetes are found. Few bacteria exist in the urethra and the urine in the bladder is sterile in health. The main inhabitants of the adult vagina are the group of lactobacilli known as Döderlein's bacilli. These organisms break down the glycogen produced by the vaginal epithelium with the production of acid, of which they are highly tolerant. Fungi which are highly tolerant of acid are also usually present, but other organisms are found irregularly and in small numbers. As the accumulation of glycogen in the vaginal wall is due to ovarian activity, glycogen is not present before puberty or after the menopause. Consequently at these times the flora is mixed rather than predominantly lactobacillary in type.

The relationship between the commensal bacteria and their animal host is a symbiotic one; the advantages of this relationship to the bacteria are obvious. But there are, possibly in no less degree, also advantages to the host.

1. The bacteria serve as scavengers assisting in the disposal of waste material.

2. In the case of the intestinal bacteria they undoubtedly play a part in the nutrition of the host. Many of the intestinal bacteria can synthesize the major B group vitamins, and some can also synthesize vitamins E and K. These syntheses are believed to make a significant contribution to the vitamin requirements of the host.

3. By their presence they tend to exclude pathogenic bacteria, and in this way serve to protect the host against disease. This exclusion may be by simple competition with the pathogen for nutrition, or it may be by the production of substances that are inhibitory to the growth of the pathogen. Thus, the acid

produced by the lactobacilli of the adult vagina protects the vagina from infection with the gonococcus and other pyogenic organisms. Certain of the mouth streptococci produce hydrogen peroxide which may play a part in the exclusion from the mouth of peroxide sensitive pathogens. Many strains of *E. coli* produce colicines which may protect the intestinal tract from other pathogenic enterobacteriaceae such as the shigellae which are sensitive to them.

The Basis of Bacterial Pathogenicity

The capacity of an organism to produce disease is known as its *pathogenicity* or *virulence*. With the exception of the cholera vibrio and the organisms responsible for bacterial food poisoning, bacteria can produce disease only if they invade or gain access to the tissues. In order to do this they must pass through the surface covering of the body—the skin or mucous membranes. It is doubtful whether any bacteria can penetrate the skin unless there has been some degree of trauma, e.g. by wounds, abrasions, or insect bites. The mucous membranes are, however, much more permeable and many bacteria appear to be able to pass readily through them.

Invasions of the tissues both through the skin and mucous membranes are of frequent occurrence. The majority of these invasions, however, do not result in disease, as the organisms that have gained entry are rapidly disposed of by the tissue defences. The invading organisms can cause disease only if, after invasion, they can multiply. The capacity to multiply in the tissues is known as *aggressiveness*. The term *invasiveness* is also used, although not strictly correctly as being roughly synonymous with aggressiveness. Finally, the mere multiplication of bacteria in the tissues does not by itself produce disease unless the bacteria can in some way damage the tissues. The capacity of bacteria to damage the tissues is known as *toxicity*.

Aggressiveness and *toxicity* are largely distinct characters and can compensate for each other to a considerable extent. Thus some organisms, such as the pneumococci, are markedly aggressive but little if at all toxic. Others such as *Str. pyogenes* are highly aggressive and moderately toxic while a few such as *Cl. tetani* and *C. diphtheriae* are highly toxic but only slightly aggressive.

Factors Contributing to Aggressiveness

On the whole our knowledge of the properties of bacteria that permit them to maintain themselves and to flourish in the tissues is slight. In some cases avirulent mutants derived from parent virulent strains are known which differ from the parent strains in no property so far demonstrable other than that of being unable to multiply in the body. It is possible that in such cases the properties of the virulent organism are such that it is capable of multiplying in the biochemical environment provided by areas of inflammation, but our detailed knowledge of this environment is insufficient to allow us any insight into what these properties might be.

As soon as a micro-organism gains access to the tissues it is confronted with a mobilization of the defensive machinery of the host. It is obvious, therefore, that in order to establish itself or to multiply it must in some way be able to overcome the host defences. The single most important component of the host's defence against invading bacteria is undoubtedly phagocytosis. Bacteria which are to survive for any time in the tissues must therefore possess some mechanism of defending themselves against this; different bacteria may do so in different ways. They may, as in the case of *Staph. aureus* and *Str. pyogenes*, produce toxins known as leucocidins which actually kill the leucocytes. Only a few bacteria however produce such substances. Many possess surface components which confer a resistance to phagocytosis. The best known of such components are the capsules of capsulated pathogenic organisms such as the pneumococcus. These are presumed to confer resistance to phagocytosis by rendering the surface of the organism sticky or mucoid so that it is not readily ingested by the phagocyte, but non-capsular surface components can also confer resistance to phagocytosis. Important examples of such components are the Vi antigen of *Salm. typhi* and the type-specific or M proteins of *Str. pyogenes*. The precise mechanisms by which these substances confer resistance to phagocytosis is not known, but it is due, possibly, to the fact that they give the bacterial surface a strongly negative charge which allows it to repel the negatively charged phagocyte.

A unique method of preventing phagocytosis is exhibited by the staphylococcus. This organism produces an enzyme—coagulase—whose activity results in the deposition of a coating of fibrin on, or around its surface. Organisms on whose surfaces fibrin has been deposited in this way, appear to be extremely difficult for the phagocyte to ingest. In general it can be said that resistance to phagocytosis is an important component of virulence, but certain bacteria, notably tubercle bacilli and brucellae, although resistant to phagocytosis by polymorphonuclear leucocytes, are readily phagocytosed by histiocytes, and appear to owe their virulence to the fact that they can multiply inside the phagocyte, as well as resisting intracellular destruction.

It is also reasonable to assume that pathogenic bacteria are much more resistant than non-pathogenic bacteria to the killing action of complement and of other normally occurring bactericidal substances that may be present in the tissue fluids. It has been known, for example, that plague bacilli contain substances that possess a complement inhibiting effect, and that coagulase appears to play some part in protecting staphylococci against the bactericidal powers of normal serum. The possession of such mechanisms plays a part in determining virulence but has not been investigated in any great detail.

By the liberation of antigens into their environment which can combine with antibody, bacteria can reduce the opsonizing and bactericidal effects of the latter (Chapter 7). These soluble antigens are probably the substances described by early workers as *aggressins*.

Some bacteria produce substances which facilitate their rapid spread through the tissues and which thereby contribute to aggressiveness. *Str. pyogenes* secretes streptokinase, a substance which activates a plasma protease precursor. The activated protease in turn breaks down the fibrin formed by the tissues as a method of localizing the infection. *Cl. perfringens*, many strains of *Staph. aureus*, and some strains of *Str. pyogenes* produce an enzyme hyaluronidase which breaks down hyaluronic acid—the intercellular cement substance of the tissues. This results in a reduction in the viscosity of the latter and therefore permits more rapid spread of the organism. *Cl. perfringens* also produces collagenase—an enzyme capable of decomposing collagen. This enzyme plays an important role in the spread of *Cl. perfringens* through infected muscle.

Toxicity

There are numbers of possible mechanisms by which bacteria may cause damage to the tissues.

1. Action of Metabolic End Products

As a result of their growth a number of metabolic end products, e.g. lactic acid and various protein degradation products, which may have some local toxic effect, are produced. The part played by such substances in the toxaemia of infection is probably small.

2. Allergic Reactions

In tuberculosis the production of significant damage to the tissues depends on the existence of allergy to tuberculin. Tuberculin is not itself a toxic substance but can damage the cells of animals previously sensitized to it (Chapter 26). Allergy probably plays an important part in determining the amount of tissue damage occurring in a number of infections, but its role in this respect is most clear in tuberculosis.

3. Interference with the Nutrition of the Host Cell

It might be expected that extensive growth of bacteria in the tissues at the expense of nutrient material utilized also by the host cell might result in damage to the latter by interfering with its nutrition. There is reason to believe that this type of damage occurs in the lung in cases of pneumococcal lobar pneumonia and makes an important contribution to the apparent toxaemia of the condition. It is not known, however, whether, or to what extent, a similar effect occurs in other bacterial infections.

4. Bacterial Toxins

These are substances produced by or present in bacteria, which have a direct toxic action on tissue cells.

Our knowledge of bacterial toxins is confined almost entirely to substances produced under the conditions of laboratory culture. It is, however, possible that an organism might produce a toxic substance as a result of its growth in the body which it does not produce under the artificial conditions of laboratory culture. This appears to be the case with the anthrax bacillus (Chapter 27), and possibly occurs to some extent with other organisms as well.

PROPERTIES OF BACTERIAL TOXINS

Exotoxins	Endotoxins
Protein	Function of somatic antigen lipopoly-saccharide
Secreted into medium from cell cytoplasm	Present in cell wall. Released only on disruption of cell
Heat-labile	Heat-stable
Converted by H.CHO into toxoid	Cannot be toxoided
Strongly antigenic	Poorly if at all antigenic
Highly specific for particular tissues (e.g. tetanus toxin for CNS)	Non-specific in action
Very high potency (1 mg tetanus toxin = MLD for 1000 tons of guinea-pigs)	Low potency (about 1 mg extracted somatic antigen = MLD for one mouse)
Produced mainly by Gram positives—clostridia, diphtheria bacilli, streptococci, staphylococci	Produced by Gram negatives—salmonellae, shigellae, brucellae, coliforms

Bacterial toxins are conveniently divided into two groups.

(a) *The Exotoxins*

These are toxins which diffuse freely from the bacteria into the surrounding medium and can be obtained in cell-free filtrates.

(b) *The Endotoxins*

These are substances present in the body of the organism and not secreted to a significant extent into the surrounding medium. They may be obtained from the bacterial cells by physically disintegrating them or by various forms of chemical extraction and are liberated to a varying extent under natural conditions by autolysis. The distinction between exo- and endotoxins is, however, not absolutely sharp. Appreciable exotoxin is released by autolysis of the cell and some endotoxin is usually demonstrable in culture filtrates.

A number of exotoxins have been obtained in a highly purified form and have been found to be proteins; it is probable that all the typical exotoxins are proteins. The organisms producing exotoxin are *C. diphtheriae, Cl. tetani, Cl. botulinum, Sh. dysenteriae, Staph. aureus, Str. pyogenes,* and the gas gangrene clostridia. With the exception of *Sh. dysenteriae* (type 1) all the exotoxin-producing organisms are Gram positive.

Endotoxins isolated from the Gram negative bacilli, viz.: salmonellae, shigellae, *Vibrio cholerae,* coliform bacteria, brucellae and the neisseriae, are present in the organism as components of the somatic or O antigens (p. 96). Endotoxins obtained from *Pasteurella pestis* and *Bordetella pertussis* species are not of this type and have properties closely resembling those of the typical exotoxins.

The typical exotoxins differ in a number of respects from the typical endotoxins.

(a) The exotoxins are highly antigenic. The endotoxins are little if at all antigenic. Endotoxins are, however, partially neutralized by antibody to the corresponding somatic antigen. This is presumably a steric effect resulting from combination of antibody with the polysaccharide component of the antigen.

(*b*) The exotoxins are as a rule more readily inactivated by heat, most of them being destroyed at 65° C in a few minutes.

(*c*) The exotoxins are much more specific in action. Some, e.g. the toxins of *Cl. tetani*, *Cl. botulinum* and *Sh. dysenteriae* (type 1), have a specific neuro-toxic action. Another important group have considerable haemolytic properties. The endotoxins on the other hand are relatively non-specific in action; all have the same general toxic effect irrespective of the species of organism from which they are obtained. On injection into animals they give rise to inflammation, swelling at the site of inoculation and pyrexia. There is reason to believe that pyrexia produced by the endotoxins is due to the local liberation of a pyrogen-inducing substance from the tissues rather than to a remote direct effect of the toxin on the central nervous system.

(*d*) The exotoxins are as a rule much more potent than the endotoxins. The exotoxins of *Cl. tetani*, *Cl. botulinum* and *Sh. dysenteriae* are in fact the most toxic substances known. It has been estimated that 1 mg of purified preparations of these toxins constitutes a lethal dose for about 1000 tons of guinea-pigs. The lethal dose for a mouse of a typical endotoxin by contrast is about 1 mg.

(*e*) Most of the exotoxins can be converted into an inactive form by treatment with a number of agents, e.g. formalin, which are capable of combining with free amino groups. This inactive form is known as *toxoid* and, although non-toxic, is fully antigenic; it can therefore safely be used for immunization.

Variations in Virulence

Virulence for one species does not necessarily imply virulence for another. Man is not naturally susceptible to many of the organisms causing disease in animals and similarly animals are not susceptible to many of the organisms infecting man. In some cases it has been shown that an animal is not susceptible to an organism because its cells are not susceptible to the toxin of that organism; thus the rat is not susceptible to the diphtheria toxin and cold-blooded animals are not suscept-ible to the tetanus toxin. In most cases, however, the differences in the suscept-ibility of different species to a particular organism must be due to the fact that the properties of the organism are such that it can establish itself in the parti-cular tissue environment of one species but not in that of another. We are, however, ignorant of both the host factors and the bacterial properties involved.

Not only is virulence a property which can only be defined in relation to a particular animal species but it is also a property which can in the last resort be defined only in relation to a particular strain of bacterium. Even within pathogenic species we find wide variations in virulence. Some strains possess a high virulence, others, although still capable of infecting are less virulent and an occasional strain is completely avirulent. Although as a general rule, the viru-lence of bacteria tends to decrease on prolonged laboratory culture, it is by no means safe for the bacteriologist to assume that cultures of pathogenic species which have been maintained for many years in the laboratory can be handled with abandon. In the case of animal pathogenic species the virulence of strains which have been attenuated by artificial culture can usually be increased by passage in an appropriate experimental animal.

It is reasonable to assume that in nature, as in the laboratory, bacterial virulence can, in the course of time, be considerably modified either in the direction of enhancement or of diminution in virulence. There is reason to believe for example that over the last twenty-five years the virulence of *Str. pyogenes* has been decreasing. Quite apart from the introduction of chemotherapy, infections due to this organism appear to be much less severe now than they once were. On a longer time scale it has been suggested that the spirochaete of syphilis has over the last four or five hundred years shown a great diminution in virulence. In the Middle Ages syphilis appears quite frequently to have been an acute and grave infection. This is in considerable contrast to the more prolonged chronic infection caused by the *Treponema* in the twentieth century. It is possible, of course, that in this particular case modern European populations have, as a result of natural selection, somewhat higher resistance to the *Treponema* than their ancestors.

It has frequently been suggested that the development of epidemics may be due to the emergence of organisms possessing an enhanced degree of virulence. Although no laboratory evidence has been produced to support this view, epidemiological evidence suggests that at least in the case of outbreaks of meningococcal meningitis the emergence of virulent variants of the organism is a necessary preliminary to the initiation of an epidemic. Many virologists believe that also the great influenza pandemic of 1918 to 1919 was due to the emergence of an influenza virus of enhanced virulence. By analogy with results obtained from experimental animals it might be thought possible that the virulence of bacteria may become enhanced during the course of an epidemic, but so far such speculation has received no laboratory support.

It should be noted that, as already stated at the beginning of this chapter, the acquisition by a bacterial strain of a high degree of virulence is not necessarily an asset. It is to the advantage of the organism to establish a relationship with the host which results in mild, rather than severe disease. Thus, although virulent variants may be of considerable importance in the initiation of epidemics, they tend ultimately, by a process of natural selection, to disappear from the population, and strains of lesser virulence better adapted for survival will ultimately re-establish themselves.

Lesions Produced by Bacteria in the Body

Whether an invasion of the tissues will lead to overt infection depends not only on the virulence and numbers of the invading organisms but also on the resistance of the host. If the resistance of the host is low, an organism of relatively low virulence may readily establish a progressive infection, whereas if the resistance of the host is high, an organism even of quite a high degree of virulence may fail to do so. The resistance of the host is known as *immunity* and will be considered in more detail in Chapter 8.

The degree of immunity a person possesses against a particular infection determines not only whether he will become infected, but also the extent to which infection progresses once it has become established. If the patient's resistance in relation to the virulence of the organism is low he may be unable to control the infection and may die. The normal level of resistance in relation to most pathogenic organisms, however, is such that the patient usually recovers. This is due to the development, as a result of prolonged association over many generations, of an equilibrium between host and parasite populations which may of course from time to time be temporarily upset.

If his resistance is high, the infection will pursue a mild course and will frequently be insufficient to produce overt clinical symptoms. The latter is known as *subclinical* or *latent* infection and is of very great importance in stimulating immunity.

Most pathogenic bacteria can give rise to latent or subclinical infections, and in communities in which such organisms are endemic overt clinical cases are always accompanied by variable numbers of symptomless infections which can be detected only by serological tests. Some organisms, however, are unable to do so. Outstanding examples of such organisms are *Treponema pallidum* and the gonococcus; these, when present in the body, invariably appear to produce disease.

In most bacterial diseases the main features of the disease are due to the damage produced by the bacteria in the area of the body which is the site of the initial invasion. The characteristics of this local lesion vary with the type of infecting bacterium, on its virulence, on the susceptibility of the host and on the particular tissue of the body affected. Exceptionally, as in gas-gangrene, the changes produced may be of a rapidly destructive nature, providing little opportunity for a defensive response on the part of the host. In most cases, however, the damage caused by the bacteria stimulates a defensive response from the host which is known as the *inflammatory reaction*. The cardinal signs of this reaction—heat, redness, swelling and pain—are often more obvious to the patient and observer, than the direct damage caused by the bacteria.

Some species of bacteria stimulate an *acute* inflammatory reaction; this type of reaction is characterized in its early stages by vascular dilatation, a marked exudation of plasma into the tissues, and the accumulation of large numbers of polymorphonuclear leucocytes. At a later stage in such reactions pus accumulates; because of this the organisms responsible for this type of lesion, e.g. *Staph. aureus* and *Str. pyogenes*, are described as *pyogenic* organisms. In addition to living and dead polymorphonuclear leucocytes and bacteria, pus contains a considerable amount of desoxyribonucleoprotein derived from the nuclei of the dead leucocytes. It is this substance which gives it its viscous consistency.

If the acute inflammatory reaction fails to check the spread of the infection, the lesion may extend locally in the tissues producing cellulitis. The lymph channels may be involved with the production of a lymphangitis and on reaching the local glands a lymphadenitis; if the infection is not arrested at this stage, the bacteria gain access to the blood stream and may as a result be widely spread throughout the body. This last condition is known as *septicaemia*. The blood may also be invaded as a result of the direct involvement of veins and venules in the inflammatory process.

The degree of local damage caused by the invading bacteria may not be sufficiently great to stimulate an acute inflammatory reaction and in this case the reaction is of chronic type, which may be exemplified by the response to the tubercle bacillus. In infections with such organisms the stage of leucocyte accumulation is of short duration and the inflammatory cells present are predominantly of mononuclear type. In chronic inflammation, as a result of the indolent nature of the lesion, processes of repair and of inflammation are frequently found hand in hand, giving rise to the histological picture known as granuloma.

When infection is due to organisms which produce potent exotoxins these may cause considerable damage at sites remote from the initial lesion without very much evidence of local reaction. This occurs *par excellence* in tetanus where the essential feature of the disease is the spread of toxin from an infected wound to the central nervous system. The growth of the organism in the wound is negligible and produces no obvious local effect.

A limited number of organisms, e.g. those of typhoid fever, relapsing fever, undulant fever and Weil's disease, produce little or no lesion at the initial site of invasion. Under these conditions there is, following invasion, a bacteraemia with secondary involvement of various organs and tissues. Haematogenous spread with secondary multiplication remote from the site of initial invasion is a common feature of virus infections.

Epidemics

A disease which is continuously and normally present in the community is referred to as *endemic*. A disease which only occurs when introduced from outside the community is referred to as *exotic*. An undue significant increase in the frequency of overt infection with an endemic disease, or the introduction of an exotic disease, constitutes an *epidemic*. Under modern conditions epidemics occur much more frequently in relation to viral than to bacterial infections. Epidemics on a world-wide scale are referred to as *pandemics*. It should be noted that the terms endemic and epidemic should not be used in respect of animal populations for which the corresponding terms are *enzootic* and *epizootic*.

On first principles, the development of epidemics of diseases normally endemic in a population may be due to one or other of three factors.

1. To a change in the resistance of the population of such an extent that the endemic pathogen can initiate an epidemic. The classic work of Topley on the production of experimental epidemics with *Salm. typhimurium* in mice showed clearly the existence of a critical density of susceptibles as a prior condition for the development of an epidemic wave. The importance of the resistance of the population as a whole—*herd immunity*—in relation to the spread of human infections is considered more fully later (p. 165).

2. Occasionally, it is possible that an epidemic may occur without any change in the immunity status of the population, as a result of an increase in the virulence of the organism responsible. On the whole this is probably a factor of minor importance in the initiation of epidemics (p. 80).

3. The abnormal dissemination of an endemic pathogen in a susceptible population is responsible, for example, for epidemics of enteric fever, bacterial food poisoning, cholera, plague and yellow fever. Under modern conditions, epidemics of these diseases have been the result of a breakdown in public health control measures.

Seasonal factors are of considerable importance. As a general rule diseases spread by the respiratory route tend to be commoner in the colder months—increased contact indoors is probably an important factor in this but there may also, during the colder months, be some lowering in the local resistance of the respiratory tract. Diseases spread by the gastro-intestinal route tend, per contra, to be more prevalent during the summer months—probably because of the greater capacity of the parasite to survive or multiply at higher ambient temperatures. Diseases spread by arthropod vectors occur maximally at a time determined by the life history of the responsible vector and/or its normal host population. However, there are considerable and unexplained differences in the seasonal prevalence of different diseases. Diphtheria epidemics when prevalent tended to occur mainly in the autumn and winter; measles shows a maximal incidence in the spring, poliomyelitis in the late summer and autumn, pertussis in the spring and early summer, and in Europe and Australia bacillary dysentery, although a bacterial gastro-intestinal disease, occurs regularly throughout the year.

Sources of Bacterial Infections

Bacterial infections can be classified as *endogenous*, due to organisms of the normal flora, and *exogenous*, due to organisms derived from a source outside the body.

Endogenous Infections

These are sometimes referred to as auto-infections. The organisms of the normal flora are normally innocuous, and as we have seen, appear to be of distinct value to the host. Occasionally, however, they may give rise to infection. The most important auto-infections are from *E. coli* and *Str. faecalis* causing infections of the urinary tract, and subacute bacterial endocarditis due to the viridans streptococci. In both these examples two conditions are fulfilled: (1) The organism initiating the infection does so in an area of the body remote from its normal habitat. (2) The infection develops only where there is some tissue abnormality causing a lowering of local tissue resistance. Thus urinary tract infections are commonly associated with local renal abnormalities such as the presence of stone, congenital malformation, tuberculosis or back pressure through ureteric or prostatic obstruction. Subacute bacterial endocarditis occurs only in hearts damaged by previous congenital effect or previous rheumatic heart disease.

Exogenous Infections

The great majority of infections are exogenous in origin. In a few instances the primary source of infection is the soil. This is the main source of infection in tetanus and gas-gangrene although it is possible that the ultimate source of soil clostridia may be the intestinal tracts of animals in which these organisms are normally present. The soil is also the source of certain fungal infections (Chapter 43).

Lower animals, either directly or indirectly, are the source of a number of infections. As might be expected, animals which live in close association with man are the greatest danger—cattle being of particular importance. Wild animals, however, especially wild rodents and monkeys, are the source of certain human diseases. They are of particular importance as constituting reservoirs of infection which are extremely difficult to control. Many of the diseases spread from wild animals to man are transmitted by insect vectors.

Man himself, however, is by far the most important source of infection for his fellows. The most obvious human source of infection is the patient suffering from overt or clinically apparent infection. Infection is also frequently transmitted by *carriers*, a carrier being defined as a person who harbours a pathogenic organism in his body but who is not suffering from overt disease. Carriers usually excrete fewer organisms than cases but since they are more in contact with the normal uninfected population and since in many infections they are more numerous than overt cases they are for many diseases equally if not more important as sources of infection. The carrier state is usual during the period of convalescence from most bacterial infections but is not normally of more than a few weeks duration. In certain instances, however, of which typhoid is an outstanding example, the carrier state may be very persistent continuing for many years and in some cases for life. Persons who carry pathogenic organisms for long periods are known as *chronic carriers*. The term *precocious carrier* is applied to people who carry the causative organism of a disease during the incubation period of the disease before they themselves develop a clinical attack. During the course of epidemics of many infectious diseases, e.g. poliomyelitis, many become infected and carry the causative organism without developing clinical symptoms. These infections are known as *latent* or *subclinical* infections; as a rule they can only be recognized by showing that the patient has developed antibody against the causative organism. Persons suffering from latent or subclinical infection are very important sources of infection, particularly when, as in poliomyelitis, they may greatly outnumber the overt clinical cases. Carriers of this type are frequently known as *contact carriers*.

Transmission of Infection

For the spread of infectious disease from one person to another to occur three conditions must be fulfilled.

1. The organism must leave the body of the infected host. In the case of organisms responsible for lesions of the skin or those which produce infections of surface wounds this occurs very readily. Organisms infecting or present in

the mouth and respiratory tract are disseminated in the environment of the patient by droplets of salivary, bronchial and nasopharyngeal secretion. The most extensive dissemination occurs through violent expulsive efforts, e.g. in coughing and sneezing. Sneezing is particularly dangerous, and it is estimated that a vigorous sneeze may expel as many as 10^5 to 10^6 bacteria-laden particles. Contamination occurring from normal conversational efforts, although there are exceptions to every rule, appears to be negligible. The great majority of the organisms present in droplets expelled in this way are undoubtedly derived from the mouth, bacteria from lower parts of the respiratory tract being present in relatively small numbers. In infectious diseases of the lung itself, e.g. in pulmonary tuberculosis, sputum, in which the causative organisms are often present in large numbers, is a much more important source of infection than droplets. Droplets must, of course, constitute the main source of infections for diseases affecting the upper part of the respiratory tract, viz. pharynx, nasopharynx and mouth.

The fate of the expelled droplets depends on their size. The larger droplets, i.e. those greater than 100μ in diameter, fall rapidly and in so doing contaminate the clothing and bed clothes of the patient, objects in his immediate vicinity and the floor. Here the droplets dry up and mingle with the dust but the organisms present in them may remain viable for long periods. Of the pathogens, streptococci and tubercle bacilli are capable of surviving for a particularly long time in dust. Droplets smaller than 100μ in size evaporate almost immediately but their contained secretions and any organisms that may happen to be present remain suspended in the air as *droplet nuclei* for a considerable time; ultimately these too fall to the ground.

In diseases of the intestinal tract notably the enteric fevers, cholera, bacillary dysentery, poliomyelitis and infectious hepatitis, the causative organisms are excreted in the faeces. Some organisms—typhoid bacilli, *Leptospira icterohaemorrhagiae* and possibly a number of viruses causing systemic virus infection —are excreted in the urine. The urine however is not a common source of infection. In certain diseases, however, the organisms are deeply situated in the tissues and cannot spontaneously reach the exterior; most of these diseases are spread by insect vectors.

2. The organisms must be transferred by some agency to the victim. In some cases this may be by direct physical contact. In the majority, however, some *vehicle* of infection is required. This may be the air, water or food or inanimate objects, e.g. clothing, with which the patient is in close contact and which have been contaminated by him. The latter in their role as agents of infection are referred to as *fomites*.

3. The organisms must gain entry to the body of the new host. There are four ways in which this may occur; across the placenta from the maternal to the foetal circulation, through the respiratory tract, through the intestinal tract or through the surface epithelium—viz. skin, conjunctiva or genital mucosa.

Spread across the Placenta

This is not a common route of infection. It is however fairly frequent in syphilis giving rise to the congenital variety of the disease, but has not been clearly established for any other bacterial infection. However, a number of virus infections, notably rubella and cytomegalic inclusion disease, are spread by this route.

Respiratory Route

This is firstly the route of infection for bacteria and viruses which cause infections of the respiratory tract itself, but it is also of importance as the route of infection for certain viruses, e.g. smallpox, measles and mumps, which cause generalized or systemic infections. Except in the case of smallpox, in which infection may occur from virus present in skin lesions, these infections are caused by material expelled from the respiratory tract of a patient or carrier. Dust and dried secretions present on clothing or bed clothes or other environmental objects contaminated by the patient appear to be the main sources of infection for bacterial respiratory pathogens. Droplet nuclei appear only rarely to be the source of such infections as the likelihood that they contain pathogenic bacteria is very slight. They are almost certainly of considerable importance, however, in the spread of virus infections. Larger droplets fall rapidly to the ground and—except in cases of very close proximity as during a violent cough or sneeze—will only rarely be direct sources of infection.

Alimentary Route

This is the route of infection for diseases affecting the intestinal tract— enteric fevers, bacterial food poisoning, dysentery, cholera and intestinal tuberculosis. It also appears to be the primary route of infection for the enteroviruses and for the virus of infective hepatitis. The sources of these diseases are the faeces of patients or of carriers. In the case of the enteric fevers urine may be a source of infection. There is good reason to believe that also pharyngeal secretions are important sources of infection for the enteroviruses and the virus of infective hepatitis. Alimentary infection may occur in three ways: (*a*) By the contamination of water supplies with excretal material. This was at one time much the commonest method of spread of the enteric fevers and cholera. Nowadays however water-borne epidemics of intestinal diseases are very uncommon except in underdeveloped communities. Their elimination has been due to the introduction of satisfactory systems of excretal disposal, particularly by water carriage, and of modern methods of water purification. (*b*) By the contamination of food. Most epidemics of the enteric fevers occurring in modern urban communities are now spread in this way—the source of infection usually being a carrier involved in the handling or preparation of the food. Under more primitive conditions where there is not a satisfactory system of excretal disposal the food may be infected by flies which feed first on excreta and then transfer the organisms to the food. (*c*) By the contamination of environmental objects by cases or carriers either directly or by the agency of the hands. It is difficult to eliminate this type of contamination completely but it can be considerably reduced by punctilious personal cleanliness and hygiene. It is probably the method of contamination mainly responsible for the spread of poliomyelitis and of dysentery.

Infection through the Body Surface

Diseases in which the organism gains access through the outer surface of the body may conveniently be classified according to the precise way in which the infection is transmitted.

1. Infections which are spread primarily by direct physical contact. This group to which the term *contagious* is applied is best exemplified by the venereal diseases—syphilis, gonorrhoea and lymphogranuloma venereum; in these the organism is transmitted mainly by genital contact. Other important examples of contagious diseases are trachoma, herpes simplex, impetigo, the common wart, yaws and leprosy. Contagious diseases may also be transmitted, though with less certainty, by indirect contact, i.e. through the intermediary of inanimate objects contaminated by the infected individual. Infection by indirect contact is, however, extremely rare in the common venereal diseases—syphilis and gonorrhoea— because of the low viability of the causative organisms outside the body.

2. Infections transmitted by blood-sucking arthropods. This mode of transmission is more frequent in viral and rickettsial than in bacterial infections. Mosquitoes transmit infections due to the arbo group of viruses. Ticks transmit some arbo group virus infections, some rickettsial infections and the tick-borne variety of relapsing fever. Lice transmit epidemic typhus, trench fever and louse-borne relapsing fever. Fleas transmit bubonic plague and murine typhus. Mites transmit scrub typhus and rickettsial pox. Sandflies transmit sandfly fever and Oroya fever.

Many arthropod transmitted infections occur primarily in nature as infections of animals and man is only an incidental host. As a rule man is infected by the vector responsible for transmission of the disease amongst animals. Occasionally however a second vector is required as in the African variety of jungle yellow fever which is transmitted amongst animals by *Aedes africanus* and from animals to man by *Aedes simpsonii*. For most insect-borne infections of this kind man is epidemiologically a dead end and further transmission amongst the human population does not occur owing to the absence of a vector parasitic on man and capable of transmitting the infection. In the case of yellow fever, however, such a vector is available and the disease once having been initiated in man is spread amongst the human population by *Aedes aegypti*. In a limited number of insect-transmitted infections man is the primary host and there is no animal reservoir of infection. This is so of epidemic typhus, louse-borne relapsing fever, trench fever and sandfly fever.

Insects normally become infected by biting a human or animal host in whose blood the causative organism is present. After this there is in most cases an interval, known as the extrinsic incubation period, during which the insect is incapable of transmitting the infection. During this time the organisms are multiplying in the insect's body. The duration of the extrinsic incubation period depends on temperature—being as a rule shorter at high than at low temperatures. Ticks which transmit certain rickettsial and arbovirus infections (p. 467), and trombiculid mites which transmit scrub typhus are unusual in that the infective agent can be transmitted from one generation of insect to the next through the ovum. This is known as transovarial transmission. Whether transovarial transmission is a fortuitous by-product of the anatomy of the insect or whether it indicates that diseases which can be transmitted in this way may at one time have been solely diseases of the insect vector is a matter for speculation. In relation to the latter hypothesis the animal reservoir population has been described as an *amplifier* population. There is little doubt, however, that transovarial transmission is much less important for the perpetuation of the parasite than is the presence of an animal reservoir.

Arthropods may transmit infection in four ways. (*a*) The infective agent gains access to the salivary glands of the insect and the wound is directly contaminated during feeding. This is apparently the mechanism mainly responsible for the transmission of viral insect-borne infections. (*b*) The infective agent multiplies in the intestinal tract of the insect and during feeding is regurgitated into the wound. This is the method involved in the transmission of bubonic plague by the flea. (*c*) The agent multiplies in the intestinal tract and is excreted in the faeces; these are deposited by the insect beside the wound when it bites and are inadvertently scratched by the victim into the wound. This mode of infection is common in the rickettsial diseases. (*d*) The agent multiplies in the coelomic cavity of the insect and infection is due to contamination of the bite wound with the coelomic fluid of an insect that has been crushed in its vicinity. This type of infection occurs in louse-borne relapsing fever.

The prevalence of arthropod-borne diseases is markedly dependent on climatic conditions; these operate mainly through their effect on the size of the vector population. Climatic factors are of particular importance in relation to diseases transmitted by mosquitoes, which are virtually restricted to tropical countries. Climatic factors will also affect movements of the animal reservoir population in relation to the human population. This effect is particularly clearly seen in the case of Murray Valley encephalitis (Chapter 33).

3. Infections which are the result of the contamination of wounds. The most serious of these are rabies which are due to the bite of a rabid animal, usually a dog, and gas gangrene and tetanus which are the result of the contamination of severe wounds by clostridia, usually derived from the soil. Of greater practical importance, because they are more frequent, are infections of superficial wounds and burns by staphylococci, streptococci and other pyogenic organisms. The infection of wounds—particularly of operation wounds and burns—during the course of hospital treatment has become a very serious problem since the introduction of antibiotics because the organisms responsible are frequently antibiotic resistant. In some of these cases the infection is due to air-borne spread from the infected wounds of other patients, but in many it is caused by organisms present in the nose or throat of the patient himself or of attendant nurses and doctors. *Staphylococcus aureus* is particularly important as a cause of hospital wound infection. Its role in this type of infection is considered in more detail in Chapter 8.

4. Infection artificially transmitted by injection. It is probable that a con-

siderable number of diseases could be spread by injection, but in practice this mode of transmission is only a risk with syphilis and homologous serum jaundice. The organisms responsible for these conditions may be inadvertently introduced by the injection of plasma, serum, or whole blood obtained from an infected patient. The risk of transmitting syphilis in this way is virtually eliminated if the plasma, serum or blood is stored for at least 24 hours before it is administered. This will not, however, prevent transmission of homologous serum jaundice. Numerous epidemics of serum jaundice have also occurred through improper sterilization of syringes (Chapter 38).

Methods Used to Control the Spread of Infectious Disease

1. By Isolating or Eliminating the Source of Infection

In the case of diseases spread from animals to man it may be possible to control these by destroying the infected animals, particularly if this can be followed by adequate quarantine measures to prevent reintroduction of the disease. These procedures have been successful, for example, in almost eliminating rabies from the British Isles.

Isolation of human cases of infectious diseases has long been practised as a method of controlling spread. Its value is greatest in relation to those organisms which usually give rise to overt infection.

Organisms which frequently give rise to subclinical or latent infection are less effectively controlled by isolation procedures. In certain cases, e.g. smallpox and diphtheria, a quarantine may also be imposed on contacts as an additional precaution.

2. By Interrupting the Route of Spread

In all cases of infectious disease infectious exudates and excreta should be disinfected and disposed of. For the control of diseases spread by the intestinal route the essential preventive measures are: a satisfactory system of excretal disposal, wherever possible by water carriage; the purification and protection of water supplies destined for human consumption; the pasteurization of milk; and the hygienic preparation and manipulation of food. In relation to the latter it is of particular importance that carriers of organisms which can be spread by food should not be allowed to take any part in food preparation. The control of air-borne infection is more difficult. Good ventilation which will serve to dilute out the organisms present in the air is a simple measure which might be expected to be valuable in offices, lecture halls, theatres or wherever else large numbers of people may congregate. It is probably wise to avoid crowded rooms at times when respiratory diseases are prevalent but there is obviously a limit to the extent to which social contact can be restricted in this way. Overcrowding in dormitories and hospital wards should be avoided. Ultra-violet irradiation and the spraying or vaporization of aerosols—disinfectants such as sodium hypochlorite, hexylresorcinol and triethylene glycol—have been used for the disinfection of air in offices, hospitals and doctors' consulting rooms, but their value in the control of respiratory infection is still in doubt.

The prevention of cross-infection in hospital, particularly the infection of clean surgical wounds, is a problem to which a great deal of attention has been given in recent years. It would be impossible to consider the subject in any detail here, not only because of its complexity due to the multiplicity of factors which must be controlled, but also because the value of many of the procedures which have been advocated from time to time has not been established decisively. The essential principles in the control of these types of infection are:

(a) The exclusion from contact with the patient, both in the operating theatre and in the ward, of all persons with septic lesions of the skin, sore throats or who are known to be carriers of *Staph. aureus* or *Str. pyogenes*; this applies particularly to surgeons and nurses and others directly attendant on the patient. Nasal creams or sprays containing antibiotics not generally used systemically appear to be of considerable value in controlling the staphylococcal carrier state. Particularly good results have been reported for a spray containing framycetin and gramicidin. If possible, patients with established wound infection or other infections, e.g. staphylococcal pneumonia from which wounds might possibly become infected, should wherever possible be isolated from non-infected patients.

(b) The maximum control of environmental contamination in wards and theatres. In the operating theatre this has been traditionally achieved in the first place by insisting that everyone entering the theatre should wear sterile gowns, caps and masks. Ideally, all persons permitted access to the operating theatre should be required to change into clean theatre uniforms. Unsterilized bedding should be excluded from the theatre suite, and all movement into or out of the theatre, and in fact within the theatre, should be reduced to a minimum. If possible, positive pressure ventilation using filtered outdoor air should be employed to reduce the risk of aerial contamination. In hospital wards the control of dust is of particular importance. A considerable amount of the dust in a hospital ward is undoubtedly contributed by the bed clothes. The vigorous shaking of bed clothes should therefore be avoided. At one time the oiling of blankets to prevent dissemination of dust was widely practised. According to Rubbo, however, this is not a satisfactory procedure, because, although it undoubtedly diminishes the extent of dissemination of dust and therefore of the micro-organisms contained therein, it concentrates these organisms at the surface of the blanket and increases the risk of contact infection.

(c) Impeccable efficiency in, and continual surveillance of, the procedures for the sterilization of instruments and dressings. In many hospitals most of the sterilization is now carried out in a central sterile supply department.

(d) The employment of a completely rigid aseptic technique both during operations and during the dressing of wounds.

(e) A full investigation of all cases of hospital infection, with the object of determining the source of the infection and, if possible, how the patient became infected. In the case of staphylococcal infection, phage typing (p. 561) is particularly valuable for this purpose. The administrative complexity of the control of hospital infection is such that it is now recognized that it can only be satisfactorily achieved if it is made the responsibility of a hospital epidemiologist or infection control officer.

3. By Increasing the Resistance of the Individual

It is possible to increase the resistance of the individual against a number of diseases by various immunization procedures (Chapter 8).

In certain circumstances antimicrobial drugs may be given as prophylactics against infection—a procedure known as *chemoprophylaxis*. The administration of chloroquine to give protection against malaria is a particularly important example. The antibiotics and sulphonamides have a definite, though limited, value as prophylactics (p. 202). Their general use as such, however, is not justified because of the danger of increasing the prevalence of drug-resistant strains and of producing allergic sensitization.

At the time of writing the major indications for systemic chemoprophylaxis are for the protection against streptococcal infections of patients who have had acute rheumatism (p. 258), in those with severely traumatized wounds (p. 390), and as cover for certain operative procedures.

CHAPTER 6

ANTIGENS AND ANTIBODIES

Despite the number and complexity of the substances found in them, the chemical composition of the tissues of the body is remarkably constant. If any unwanted substance should gain entry to the tissues, efforts are made to remove it as speedily as possible. Simple substances are removed from the site of their introduction by the blood and lymph and are eliminated from the body by the kidneys. More complex substances, and particularly those with large molecules, are removed from the tissues in the same way but they cannot be so easily eliminated from the body. For their disposal a different technique is called into play. This is the production of a substance—*antibody*—which can combine with foreign material, neutralize it if it is toxic and generally facilitate its disposal.

Substances which can stimulate antibody production are known as *antigens*. As will be seen later, the relationship between antibody and antigen is highly specific. Furthermore, the combination of antibody and antigen can be detected only if it produces some demonstrable reaction. We may therefore define an antigen as *a substance which, when introduced into the tissues, stimulates the production of an antibody and which can combine specifically and react demonstrably with the antibody so produced.*

Whether they are produced against an infecting micro-organism or against antigen introduced into the tissues by injection, antibodies appear in the blood plasma and in the tissue fluids. For the study of antigen–antibody reactions the normal source of antibody is serum. Consequently the study of antigen–antibody reactions is usually referred to as serology. Antibodies can be obtained from serum in a highly concentrated and purified form but for most purposes crude serum is perfectly adequate. When serum containing a specific antibody is mixed with its homologous antigen various types of observable reaction occur, the particular type of reaction depending on the environmental conditions. These reactions are known as antigen–antibody reactions. Of these the most important for serological study are agglutination and precipitation.

ANTIGENS

From what has been said of the function of antibodies it can be seen that, in order to be antigenic, a substance should have two major properties.

1. It should be large enough not to be disposed of by normal physiological means. In practice, the minimum molecular weight consistent with antigenicity

is about 5000. Four groups of naturally occurring substances fulfil this requirement of high molecular weight—proteins, polysaccharides, lipids and nucleic acids. Of these, however, only proteins and polysaccharides have been shown to be capable of stimulating antibody production in pure form. Proteins are in general considerably more effective in stimulating antibody production than are polysaccharides. An outstanding exception to the high antigenicity of protein is gelatin which is hardly, if at all, antigenic. It is thought that this is due to its particularly low content of the amino acid tyrosine, resulting in a relatively non-rigid structure. Why proteins are more effective than polysaccharides in stimulating antibody production and why lipids and nucleic acids appear, by themselves, to be completely incapable of doing so is at present unknown.

Many substances which are unable to stimulate antibody production by themselves, however, can do so when combined with protein, or if present in intact cells, e.g. in bacteria, or if adsorbed onto inert particles such as collodion. These substances appear to act as carriers which ensure the retention in the body of the foreign material for sufficiently long to allow antibody production to occur. Substances which can produce antibody only when combined in this way are known as *partial antigens* or *haptens*. Nucleic acids, certain polysaccharides, e.g. the C substances of the streptococci, and at least one bacterial lipid—Wassermann reagin or cardiolipin are examples of large molecular weight haptens. They can be precipitated by antibody and are frequently referred to as *complex haptens*. In general the antigenicity of bacterial polysaccharide, which as we have seen is much lower than that of proteins, is greatly enhanced when—as in the intact cell—it is a component of a larger complex, e.g. the lipoprotein polysaccharide complexes of the Gram negative bacilli. The teichoic acids of Gram positive cell walls, which have also been shown to possess serological specificity, probably fall into this class of complex haptens, although the production of antibody in response to purified teichoic acid has not so far been reported.

In addition, when combined with protein, a variety of low molecular weight compounds, e.g. p-aminobenzoic acid, tartaric acid, simple sugars and picric acid, will function as antigens. Such low molecular weight compounds are not precipitated by antibody, and are known as *simple haptens*. Combination with antibody may, however, be shown by their capacity to inhibit the ability of the antibody to precipitate the hapten protein complex or complete antigen.

2. A second major property of an antigen is that it should be recognizable as a foreign substance by the animal producing the antibody. As will be seen later, it is necessary to define the word foreign, as used in this context, rather carefully. For the moment, however, it will be sufficient to note that for an animal to produce antibody consistently against its own tissue components would be an unnecessary act of biological self-annihilation.

In recent years an enormous amount of work has been carried out on the chemical characterization of naturally occurring antigens, and on the identification of the particular groups responsible for antigenic specificity. The identification of the latter depends on inhibition reactions in which completely characterized components of the antigen or haptens of known composition, inhibit the capacity of the antibody to precipitate the complete antigen. Thus, the finding that precipitation of a streptococcal antigen is specifically inhibited by α-glycerophosphate indicates that α-glycerophosphate residues are important for determining the antigenic specificity of the antigen.

Knowledge of chemical structure is most complete in respect of polysaccharide antigens, and for many of these not only has the structure been determined but also the nature of the groups conferring antigenic specificity identified. Thus it has been shown by McCarty that the component responsible for the specificity of the Lancefield group A antigen of *Streptococcus pyogenes* is a polymer of rhamnose and N-acetyl glucosamine, the antigenic specificity depending on the N-acetyl glucosamine residues protruding as side-groups from a rhamnose backbone. The completely antigenically distinct group C polysaccharide, is a similarly constructed polymer of rhamnose and N-acetyl galactosamine, with its specificity determined by side-chains of N-acetyl galactosamine.

Probably the most intensively studied of all polysaccharide antigens have been the pneumococcal capsular polysaccharides. These are complexes of various amino sugars, hexoses and uronic acids, and are much more complex than the streptococcal antigens referred to above. Thus the type 3 pneumococcal polysaccharide is a polycellobiuronic acid chain containing alternate glucose and glycuronic acid residues. The type 8 polysaccharide also contains polycellobiuronic acid but with a different linkage between the glucose and glycuronic acid and with glucose and galactose residues in the cellobiuronic acid units. Type 8 and type 3 polysaccharides cross-react serologically because of the presence in each of cellobiuronic acid but they differ because of the different linkages involved and because of the additional residues in the type 8 determinant. The importance of the ways in which sugar residues are linked together in determining the specificity of naturally occurring antigens is also shown in the dextrans or polyglucoses, polymers which show different types of linkage being clearly distinguishable serologically.

With naturally occurring protein antigens the situation is more difficult as the complete structure of only very few proteins has so far been determined. It is therefore not yet possible to relate the details of protein structure to antigenic specificity. Nevertheless, the antigenic specificity of protein clearly depends on its surface configuration, which is in turn imposed by the nature and arrangement of its constituent amino acids. Thus proteins whose tertiary structure has been altered by denaturation, e.g. by rupture of —S—S— and H bonds, acquire a new antigenic specificity. The immunological role of the amino acids in protein specificity is shown in a number of ways. Gelatin, which in itself is non-antigenic, can be rendered antigenic by the introduction of tyrosyl residues. The antigenic structure of natural proteins can be altered by attaching small peptides to their free amino groups. Such complexes have been found to elicit antibodies of three distinct specificities: (a) towards the carrier protein; (b) towards the attached peptide; and (c) towards a combination of the peptide and protein. A variety of synthetic peptides have now been produced which are in themselves fully antigenic. Many of them have been composed of only two or three different types of amino acids, with at least one compound—synthetic poly-L-proline—comprising only one type of amino acid. The minimum size for these antigenic polypeptides appears to be about 20 amino acid residues. So far, however, no synthetic peptide has been prepared possessing an antigenic specificity identical with that of the determinant group of any known protein, even when, as with collagen, the peptides are built up from the major amino acids—in this case proline and glycine—present in the native protein.

Although a large molecular size is essential for antigenicity the reactive site, which combines with antibody and determines antigenic specificity, is in fact quite small. Thus in the case of silk fibroin it has been estimated by Kabat that the antigenic determinant group consists of about 10 amino acids. This is very probably an average size for the determinant group of a native protein. In certain synthetic polypeptides it in fact appears to be rather smaller. When one takes into account that 20 amino acids commonly occur in proteins it is clear that with determinant groups of this magnitude an enormous number of antigenically distinct proteins are possible.

The number of determinants which any particular antigen possesses depends on the size of the antigen. Thus for large protein antigens such as the haemocyanins it has been estimated that each molecule can combine with over 100 molecules of antibody. Such molecules usually carry determinants of more than one antigenic specificity. For smaller antigens such as albumen, with molecular weights around 40,000, the number of antibody molecules with which the antigen could combine is, of course, much less but would still be appreciable. In these cases it is obvious that antibody–antigen precipitates must consist largely of antibody.

Natural Occurrence of Antigens and Haptens

Antigenic and haptenic substances are present in all living organisms, occurring either as structural components or as free compounds in the extracellular fluids. Although all species possess serologically distinct antigens, some antigens are widely distributed, the same compound occurring in a variety of species. Antigens of this type are known as *heterophile* antigens. The most studied of the heterophile antigens is the Forssman antigen which is found in the tissues of a variety of animal species as well as in many bacteria. The Forssman antigen is chemically a glycolipid owing its specificity to amino sugar residues.

The naturally occurring antigens and haptens of most importance to medicine are (1) those found in human tissues and cells and (2) those present in and produced by bacteria and other micro-organisms.

1. Of the antigens occurring in human tissues those present in the red cells, especially those responsible for the ABO blood groups, have been most studied. These antigens are polysaccharide in nature, possibly occurring in the cells as glycolipid, and owe their specificity to sugar and amino sugar residues. There is now considerable evidence that the ABO antigens are all derived from a basic

structure resembling that of the pneumococcus type 14 polysaccharide, by addition of appropriate determinant groups. In this process the antigen responsible for group O specificity appears to be an intermediate, from which, in the presence of the appropriate genes either the A or B substances may be derived.

The increased importance of tissue transplantation and the recognition of diseases associated with autoimmune responses (p. 121) have in recent years led to an intensive study of tissue antigens. In addition to species-specific antigens or isoantigens these include antigens which are specific for individual organs. Many organ-specific antigens are non-species specific but some are specific for the organ of a particular species. The study of tissue antigens has been enormously facilitated by the application of the fluorescent antibody technique (p. 39). The antigens which stimulate the rejection of tissue grafts are known as histocompatibility antigens. Many if not most of these are present on leucocytes as well as on tissue cells.

2. Bacterial antigens are either (*a*) excreted by bacteria into their environment or (*b*) present as structural components of the bacterial cell. The antigens excreted by bacteria are the exotoxins and various extracellular enzymes; these are protein in nature. The bacterial cellular antigens are:

1. Capsular antigens and haptens. In most cases these are complex mucopolysaccharides which in the pure state are poorly if at all antigenic but which are strongly antigenic in the intact cell. At least one capsular polysaccharide—hyaluronic acid—found in the capsules of group A streptococci, is non-antigenic even in the intact cell. This is possibly because of a tolerance (p. 119) induced by its wide distribution in animal tissues. The *Bacillus* genus is exceptional in that certain species, including the anthrax bacillus, possess capsular antigens composed of a glutamyl polypeptide. Some bacterial species possess surface antigens distributed in a layer too thin to be seen as a visible capsule and which are consequently referred to as microcapsular antigens (p. 5). Such are the M proteins of *Streptococcus pyogenes* which can be inactivated by tryptic digestion and the Vi antigen of *Salmonella typhi* and certain other salmonellae.

2. Somatic antigens. By definition somatic antigens are antigens present in the body of the organism as opposed to antigens present in flagella and capsules. In practice the term is used principally for antigens present in the cell walls of Gram negative bacteria, particularly the enterobacteriaceae. These are polysaccharide phospholipid protein complexes the serological specificity of which resides in the polysaccharide component. The most superficial determinants of the somatic antigen complexes are known as O antigens. These may be lost by mutation. In this case other deeper lying determinants, whose reactivity is masked by the normal surface determinants, are revealed. This antigenic loss is associated with a change in colony appearance from smooth to rough and the variation is therefore known as S → R variation.

Polysaccharides are also of considerable importance as antigenic or haptenic components of the cell walls of Gram positive organisms. Thus in the streptococci they constitute the Lancefield group determining or C substances. In Gram positive organisms the cell wall teichoic acids (p. 5) also possess serological specificity. The differences in serological behaviour between different teichoic acids appears to be determined by the nature of the sugar residues which they contain. The glycerol teichoic acids also appear to possess a specificity due to the presence of glycerophosphate and alanine residues.

3. Flagellar antigens. All flagellar antigens which have been investigated chemically have been found to be protein but appear to be incomplete proteins in the sense that they do not contain a full range of amino acids (p. 9). Flagellar antigens are frequently referred to as H antigens. Occasionally flagellated bacteria lose their flagella by mutation—a loss often referred to as H → O variation. The variants are non-motile and inagglutinable by O anti-sera. No other properties of the bacteria are affected.

4. Fimbrial antigens. The composition of these antigens does not appear to have been studied in detail. Since the normal fimbrial antigens of the enterobacteriaceae are heat labile they are probably protein in nature. The specific F antigens on the sex pili of *E. coli* K12 is, however, probably carbohydrate since the capacity of F plus strains to adsorb male-specific bacteriophage is eliminated by exposure to periodate.

SPECIFICITY OF ANTIGENS AND ANTIBODIES

The reaction between antibody and antigen is highly specific, an antibody being capable of reacting only with the antigen responsible for its production or a closely related one. The specificity of the relationship between antibody and antigen was shown by Landsteiner in a series of classic experiments to be based on the chemical structure of the antigen.

Landsteiner found that he could attach various groups to an aromatic amine such as aniline, and following treatment with nitrous acid the diazo compound so produced could be coupled with protein. The complex thus formed is known as a *conjugated antigen* or *azoprotein*. When such an antigen is used for immunization, antibodies to both the introduced group and the protein bearer are produced. By using one type of protein for the preparation of the conjugated antigen used in immunization and a second type of protein which did not cross-react serologically with the first for the preparation of the antigen used for testing, Landsteiner was able to investigate the specificity of the antibody directed against the introduced haptenic group.

His results showed a very close dependence of serological specificity on chemical structure. Thus serum prepared against a conjugated protein containing a p-aminobenzoic acid hapten gave no cross-reactions with conjugated proteins in which the haptens were aniline, p-aminobenzene sulphonic acid or p-aminophenyl arsonic acid. Sera prepared against azoproteins in which any one of these substances was the introduced hapten gave little or no cross-reactions with any of the others. Each of these compounds is therefore serologically distinct.

The spatial distribution of the radicles incorporated in the molecule were also found to play an important part in determining specificity. Thus ortho-, meta- and para-aminobenzoic acids were found to be completely distinct antigenically.

Landsteiner found also that antigenic specificity extended to stereoisomers. Thus, e.g. serum prepared against laevo-tartaric acid gave negligible reactions with meso- and dextro-tartaric acids. Similarly Avery and Goebel found it was possible to distinguish by serological reactions between α- and β-glycosidic linkages.

We must now consider how the antibody molecule reflects the differences in structure of the antigen in such a way as to combine specifically with it. At the moment our knowledge of the nature of the groups on the surface of the antibody molecule which combine with antigen is extremely limited. We do, however, have some information.

1. There is considerable evidence that each antibody molecule possesses two antigen combining sites of identical specificity.

2. The antigen combining site probably contains about 10 to 20 amino-acid residues. Estimates of this order of magnitude have been obtained for antibodies to certain synthetic haptens and for dextrans, and would appear to be about the right size to reflect the antigenic determinants of proteins (p. 95). It is obvious that a combining group of this size makes possible the occurrence of a very large number of antibody molecules of different specificities.

To explain the specificity of the relationship between antibody and antigen it is assumed that the combining group of the antibody molecule has a shape which is complementary to that of the reactive area of the antigen molecule. This shape is a function of the tertiary structure of the antibody and is directly dependent on the pattern of amino acids which constitute the combining site. As a result of this physical complementarity when antigen and antibody come together their reactive sites fit snugly together, a relationship which is often described as resembling that of a lock to its key. Combination between antibody and antigen can then occur through the operation of short-range intermolecular forces. Of these, undoubtedly the most important are the non-specific intermolecular forces between instantaneous dipole moments known as van der Waal's forces. These only become effective when the two molecules are very close together, their strength varying inversely as the sixth power of the intermolecular distance. Other intermolecular forces, which also take part in antigen–antibody combination, are Coulomb or electrostatic forces and hydrogen bonds. The latter are bonds formed by the attraction which hydrogen and the electronegative atoms oxygen, nitrogen or sulphur together exert on the unshared electrons of an electronegative atom in another molecule. Coulomb or electrostatic forces are forces which operate between oppositely charged positive and negative groups, e.g. between ionized acidic groups in the antigen; instances of these are the carboxyl groups of the dicarboxylic amino acids of proteins, antigens and ionized NH_3^+ groups of diamino acids on the surface of the antibody and vice versa. There is some doubt as to the precise role of Coulomb forces in antigen–antibody combination. In reactions involving uncharged haptens and antigens they obviously play no part.

Recently considerable attention has been given to the contribution made by hydrophobic interactions between apolar groups to antigen–antibody combination. In the aqueous environments in which antigen–antibody reactions must occur these interactions are presumed to be of greater importance than hydrogen bonding and electrostatic interactions. Under these conditions the water molecules should themselves form hydrogen bonds with antigen and antibody; and water, being of high dielectric constant, would diminish the strength of the electrostatic attraction between oppositely charged antigen and antibody groups.

As a result of the operation of these various forces the antigen–antibody union is a very firm one, and the complex is not readily broken down. Under certain conditions, however, the union is reversible. Dissociation of antibody from antigen may occur on dilution of the mixture or on addition of fresh antigen to an antigen–antibody complex. Antibodies prepared in different animals or on different occasions in the same animal may vary considerably in *avidity*, i.e. in the firmness with which they bind antigen. In some cases low avidity may be due to a low degree of complementarity resulting in a poor fit between antibody and antigen-combining groups. This probably explains the low avidity of the so-called 'natural' antibodies (p. 156). Antibodies produced by prolonged immunization are usually more avid than those produced early in immunization. In this case the greater avidity of the later antibodies may be due to the fact that their combining groups reflect a larger area of the antigen surface, so permitting a greater degree of binding between antibody and antigen. This explanation is supported by the finding that such antibodies are usually considerably less specific than less avid ones, since if the antibody reflects a larger area of the antigen surface it is more likely to possess combining groups, reacting with determinants shared by the antigen with other antigens.

PROPERTIES OF ANTIBODIES

Chemically, antibodies are globulins, i.e. proteins possessing a low solubility in water and completely precipitated from serum by half saturation with ammonium sulphate. They may be more precisely characterized, as first shown by Tiselius and Kabat, by their electrophoretic mobility. On electrophoresis they are found in the gamma globulin fraction—the fraction with lowest mobility towards the positive electrode, and therefore the fraction possessing the lowest negative charge at physiological pH. This fraction accounts for about 1 per cent of the total serum protein and contains three major antigenically distinct components—IgG, IgA and IgM, known collectively as *immunoglobulins*. Two minor components γD and γE have recently been described, but so far little is known of their properties or function. There is some evidence that γE may contain the reaginic antibodies responsible for immediate type hypersensitivities (p. 174).

For the purification of the immunoglobulins chromatography on ion exchange resins such as DEAE cellulose, gel filtration on Sephadex columns, electrophoresis and ultracentrifugation, which will sediment IgM antibodies, are the methods principally employed. The critical separation of the different classes of immunoglobulin requires the combined use of a number of such procedures. For the purification of antibody with a specific combining affinity, however, the antibody must be recovered from specific antibody–antigen complexes. These may be obtained as precipitates or by the combination of antibody with antigen which has been chemically linked to a solid supporting medium such as red cells, cellulose and various ion exchange resins. Various methods have been used to separate antibody from these complexes, viz. by heating, adjustment of pH, treatment with salts or enzymic destruction of the antigen, the particular method which is effective depending on the antibody–antigen system involved. These methods are not suited to antibody purification on a large scale.

Some of the principal properties of the immunoglobulins are presented in the

PROPERTIES OF HUMAN IMMUNOGLOBULINS

Class	IgG	IgA	IgM
Ultracentrifuge*	7S	7–15S	19S
M.W.	160,000	400,000†	900,000
Carbohydrate (per cent)	2·6	10·7	12·2
Concentration in plasma (g per cent)	1·2	0·4	0·1
Capacity to cross placenta	+	–	–
Capacity to fix to guinea-pig skin‡	+	–	–
Capacity to bind complement	+	–	+
Gm factors	+	–	–
InV factors	+	+	+

* Given as Svedberg units.
† Dimer form.
‡ Can be demonstrated by passive cutaneous anaphylaxis (PCA).

table. Of the three groups IgG is the most important, accounting for about 70 per cent of the total immunoglobulin. It has a sedimentation constant of 7S in the ultracentrifuge and a molecular weight of 160,000. On immuno–electro-phoresis it is the most heterogeneous of the immunoglobulins, comprising a family of molecules which exhibit a very wide range of electrophoretic mobility. IgA is a globulin of relatively fast electrophoretic mobility. It occurs mainly as a dimer of two 7S subunits which have however a considerable tendency to polymerize and dissociate. IgM is a much larger molecule than either of the preceding, with a molecular weight of 900,000 because of which it is frequently referred to as *macroglobulin.* It appears to be a polymeric complex of five 7S molecules bound together by disulphide linkages. These linkages are readily ruptured by exposure to reducing agents such as mercapto-ethanol. This, however, destroys antibody activity. IgM appears to be metabolized much more rapidly than the other two immunoglobulins, and probably as a result of this, occurs to a relatively slight extent in the extravascular fluid.

On the basis of various fractionation procedures it has been established that each 7S antibody molecule consists of four polypeptide chains. Two of these are 'heavy' chains with a molecular weight of approximately 50,000, and two are 'light' chains with a molecular weight of approximately 20,000. The chains are bonded together by non-covalent linkages and by interchain disulphide bonds of which there appear to be three per molecule. On the basis of physical data obtained from measurements of agglutinated particles in electron micrographs IgG appears to be a spindle-shaped molecule 250 to 300 Å long by 40 Å wide. Each such molecule possesses two combining sites, almost certainly located at opposite ends of the spindle. The most acceptable model, which is that proposed by Edelman and Gally, is shown in Fig. 10. The IgM molecule is probably spherical. This is not surprising in view of its polymeric character.

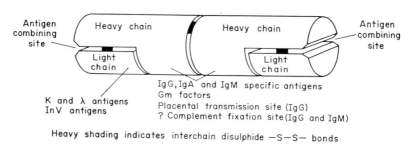

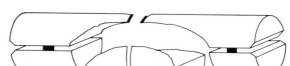

FIG. 10. MODEL OF 7S IMMUNOGLOBULIN MOLECULE

The IgG molecule may be broken down in two principal ways.

1. By reduction with mercapto-ethanol followed by dialysis against acetic acid. This results in a liberation of the light and heavy chains.

2. By the action of proteolytic enzymes. When treated by papain in the presence of cysteine—as first shown by Porter—the molecule yields three approximately equal fragments. These are two similar fragments (Fab) of molecular weight 45,000, each containing a light chain and part of a heavy chain, and one fragment (Fc) of molecular weight 55,000, containing the remainder of the heavy chains. When digested by pepsin in the absence of cysteine, as in the commercial preparation of diphtheria antitoxin (p. 165), one 5S fragment, approximately equivalent to the two papain fragments is obtained. The remainder of the molecule is completely degraded by pepsin treatment.

The three classes of immunoglobulins can be readily differentiated by immuno-electrophoresis (p. 133), giving distinct precipitin bands with specific immune sera. This differentiation is possible because each of the classes IgG. IgA and IgM possesses determinants specific for that class. When the antibody molecule is broken down into its constituent peptide chains these determinants are found to be associated with the heavy chains. In addition to these specific determinants the different immunoglobulins possess antigenic determinants common to all three classes. The common determinants of human gamma globulins are located on the light chains. Two antigenic varieties of light chain have been distinguished—κ and λ. About 60 per cent of antibody molecules possess κ type chains, and about 30 per cent λ type chains. κ and λ chains are apparently never found on the same molecule. The antigenic composition of the light chains of the remaining 10 per cent of antibody molecules has not been determined. Antigenic differences have also been demonstrated amongst IgG heavy chains on the basis of which four antigenic subclasses γ2a, γ2b, γ2c and γ2d or Ne, We, Vi and Ge respectively, have been defined.

In addition to the types of heterogeneity described above, both light and heavy chains of IgG—and this is presumably true of other immunoglobulins—have been found to show considerable electrophoretic heterogeneity. Light chains of both κ and λ type have yielded 8 to 10 distinct bands on electrophoresis in polyacrylamide gel, and recently a similar banding has been found in heavy chains. These differences undoubtedly reflect variations in the amino acid sequences of individual chains. Sequence analysis of light chains from myeloma proteins and of rabbit heavy chains have revealed considerable variability in the sequences in the N-terminal ends of the chains, while the sequence in the C-terminal end appears to be relatively constant for each chain type. Analysis of rabbit and myeloma heavy chains have shown also the occurrence of pyrrolidone carboxylic acid—probably derived from glutamine at the N-terminal ends of the heavy chains. The function of this compound is at present unknown.

Allotypes

In the rabbit, gamma globulin antigenic subtypes or allotypes can be demonstrated by using immune sera prepared in other rabbits. Rabbit allotypes are controlled by two genetic loci, a and b, for each of which 3 allelic genes have been identified, giving a total of 6 rabbit allotypic determinants. Light chains carry only b determinants but heavy chains appear to carry both a and b. As all the rabbit allotype antigens may occur on any class of immunoglobulin, rabbit heavy chains must contain both common antigens and antigens specific for each immunoglobulin class. This has suggested that the heavy chain may in fact consist of two subchains.

Human gamma globulin allotypes were first demonstrated by Grubb and Laurel who showed that sera of patients suffering from rheumatoid arthritis (p. 125) frequently contained, in addition to the rheumatoid factor, antibody-like substances capable of reacting with antigenic determinants present on the gamma globulins of some individuals but not of others. The antigens involved are known as Gm antigens and appear to be confined to IgG molecules, in which they occur on the Fc part of the heavy chains. Some 20 Gm antigens have been identified. They appear to be controlled by alleles at more than one locus and to show some relationship in distribution to the antigenic subclasses which have been identified in the heavy chains.

Antibodies capable of identifying Gm groups may occasionally be found in the sera of normal persons, providing so-called SNagg reagents. There is evidence that these antibodies are produced either as a result of immunization of the foetus with maternal gamma globulin of different Gm type, or by immunization following blood transfusion or the injection of gamma globulin. Under these conditions, gamma globulin allotypic antibodies seem to be produced only in children. Gm groups are determined by haemagglutination inhibition tests which ascertain the capacity of the individual's serum or gamma globulin to inhibit the agglutination of Rhesus positive (D positive) red cells coated with non-agglutinating anti-D serum by the Gm reagent. If, for example, in such a test the anti-D serum is Gm a^+ the agglutination of the coated red cells by the Gm reagent will be inhibited by any Gm a^+ serum or gamma globulin. By the use of SNagg reagents a second allotype specificity, InV, has been identified; associated with the light chains, this allotype is controlled by three allelic genes at a single locus.

There is reason to believe that further allotypic specificities may be demonstrable in human gamma globulin. Thus heterogeneity in κ type light chains has been demonstrated by the use of monkey antisera, and in human IgM by using rabbit antisera. There is also evidence that antibodies of different combining specificity isolated from immune precipitates are antigenically distinct. However, it is not known whether this distinction can be regarded as an allotypic specificity determined by the genome of the individual, or whether it is a specificity associated with the combining groups of the antibody and therefore dependent on the nature of the antigen.

It has been clearly demonstrated, and this is an essential requirement of the lattice theory of agglutination and precipitation (p. 133), that each IgG molecule carries two combining sites. These are presumed to be located at opposite ends of the molecule. In reduced IgG preparations antibody activity is found only in association with the heavy chains. Only about 20 per cent of the total antibody activity has, however, been recovered in heavy chains alone. It is therefore possible that the antibody site involves the participation of both the heavy and the light chains. This possibility is also suggested by the fact that in the guinea-pig, antibodies of different specificity have been shown by Edelman and Poulik to yield light chains with different patterns of electrophoretic mobility. It is possible in fact to reconstitute an antibody from suitably prepared light and heavy chains. Maximum antibody activity, with recoveries of about 60 per cent, are achieved when the molecule is reconstituted from specific heavy and specific light chains. When specific heavy chains are combined with non-specific light chains, i.e. with light chains from antibody with a different specificity the antibody recovery is about 35 per cent. When non-specific heavy and specific light chains are employed no activity is recoverable. These results clearly support the view that although the heavy chains are the major determinants of specificity, it in fact involves a co-operative activity of both chains.

Since antibody activity is demonstrable in Fab fractions free of detectable carbohydrate the latter is presumed to make no contribution to the antigenic site. Its specificity is therefore presumed to be due to the configuration imposed by the constituent amino-acid residues. Since the configuration or tertiary structure of a protein is probably inherent in its amino acid sequences it might be expected that differences in amino acid content or sequence could be related to antibody specificity. The great heterogeneity of antibody structure which has been found to exist quite independently of antigen-combining specificity must obviously be clarified, however, before it will be possible to relate antibody specificity to the sequence of amino acid residues on the surface of the antibody molecule. The position is further complicated by the fact that antibodies combining with single well-defined antigens may be quite heterogeneous in their affinity for antigen, and therefore also presumably in the composition of their combining sites. The technical problem is rendered much more difficult by the fact that the antigen-combining site accounts for only about one per cent of the entire antibody molecule.

FUNCTIONAL HETEROGENEITY IN ANTIBODIES

As well as being structurally dissimilar, antibodies are functionally heterogeneous in relation to their biological properties. In some instances differences in function are associated with variations in structure and a particular immunoglobulin class is characterized by the presence or absence of a specific property. In other instances a correlation between structure and function has not so far been established.

Heterogeneity is expressed in the following ways.

1. Differences in immunological specificity. This is the most fundamental way in which antibodies differ, and its structural basis has already been considered. There is no reason to believe that any particular type of antigen stimulates the production of antibody of a particular immunoglobulin class, but there is evidence that the physical state of the antigen is important, particulate antigens tending to elicit the production of IgM antibodies. This is consistent with the finding that most haemagglutinating antibodies are macroglobulins. In general, regardless of the nature of the antigen, IgG antibodies are produced by strong antigenic stimuli and by prolonged antigenic stimulation.

2. Antibodies of the same specificity may differ in *avidity*. This term is used to describe the firmness with which antibody combines with antigen (p. 99), and may be measured by estimating the readiness with which the antibody may be dissociated from antigen–antibody complexes. Avid antibodies combine firmly with antigen and are not readily dissociated. Methods which have been used for dissociating antigen–antibody complexes are: (*a*) dilution, or (*b*) the addition of isotopically labelled antigen to unlabelled complexes of antibody and antigen. In general the avidity of antibody appears to increase with time after immunization quite regardless of antibody class. Because of this it is not at present possible to associate intrinsic differences in avidity with any particular class. There is, however, evidence that IgG is the most effective immunoglobulin in toxin neutralization.

3. Antibodies differ in their capacity to produce observable antibody–antigen reactions in vitro.

(*a*) Differences in precipitating power. The existence of antibody of low precipitating power was first shown by Heidelberger and Kendall who found that a rabbit antibody to serum albumen could not be removed by successive additions of antigen, but was nevertheless precipitated on adding a large amount of antigen in a single moiety. In man the reaginic antibodies involved in the idiosyncrasies (p. 174), are non-precipitating, and non-precipitating diphtheria antitoxin has been demonstrated in persons immunized with diphtheria toxoid. In general IgG antibodies appear to be much more effective precipitins than IgM or IgA.

(*b*) Differences in agglutinating power. Antibodies deficient in agglutinating capacity were first recognized in cases of human immunization against Rhesus red cell antigens. So-called non-agglutinating antibodies are only relatively deficient in agglutinating power. They agglutinate red cells in media of high protein content or after digestion with papain or trypsin, but fail to agglutinate untreated cells in saline solution. Non-agglutinating Rhesus antibodies are 7S antibodies, in contrast to saline agglutinating antibodies of the same specificity, which are 19S. In other systems, however, 7S antibodies contain both agglutinating and non-agglutinating varieties. The precise basis for the low agglutinating capacity of certain antibodies is unknown, but it has been suggested that they possess only a single combining group, as a result of which they are unable to build up a red cell agglutination lattice. Such an explanation seems unlikely, however, since their deficiency in agglutinating ability is not absolute. An alternative view is that these antibodies are shorter in their long axis than normal agglutinating antibodies and are therefore incapable of clearing projections on the cell surface sufficiently to make effective contact with adjacent cells.

(*c*) Differences in complement fixing ability. Non-agglutinating anti-Rh antibodies and the reaginic antibodies referred to above are deficient in this respect. Certain non-agglutinating antibodies to red cell antigens which do fix complement have been described, however. In the rabbit, 19S antibodies appear to be much more efficient than 7S antibodies in sensitizing sheep red cells to lysis by guinea-pig complement. IgA, however, appears to be devoid of complement fixing power.

4. Differences in the capacity to traverse natural barriers. Because of their larger size, IgM antibodies diffuse through the vascular endothelium much less readily than IgG antibodies. Consequently a very small amount of IgM is normally found in extravascular tissues though it is probable that much more can diffuse through the walls of blood vessels in areas of inflammation. The amount of IgG in extravascular tissues, however, is equal to that in the blood stream, and it has been estimated that about 25 per cent of the circulating gamma globulin exchanges between the intravascular and extravascular pools each day. Only IgG is capable of passing through the placenta from the maternal to the foetal circulation. This explains why saline anti-Rh agglutinins are not found in the foetal circulation in cases of maternal Rh immunization, and why in cases of ABO incapatibility between mother and foetus, iso-agglutinins—which

are 19S antibodies—do not cross the placenta from the maternal to the foetal circulation. If such transfer did occur, it would undoubtedly set up a severe haemolytic reaction in the foetus. The placenta is a barrier not only to IgM but also to IgA and reaginic antibodies (p. 174).

The failure of IgA antibodies to cross the placenta indicates that placental transfer is not simply a function of antibody size. Evidence has in fact associated this transfer with the presence of a specific placental transfer site on the Fc section of the heavy chains. Removal of this part of the molecule by papain, or pepsin digestion, renders the IgG molecule incapable of placental transfer. Because of this enzyme refined diphtheria antitoxin (p. 101) will not be transmitted from the mother to the foetus. Recent evidence suggests that IgA antibodies tend to be concentrated in certain secretions, namely colostrum, nasal mucus and saliva. It is possible however that this is due to local synthesis rather than to selective transfer.

5. Differences in capacity to elicit the reactions of immediate-type hypersensitivity. These disparities, which depend in the first instance on differences in capacity for non-specific fixation to tissue cells, are considered in more detail in Chapter 9 (p. 169).

PRODUCTION OF ANTIBODIES

Antibodies are produced by the cells of the reticulo-endothelial system—the sites of maximal formation being the lymph nodes, from which antibody is carried by the lymph to the blood, and the spleen. The spleen appears to be the main site of antibody production when antigen is introduced by the intravenous and intraperitoneal routes. After intramuscular and subcutaneous injection antibody production occurs mainly in the draining lymphatic glands.   All of these tissues have been shown, when removed from animals which had been antigenically stimulated in vivo, to produce considerable amounts of antibody when subsequently exposed to the antigen in vitro. The in vivo role of the spleen has been demonstrated by the finding that splenectomized animals produce little or no antibody when the antigen is injected into the blood but produce it normally when the antigen is injected by other routes. The in vivo role of the lymph nodes has been shown by the demonstration after antigenic stimulation of a high concentration of antibody in the efferent lymph.

There is some evidence suggesting that antibody can be produced locally in the tissues at sites of contact with antigen. This is particularly likely to occur when the antigen is injected with an adjuvant (p. 101) which results in the production of a local granuloma. Apart from this antibodies can be demonstrated in faeces, urine, mucous secretions and milk. There is no clear proof, however, that these antibodies have in fact been produced locally by tissue cells. It is probable that they originate from antibody-producing cells which have migrated to the site of contact with the antigen or that they represent a spillover from the blood.

In general the capacity to produce 19S antibodies appears at an earlier stage in development than does the capacity to produce 7S antibodies. This applies both at the level of individual development—the antibodies produced by the infant are mainly IgM—and at the level of evolutionary development, the capacity to produce 19S antibodies being found in certain of the elasmobranch fishes which do not produce 7S antibodies. More primitive vertebrates and invertebrates are devoid of antibody-producing capacity. In view of the fact that 19S antibodies appear to be complexes of 7S antibodies, although antigenically different, these findings are surprising. Why 19S antibodies should appear earlier both phylogenetically and ontogenetically is unknown. In addition the sequence of appearance of antibodies following first contact with antigen seems invariably to be IgM followed by IgG.

Antigens will stimulate antibody production only if they gain access to the tissues either spontaneously or because they have been deliberately introduced. Soluble antigens, may, from time to time, gain access to the tissues spontaneously—from the respiratory and intestinal tracts and on occasion through the skin. Bacteria and other organisms gain access to the tissues spontaneously during the course of infection, and infection invariably stimulates antibody production.

The deliberate introduction of antigen into the tissues is known as *immunization* (Chapter 8). The antigen may be introduced by the intravenous, intraperitoneal, intramuscular, subcutaneous or intradermal routes; of these the intravenous route is the most effective in stimulating antibody production and is that normally chosen in the immunization of experimental animals. Intraperitoneal inoculation is also highly effective, but the intramuscular and subcutaneous routes, which are those used in the immunization of man, are less so. The intradermal route is mainly used for the inoculation of living organisms.

The rapidity with which antibody appears following the introduction of antigen, the amount of it that is produced, and the time for which it persists differs considerably with different antigens, and with different animal species. In general, although different individuals of the same species may show appreciable variation, the pattern of response in any particular species to the same antigen is much the same.

The response of the body to a first injection of antigen is quite different from its response to a second or subsequent injection. The difference is most marked in relation to soluble antigens, e.g. the exotoxins. Following a first injection of such an antigen, there is a latent period of from some days to a few weeks during which no detectable antibody is produced; the antibody level then slowly increases to reach a low maximum titre. This titre is maintained for a variable time and then gradually falls to a negligible level. If, at this stage, a second injection of antigen is given, the response is quite different. Antibody is produced much sooner than after the first injection, reaches a higher level and persists for a longer period. The level of antibody attained can be increased by further injections until the maximum level attainable in that animal is achieved. When, instead of a soluble antigen, a suspension of bacteria is used as antigen, the difference between the response to the first and second injection is not so marked, the animal giving what appears to be a secondary response to the first injection. This is probably so because the animal has had a prior experience of the same or related antigen, and the response is in fact secondary. In recent years the response to polio antigens has been studied in considerable detail and with these a very clear differentiation between the first and subsequent injections has also been observed.

The relatively weak reaction to the first injection of antigen is known as the *primary response* and the strong reaction to the second and subsequent injections as the *secondary response*. The first contact with an antigen apparently conditions or educates the reticulo-endothelial system so that, on subsequent contact with the same antigen, it responds much more promptly with the production of antibody. This conditioned state of the antibody-producing cells is sometimes referred to as *potential immunity*. In man, after immunization with certain antigens, a state of potential immunity persists for several years, and possibly in some cases for life.

Following the first appearance of antibody in the circulation its concentration increases gradually to a maximum. The rate of antibody increase is exponential suggesting that there may be concomitant proliferation of antibody-producing cells. Having attained a maximum the titre gradually falls due to a gradual destruction and elimination of the antibody. Since the rate of fall is much less than that found when preformed antibody has been passively introduced it is apparent that even during the phase of decline antibody must still continue to be produced—the actual level found representing a balance between the rates of destruction and elimination and that of the production of new antibody.

Animals which have been immunized with certain antigens may apparently produce antibody in response to various non-specific stimuli, e.g. bleeding, the injection of unrelated antigens and of other substances and the administration of ACTH. This non-specific response is sometimes, though erroneously, known as the *anamnestic reaction*. The amount of antibody produced in these circumstances, however, is small and it persists for only a short time. Anamnestic responses are probably the result of some unknown physiological effect of the stimulus which leads to antibody release rather than to antibody formation.

It has been claimed that similar anamnestic responses may occur in man—in particular, that persons who have been inoculated with typhoid vaccine may produce a considerable amount of antityphoid antibody during the course of infections other than typhoid fever. This type of response is of considerable importance in its bearing on the interpretation of the results of diagnostic serological tests such as the Widal reaction but, unfortunately, the problem has not been fully investigated. It is probable that, as in animals, it is slight and irregular in occurrence.

Factors Affecting Antibody Production

The production of antibody in response to antigenic stimulation is influenced by a number of factors.

1. Age of the animal. At birth the antibody-producing machinery is immature in its capacity to respond to antigenic stimulation. Nevertheless the new-born infant can clearly respond to antigenic stimulation, and with a particularly potent antigen this response may be quite considerable. It is not yet possible to

identify precisely the stage in embryological development at which antibody synthesizing capacity first appears. In sheep, antibody responses to certain antigens have been found by Silverstein half-way through the gestation period. There is evidence that the human foetus, too, can make an antibody response. (1) Plasma cells have been demonstrated in foetuses at 5 months' gestation. (2) Children suffering from the rubella syndrome due to intra-uterine infection during the first 3 months of pregnancy (p. 523), have been shown to have considerably higher antibody levels than cohort controls at ages of up to 10 years when all maternally transmitted antibody must have long since disappeared. (3) 19S *Toxoplasma* antibody has been identified in foetal serum at the 28th week of gestation. Since 19S antibodies do not pass through the placenta this antibody must have been produced by the foetus.

After birth there appears to be a rapid improvement in the efficiency of the antibody-producing machinery and this improvement, as shown by the response to poliomyelitis vaccine, continues at least up to the age of 1 year. As measured by the response to diphtheria toxoid the rate of improvement appears to be maximal in the immediate postnatal period. As the rate is the same for premature as for normal infants, it is presumably not a function of the developmental age of the antibody-producing system but instead must be related to the infant's exposure to the extra-uterine environment.

From a variety of studies it is clear that the first antibody produced in response to antigenic stimulation is of the 19S variety. It is not surprising, therefore, that 19S antibodies predominate in the infant's antibody response. There is evidence that the production of 19S antibodies is not associated with the acquisition of immunological memory. This fact combined with the evidence for a general immaturity of the antibody synthesizing machinery immediately after birth would support a policy of deferring active immunization wherever feasible until the age of at least 6 months.

2. Animals whose blood contains preformed antibody, present either as a result of passive transfer from the mother across the placenta, or as a result of passive immunization, respond poorly to immunization with the homologous antigen. In children, maternally transferred antibody prevents production of circulating antibody following antigenic stimulation but nevertheless appears to permit some conditioning of the cells so that the secondary response is observed on subsequent stimulation. The extent of the secondary response appears, however, to be appreciably less than in the animal lacking passively transferred antibody.

3. The production of antibodies may be diminished or abolished by the administration of various immunosuppressive agents. These agents are of considerable clinical importance as they may be used to suppress the homograft reaction (p. 117). They may be divided into two groups: (a) X-rays and cortisone, which are effective only if given before the introduction of the antigen. Both have a generally depressing effect on lymphoid tissues, and if this explains their inhibition of antibody production it follows that the cells which have already become conditioned to produce antibody must have acquired resistance to them. (b) Agents which are maximally effective only if introduced after injection of the antigen. They include purine and pyrimidine analogues, nitrogen mustards, the

folic acid antagonist methopterin, methotrexate, which inhibits the action of the enzyme folic reductase, actinomycin D which inhibits the synthesis of RNA on a DNA template and cyclophosphamide. The latter compound has been found to be particularly effective in suppressing antibody production in relatively non-toxic concentrations.

4. The degree of antibody response depends, within limits, on the amount of antigen introduced on primary stimulation (p. 108). Very small amounts of antigen will not stimulate any demonstrable antibody production although they may be able to induce some degree of potential immunity. At the upper end there is a limit beyond which increases in antigen dose do not result in increased antibody production. In fact, very large doses of antigen may inhibit antibody production. This has been observed in mice immunized with pneumococcal polysaccharide, and in rabbits immunized with large doses of heterologous protein. This inhibition of antibody response by large doses of antigen is known as *immunological paralysis*. It is obviously very similar, and possibly identical, to the condition of immunological tolerance (p. 119).

5. The antibody response to an antigen can be increased considerably by the injection together with the antigen of substances known, because of their stimulating effect on antibody production, as *adjuvants*. The most potent adjuvant so far described, and that which has been most studied in experimental animals, is the *Freund* adjuvant. The complete Freund adjuvant is a mixture of mineral oil, emulsifying agent and killed mycobacteria. In addition to enhancing antibody production against both exogenous and autogenous antigens (p. 125), the Freund adjuvant is extremely potent in stimulating delayed type hypersensitivity (p. 179). The adjuvant stimulates the formation of a granuloma at the site of injection, and of secondary granulomata in the draining lymphatic glands. There is also evidence of a widespread stimulation of the reticulo-endothelial system. Because of the severe granulomatous reaction it produces the complete Freund adjuvant is unsuitable for administration to man. Incomplete adjuvants containing only mineral oil and emulsifier, and producing only local granulomata have, however, been used in man, e.g. in emulsified influenza vaccine, but antigens of this type have not so far been generally adopted for human immunization.

The mechanism by which these adjuvants enhance antibody production is not completely understood. There is little doubt that it is in part due to the retention of antigen locally in the granuloma. This delays its destruction and therefore provides a more persistent antigenic stimulus. Some antibody production also occurs in the granuloma itself. The active agent in the mycobacterial suspension of the complete Freund adjuvant appears to be a *peptidoglycolipid*. Precisely how this acts is unknown. It may stimulate phagocytic cells directly, or combine with the antigen in such a way as to delay its destruction or combine with antibody to form a complex which in some way derepresses antibody synthesis.

Although Freund type adjuvants have been most studied experimentally, aluminium salts have been the adjuvants most widely used for active immunization in man, e.g. in alum-precipitated diphtheria toxoid, at one time the main antigen employed for immunization against diphtheria. Aluminium salts are presumed to act in a manner similar to the incomplete Freund adjuvant.

The capacity of pertussis vaccine to enhance the antibody response to diphtheria toxoid is well established. The effect appears to to be due to the endotoxin of the organism, and purified endotoxins of a variety of Gram negative bacteria have been shown to have a marked adjuvant effect on the response to protein antigens. There are two main ways in which endotoxins might produce an adjuvant defect: (a) As stimulants of the reticulo-endothelial system. (b) By a disruptive effect on lysosomes—structures which appear to be the main centres of hydrolytic enzyme activity in the cell, and which may play an important part in the natural disposal of antigen. If lysosome function is depressed the antigen may possibly persist for a much longer time than in the normal cell.

6. There is some evidence that if a number of antigens are introduced into an animal at the same time the antibody response to each may be less than if the antigens are introduced separately. This competition of antigens appears to be most marked when an animal has already been immunized against one of the antigens in the combination, in which case the antibody response may be mainly directed against this antigen.

The Antibody-producing Cells

There is now convincing evidence that the principal antibody-producing cell is the plasma cell. This cell is not a normal body cell but appears to develop specifically in response to antigenic stimulation. Plasma cells have a strongly basophilic cytoplasm due to a high concentration of RNA. Because of this they stain intensely with pyronin which combines specifically with RNA, and are as a result known as *pyroninophilic* cells. The mature plasma cell possesses a small eccentric nucleus with an irregular distribution of chromatin around the periphery of the nucleus, giving the latter the appearance of a clock face. To one side of the nucleus is a clear bean-shaped area corresponding to the site of the Golgi apparatus. In addition an extensive endoplasmic reticulum—a sine qua non of protein secreting cells—is demonstrable on electron microscopy.

The evidence in support of the plasma cell as the main antibody-producing cell is as follows: (1) The concentration of plasma cells in the medulla of the lymph nodes and spleen shows a sharp increase following antigenic stimulation. (2) The tissues of patients suffering from hypogammaglobulinaemia (p. 116) are markedly deficient in plasma cells. (3) Antibody may be demonstrated directly in plasma cells by a modification of the fluorescent antibody technique in which the cells are exposed to antigen, then washed and exposed to a fluorescent antibody specific for the combined antigen. During antibody production accumulations of antibody can be seen as hyaline amorphous masses in pockets of endoplasmic reticulum in haematoxylin-stained preparations. These collections, known as *Russell* bodies, can be seen also in electron micrographs.

By using the fluorescent antibody technique each of the classes of immunoglobulin has been identified in plasma cells. In this connexion it is of interest, however, that plasma cell tumours or plasma cell myeloma produce IgG and IgA, but not IgM immunoglobulins. Conversely, macroglobulinaemia or Waldenström's disease shows no excess of IgA or IgG, and is characterized histologically by lymphoid cell hyperplasia. There is some conflict of evidence as to whether under normal conditions individual plasma cells can produce more than one type of immunoglobulin. Fluorescent antibody-staining indicates, however, that only one immunoglobulin type is demonstrable in the majority of cells, similarly the majority of cells produce light chains of either κ or λ types but not of both.

A substantial body of evidence links the plasma cell with the small lymphocyte and suggests that the latter is the precursor of the former.

1. A striking feature of the cellular response to antigenic stimulation is the production of *germinal centres*, whose major function is the production of lymphocytes, in the lymph nodes and spleen. The increased production of lymphocytes in lymph nodes following antigenic stimulation is readily demonstrable by lymphocyte counts in the efferent lymph.

2. Lymphocytes are capable of *restoring immunological functions* to animals deprived of such function, whether this deprivation be by X-irradiation, by neonatal thymectomy, by the use of immunosuppressive drugs or by the induction of immunological tolerance. This restoration of function occurs not only with cellular immune reactions (p. 117), but also for antibody production. Thus, Gowans and McGregor showed that in rats depleted of small lymphocytes by drainage of lymph through a thoracic duct fistula, and which were as a result unable to produce antibody to tetanus toxoid or sheep red cells, the capacity to produce antibody could be restored by injecting small lymphocytes.

3. Further evidence for this view has been obtained by Elves who showed that the lymphocytes of sensitized animals could be induced on exposure to phytohaemagglutinin obtained from the kidney bean, to undergo transformation into *blast cells* (PHA cells), in which gammaglobulin could be demonstrated by the fluorescent antibody technique. A similar transformation could be induced by exposure to a specific antigen. Moreover, it was found that in patients with hypogammaglobulinaemia—a condition in which there is a gross deficiency in plasma cells—the small lymphocytes could not be transformed by exposure to phytohaemagglutinin. These observations suggest the identity of the blast cells produced by lymphocyte transformation with the presumptive blast cell precursor of the plasma cell.

Although plasma cells are the primary antibody producers, there is no direct evidence that they take up antigen following introduction of the latter into the tissues, or that antibody production is the sequel to a direct contact of plasma cell with antigen. The cells that are principally concerned in the uptake of antigen are macrophages and endothelial cells, in which antigen can be readily demonstrated by the fluorescent antibody technique. Macrophages and endothelial cells do not produce antibody, and since plasma cells—the main antibody producers—are not involved in the uptake of antigen, a two-stage theory of antibody production has been suggested, notably by Fishman (p. 114). This theory postulates that the antigen is processed by the macrophage, and that the processed antigen or a fragment of it, or some informational macromolecule is transmitted from the macrophage to the plasma cell. The fact that macrophages and endothelial cells are principally involved in the uptake of antigen does not, however, imply that they must necessarily play a direct part in the chain of events leading to antibody production. The moiety of antigen responsible for antibody stimulation may be only a small proportion of the total amount of antigen introduced into, or gaining access to the tissues; this moiety may reach the plasma cells or their precursors directly, or possibly via the dendritic cells, noted by White and shown to contain antigen, in the germinal centres of lymph nodes and spleen exposed to antigenic stimulation.

Theories of Antibody Production

Two types of theory have been proposed to explain the mechanism of antibody production: (a) instructive, and (b) selective.

Instructive Theories

The Antigen Template Theory

This theory, first proposed by Breinl and Haurowitz, was stated in its modern form by Pauling. Its initial justification was the necessity to explain an animal's capacity to produce antibody against an apparently infinite diversity of antigens, including artificial antigens with which the animal would be extremely unlikely ever to have come into normal biological contact. The theory assumes that the antibody is synthesized as a normal globulin in so far as the incorporation of the amino acids into a polypeptide chain is concerned but that while still in an expanded or extended state the polypeptide chain is brought into contact with the antigen. During this contact the surface configuration of the antigen acting as a template determines the way in which the polypeptide chain is folded to form the reactive part of the antibody molecule. The theory implies that proteins identical in amino acid composition and sequence may nevertheless differ in tertiary structure. Whether this can occur is at the moment in doubt. It seems more probable that the tertiary structure of a protein is an inevitable consequence of its amino acid composition. In this case the antigen would be required to determine the amino acid sequence of the antibody protein during synthesis. This might occur if the antigen interfered at ribosomal level with amino acid incorporation. For example it might conceivably cause a misreading of the genetic code as has been suggested for streptomycin in bacteria (p. 194). Apart from these considerations however the antigen template theory faces some major practical difficulties.

1. An examination of the kinetics of antibody production appears to indicate that the synthesis of antibody is associated with exponential multiplication of cellular or subcellular units. This multiplication is particularly apparent in the secondary antibody response. It would be difficult to see how an antigen template could be capable of the necessary replication.

2. If, as one might expect, the antigen acting as a template were associated with ribosomes, a single plasma cell might produce a number of serologically

distinct antibodies since there would appear to be no reason why different ribosomes might not combine with different antigen molecules. In fact most, and possibly all, antibody-producing cells which have been examined under in vitro conditions produce antibody of only a single specificity.

3. So far, it has not been possible to demonstrate antigen in antibody-producing cells by either fluorescent antibody or autoradiographic techniques.

4. A crucial observation against the antigen template theory would be the continuation of antibody production after all traces of antigen had disappeared. It is undoubtedly true that antibody production does continue considerably beyond the point at which it is possible to demonstrate antibody in the circulation by currently available techniques. This finding, however, would be consistent with the persistence of sequestered or intracellular antigen, which might provide the continuing stimulus required.

5. To explain the difference between the primary and secondary response it would be necessary to ascribe two quite different functions to the antigen: (a) On first contact the antigen would be incorporated as a template, thereby priming the cell so that it became capable of producing antibody. (b) On subsequent contact the antigen would provide a stimulus to cell division which would explain the kinetics of the in vivo response. Such division has been shown to occur following in vitro stimulation of cells previously sensitized in vivo.

The RNA Template Theory

As previously indicated, the cell types primarily responsible for the uptake of antigen are the macrophages. These cells have not been shown to be capable of producing antibody nor of undergoing transformation into antibody-producing cells. If they play an essential part in the sequence of events leading to antibody production their role might be either: (a) To break down the antigen into smaller fragments acceptable to the antibody-producing cells, or (b) To produce an informational macromolecule with a structure complementary to that of the antigen so that it could function as a template for the synthesis of antibody. Fishman, the main proponent of this latter theory, has succeeded in stimulating specific antibody production in rats by injection of RNA extracted from macrophages which were previously incubated with antigen in vitro. The RNA preparations employed, however, almost certainly contained small amounts of antigen the antigenicity of which might have been in some way enhanced by complexing with RNA. The RNA template theory would be unaffected by most of the difficulties faced by the antigen template theory. There would be some difficulty, however, in explaining why most antibody-producing cells produce antibody of only a single specificity. It would in this case be necessary to assume that the antibody-producing cell could accept only one type of RNA. Moreover, the persistence of immunological memory would make it necessary to postulate a very stable type of messenger RNA.

Selective Theories

Selective theories of antibody production do not admit the possibility that the pattern of antibody synthesis is dictated directly or indirectly by the antigen. On the contrary they propose that the capacity to produce specific antibody is genetically determined and that the antigen plays only a selective role.

The Clonal Selection Theory

This theory, put forward by Burnet, is the most widely adopted selective theory. It is a modified form of a theory first proposed by Jerne and postulates that the antibody-producing machinery has an intrinsic genetically controlled capacity to synthesize globulin molecules with a large number of specific surface patterns. These globulin molecules are assumed to be present as components of the cell surface. Individual antibody-producing cells can, however, only synthesize globulin of a specific configuration. When an antigen is introduced into the body it combines with cells whose surface molecules contain globulin with the appropriate complementary pattern. This combination in some way stimulates cellular multiplication; as a result a clone of cells is formed which produces globulin of the same configuration and which continues to produce it in the absence of the antigen.

The clonal selection theory of antibody production meets all the objections to the antigen template hypothesis. It resolves the problem of the primary and secondary antibody responses by postulating only a quantitative difference between them, reflecting differences only in the numbers of antibody-producing cells present, and the problem of the persistence of antibody response in the absence of antigenic stimulation simply does not arise. The main difficulty it presents is that it requires the existence of a large number of cells each possessing a genetically predetermined globulin pattern. To minimize the number of predetermined patterns required Burnet has postulated that each cell can vary its pattern within a limited range by undergoing a somatic mutation. The existence of such mutations has not, however, been demonstrated. Even on this basis the number of cell types required must still be considerable since they must provide both for differences in pattern and immunoglobulin class, and for other types of heterogeneity (p. 104) that can be demonstrated for each specific antibody pattern. At the genetic level this must imply a situation of enormous complexity since the host cell genome would have to carry the genetic code for all the proteins required. In this case the restricted potential of different immunologically competent cells would require the repression in each such cell of the great bulk of this genetic information.

The Derepression Hypothesis

Originally proposed by Szilard, this is a selection theory which postulates the occurrence of selection at a subcellular level. It assumes the existence of toti-potential cells each capable of producing the entire range of antibodies which may possibly be required. Normally the transcription of the messenger RNA necessary for the synthesis of these antibodies is repressed but on contact with antigen the transcription of RNA required for the synthesis of the corresponding antibody is derepressed in a manner similar to the derepression of inducible enzymes (p. 30). Like the clonal selection theory, this theory requires that the host genome should embrace all possible antibody configurations. It is reasonable to wonder whether such a genetic load would be consistent with the general economy of nature. Furthermore, the derepression hypothesis does not account by itself for the cellular division which has been demonstrable under in vitro conditions following exposure of sensitized cells to antigen.

ABNORMALITIES AFFECTING ANTIBODY PRODUCTION

Hypogammaglobulinaemia

This condition, characterized by a gross deficiency in gamma globulin production, occurs in a secondary form associated with various blood dyscrasias and as a primary condition. The commonest primary form (Bruton type) is a familial sex-linked condition occurring only in males. There is a marked hypoplasia of the lymphoid tissues with an absolute deficiency of plasma cells. The thymus appears normal (p. 122). The gamma globulin concentration in the serum is less than 100 mg per 100 ml but gamma globulin is rarely completely absent. This gamma globulin deficiency affects all immunoglobulin types, IgG, IgA and IgM. As a result of this deficiency children with hypogammaglobulinaemia possess extremely low resistance to bacterial infection. They usually respond normally to virus infections, however, and to infection with the tubercle bacillus. They show no alteration in the capacity to mount delayed-type hypersensitivity reactions. As a rule they reject homografts but the rejection period is usually longer than in the normal child.

Multiple Myeloma

This condition in which multiple tumours composed of plasma cells appear in various tissues is, not surprisingly, associated with considerable excess of gamma globulin in the blood, the excess gamma globulin showing as a sharp peak in one part of the electrophoretic spectrum. The precise position of this peak varies from patient to patient but is constant in any one patient throughout the course of the disease. The gamma globulin may be of IgG or IgA type. The restricted electrophoretic mobility of the excess gamma globulin is consistent with its production by a neoplastic proliferation in a single clone of cells responsible for the production of gamma globulin in that particular part of the electrophoretic range. From this it is concluded that in normal health, individual clones of plasma cells are responsible for the production of gamma globulin of different specific mobilities. No antibody function has so far been ascribed to the abnormal gamma globulin. In general these patients are poor producers of antibody and in consequence have a low resistance to bacterial infection. About 50 per cent of multiple myeloma patients excrete considerable amounts of an abnormal protein—the Bence–Jones protein—in their urine. This protein is precipitated when the urine is heated to between 50 and 60° C, going into solution again at 80° C. The abnormal protein consists in fact of the light chains of gamma globulin. The production of Bence–Jones protein is due to a disorganization in gamma globulin production, leading either to an excessive production of light chains or to an asynchronous production of heavy and light chains.

Macroglobulinaemia

In this condition, first described by Waldenström, the patient's serum contains a large amount of macroglobulin (IgM) and is viscous at room temperature. IgG and IgA are usually decreased. The condition is associated with considerable hyperplasia of the lymph nodes, which contain large numbers of cells intermediate in character between lymphocytes and plasma cells. Frequently the cell type changes during the course of the disease to that of a typical plasma cell. Macroglobulinaemic patients appear to have a normal resistance to infection.

CELLULAR IMMUNE RESPONSES

So far we have been concerned only with immune responses to antigenic stimulation characterized by the production of humoral antibodies. There is, however, a large body of evidence to suggest that on contact with an antigen the animal body may mount a cellular response which is immunologically specific and independent of circulating antibody. The cell primarily involved in this response is the small lymphocyte, which behaves as if it were the carrier of immunological specificity. The simplest interpretation of its function is that it possesses antibody-like groupings on its surface. It could therefore be described as a 'cellular antibody'. The operation of this lymphocyte mediated cellular immunity may be seen in two physically distinct, though fundamentally related phenomena—*homograft rejection* and *delayed-type hypersensitivity*. The latter will be considered in more detail in Chapter 9.

Homograft Rejection

It has been known for many years that skin grafts between different members of the same species (homografts) are normally rejected. On the other hand grafts of skin from one site on an individual's body to another (autografts) are accepted. Grafts between identical twins are also accepted and will persist indefinitely. That homograft rejection has an immunological basis has been established by the following lines of evidence.

1. The readiness with which grafts are rejected depends on the antigenic relationship between the donor of the graft and the host. The more remote this relationship the more vigorously is the graft rejected.

The antigens in the graft against which the host reacts are known as *histocompatibility antigens*, and are under the control of distinct histocompatibility genes. Thirteen of such genes have so far been recognized in mice. By continuous interbreeding between brother–sister pairs, strains of mice of virtually identical genetic and antigenic constitution have been derived. Individual mice of each of these strains possess identical histocompatibility antigens and will normally accept grafts from one another. Grafts between individuals of such inbred lines, and between identical twins in man are described as *syngeneic*. Grafts between genetically distinct individuals of the same species are described as *allogeneic* or *isogeneic*; they are frequently referred to simply as homografts. Grafts between individuals of different species are known as *heterogeneic* or as *xenogeneic*.

2. When a skin graft has been rejected, a second graft from the same donor is rejected much more rapidly. This accelerated rejection shows a high degree of specificity for the donor species from which the graft was obtained.

Mechanism of Graft Rejection

There is now virtually conclusive evidence that homograft rejection is mainly, if not exclusively, due to lymphocytes which have been conditioned by the graft tissue towards which they have developed a serological specificity.

1. Rejection is greatly inhibited by any procedure which results in a fall in the lymphocyte population, e.g. thymectomy, X-irradiation, the administration of antilymphocyte serum and drainage of the thoracic duct. Animals which have lost their capacity for graft rejection by lymphocyte depletion, regain this capacity following injection of lymphoid tissues from syngeneic animals. The capacity for graft rejection may be restored to thymectomized animals by grafting a portion of the thymus of a normal animal.

2. In the case of skin homografts lymphatic channels are necessary for the development of the rejection mechanism. In anatomical situations where such vessels are absent, as in hamster pouch skin, graft rejection does not occur. By the use of lymphoid cells labelled with tritiated thymidine it has been possible to show that these cells migrate in large numbers from the regional lymph node to the graft.

3. More direct evidence of the role of the sensitized lymphocyte has been obtained by the demonstration of a cytotoxic effect on allogeneic donor cells in tissue culture, in the absence of antibody and complement. The 'immune lymphocyte transfer reaction' of Brent and Medawar points to the same conclusion. In this reaction sensitized lymphoid cells from a graft recipient produce an acute inflammatory reaction when injected intradermally into the graft donor.

The extent to which humoral antibody contributes, if at all, to graft rejection cannot at the moment be precisely defined. Following graft rejection, the development of antibodies capable of agglutinating donor red cells has been demonstrated, together with antibodies which have a cytotoxic effect on donor leucocytes in tissue cultures. Graft rejection is not enhanced, however, by the injection of serum from a sensitized animal. This finding would indicate that humoral antibody must play at most a minor role in graft rejection.

Graft Versus Host Disease

This is a condition which develops when an animal is injected with lymphoid tissue from a donor lacking one or more antigens present in the recipient. Under these circumstances the donor's lymphoid cells can mount an immune reaction against the antigens of the recipient which are not present in the donor. The condition does not develop if the graft contains antigens absent from the recipient, and against which the latter can mount an immune response resulting in the graft being rejected. Graft versus host disease was first observed in young mice in which it assumes a characteristic form known as 'runt disease'. The affected animals fail to thrive, die within a few weeks and at autopsy show a marked atrophy of their lymphoid tissues.

Graft versus host disease occurs only under one of the following conditions; (a) The recipient is very young and is injected with a foreign lymphoid tissue to which it can develop tolerance. (b) In adult animals which have been rendered tolerant to the graft antigens in early life. (c) In animals that are genetically disqualified from reacting with the graft tissue. An animal will accept tissue from its parents but parents will reject tissue from their offspring. (d) When the normal immunological responses have been inhibited by immunosuppressive agents (p. 109).

It has been established beyond all reasonable doubt that, as in homograft rejection, the cell type which is responsible for graft versus host reactions is the small lymphocyte. In fact, Gowans has demonstrated the migration of small lymphocytes from the graft into the lymphoid tissues of the host, and their transformation there into pyroninophilic cells similar to those found in local lymph nodes during homograft rejection.

IMMUNOLOGICAL TOLERANCE

As we have seen, the capacity of an animal to respond to antigenic stimulation can be inhibited by the administration of immunosuppressive agents. These act in an entirely non-specific fashion, destroying or inhibiting the capacity of the animal to respond to any antigen. The capacity of an animal to respond to a specific antigen can, however, be inhibited while allowing it to respond to other antigens, if the animal is exposed to the antigen in early life, or exposed at a later stage to *a very large amount* of the antigen. This induced inability of the animal to respond to antigens to which it would be expected to respond normally is known as immunological tolerance.

The far-reaching immunological implications of this phenomenon were first realized by Burnet and Fenner who saw in it a vital clue to the mechanism by which animals are rendered non-reactive to antigens present in their own tissues. They postulated that if an animal were exposed to an antigen during the course of embryological development and before the effective establishment of its immunological machinery, the capacity of the animal to respond to that antigen in later life might be suppressed. Decisive experimental support for this hypothesis was obtained by Medawar and his associates who showed: (1) That each member of a pair of synchorial cattle twins was capable of accepting a skin homograft from the other twin. Skin grafts between twins which had not exchanged erythropoietic tissue during intra-uterine development were rejected in the normal fashion. (2) When embryonic or new-born mice were injected with tissues of mice from an unrelated (allogeneic) strain they were able in later life to accept skin grafts from that strain. They had acquired, as a result of the injection, a tolerance to the donor cells. In addition to failing to reject homografts, the animals were also found to be incapable of producing antibody against the graft cells. In general, the extent to which tolerance can be induced against donor cells depends on the genetic relationship between the donor and the host. If these are closely related, tolerance is much easier to induce than otherwise.

Although at first it was thought that tolerance to homografts could be induced only in the immature animal, it has now been clearly established that this is not the case. Tolerance can be induced in the adult animal, but only to tissues derived from donors that are closely related genetically to the recipient. Genetic barriers are in the adult much more difficult to surmount than in the neonate. In addition much larger doses of antigen are required. The ease with which tolerance can be induced in the adult can be very substantially increased by the use of immunosuppressive agents.

Tolerance can also be induced to soluble antigens. Thus, as has been known for a long time, it is possible to induce tolerance to pneumococcal polysaccharide in adult mice by injecting large doses of antigen (p. 110). The polysaccharide is not broken down by the mouse tissues, and therefore persists to provide a tolerance inducing stimulus for a long period. It was at one time thought that the apparent failure to produce antibody was due to a neutralization of any antibody which might be produced by the excessive amount of antigen present in the circulation. The use of the fluorescent antibody technique has, however, failed to reveal the presence of any antibody in the cells of the tolerant animal. In this respect, therefore, the phenomenon resembles the tolerance that can be induced to tissue homografts in young animals.

The above example is the only instance of the induction of tolerance to polysaccharide antigens. Tolerance to protein antigens is, however, readily produced in a variety of animals. The tolerance induced in the rabbit to protein antigens such as human or bovine serum albumen and globulin, has in recent years been the most widely used experimental model. This tolerance has been shown to be highly specific for the inducing antigen, and unlike tolerance to homografts, is not of permanent duration—presumably because of the non-persistence of the antigenic stimulus necessary to maintain the tolerant state. After the antigen has been completely eliminated the normal non-tolerant state returns. It has been apparent, however, that the persistence of antigen, demonstrable in the circulation, is not necessary for the maintenance of the tolerant state. This would seem to indicate that the tolerance inducing antigen is antigen which persists in an intracellular location.

Although at one time a distinction was drawn between tolerance induced in the neonate, and tolerance or immunological paralysis in the adult, most workers now consider that the mechanism operating in both is the same. In both, the tolerance inducing dose is several times the dose required to immunize. The greater difficulty in producing tolerance in the adult may arise from the much larger number of immunologically competent cells, or because they are less prone to destruction or suppression by antigen. There is evidence that if the foetus is injected with a small amount of an antigen which in higher concentration will induce tolerance, antibody is developed against it. All the evidence therefore tends to equate immunological non-reactivity, whether this occurs in the adult or in the infant.

An explanation of tolerance on the basis of the clonal selection theory has been proposed by Burnet. This postulates that contact of antigen with immunologically competent cells at an early stage in development results in the death of the homologous antibody-producing cells. With the destruction of these cells the animal loses the capacity to produce the corresponding antibody until such time, if ever, as it regains the capacity to produce cells with the same immunological potential. The hypothesis can be readily extended to cover the induction of tolerance in the adult, by presuming a very much lower susceptibility of adult antibody-producing cells to the lethal effects of excess antigen—a correspondingly larger dose of antigen being required. The mechanism by which excess antigen kills immunologically competent cells is unexplained, but might, for example, be by a lethal deviation of protein synthesis from the production of essential cellular components.

An alternative explanation which presumes the two-stage theory of antibody formation is that antigen gains access to the antibody-producing cell, and blocks the transmission of an informational macromolecule-RNA, on Fishman's theory, from the macrophage involved in the processing of the antigen to the ultimate antibody producer.

The way in which tolerant cells lose their tolerance and regain the capacity to produce antibody, which they will eventually do in the absence of antigenic stimulation, is relevant to this problem. It would seem that the reacquisition of immunological reactivity is not due to a loss of tolerance consequent on the loss of antigen by the tolerant cells but is the result of the formation of new non-tolerant cells from appropriate precursors. This explanation would also readily account for such spontaneous loss of tolerance failing to occur in thymectomized animals, and occurring much more rapidly in the young than in the older animal, completely irrespective of the duration of previous exposure to the antigen.

Apart from immunological paralysis induced by pneumococcal polysaccharide in mice it has not so far proved possible to produce immunological tolerance to a bacterial antigen. This is presumably because the antigenic difference from the host is much too great to be surmounted by the tolerance inducing machinery. There is, however, one known instance of the spontaneous development of tolerance to an infecting micro-organism. This is the tolerance induced in mice by the virus of lymphocytic choriomeningitis (p. 477). This virus is of low virulence for mice, and in infected colonies causes a persistent asymptomatic infection. Mice readily become infected in utero or during the neonatal period from their mothers. Following such neonatal infection the virus is demonstrable in the brain, blood and other tissues. Despite this, the mice do not make antibody against or develop hypersensitivity towards the virus.

When, as is normal, a foetus is the result of the mating of genetically dissimilar parents, it has the essential properties of a homograft. The mother does not, however, mount an immunological response against it. Although foetal white cells and red blood cells can stimulate the production of antibodies in the mother the foetus itself is not rejected. This might be because the mother has, during pregnancy, a fundamental incapacity to mount a response against foetal antigens, or because—despite such a response—the placenta may not provide a suitable environment for the operation of the rejection mechanism. At the moment it is not possible to decide between these alternatives. It has been suggested that the final separation of the placenta on the termination of pregnancy is due to the homograft rejection mechanism. The occurrence of placental separation in matings between genetically identical parents is, however, strong evidence against this view.

It is reasonable to ask why animals should have the capacity for homograft rejection at all, since grafting is a completely artificial phenomenon. One extremely plausible theory proposes that the mechanism has evolved as a method of eliminating malignant mutants of normal tissue cells. In this case the development of malignancy might conceivably be the result of a breakdown in a normal immunological responsiveness.

ROLE OF THE THYMUS

It is tempting to consider a unitary hypothesis of cellular and humoral immune responses, viz. that the same cell can mediate both types of response and that the particular type of response elicited depends on environmental factors. The evidence available, however, favours the alternative hypothesis that although cells which are morphologically small lymphocytes, are involved in both types of response they comprise two distinct functional types, one which has been conditioned to differentiate to antibody production, and the other to become the vehicle of a cellular response. The situation is clearest in the fowl—for which Good and his colleagues have shown that the thymus conditions lymphocytes to cellular responses, and the bursa of Fabricius in the hind gut to antibody production. Thus, it has been found possible by removal of one of these organs to eliminate the corresponding type of immune response. In man the position is not quite so clear-cut as in the fowl. There is evidence that the lymphoid tissues of the adenoids, tonsils and Peyer's patches of the intestinal tract are bursa equivalents but that in man and higher animals generally the thymus also exercises some control over antibody production.

Evidence for the immunological function of the mammalian thymus has been obtained principally from the results of thymectomy in mice, which when carried out in the neonatal animal is followed by:

1. A marked decrease in the number of circulating lymphocytes, with evidence of severe lymphoid hypoplasia in the lymphoid tissues.

2. Loss of the capacity to reject homografts.

3. Loss of the capacity to develop delayed-type hypersensitivity.

4. Considerable impairment of antibody-producing capacity. The degree of

impairment, however, has been found to vary considerably in different animals, and antibody production is clearly less affected by thymectomy than the capacity to develop delayed-type hypersensitivity.

5. The development of a wasting disease very similar to runt disease (p. 119), or to secondary disease in X-irradiated animals. Wasting disease has not been found to occur in thymectomized animals maintained in a germ-free state. This suggests that the condition might be due to a breakdown in the immunological defences against environmental parasites. As against this interpretation, however, is the fact that the condition cannot be prevented, in mice at any rate, by injection of the serum of a normal animal.

6. The lymphocytes of thymectomized mice have much less capacity to produce graft versus host reactions (p. 118) than those of normal mice.

The dramatic effects of thymectomy in the neonate are not found in the adult. Although there is some fall in the number of circulating lymphocytes, immunological function suffers no obvious interference. Under special conditions, however, certain immunological defects can be demonstrated. (a) Irradiated thymectomized mice injected with normal marrow fail to show the recovery in immunological capability, as demonstrated by the capacity to reject skin homografts, which occurs in marrow-protected irradiated but non-thymectomized mice. (b) Thymectomized animals show a much slower spontaneous recovery from induced immunological tolerance than non-thymectomized animals when the tolerance inducing antigen is withdrawn.

Immunological function can be restored to thymectomized animals in two ways: (1) By injecting lymph node suspensions from normal animals; the responsible cells are presumed to be lymphocytes. (2) By grafting thymus tissue from another animal. There is considerable evidence that such grafts are invaded by lymphoid cells of host origin, and that these cells gain immunological competence in the graft, returning again to the host lymphoid tissues. It has also been shown that thymus tissue can restore immunological function to thymectomized animals under conditions where cellular migration to and from the thymus cannot occur. Thus, Miller has found recovery of function after thymus tissue has been implanted in millipore membranes, in the peritoneal cavities of young mice thymectomized at birth. However, it has not been possible to restore immunological function by the injection of thymic extracts.

From these results it is clear that the thymus plays a major role in the establishment of immunological function in the young animal, and more particularly in the establishment of a population of immunologically competent lymphocytes. Some part of this role—particularly in the conditioning of cells destined to produce antibody—is probably carried out by lymphoid tissues associated with the alimentary tract; these would therefore be the equivalent of the bursa of Fabricius in the fowl. This would explain the rather irregular failure in antibody-producing capacity following thymectomy.

The fundamental importance of the thymus in man is seen in the so-called Swiss type of congenital agammaglobulinaemia (SAG), in which there is marked thymic aplasia together with a virtual absence of lymphoid tissue and of plasma cells from the alimentary tract. These changes are associated with a total lack of both cellular and humoral immune responses and are incompatible with survival, no child affected having survived past $2\frac{1}{2}$ years of age. The condition has many of the features of runt disease (p. 119), and some cases have been shown to be associated with a colonization of the foetal tissues by lymphoid cells of maternal origin. Such cases were presumably examples of a graft versus host reaction (p. 118).

There are three main ways in which the thymus might exercise immunological control.

1. It might be responsible for the initial seeding, during immunological development, of lymphoid tissues with lymphocyte precursors. The high rate of lymphocyte production in the thymus in the young animal is consistent with this role. The low immunological competence of the thymus lymphocyte, and the demonstration that the lymphocytes of thymus grafts are of host origin are however in conflict with it.

2. Lymphocyte precursor or stem cells may be transformed into cells with immunological capacity by migration through the thymus, where they undergo transformation through the action of a hormone secreted by the thymic epithelial reticular cells.

3. Lymphocyte precursor or stem cells may be transformed by thymic hormone in situ in lymphoid tissues, without the necessity for migration through the thymus. The evidence available at the moment admits the possibility that both these latter mechanisms may be operative.

There is some reason to believe that the thymus plays a part in the maintenance of immunological tolerance. This function was first proposed by Burnet who attributed to the thymus the role of eliminating clones of immunologically competent conditioned host lymphocytes reacting with host tissues. That the thymus must have some function in relation to the maintenance of tolerance is suggested by the finding that a spontaneous auto-immune haemolytic anaemia in mice is accompanied by thymus hyperplasia, and that thymus hyperplasia is also found in human cases of myasthenia gravis—a condition, possibly of auto-immune origin, in which antibodies reacting with striated muscle are frequently found. Myasthenia gravis is also found in association with systemic lupus erythematosus, a condition marked by the development of several varieties of auto-immune antibodies.

AUTO-IMMUNIZATION

So far the immune response has been considered as a mechanism whose essential function it is to dispose of foreign material that may have gained access to the tissues. It was early found however that an animal could form antibodies not only against foreign substances but also against certain substances present in its own body. This process is known as auto-immunization and the antibodies so formed are known as auto-antibodies. The first demonstration that a normal animal could produce antibodies against components of its own tissues was Metalnikoff's finding that rabbits could be immunized against their own spermatozoa. Shortly afterwards it was shown by Uhlenhuth that rabbits could produce antibodies against their own lens protein. More recently the range of tissue antigens against which animals may be stimulated on injection to produce auto-antibodies has been extended to include thyroglobulin and antigens present in brain, adrenals and uveal tract. In general the production of auto-antibodies is considerably enhanced if the antigen is incorporated in Freund's adjuvant. In all of these cases the antigen responsible for immunization and against which the antibody is directed possesses organ specificity—the same antigen being present in the corresponding organs of other animal species.

Although it has been clearly demonstrated that animals can produce antibody reacting with certain components of their own tissues the number of such components which have been proved capable of stimulating the production of auto-antibodies in the normal animal is limited. It may in fact be assumed that the possession by the animal body of a general capacity to develop antibody against its own tissue components would not be compatible with life—a concept which was early entrenched in immunological thinking and was given formal statement by Ehrlich in the expression *horror autotoxicus*. The animal body must therefore possess some mechanism whose function it is to prevent such auto-immunization. It is tempting to assume that the restrictions imposed on the normal animal's capacity to produce antibody to antigens in its own tissues is due to the same mechanism as that responsible for induced immunological tolerance. Since such antigens are continually present during embryological development ideal conditions for the development of tolerance would be present. The failure to establish tolerance in relation to certain tissue antigens, e.g. lens protein, thyroglobulin etc., might in this event be due to the fact that these antigens do not gain access to the circulation in such a way as to establish tolerance.

In recent years the phenomenon of auto-immunization has attracted considerable attention because of the fact that on occasion auto-antibodies against certain tissue antigens have been found to develop spontaneously in man frequently in association with lesions in the corresponding tissues. The more fully documented syndromes found to be associated with the production of auto-immune antibodies are: chronic thyroiditis, disseminated lupus erythematosus and acquired haemolytic anaemia. In chronic thyroiditis the antibodies found react with thyroglobulin and with antigens present in the microsomes of the secretory cells of the acinar epithelium. In disseminated lupus erythematosus the antibodies found are specific for the desoxyribonucleoprotein of leucocytes and other tissue cells. In acquired haemolytic anaemia antibodies demonstrable by the Coombs antiglobulin test can be shown to be adsorbed in vitro on to the surface of the patient's red cells. Other conditions which have been found to be associated with what appear to be auto-immune reactions are certain types of cirrhosis of the liver, idiopathic Addison's disease, rheumatoid arthritis, male sterility and ulcerative colitis.

The precise relationship between humoral auto-antibodies and the disease processes with which they may be associated is not at the moment clear. That antibodies against tissue cells can cause serious tissue damage is shown clearly in two experimental models: (1) Guinea-pigs may be killed by the injection of antiserum containing antibody to the Forssman antigen (p. 95) which is widely distributed in their tissues. (2) As first shown by Masugi, it is possible to produce nephritis in rats by injection of duck anti-rat kidney serum. The pathogenesis of this condition is of interest. If the serum injected is of high titre, nephritis develops rapidly but if the serum is of low titre, nephritis develops more slowly and is associated with appearance of a rat antibody to duck gamma globulin. This antibody presumably combines with and potentiates the action of the duck antibody combined with the renal tissue. Recent evidence indicates that in both cases the glomerular basement membrane is the site of attack, and is probably damaged and its permeability affected by the adsorption of complement the presence of which can be demonstrated by the fluorescent antibody technique.

In most of the experimental auto-immune conditions mentioned above, and which have been produced in animals following injection of testicular, uveal, brain and renal tissue with Freund adjuvant, lesions have been found in the homologous organ. In none of these cases, however, has it been possible to incriminate humoral antibody as the cause of the lesions. These are much more likely to be due to the delayed-type hypersensitivity which the Freund adjuvant so readily induces. In general passively transferred antibody has been found in animals to be without tissue damaging effect, though in the presence of complement such antibodies have been found to be damaging in vitro.

In man the clearest evidence for a destructive role of an auto-immune antibody has been obtained in acquired haemolytic anaemias. In cases of haemolytic anaemia associated with so-called 'cold' type auto-antibody, there seems little doubt that intravascular haemolysis occurs as a result of the adsorption of complement to antibody-sensitized cells. In addition, auto-antibody almost certainly facilitates destruction of the sensitized cells by the spleen. Auto-antibodies may also play a part in the pathogenesis of Hashimoto's disease, since the cytotoxic effect of an antibody believed to be directed against the microsomal antigen has been demonstrated—by Pulvertaft—in tissue cultures of thyroid cells. There is evidence suggesting the possible participation of humoral antibodies in the aetiology of thyrotoxicosis and myasthenia gravis in the observations that: (a) babies born to mothers with these conditions may exhibit similar symptoms for a period after birth, while the passively transferred maternal IgG persists in the infants' circulation, and (b) that symptoms of both conditions can be produced in experimental animals by the injection of patients' sera. In many cases of postulated auto-immune disease in man, the humoral antibodies identified, however, may be the concomitants or the results of the disease rather than its cause. In some cases the disease may be the result of cellular immune reactions of delayed-type hypersensitivity. Thus, tissue cultures of lymphoid cells from patients with ulcerative colitis and rheumatoid arthritis, have produced cytotoxic effects on cells of the small intestine and on fibroblasts. In some cases there could well be a combined effect of sensitized cells and humoral antibody.

There are two main ways in which spontaneous auto-immunization might occur. (1) In the case of antigens, e.g. thyroglobulin and antigens present in the testis, lens, brain, adrenals and uveal tract, against which tolerance does not appear to be acquired in foetal life and which will stimulate antibody production in normal animals, auto-immunization simply requires that the antigen should gain access to the circulation, from which it is normally excluded, and thereby eventually reach the reticulo-endothelial system. (2) As a result of a breakdown of the tolerance mechanism, possibly as a result of a somatic mutation in antibody-producing cells, so that antibodies whose manufacture is normally forbidden are produced. This may prove to be the mechanism involved in the development of auto-immune antibodies against antigens, e.g. desoxyribonucleoprotein, to which tolerance is normally established in embryonic development.

CHAPTER 7

ANTIGEN–ANTIBODY REACTIONS

In this chapter we will be concerned with the types of reaction which may result from the combination of antibody and antigen. The more readily demonstrable results of such combination are agglutination, precipitation, complement fixation, killing and lysis, capsule swelling, phagocytosis and neutralization.

It was at one time thought that each of the different antigen–antibody reactions required a different type of antibody. Consequently antibodies were given different names—agglutinin, precipitin, lysin, opsonin—according to the different types of reaction observed. It was soon found, however, that the same antibody may produce a number of effects. Thus antibody to bacterial cellular antigens capable of agglutinating a suspension of the bacteria and of precipitating a soluble preparation of the homologous antigen, may also render the cell susceptible to phagocytosis in the presence of polymorphonuclear leucocytes, and to lysis and killing in the presence of complement.

Such observations led to the formulation of the *unitarian theory* of antigen–antibody reaction. This theory postulates that a single antigen can stimulate the production of only a single type of antibody and that the effect of this antibody depends only on the physical state of the antigen and the environmental conditions under which the reaction occurs.

In its insistence that each demonstrable type of antigen–antibody reaction did not require a separate type of antibody, the unitarian theory was correct. The theory must be reformulated, however, since—as we have seen—the antibody response to a single antigen may be heterogeneous. Some antibodies, while combining with antigen, are incapable of carrying out the classical in vitro antigen–antibody reactions of agglutination, precipitation and complement fixation. Others, efficient in agglutination and precipitation, have poor complement fixing activity. Some antitoxic antibodies, although actively precipitating toxin, are relatively inefficient in protecting animals against the effects of the toxin. We may say, therefore, that although antibody to a particular antigen may exhibit a range of activities and may produce a number of demonstrable antigen–antibody reactions, particular antibodies may be deficient in the capacity to carry out some of these reactions.

THE AGGLUTINATION REACTION

Agglutination is the clumping that occurs when particulate antigens, e.g.

bacteria and red cells, are mixed with homologous antiserum. It can only occur if the latter contains antibody to antigens located on the surface of the particle, and only in the presence of electrolyte. Agglutination can only be demonstrated satisfactorily if the antigens used are stable in suspension prior to addition of the antiserum.

Agglutination tests are of two types.

1. Direct Agglutination Tests

The antigens involved in these tests are structural components of the surfaces of cells, e.g. of bacteria or red cells.

Direct bacterial agglutination tests may be carried out by *slide* or *tube* methods. Slide methods are merely qualitative, or, at most, semi-quantitative procedures. They are usually carried out with living organisms taken from colonies on plates or from the growth on an agar slope, and are of considerable value in the preliminary identification of certain bacteria, notably *Salmonella*, *Shigella*, *Vibrio* and *Brucella* species. Tube tests are more precise and are normally carried out as quantitative procedures. Killed bacterial suspensions are generally used, the method of killing depending on the antigen required for the test. Serial dilutions of the serum are made, and the highest dilution capable of agglutinating the organism under standard defined conditions is determined, this dilution is known as the *titre* of the serum. Tube agglutination tests are of great importance in confirming the results of slide agglutination tests for the purpose of bacterial identification, and in the estimation of the antibody content of a patient's serum (p. 230).

2. Passive Agglutination Tests

In these the antigens are adsorbed or otherwise attached to the surfaces of carrier particles which are then agglutinable by antibody to the adsorbed or attached antigen. The most generally useful carrier particles are undoubtedly red blood cells, human and sheep red cells having been particularly used. Many bacterial polysaccharide antigens readily adsorb to untreated cells. Adsorption is more effective at 37° C than at lower temperatures, and is often considerably enhanced following pretreatment of the antigen by boiling or by exposure to dilute alkali. Several serologically distinct polysaccharide antigens can be adsorbed to the same red cells, apparently without mutual interference, and adsorbing, presumably, to different receptors on the cell surface. Adsorption of bacterial antigen may on occasion mask certain of the surface groupings of the red cell. Thus adsorption of *Salm. typhi* Vi antigen to human red cells reduces agglutinability by anti-A and anti-B antibodies, and adsorption of certain *Klebsiella* capsular antigens blocks the adsorption of influenza virus.

Passive haemagglutination tests have been found to be of considerable value for the estimation of antibody to Gram negative bacillary somatic antigens (p. 96), and in the identification of a variety of streptococcal antigens which have been found to be capable of causing red cell sensitization. Certain antigens capable of sensitizing red cells can also occur in a non-sensitizing form, which may be demonstrated by their capacity to combine with antibody, thereby inhibiting the capacity of the latter to agglutinate appropriately sensitized cells. The non-sensitizing antigens, although possessing the serological specificity of the sensitizing antigens, may lack the groups necessary for combination with the red cell surface.

Generally, protein antigens adsorb poorly to untreated red cells, but as shown by Boyden, strong adsorption occurs if the cells are first treated with low concentrations of tannic acid. The precise nature of the change that tannic acid produces in red cells is unknown. Protein antigens may also be coupled to red cells by chemical means, e.g. through the intermediary of bis-diazotized benzidine which links the protein to a substrate, possibly another protein, on the red cell surface. Coombs has described an ingenious coupling technique in which the protein is first linked by bis-diazotized benzidine to a non-agglutinating anti-D serum, and the former adsorbed by antibody antigen union to D-positive red cells.

A number of antigens will adsorb to particles of polystyrene latex and of bentonite. So far, however, these carriers have been used mainly for the demonstration of the rheumatoid factor—found in the sera of patients with rheumatoid arthritis—which behaves as if it were an antibody to human gamma globulin.

Antiglobulin or Coombs's Technique

As previously indicated, some antibodies, because of an unknown structural property, are unable to cause agglutination in saline media. They may be demonstrated by Coombs's antiglobulin technique. This technique was first introduced for the demonstration of non-agglutinating anti-Rh antibodies in cases of human Rhesus immunization, but it has also been used to demonstrate non-agglutinating antibody to *Salmonella*, *Shigella* and *Brucella* antigens in human sera. The relative concentration of agglutinating and non-agglutinating antibodies in human sera have been found to vary independently. Some immune sera may contain only low titres of agglutinating antibody but very high titres of non-agglutinating antibody.

THE PRECIPITIN REACTION

When the antigen is in solution and provided antibody and antigen are present in suitable proportions, the antigen–antibody complex is precipitated. Like agglutination, precipitation can occur only in the presence of electrolyte.

The precipitin reaction may be applied to the detection of either antibody or antigen, but is not as extensively used in bacteriology for either of these purposes as the agglutination reaction. Although of relatively limited practical value it is, however, of great theoretical importance, and its investigation has thrown considerable light on the nature of antigen–antibody reactions in general. Its main use in the detection of bacterial antigens is in the Lancefield grouping of streptococci and in the identification of antigenic components, e.g. of *Bacillus anthracis* and *Pasteurella pestis* in the tissues of infected animals. Its only important application in the demonstration of antibody is in the Kahn and other flocculation tests used in the diagnosis of syphilis.

The precipitin reaction is more dependent than the agglutination reaction on the relative amounts of antibody and antigen present. Inhibition of precipitation may occur through the presence of excess antigen or of excess antibody. In both cases soluble non-precipitating antigen–antibody complexes are formed. Inhibition of precipitation in the presence of excess antigen is the greater difficulty and is shown by all precipitating antisera. Inhibition of precipitation because of antibody excess is shown only by certain sera, notably those prepared by immunization of horses with protein antigens.

Precipitation Techniques

Ring Test

This is the method normally used when the precipitin reaction is employed for the detection of antigen.

A small amount of antiserum is placed in the bottom of a precipitin tube (a very small test tube) and the antigen solution carefully layered on top of it. The precipitate forms as a narrow ring at the junction of the two fluids. The ring test is not significantly affected by inhibition due to antigen excess. This is because at the zone of junction the two fluids diffuse into each other and at some point in this zone the optimal relative concentrations of antibody and antigen necessary for precipitation will be present.

Simple Mixture

In this procedure the antigen solution and serum are mixed, incubated and then observed for precipitation. Since inhibition of precipitation in the region of antigen excess is frequently found, it is usual to set up a number of tubes each containing different dilutions of antigen but a constant amount of serum. The simple mixture technique is employed in the Kahn and other flocculation tests used for the diagnosis of syphilis. It may also be used for the estimation of the amount of antibody in serum by a serial dilution procedure analogous to that employed in agglutination tests; for this purpose a low concentration of antigen must be employed.

Optimal Proportions Technique

If a series of tubes are set up each containing the same amount of antibody but varying amounts of antigen it will be found that a precipitate forms first with one of the dilutions of antigen. The ratio of antigen to antibody present in this tube is known as the *constant antibody optimum ratio*. This optimum ratio is the same for all dilutions of antibody. This procedure can readily be applied to the estimation of antibody and will allow a comparison of the amount of antibody in an unknown serum with that in a standard serum. The method can also be adapted for the estimation of antigen.

With certain sera, a *constant antigen optimum ratio* can also be demonstrated. If varying amounts of antibody are mixed with a constant amount of antigen, the antigen–antibody ratio giving optimal flocculation is the same for all dilutions of antigen. This procedure is used commercially in the preliminary assay of diphtheria antitoxin. The constant antigen optimum ratio can be determined only for sera which show an inhibition of precipitation in the presence of antibody excess (p. 131).

The constant antibody and constant antigen optimum ratios are not identical. In the constant antibody titration at the optimum ratio all antibody and antigen is precipitated. In the constant antigen titration on the other hand optimum precipitation occurs in the presence of some excess antibody.

Absolute Quantitative Methods

When any of the methods so far described are used for the estimation of antibody only a relative indication of the concentration of antibody is obtained. The results therefore give no indication of the amount of antibody protein present and only permit a comparison of the antibody content of an unknown serum with that of a known serum. An absolute estimation of the antibody content of a serum in terms of antibody protein can be obtained by precipitating all the antibody with antigen and determining the amount of antibody nitrogen present in the precipitate by chemical methods. The results obtained by this method in the estimation of both antibody and antigen have a degree of accuracy unattainable with other procedures.

Gel Diffusion Techniques

These are modifications of the precipitin technique in which the reactions are allowed to occur in agar. In the Ouchterlony technique antigen and antibody

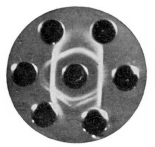

FIG. 11. OUCHTERLONY AGAR GEL DIFFUSION TECHNIQUE FOR THE PRECIPITIN REACTION

Centre well contains antiserum. Peripheral wells contain different antigen solutions. The antiserum possesses three distinct antibodies. Note reactions of identity (fusion of lines) and of non-identity (crossing of lines).

are allowed to diffuse towards one another from wells cut in an agar plate, a line of precipitate which usually takes 24 hours or longer to develop forming in the zone between the wells. If more than one antigen reacting with the antiserum is present each will give rise to a separate precipitate line and the method can therefore be used to show the mimimum number of antigens present in a solution. The Ouchterlony method may also be used to determine the relationship between the antigens present in different antigen solutions precipitating with the same antiserum or the relationship between the antibodies present in different antisera precipitating with the same antigen solution. If, in the first case, the antigens in each solution are identical they will give lines of precipitate which fuse together; this is known as the *reaction of identity*. If the antigens are different they will give lines of precipitate which intersect each other; this is known as the *reaction of non-identity*. In the reaction of *partial identity* the two precipitate lines join but one forms a 'spur' projecting beyond the other; this occurs when the antigens have a common structure but that forming the spur contains an additional antigenic determinant.

Immuno-electrophoresis

The status of electrophoresis as one of the most powerful tools of biochemical research, permitting the separation of macromolecules carrying different electrical charges is now well established. By combination with the agar gel double diffusion precipitin technique, the sensitivity and discrimination of the procedure are enormously increased allowing the differentiation of antigens both on the basis of serological specificity and electrophoretic mobility. The reaction is usually performed in thin layers of agar gel on glass slides, and is carried out in two stages. In the first, the antigen mixture is introduced into a small well cut into the agar, and electrophoresed, the different components of the mixture separating according to their electrophoretic mobility. When the electrophoretic run is complete a gutter is cut along the length of the slide, and antiserum containing antibody to the antigens present in the mixture pipetted into it. The slides are then kept at room temperature in a closed container to minimize evaporation. After about 24 hours precipitin lines develop in the agar, the centre of each coinciding with the area of maximum concentration of the corresponding antigen. This technique has proved especially valuable for the identification and differentiation of serum proteins—some 75 of which have been distinguished by its use. It has been of particular importance in the differentiation of the immunoglobulins and of the components of complement, and has been widely used for the separation of a variety of bacterial and viral antigens.

MECHANISM OF AGGLUTINATION AND PRECIPITATION

Two main theories as to the way in which agglutination and precipitation occur have been proposed but there is as yet no decisive evidence in favour of either. Marrack has proposed that each antibody molecule forms a bridge between two antigen molecules by combining with both at the same time. Since antigen being multivalent can combine with a number of antibody molecules this mechanism would permit the building up of a multimolecular lattice of antibody and antigen. This theory, which is known as the *lattice* hypothesis, requires that antibody should be at least divalent.

The second theory postulates that precipitation and agglutination are both non-specific reactions and are to be explained as phenomena of colloid chemistry. It is proposed that the reactions occur in two stages, the first stage being the specific combination of antibody and antigen. The theory postulates that as a result of this combination the lyophilic groups on the surface of the antigen are masked by antibody, and that in consequence the antigen–antibody complex behaves like a hydrophobic colloid which can be flocculated if its surface potential is reduced. Evidence in support of this theory is provided by the fact that electrolyte, e.g. sodium chloride, is capable of lowering the surface potential of bacteria and is found to be essential for both agglutination and precipitation reactions.

It is possible that both of these mechanisms might operate. In this case the first stage in precipitation or agglutination might be the formation of small aggregates by the lattice mechanism. The formation of larger aggregates from these might then be due to the second mechanism described.

COMPLEMENT AND ITS ACTION

The term complement is applied to a group or complex of substances occurring in the serum of man and other animals, which can combine with antigen–antibody complexes, and which also mediate the lysis of red blood cells and other cells sensitized by antibody. Complement does not combine with either antibody or antigen alone, but only with the complex formed by their combination. Combination of complement with antibody–antigen complexes is known as *complement fixation* or *complement deviation*. When the antigen component of the complex is present on an intact cell, the adsorbed complement may initiate or lead to damage to the cell surface. The model which has been studied most is that of the sensitized red cell. In this case, complement adsorption, by an enzymic reaction, leads to the production of holes in the membrane of the cell, as a result of which the cell undergoes haemolysis—usually referred to as *immune haemolysis*. With bacteria susceptible to its action, complement adsorption results in killing and often in lysis of the cell.

Composition of Complement

Although some of the individual components of complement are heat-stable, complement as a whole is heat-labile, the complement activity of fresh serum being destroyed by exposure to a temperature of 56° C for half an hour. Like antibody, complement activity is recoverable in the globulin fraction of the serum. The individual components which have been identified immuno-electrophoretically have however the mobility of β globulins. Moreover, complement differs sharply from antibody in that its concentration is not increased by immunization. All adults of the same species show much the same complement levels.

For many years, four distinct complement components have been distinguished on the basis of inactivation by various reagents—$C'1$, $C'2$, $C'3$ and $C'4$.

$C'1$, the first component to combine with sensitized cells, constitutes the main bulk of complement adsorbed to antigen–antibody complexes. It is heat-labile, being destroyed when exposed to 56° C for 30 minutes, and is found in the euglobulin fraction of the serum, i.e. the fraction precipitated by removal of electrolyte. C'1 is the precursor of an esterase which is activated on combination with antigen–antibody complexes. Its esterase activity may be demonstrated in vitro by its action on synthetic substrates, viz. p-toluenesulphonyl-L-arginine methyl ester for guinea-pig C', and N-acetyl-L-tyrosine ethyl ester for human complement. C'1 can be dissociated by EDTA into three components: C'1q—the component combining directly with the antigen–antibody complex, C'1r and C'1s, which has been identified as the proesterase. In the presence of calcium ions the three components are associated to form the C'1 macromolecule.

C'2 is a heat-labile component found in the pseudoglobulin fraction of serum—occurring in the soluble fraction after dialysis against water.

C'3 was originally defined as a heat-stable component found mainly in the euglobulin fraction of the serum. It was originally distinguished from other complement components by its capacity to combine with yeast cell walls (zymosan), and by its susceptibility to cobra venom. Recent work has however identified at least six subcomponents, separable by column chromatography, in the classical C'3 complex. These have been designated by Müller–Eberhard, following their apparent order of fixation, as C'3, C'5, C'6, C'7, C'8 and C'9. This nomenclature will be followed here.

C'4 is found mainly in the pseudoglobulin fraction of serum. It is heat-stable and distinguished from other complement components by its susceptibility to inactivation by ammonia.

Immune haemolysis

Immune haemolysis is of practical importance for the following reasons: (a) As a convenient model for the study of the mechanism of complement action. (b) It provides the simplest system for the assay of complement and complement components. (c) It is of very great value as an indicator system in complement fixation reactions. To demonstrate immune haemolysis three reagents are required:

1. Red cells. These are normally obtained from the sheep.

2. Antibody to sheep red cells. This is usually prepared in the laboratory by immunization of rabbits. It is sometimes referred to as *immune body* and sometimes as *haemolysin*. The latter designation is unfortunate since it incorrectly represents the role of the antibody in the production of lysis. The haemolytic serum must be heated to 56° C for half an hour to destroy any complement present.

3. Complement. The normal source of complement for laboratory tests is fresh guinea-pig serum which has a balanced content of all the complement components. Complement is a highly labile reagent, and its activity disappears rapidly on storage. This loss may be minimized by preservation in the frozen state, or better still, by lyophilization. A special preserving solution containing sodium azide and a high concentration of salt will permit storage at 0 to 4° C for considerable periods.

Using these reagents the basic features of complement action can be readily demonstrated:

1. Both complement and antibody are necessary for lysis.

2. Cells which have been sensitized by antibody absorb complement.

3. Cells which have not been sensitized by antibody do not absorb complement.

The union of antibody with cells occurs rapidly even at temperatures as low as $0°$ C. The union is a firm one—the cells retaining their adsorbed antibody even when repeatedly washed in saline. Union of complement with sensitized cells is much less rapid. Although it also occurs at a low temperature no lysis is apparent below $15°$ C; lysis is maximal at $37°$ C. Both the fixation of complement and complement lysis will occur only in the presence of low concentrations of calcium and magnesium ions.

The components of complement are fixed to the sensitized cell in the order $C'1, 4, 2, 3$, the fixation of each component being dependent on the fixation of the component immediately prior to it in the reaction sequence. Fixation can, by appropriate manipulation of the environmental conditions, be blocked at each stage, to yield intermediate complexes. These complexes are of considerable value in research on the mechanism of fixation, and are also employed for the quantitative estimation of the next component in the series. Complexes are indicated by a formula comprising the letters SA denoting an antigen site combined with antibody, followed by the symbols of the particular complement components adsorbed.

Adsorption of $C'1$ occurs only in the presence of calcium ions. It results in the activation of $C'1s$ proesterase to $C'1$ esterase or $C'1a$, to give the complex $SAC'1a$. Normal serum contains an inhibitor of $C'1$ esterase; this has no action, however, on the esterase activity of fixed $C'1a$. Esterase activity of $C'1a$ appears to be necessary for the coupling of $C'4$—the next component to be adsorbed—to $C'2$. As a result of this enzymatic coupling, an inactive fragment $C'2i$ is released, the fragment which binds to the complex being designated $C'2a$. This reaction can only occur in the presence of magnesium ions. The resulting complex $SAC'1a$, 4, $2a$ is unstable and spontaneously undergoes degradation to $SAC'1a$, 4. Once coupling of $C'4$ and $C'2$ has occurred, $C'1a$ is expendable, and can be eluted from the cell without affecting subsequent haemolysis.

The final stages in the reaction sequence are not fully understood. Two phases appear however to be distinguishable. In the first phase, as shown by Müller–Eberhard for human complement, the unstable intermediate $SAC'1a$, 4, $2a$ is converted into a stable complex by fixation of the subcomponents $C'3$, $C'5$, $C'6$ and $C'7$. In the second phase fixation of $C'8$ and $C'9$ leads to the membrane lesion which is the immediate cause of lysis.

Red cells can be sensitized to complement lysis both by antibody to antigens which occur as components of the red cell surface, and by antibodies to antigens, for example, bacterial polysaccharides which have been passively adsorbed onto the red cell surface (p. 129). Certain red cells can also be non-specifically sensitized to lysis by treatment with low concentrations of tannic acid or polyethylene glycol. These substances presumably act by permitting the non-specific adsorption of gamma globulin.

For the sensitization of sheep red cells to complement lysis, it has been shown by Humphrey that 19S antibody is about 1000 times more efficient on a molecular basis than 7S antibody. This finding lends support to the proposal, originally made by Weinrach and Talmage, that 7S antibodies could only sensitize to lysis if two antibody molecules were combined with adjacent antigenic sites on the cell surface. Under these circumstances evidence presented by Ishizaka and Campbell suggests that the adjacent gamma globulin molecules interact to produce some mutual denaturation. In this case, the greater sensitizing efficiency of 19S antibodies may be due to the ability of the 19S molecule to combine by itself with a number of adjacent sites. It is conceivable that this might lead to some internal denaturation of the molecule.

There is now unequivocal evidence that the specific event leading to the lysis of the cell is the production of holes in the cell membrane, which permits the haemoglobin to escape. These holes have been clearly seen in electron micrographs. The nature of the cell substrate disintegrating to produce the hole is unknown. It has been suggested that the holes are produced by a lysolecithin-like substance, released or produced by the adsorbed complement complex. There is, however, no decisive evidence in favour of this view.

Bactericidal Effects of Complement

Many Gram negative bacteria are killed and lysed by complement in the presence of specific antibody. The cholera vibrio is particularly susceptible, as first noted by Pfeiffer. Gram positive bacteria, on the other hand, are highly resistant. The complement components involved in immune bacteriolysis appear to be identical with those involved in immune haemolysis. That the site of complement reaction is the cytoplasmic membrane is shown by the fact that spheroplasts derived from Gram negative bacilli are lysed, in contrast to protoplasts of Gram positive organisms which are insusceptible to complement. In the intact cell, complement damage to the cell membrane follows sensitization of the cell by antibody to cell wall antigen. In this respect the situation is analogous to that of red cells sensitized with passively adsorbed antigen. In general, smooth organisms (p. 305) are less susceptible to lysis than are rough organisms and cells with surface antigens external to the O antigen, e.g. the *Salm. typhi* Vi antigen, are less susceptible to lysis than non-Vi forms. These findings suggest that the closer the antigen site is to the cell membrane the more likely is lysis to follow complement adsorption.

There is considerable evidence that the bacteriolytic effect of complement requires the activity of lysozyme, present with complement in fresh mammalian sera. It might therefore be expected to play an important part in complement lysis under in vivo conditions. Without lysozyme, complement can only have a bacteriostatic or a bactericidal effect. The precise role of lysozyme in complement lysis is not clear but presumably involves action on the mucopeptide layer of the cell wall (p. 5).

Conglutination

Since the turn of the century it has been known that the fresh, unheated serum of certain animals, notably the horse, can render red cells agglutinable by normal bovine serum. This agglutination is due to the combination of a substance—known as *conglutinin*—in bovine serum, with horse complement components adsorbed to the red cells sensitized by natural antibody present in the bovine serum. From the available evidence there can be little doubt that the agglutinable complex is SAC'1a, 4, 2a, 3. Conglutinin almost certainly combines with the C'3 component, but only when the latter is fixed on sensitized cells. Horse serum is relatively deficient in the later components, and therefore has slight haemolytic potency. Because of this, it is of particular value for the production of the intermediate complex required for conglutination. Conglutinin is a euglobulin of molecular weight 750,000, and the electrophoretic mobility of a β globulin.

Bovine conglutinin also combines with yeast cell walls, or zymosan, the receptor in which appears to be a mucoprotein. Combination of conglutinin both with zymosan and C'3 requires the presence of calcium ions; these appear to constitute the bond between conglutinin and the conglutinable complex. It is presumed, though not definitely established, that the receptors for conglutinin in zymosan and in C'3 are identical.

Like complement lysis, the conglutination reaction can be used as an indicator reaction in complement fixation tests—the fixation of complement by an antigen–antibody complex being shown by demonstrating its non-availability for the sensitization of red cells to conglutination.

Immunoconglutinin

Conglutinin is not an antibody, and its concentration in serum does not increase as a result of immunization. An antibody to adsorbed complement with somewhat similar reactivity to conglutinin can, however, be produced by immunization. This may be achieved in two ways: (1) By heterostimulation. The animal is injected with an antigen–antibody complex to which a heterologous complement has been adsorbed. (2) By autostimulation. Following injection of large amounts of bacterial vaccine the animal produces antibody to its own complement which has adsorbed to the bacterial antigen. Autostimulation may also occur as a result of natural bacterial infection. Heteroconglutinin is a 7S antibody reacting with fixed C'3. Autoconglutinin is predominantly a 19S antibody which reacts also with the fixed C'3 component. The two antibodies differ from one another in specificity, and since they do not react with zymosan, differ too, in specificity from bovine conglutinin. Unlike conglutinin, their combination with C'3 is not mediated through calcium ions.

Immune Adherence

Complement also plays an important part in the phenomenon of immune adherence, in which bacteria or other particulate antigens sensitized by antibody are found to adhere to the red cells of primates, or to the platelets of a variety of animal species. The phenomenon can be used as a basis for the demonstration of either antibody or antigen, and appears to possess a high

degree of sensitivity. Immune adherence requires the adsorption of the complement components $C'1, 4, 2, 3$; the further components of the $C'3$ complex are
not required. The capacity of human red cells to participate in immune adherence is destroyed by proteolytic enzymes. It is possible that the immune
adherence phenomenon might be a valid model for the initial stages of contact
between bacteria and leucocytes or macrophages in phagocytosis.

PHAGOCYTOSIS

Phagocytosis is the ingestion of bacteria or other particles by phagocytic cells.
The latter, which are of fundamental importance in the defence of the body
against infection, are of two types: (1) Large phagocytic cells—the macrophages and monocytes—of the reticulo-endothelial system. (2) The polymorphonuclear leucocytes of the peripheral blood. The role of phagocytosis in the
defence of the body and the fate of the ingested cells is considered in more
detail on page 147. Here we will be concerned only with the participation of
antibody and/or complement in the process.

The phagocytosis of bacteria by polymorphonuclear leucocytes can sometimes be seen in films from pus and is particularly striking in urethral pus
obtained from cases of gonorrhoea. It may be demonstrated readily in vitro
using as a source of leucocytes the top or buffy layer obtained on centrifuging
citrated or heparinized blood. The stages in phagocytosis can be observed
microscopically in films stained with Leishman's or other blood stain. In these
the phagocytosed bacteria are seen in the cytoplasm of the leucocytes where they
frequently show marked degenerative changes with loss of their normal staining
properties.

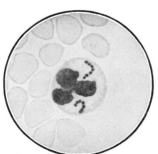

FIG. 12. PHAGOCYTOSIS OF
STREPTOCOCCI BY POLYMOR-
PHONUCLEAR LEUCOCYTES

It is convenient to consider first phagocytosis as it occurs in free suspension
in a fluid environment. For the phagocytosis of avirulent bacteria, and this
applies also to inert particles, antibody is not required. In general, however,
antibody is essential for the phagocytosis of virulent bacteria. The role of antibody can be traced clearly to an effect on the bacteria, and not to an effect
on the phagocyte. As a result of the adsorption of antibody to the bacteria, the

latter are rendered more palatable to the phagocytes. This process is known as *opsonization*. Both IgM and IgG antibodies appear to be effective. Bacteria can also be opsonized by normal serum but to very much less extent than by immune serum. It seems likely that the capacity of antibody to sensitize to phagocytosis is due to neutralization of the normal negative charge of the bacterial surface, the bacteria having a less repulsive effect on the negatively charged phagocytes.

Even though the precise role of complement needs clarification, there seems to be little doubt that its adsorption greatly increases the efficiency of opsonization. This is particularly noticeable in opsonization by normal serum, the opsonizing capacity of which is by itself very low, due to its low antibody content. The potentiating effect of complement on phagocytosis is presumed to be a non-specific result of the adsorption of further protein to the bacterial surface.

Although the opsonic effect of antibody is exercised solely on the bacteria, there is some evidence that high concentrations of serum or plasma may increase the phagocytic efficiency of the white cell. This may be due to neutralization of toxic substances, viz. end products of leucocyte metabolism, to colloid osmotic effects, or to some, as yet undetermined factor. The salt concentration of the environment has an appreciable effect on phagocytosis; divalent cations, e.g. calcium, seem to be necessary, and the process appears to occur most efficiently in media of low tonicity.

The capacity of antibody to render bacteria susceptible to phagocytosis may be used as the basis of a method for the estimation of antibody concentration. Tests of this type are known as opsonic tests and were at one time used extensively as an index of immunity. Since in most cases, however, they measure antibodies which are more readily demonstrable by the simpler agglutination technique opsonic tests are no longer used—except, rarely, in the case of *Brucella* infection, as standard serological procedures. In brucellosis, their value is due to the fact that the serum of the patient may contain a high concentration of antibody capable of sensitizing brucellae to phagocytosis in the absence of demonstrable agglutinating antibody.

It has been shown by Wood that, although little phagocytosis occurs in the absence of serum or plasma when bacteria are incubated with leucocytes in a fluid medium, the degree of phagocytosis is greatly increased if the mixture is made on a rough surface such as paper or cloth. In these circumstances, the leucocytes can apparently 'pin' the bacteria against surface irregularities and can then ingest them more readily. This type of phagocytosis is known as *surface phagocytosis*. It is believed to be an important mechanism in the tissues where there are many irregularities against which bacteria may be pinned by leucocytes.

NEUTRALIZATION

When an antigen has a demonstrable in vivo or in vitro effect, this effect can often be neutralized by antibody. Tests in which this is demonstrated are known as neutralization tests.

Toxin Neutralization

Bacterial exotoxins (p. 78) are highly antigenic and their activity may be completely neutralized by appropriate concentrations of antibody. Antibody to bacterial exotoxins is usually referred to without qualifications as *antitoxin*. Bacterial endotoxins, at least of the type found amongst the enterobacteriaceae, are poorly if at all antigenic and their toxicity is incompletely neutralized by antibody (p. 78). Such antibody, whose specificity is directed against the polysaccharide component of the somatic antigen complex, is not usually referred to as antitoxin.

The neutralizing capacity of an antitoxin can be assayed by neutralization tests in which mixtures of toxin and antitoxin are injected into susceptible animals. The most widely used indicator of toxin activity in such tests is the lethal effect of the toxin on the animal, the concentration of an antitoxin being estimated by determining its capacity to neutralize this lethal effect. With toxins, such as the diphtheria toxin, which produce reactions in the skin, these can be used as indicators of toxin activity. This phenomenon is the basis of the Schick test used for the demonstration of immunity against diphtheria (p. 287), and can also be applied to the assay of diphtheria antitoxin, using the guinea-pig as test animal.

If a toxin has a demonstrable in vitro effect, this effect is neutralized by antitoxin. Thus antitoxins to haemolytic toxins neutralize the haemolytic action of the toxin. This neutralization can be made the basis of an in vitro method of assaying the antitoxin. The only procedure of this type of clinical importance is the estimation of the antibody to streptolysin O (antistreptolysin O). This antibody is significantly increased in patients with acute streptococcal infection and in those suffering from acute rheumatism (Chapter 14).

The specific neutralization of toxin by antitoxin is utilized in the Nagler reaction used for the identification of *Clostridium perfringens*. The test depends on the capacity of antitoxin to neutralize the lecithinase activity of *Cl. perfringens* and is usually carried out in plate cultures (Chapter 29).

Toxin is not destroyed by combination with antitoxin. By certain procedures, for example by treatment with dilute acids, by freezing and thawing or even by simple dilution, toxin may be dissociated from combination with antitoxin; the liberated toxin is fully active. Toxin antitoxin mixtures are therefore quite unsuitable as immunizing agents.

Neutralization of Enzyme Activity

Antibodies to enzymes can inhibit the enzymic activity of the enzyme. As in the case of toxins the enzyme may be dissociated from the enzyme-antibody complex in a fully active form. The mechanism of neutralization is not fully understood, but may be due either to neutralization of the active group of the enzyme by the antibody, or by combination of antibody with determinants on the enzyme distinct from the active group. Such combination may interfere with the effective binding of the enzyme to its substrate by a steric effect, or by inducing a conformational change in the surface of the enzyme. In some cases, however, the activity of an enzyme may increase by combination with antibody; this appears to occur particularly when the enzyme combines with low molecular weight substrates. An interesting example of such enhancement was the demonstration by Pollock that the activity of a pencillinase, produced by *Bacillus licheniformis*, against benzyl penicillin and cephalosporin C was inhibited by antibody to the enzyme, but that its activity against methicillin was enhanced. These findings lend support to the view that the primary effect of antibody is the production of conformational changes in the enzyme surface. These changes may diminish the affinity of the enzyme for one substrate while increasing its affinity for others.

CHAPTER 8

IMMUNITY

By immunity we mean the resistance which the animal body possesses against micro-organisms and their products. The mechanisms responsible for this resistance are the subject matter of the science of immunology. Immunity is of two main types—*innate* or *basic*, and *acquired*. Innate immunity is that which the individual possesses by virtue of his constitutional and genetic make-up. Acquired immunity is the immunity which he acquires during the course of his life and which develops as a result of contact with micro-organisms or their products.

INNATE OR BASIC IMMUNITY

In general, individuals of the same species show a uniform pattern of genetically determined susceptibility to different bacterial species. Considerable differences exist however in the innate susceptibility of different animal species to many bacteria. Thus man is immune to many infections of animals, and animals are immune under natural conditions to most human infections. A particularly interesting example of such a difference in species susceptibility is shown in the contrasting responses of mice and men to two pathogenic micro-organisms of very similar properties—*Salm. typhi* and *Salm. typhimurium*. In man, *Salm. typhi* produces a serious invasive disease whereas *Salm. typhimurium* produces a relatively mild, localized infection of the gastro-intestinal tract (Chapter 20). In mice the position is reversed, *Salm. typhimurium* producing invasive disease, and *Salm. typhi* being non-pathogenic under natural conditions of infection by the alimentary route. The reasons for these differences are not known. Genetically determined differences in susceptibility also occur within individual species. Perhaps the most dramatic example of such intraspecies differences is the high resistance of Algerian sheep, as compared with European sheep, to anthrax. In man similar genetically determined differences in susceptibility have, however, been more difficult to demonstrate. It has been thought, for example, that Africans and American Indians are intrinsically much more susceptible to tuberculosis than Caucasians. In comparing different social and racial groups, however, it is extremely difficult to distinguish genetic from social and environmental factors. More conclusive evidence of genetically determined differences in susceptibility to tuberculosis has been obtained from a study of the incidence of the disease in homozygotic and heterozygotic twins. Thus if one twin develops tuberculosis, the chance that the second twin, too, will develop tuberculosis is much higher if the twins are homozygotic than if they are heterozygotic.

Surface Defences

In Chapter 5 we saw that, in most cases, in order to produce disease, bacteria must gain access to the tissues. They are prevented from doing so by the surface defences of the body. The chief of these is the integrity of the investing layers of epithelium—skin and mucous membrane.

The skin, as long as it is intact, is an almost complete barrier against bacterial invasion. The mucous membranes are more permeable than the skin, and some bacteria appear to be able to penetrate them fairly readily; their integrity is nevertheless of considerable importance in preventing invasion.

Next we have the various secretions and excretions which bathe the skin and mucous membranes—sweat, tears, mucus, saliva, gastric and intestinal juices and urine. These act mechanically by washing off bacteria which have adhered to the surface and, in the case of some of the mucous membranes, are aided by the action of cilia which create currents directing bacteria away from deeper structures. In addition they contain dissolved bactericidal substances, the most widely distributed of which is probably lysozyme, an enzyme which acts on bacteria by hydrolysing glycosidic linkages in the cell wall mucopeptides (p. 5). The skin secretions—sebum and sweat—contain saturated and unsaturated fatty acids, substances which have distinct microbicidal effects and are responsible for the low pH of the skin. The hydrochloric acid of the gastric fluid has considerable sterilizing effect and is responsible for the virtual absence of bacteria from the stomach and duodenum.

The commensal organisms, particularly those of the mucous membranes, appear to play an indirect role in the defence of the body. Some of them are known to produce substances inhibitory to other organisms. Thus some of the mouth streptococci produce hydrogen peroxide which is inhibitory to many species. Some of the coliform bacteria produce *colicines*; these are substances which will kill certain other coliform bacteria and shigellae. The lactobacilli of the vagina produce considerable amounts of lactic acid from the glycogen of the vaginal epithelium; the resultant acidity confers on the vagina virtually complete immunity from pyogenic infection. The propionibacteria of the skin produce propionic acid, a substance which is presumably of some importance in maintaining the acid reaction of the skin secretions. It is also possible that the organisms of the normal flora may tend to exclude pathogens by competing with them for nutrient material.

Tissue Defences

Despite the barriers outlined above, invasion does occur, probably quite commonly, but every invasion does not lead to an infection. In the tissues the multiplication of the invading bacteria is opposed by the host's defensive mechanisms. These fall into two categories: humoral and cellular.

Humoral Defences

A variety of substances possessing considerable antibacterial activity have been demonstrated in the tissue fluids, the most important being antibodies and complement. Although the capacity to produce antibodies is an innate property of the animal body, their actual production is a manifestation of acquired immunity and will be considered under that heading. As previously indicated, complement has an enhancing effect on phagocytosis (p. 140) and is in addition capable of killing and sometimes of lysing Gram negative bacteria which have been sensitized by antibody. That the bactericidal effect of the complement system is of importance in resistance to infection is supported by a number of observations: (1) In infections of experimental animals with Gram negative bacteria, a correlation appears to exist between resistance to the bactericidal action of complement demonstrable in vitro, and virulence. (2) Strains of E. coli associated with human infections are claimed to be invariably complement resistant. This is presumably due to heat-labile surface antigens which prevent complement from reaching close enough to its normal target, the cytoplasmic membrane, to cause lethal damage to the cell. The Vi antigen of the typhoid bacillus possibly has a similar effect. (3) There is some evidence of an increased susceptibility to Gram negative infection in guinea-pigs congenitally deficient in the $C'3$ component of complement. If complement is important in defence it might be expected that agencies which inactivate it or interfere with its action would thereby diminish resistance. Thus, it has been suggested that the susceptibility of the kidney to coliform infections may be due to inactivation of $C'4$ by ammonia released from amino acids by renal deaminases.

Properdin

This is a euglobulin first described by Pillemer which can adsorb to yeast cell walls (zymosan), the zymosan properdin complex being capable of fixing the $C'3$ component of complement. In the presence of complement and magnesium ions, properdin has been claimed to have a non-specific bactericidal effect, particularly on Gram negative bacilli, and to be capable of neutralizing the infectivity of certain viruses. Recent evidence suggests, however, that the bactericidal and virus neutralizing properties of normal serum are not due to properdin, but to low titred and relatively non-specific natural antibodies acting in conjunction with complement. These can be removed by absorption without affecting serum properdin levels.

β-Lysin

This is a heat-stable substance present in normal serum, which possesses considerable bactericidal activity for various Gram positive bacilli. Recent work has shown, however, that β-lysin does not exist free in plasma, but is liberated from platelets during clotting. It must be regarded as doubtful therefore, whether it plays any significant role in normal tissue defence.

Lysozyme

This enzyme is found in many body secretions, in various tissue fluids and in phagocytic cells (p. 147). Under in vitro conditions lysozyme has been found to be particularly active against members of the *Bacillus* genus. Recent evidence, however, appears to indicate an important role for lysozyme, in co-operation with complement, in the lysis of sensitized Gram negative bacteria (p. 137).

Tissue fluids also contain cellular breakdown products with significant antibacterial action, e.g. certain basic peptides and haematin compounds derived from disintegrated red cells. Lactic acid produced by glycolytic cellular metabolism has marked bactericidal properties on many bacteria. It is unlikely that the concentrations of lactic acid found normally in the tissues play a significant part in defence but the higher concentrations found in areas of inflammation probably do.

Cellular Defences

Phagocytosis is probably the single most important component in the defence of the body against invading bacteria. Two cell types are involved—the macrophages and the polymorphonuclear leucocytes (p. 139). The former are of two varieties—free and fixed. Free macrophages are present in the tissues, where they are known as tissue histiocytes, and occasionally in the blood, where they are known as monocytes. The fixed macrophages comprise the endothelial cells lining the blood sinusoids of the liver and spleen and the lymph sinusoids of lymphoid tissue, the reticular cells of lymphoid tissues and the microglia of the brain. The polymorphonuclears and tissue macrophages can be readily mobilized at the site of an invasion. They are therefore the cells responsible for the primary defence of the tissues. The fixed macrophages of the reticulo-endothelial system constitute on the other hand a clearing mechanism for organisms which have gained access to the blood and lymph.

As we have seen, the phagocytosis of bacteria under in vitro conditions in a fluid environment requires prior sensitization with antibody. The combination of antibody with the bacteria is specific but its role in opsonization is non-specific and probably principally that of diminishing the negative charge on the bacterial surface. In support of this view is the finding that negatively charged proteins such as albumen have an inhibitory effect on phagocytosis. Complement has an enhancing effect on phagocytosis, especially in the presence of the low titred natural antibodies of normal serum.

Opsonization by antibody is also essential for the efficient removal of bacteria from the blood by the fixed macrophages of the reticulo-endothelial system. This is clearly shown in the results of experimental infections in animals. Virulent bacteria, e.g. pneumococci, are rapidly cleared from the blood of immune animals but persist and in fact multiply when injected into the blood of non-immune animals. The importance of complement in this process is also shown by the reduced efficiency of the clearing mechanism in animals from whose circulation complement has been removed by the injection of antigen–antibody aggregates.

As previously indicated (p. 140) appreciable phagocytosis of virulent organisms can occur in the absence of antibody by the method known as *surface phagocytosis*. In the tissues this mechanism might be expected to be of value in the very early stages of invasion when there is still relatively little exudation of fluid. As a contribution to the total defence of the body, however, it must be of secondary importance compared with the phagocytosis of opsonized bacteria. That this is the case is shown particularly by the high susceptibility of hypogammaglobulinaemic patients to bacterial infections.

The fundamental importance of phagocytosis both by free and fixed phagocytes in immunity is shown by a number of observations.

1. There is a very great increase in susceptibility to infection with pyogenic organisms in individuals suffering from agranulocytosis.

2. Resistance to infection is lowered by procedures, for example, the administration of cortisone or the local injection of adrenaline, which interfere with migration of phagocytes to the site of invasion.

3. Individuals suffering from congenital disorders characterized by abnormal forms of neutrophil granulation are particularly susceptible to infection.

The progress of phagocytosis and the fate of the ingested bacteria have been most studied in relation to polymorphonuclear leucocytes. Ingestion by polymorphonuclears has been shown to occur, not as a result of passage of the bacteria through the cell membrane, but by an invagination of the cell membrane around the bacteria. As a result of this process the bacteria are eventually enclosed in a cytoplasmic vacuole formed from the membrane. The process is strictly analogous to pinocytosis by which tissue cells in general take in fluid material.

Phagocytosis is triggered by initial contact of the bacterium with the cell surface and requires the expenditure of energy by the cell. This energy is obtained in the case of the polymorphonuclear leucocytes and free tissue macrophages by glycolysis, which leads to the liberation of lactic acid in the environment of the phagocytic cell. The alveolar macrophages of the lung appear to be unusual in deriving their energy from aerobic oxidation. Phagocytosis by polymorphonuclear leucocytes occurs efficiently over the pH range 6 to 8, is maximal under slightly hypotonic conditions and appears to require the presence of divalent cations.

Following ingestion, the granules of the phagocytic cell, which appear to be strictly analogous to the lysosomes of tissue cells, disappear. The disappearance of the granules is due to the discharge of their contents into the phagocytic vacuole. This appears to occur as a result of fusion of the granule membrane with the membrane of the vacuole.

In many cases bacteria which have been ingested by leucocytes are rapidly killed. The precise way in which bacteria are killed by phagocytes is not at the moment clear. It can be safely presumed, however, that death is due to the action of substances released from the granules into the phagocytic vacuole. The most important of these substances are lactic acid, produced as a result of cellular glycolysis, lysozyme and *phagocytin*—a potent bactericidal substance which under in vitro conditions has a lethal effect in concentrations of the order of 1μg per ml, and which is active against a wide range of bacteria. Its mode of action is unknown. Phagocytin has not so far been purified but is believed to be a basic protein.

Other antibacterial substances that have been isolated from white cells are hydrogen peroxide and *leukin*—a protamine-like protein derived from the nuclear fraction of leucocytes, and which has been shown to be highly active against certain Gram positive bacteria. Whether these compounds gain access to bacteria within the phagocytic vacuoles is unknown, and their contribution to intracellular death cannot therefore be adequately assessed.

Most phagocytosed bacteria appear to be killed within a short period after ingestion, though some species, e.g. gonococci, can survive for a considerable time after ingestion. As a final stage in their disposal the phagocytosed bacteria are digested. Changes in staining reactions may be seen from 30 to 60 minutes after ingestion, but complete digestion requires a period of several hours. Digestion presumably occurs as a result of the action of the proteases and other hydrolytic enzymes liberated from the granules of the phagocyte.

In general, phagocytosis follows a similar pattern for both mononuclear phagocytes and polymorphonuclear leucocytes. The mechanism by which bacteria are killed within the macrophage is, however, much less clear. So far, the only substances with distinct antibacterial properties to be isolated from macrophages are lactic acid and lysozyme. These are, however, present in relatively low concentrations, except in the alveolar macrophages of the lung which are reported to have a high lysozyme content. Macrophages also contain hydrolytic enzymes but in considerably less variety than do granulocytes. A noticeable difference is the absence of alkaline phosphatase and peroxidase. The killing of bacteria by macrophages is a relatively slow process, and the organisms can be observed to persist intracellularly in a morphologically unchanged state for long periods. Certain organisms—tubercle bacilli, brucellae, *Listeria monocytogenes* and *Salm. typhi*—have considerable capacity not only to evoke inflammatory reactions in which macrophages are the predominant cells, but also to multiply within the macrophage.

The Inflammatory Reaction

When bacteria gain access to the tissues they trigger a series of events which result in the mobilization of the tissue defences. The changes occurring are known collectively as the inflammatory reaction. Although it has been studied in great detail, the precise mechanism of the inflammatory response is still imperfectly understood. In general we may distinguish two types of response, *acute* and *chronic*. The acute response is rapid in onset and characterized by the accumulation of large numbers of polymorphonuclear leucocytes. If sufficiently intense, it results in the accumulation of pus which is a mixture of fluid exudate, dead bacteria and living and dead leucocytes. The typical acute inflammatory reaction leading to the production of pus is elicited only by certain bacteria, notably the cocci and the coliform bacteria, which, as a result, are known as *pyogenic* organisms.

In contrast to the acute reaction, the chronic inflammatory reaction is of slow development and is characterized by the accumulation of lymphocytes and macrophages. It is normally preceded by a transient phase of polymorphonuclear accumulation. Organisms which characteristically produce chronic inflammatory reactions are the tubercle bacillus, *Tr. pallidum*, *Salm. typhi* and the brucellae. Why some bacteria stimulate acute inflammatory reaction, and others stimulate a chronic inflammatory reaction is not yet known. It is possibly related to the severity of the local damage produced by the bacteria. An acute inflammatory reaction may be produced if the damage inflicted is severe, and a chronic inflammatory reaction when the damage is less severe.

In the acute inflammatory reaction there is a marked increase in vascular permeability which allows the passage of plasma, bearing antibodies and complement, and of polymorphonuclear leucocytes into the tissues. Recent evidence indicates that the increase in vascular permeability occurs in two phases. In the first there is an increased permeability of the small venules, allowing the passage into the tissues of antibody and complement. This phase by itself is probably able to control many bacterial invasions. The second phase consists mainly of a migration of the polymorphonuclear leucocytes. This migration appears to occur through the walls of the capillaries, but whether the cells pass through or between the endothelial cells of the capillaries, has not been determined. The first observable event in migration is an adherence of the cells to the internal surface of the capillary wall. This adherence occurs on the side of the capillary nearest to the invading bacteria and is presumed to be the result of damage to the wall by bacterial products. The identity of these products and the precise mechanism by which they inflict damage is unknown.

Once outside the blood vessels, the leucocytes lose their random motion and move in a straight line towards the invading particle. This direct movement is known as *chemotaxis*, and is generally believed to be initiated by chemotactic substances produced at the invasion site. The identity of these chemotactic substances is unknown. There are three main possibilities: (1) That they are produced by the bacteria themselves, the leucocytes moving along a concentration gradient towards the bacterial source. (2) That they are liberated from leucocytes that have made contact with, or that have been damaged by, bacteria. (3) That they are produced from some normal component of the tissue fluid by an antigen–antibody reaction occurring as a result of invasion. Evidence for such a mechanism has been obtained by Boyden, who identified a heat-labile component in normal serum and plasma which is activated to form a heat-stable chemotactic substance by antigen–antibody complexes.

There is reason to believe that the outpouring of fluid, associated particularly with the early stages of inflammation, serves to open up the lymphatic channels, thereby facilitating the spread of bacteria which have not been disposed of in the initial phases of the reaction, to the local lymphatic glands. Here they stimulate an inflammatory response characterized particularly by the accumulation of polymorphonuclear leucocytes in the hilar sinuses at the outlets of the glands. This accumulation has been likened by Wood to 'a log jam at the outlet of a millpond', and serves to prevent the outflow of bacteria from the gland, thus giving the phagocytic cells of the latter a better opportunity for phagocytosis. Before this polymorphonuclear accumulation occurs the lymph gland is a relatively inefficient filter, bacteria readily passing through it to gain entry to the blood stream via the thoracic duct.

In addition to stimulating a local accumulation of leucocytes at the site of invasion, infection with pyogenic bacteria results in an increase in the number of leucocytes present in the circulating blood. This phenomenon is known as *leucocytosis* and is the result of an increased output of leucocytes by the haemo-poietic tissues. One of the most readily apparent clinical concomitants of pyogenic infection is fever, the production of which is usually regarded as a defensive mechanism. The mechanism by which infection produces fever has not been fully explained but in certain cases, possibly in all, it appears to be due to the production of pyogenic substances from leucocytes as a result of the action of the invading organisms.

In the past most attention has been directed to the more biological aspects of the inflammatory reaction considered above, but it is now realized that inflammation is associated with biochemical changes in the tissues which also play an important part in defence. The leucocytes which migrate to the inflamed area have a predominantly glycolytic metabolism; this leads to the accumulation of lactic acid, which has a direct bactericidal effect, at the site of infection. Thrombokinase liberated from damaged tissue precipitates the deposition of a fibrin barrier around the inflamed focus. This barrier helps to restrict spread of the infecting organisms through the tissues, but is permeable to antibodies and to leucocytes; the latter are in fact believed to be capable of creeping by amoeboid motion along the fibrin strands. Inflamed areas show an increased carbon dioxide and diminished oxygen tension. The increased carbon dioxide tension appears to enhance the bactericidal effect of lactic acid, and the fall in oxygen tension renders the tissue environment unfavourable to the growth of highly aerobic organisms. A low oxygen tension such as would be produced by trauma to the tissues is, however, of value to most organisms in the early stages of invasion.

The leucocytes are of value in defence not only when living, but also when dead. They contain considerable amounts of a haeme compound—verdo-peroxidase—which is actively bactericidal, and of lysozyme; both of these are liberated on death of the cell. Significant amounts of bactericidal haeme compounds are also derived from disintegrated red cells. Even dead tissue cells contribute to the defensive effort since they release various anti-bacterial components—notably certain lipids and basic peptides.

For the removal of bacteria which have gained access to the blood, the fixed phagocytic cells of the reticulo-endothelial system constitute a highly efficient clearing mechanism. Under experimental conditions it is possible to overload the cells of the reticulo-endothelial system by the intravenous injection of large amounts of colloidal suspensions, e.g. carbon and thorium dioxide (Thorotrast). This overloading is shown in a depression in the rate of clearance of inert material such as denatured serum albumen from the blood. There is no evidence, however, that the reticulo-endothelial system can be overloaded under the conditions of normal infection, although under certain circumstances its function may be impaired. The persistent bacteraemia of septicaemic infections is more likely to be due to a defect in opsonization coupled with a breakdown of the primary filters, viz. the local inflammatory reaction and the local lymphatic glands.

Bacteria which have gained entry to the blood are largely removed by the reticulo-endothelial cells of the liver and the spleen. In this process the Kupffer cells of the liver sinusoids appear to be particularly active. The spleen can in fact be removed—as in the treatment of acquired haemolytic anaemia—without serious impairment of resistance. Nevertheless, there is some evidence for the existence of a functional difference between the phagocytic cells of the liver and those of the spleen. Experimental evidence obtained by Mollison suggests that red cells sensitized with antibodies which are incapable of combining with complement are broken down by the spleen, whereas red cells sensitized with antibody capable of combining with complement are also broken down in the liver. Biozzi and Stiffel have found that in new-born pigs, injected salmonellae are principally removed and disposed of by the spleen. These possible differences in function between the phagocytic cells of the liver and spleen obviously require further clarification.

Alterations in Basic Immunity

The efficiency of the basic defence mechanisms may be impaired by a number of non-specific factors. Surgical lesions of the urinary tract, such as congenital anomalies and stone, predispose to infection with organisms normally parasitic in the intestinal tract. Acute alcoholism increases susceptibility to infection and does so apparently by lowering the efficiency of phagocytic cells. In diabetes there is also an increased susceptibility to pyogenic infection. It has been suggested that this is due to the accumulation of keto-acids and dihydroxyacetone, substances which are reported as being capable of antagonizing the bactericidal effect of lactic acid. The marked reduction in leucocytes found in certain blood disorders, e.g. agranulocytosis and aplastic anaemia, results in an increased susceptibility to pyogenic infections. Resistance to infection is also reduced in Addison's disease and in hypothyroidism.

Susceptibility to respiratory infection, e.g. bronchitis and pneumonia, is greatly increased in the aged; this is presumably because of a reduction in the efficiency of the local defences of the respiratory tract. With increasing age there is, of course, an increase in acquired immunity which would tend to balance any diminution in basic immunity. This possibly explains the fact that increased susceptibility to most other types of infection is not observed in the old. On the other hand, bacterial infections, when they occur, tend to be more severe in older people. This is shown particularly in typhoid fever in which the mortality increases quite sharply after the age of forty. Increased susceptibility to respiratory infections is a regular feature of influenza and the common cold. The viruses presumably prepare the way for bacterial invasion by causing local damage to the defences of the respiratory tract.

Cortisone and its analogues (corticoids) have been shown to have a marked capacity to inhibit inflammatory reactions to a variety of noxious stimuli. Moreover, they can depress the phagocytic activity of the reticulo-endothelial system, and if administered prior to injection of antigen, have a depressing effect on antibody production. As a result they can lower resistance to bacterial infection—permitting rapid multiplication and spread of infecting organisms and transforming minor invasions into serious infections. These latter effects are much more marked in certain experimental animals, e.g. rabbits, rats and mice, than in man. That they are important in man, however, has been shown by the development of tuberculosis in patients undergoing long term corticoid therapy and by the marked deterioration produced by corticoids when they have been inadvertently given to patients suffering from active pulmonary tuberculosis.

Malnutrition is commonly believed to predispose to bacterial infection. Experimental support for this view has been obtained by Dubos, who found that young mice maintained on protein deficient diets had a much higher susceptibility to various bacterial infections than mice maintained on a normal diet. Similar differences were not observed in adult mice, probably because the adult animal has a much greater nutritional reserve. In man there is, however, little clear evidence to relate nutrition to resistance except in the case of tuberculosis, susceptibility to which appears to be increased when the nutritional status of the community is lowered. This was clearly evident in Britain and Germany during both World Wars.

In experimental animals considerable, though transient, non-specific increases in resistance to infection can be produced by injection of killed Gram negative bacteria, e.g. TAB vaccine, and of live or killed mycobacteria. The active agent in Gram negative bacteria has been identified as the somatic antigen complex or endotoxin. The increased resistance following the injection of endotoxin is due to a number of factors.

1. An increase in the number of active phagocytic cells lining the liver sinusoids. There is some evidence that this increase is due to activation of pre-existing non-phagocytic endothelial cells.

2. An increase in the functional activity of the phagocytic cells both of polymorphonuclear and macrophage types. There is, however, no evidence of any increase in the intrinsic bactericidal powers of phagocytic cells following the injection of endotoxin. Evidence has been obtained, however, of an increase in the killing power of phagocytes following infection with the tubercle bacillus or with *Brucella abortus*. This increase in killing power appears to be directed only towards organisms, e.g. mycobacteria and brucellae, which can establish a state of intracellular parasitism.

3. An increase in serum opsonic and bactericidal activities due to a release of specific antibodies into the blood.

ACQUIRED IMMUNITY

As we have seen, the efficiency of the phagocytic mechanisms of the body is increased following injection of Gram negative endotoxins and of mycobacteria. It is to be presumed that such a non-specific increase in basic resistance occurs as a result of natural mycobacterial or Gram negative bacillary infection. This increase in resistance is, however, transient and non-specific. It is best thought of as an enhancement of basic immunity rather than as an acquired immunity. Acquired immunity may be defined as an *immunity specific for a particular disease which the animal acquires during the course of its life.* This immunity is in fact the consequence of the immune responses which the animal body can mount to the antigenic stimulation which were considered in Chapter 6.

Acquired immunity is of two varieties—*active* and *passive.*

Active immunity is due to the activity of the cells of the patient's own body and is mainly a consequence of the acquisition by antibody-producing cells of the capacity to produce specific antibody.

Passive immunity is due to the presence in the body of antibodies introduced into it from the blood of another animal that had been actively immunized.

Both these varieties of immunity—active and passive—may be acquired either *naturally* or *artificially.*

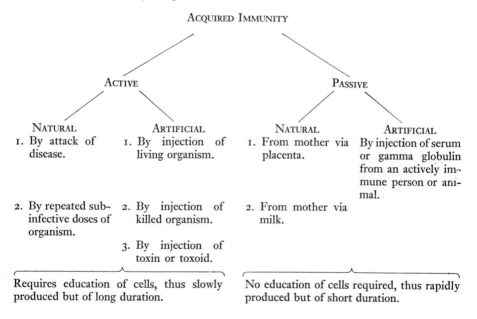

ACQUIRED IMMUNITY

ACTIVE   PASSIVE

NATURAL	ARTIFICIAL	NATURAL	ARTIFICIAL
1. By attack of disease.	1. By injection of living organism.	1. From mother via placenta.	By injection of serum or gamma globulin from an actively immune person or animal.
2. By repeated sub-infective doses of organism.	2. By injection of killed organism.	2. From mother via milk.	
	3. By injection of toxin or toxoid.		

Requires education of cells, thus slowly produced but of long duration.   No education of cells required, thus rapidly produced but of short duration.

The Role of Antibody in Active Immunity

There is now considerable evidence of the occurrence of cellular as well as of humoral immune responses to antigenic stimulation. Cellular responses are manifested in homograft rejection (p. 117), in graft versus host reaction (p. 118) and in delayed-type hypersensitivity (p. 179). The carrier of the immune response under these conditions appears to be the small lymphocyte. There is also evidence that the lymphocyte is the primary effector cell in homograft rejection and in graft versus host reactions. In addition there is reason to believe that the small lymphocytes responsible for these reactions have been conditioned as carriers of cellular immunity by exposure to some substance elaborated by the thymus (p. 122).

Since cellular immune responses as manifested by delayed-type hypersensitivity develop, during the course of infection, to a variety of bacterial and viral antigens it is reasonable to consider that they may have a role of some importance in acquired antimicrobial immunity. So far, however, there is evidence for such a role only in two types of infection: (1) In infections due to characteristically intracellular bacteria—the most important of which are the tubercle bacilli and the brucellae, and (2) in infections due to viruses. There is in fact reason to believe that in both these conditions a cellular immunity of delayed hypersensitivity type is the primary basis of acquired immunity. The most important evidence pointing to this conclusion is the finding that individuals with hypogammaglobulinaemia possess normal resistance to such infections but show a considerable impairment of resistance to infection with characteristically extracellular pathogens. In immunity against the tubercle bacillus there is evidence that the macrophage rather than the lymphocyte is the important effector cell but that its role is dependent, in some way not yet determined, on the sensitized lymphocyte. The problem is discussed more fully in Chapter 26. It seems likely that a similar situation exists in relation to virus infection. In the latter, however, another cellular factor comes into the picture. This is the production of interferon (p. 441). Interferon is, however, quite non-specific in action and the immunity it produces is of short duration. It is unlikely to play any part in specific acquired immunity of long duration. Its vital biological role lies probably in the recovery from virus infection. It is very unlikely that a cellular component plays a significant part in the development of acquired immunity to infections of which intracellular multiplication is not a characteristic feature. In the latter, therefore, we must continue to accept that antibody is the primary basis of acquired immunity.

The fundamental part played by antibody in immunity against microbial infection has been established by a number of different lines of evidence.

1. For those conditions in which the nature of the antigen responsible for the stimulation of immunity has been identified there is a clear correlation between the presence of antibody demonstrable by in vitro tests, and immunity to infection.

2. Children suffering from hypogammaglobulinaemia have a greatly impaired resistance to bacterial infection. A similar diminished resistance to infection is found in patients with multiple myeloma, a condition in which there is a malignant proliferation of what appears to be a single clone of antibody-producing plasma cells. Individuals with quantitatively normal gamma globulin levels may also possess considerably diminished resistance to infection because

their gamma globulin is qualitatively deficient. This condition is known as *dysgammaglobulinaemia*.

3. Interference with the antibody synthesizing machinery, e.g. by X-irradiation, by the administration of cytotoxic drugs, or, in the case of the young animal, by thymectomy, markedly reduces or eliminates the capacity to produce antibodies, and greatly enhances the animal's susceptibility to infection.

Naturally Acquired Active Immunity

This is the immunity which an individual develops as a result of a natural contact with a pathogenic organism. This contact may result in a major invasion with the production of clinical disease or it may result in a minor invasion without the production of clinical disease. Invasions of this latter type are known as *latent* or *subclinical* infections (p. 81). They are of primary importance in the production of immunity against many of the infections, e.g. poliomyelitis, which are normally endemic in a community.

Following infection the patient will, in most cases, be immune to further infection with the same organism for a period which varies with the particular disease. In some cases, e.g. the common cold, gonorrhoea and staphylococcal infections, the immunity produced by infection is of short duration. In others, however, e.g. after diphtheria, typhoid fever, yellow fever and smallpox, it is of long duration and may persist, to a greater or lesser extent, for life.

In general, immunity appears to be most persistent to conditions in which a bacteraemic or viraemic stage is of importance in the evolution of the infection and in which therefore the organisms are readily accessible to blood borne antibody. As a rule, conditions with a viraemic or bacteraemic stage have a long incubation period during which the infecting organism has adequate time to stimulate a secondary antibody response. In some of the conditions in which immunity appears to be of short duration the duration of the immunity may be longer than would at first sight appear since the organism responsible for the second and subsequent attacks may be antigenically different from that responsible for the first.

The immunity produced as a result of infection is serologically specific. Consequently, when an individual has been infected with an organism which belongs to a species consisting of a number of different serological types, immunity to reinfection is present only for the serological type with which he has been infected. He is therefore fully susceptible to other serological types of the same species. Thus a patient may have a number of different attacks of streptococcal throat infections, each being due to a different serological type of *Str. pyogenes*.

In most bacterial infections the development of antibody during the course of the infection appears to be the mechanism primarily responsible for spontaneous recovery from the infection. A particularly dramatic example of this association was frequently observed in pre-antibiotic days in cases of pneumococcal lobar pneumonia, the appearance of the crisis—i.e. a phase during which the patient's condition changed rapidly and dramatically for the better—being associated with a great increase in the concentration of antibody in the blood. In certain cases, however, the presence of even considerable amounts of circulating antibody does not appear to have any appreciable effect on the persistence of the infection. This is particularly true of subacute bacterial endocarditis and brucellosis probably because in these conditions the organisms are present in sites in which they are inaccessible to circulating antibody. In viral diseases antibody is less clearly related to recovery, the acute phase in the infection normally coming to an end before the appearance of detectable antibody levels in the blood. It seems probable that recovery from virus infection is due to the production by the infected cell of an agent—interferon—which has the specific effect of preventing viral multiplication (p. 154).

Our knowledge of the precise nature of the antigens responsible for the stimulation of protective antibody is in many cases incomplete. As we have seen bacteria are antigenically complex and following an infection antibodies are produced against a variety of bacterial antigens. Only a limited number of such antibodies, however, will protect against infection. In all cases the antigens involved are situated on the surface of the organism, e.g. the Vi antigen of *Salm. typhi* and the M proteins of *Str. pyogenes*. These are the antigens which confer antiphagocytic properties on the organism and which therefore are of primary importance in determining its virulence. Antibodies to flagellar antigens are not protective since combination of such antibodies with the flagella does not sensitize bacteria to phagocytosis. Immunity to organisms producing exotoxins, e.g. diphtheria bacilli and *Clostridium tetani*, is due not to antibacterial antibodies but to antitoxin. Immunity against viral infections is also produced by antibody against surface antigens but against these phagocytosis is not an important mechanism of defence. Such antibodies appear to protect by preventing the virus from invading the tissue cells (p. 444).

The sera of most individuals contain antibodies, demonstrable by in vitro tests, against organisms with which they have not been overtly infected. These are usually referred to as *natural antibodies*. Many of these antibodies are undoubtedly produced in response to subclinical infection. The role of subclinical infection in stimulating antibody production has been particularly clearly established in relation to diphtheria. Thus it has been observed that in a closed community where diphtheria has occurred many children who showed no clinical signs of diphtheria had nevertheless been stimulated to produce diphtheria antitoxin.

Many of the natural antibacterial antibodies, however, are clearly not produced as a result of subclinical infection with the corresponding organism. Some are in fact active against bacteria with which the individual is unlikely ever to have been in contact. The finding that such antibodies do not develop in animals raised under germ-free conditions would indicate that their production is stimulated by contact with commensal bacteria of the respiratory and intestinal tracts, which share antigens with pathogenic bacteria. This is also a conceivable origin for the blood group iso-agglutinins, the fact that certain blood group antigens have been identified in various bacteria suggesting that these too may have been produced by active immunization. The presence of unusual natural antibodies such as those for periodate treated red cells would, however, be more difficult to explain on a basis of natural contact. These may therefore represent accidental antibody-like by-products of gammaglobulin producing cells.

Natural antibacterial antibodies appear to be mainly 19S gamma globulins, and to be less specific and to combine less avidly with antigen than the antibodies produced in response to overt infection.

Artificially Acquired Active Immunity

By artificial active immunization we mean the deliberate stimulation of antibody production by the introduction into the animal body of living or dead micro-organisms, or their products. In some cases, notably tuberculosis, yellow fever and smallpox vaccination, the degree of immunity produced is of the same order as that produced by natural infection. In many instances, however, and this seems to be the general rule when killed vaccines are used, the immunity produced is appreciably less than that following infection or the use of live attenuated vaccines.

Active immunity requires for its development a considerable time which is to be measured in weeks or months rather than in hours or days, but, against this disadvantage, is the fact that the immunity, once developed, persists for long periods, in some cases for years. The cells once educated to produce an antibody remember the lesson they have learned and, even if it goes out of production, they can be much more rapidly stimulated to produce it again than can cells never so educated.

Living Vaccines

Man's first deliberate effort to protect himself against a disease was by voluntarily exposing himself to infection. In parts of Asia, for several centuries, material taken from a mild case of smallpox was inoculated into those desiring protection. The result was the development of smallpox often, but not necessarily, of mild type. Since, at that time, almost everyone suffered from smallpox, it was thought preferable to run the risk at a selected time with a mild form of the disease rather than to wait for chance infection.

Surprisingly, the number of fatalities was not as high as might have been expected; a contemporary account claims a mortality of less than 1 per thousand. This low mortality rate was undoubtedly due to the unusual route of contact and to the fact that the virus used was of relatively low virulence.

The next advance was due to Jenner. While practising variolation, Jenner found that inoculation did not 'take' on individuals who had had cowpox. As a result he conceived the idea that it might be possible to protect against smallpox by the deliberate inoculation of cowpox, a procedure which he called 'vaccination'. The modern technique of vaccination against smallpox stems directly from Jenner's procedure (p. 485).

The modern era in immunization was opened by Pasteur who discovered methods of *attenuating*, that is, of modifying the virulence of certain bacteria so that they could be introduced into the body without serious risk. Pasteur found that cultures of the chicken cholera bacillus (*Pasteurella septica*) maintained in the laboratory had become non-pathogenic. Fowl inoculated with these cultures, however, were immune to infection with virulent chicken cholera bacilli. Pasteur's most dramatic demonstration of the capacity of attenuated organisms, i.e. organisms of diminished virulence, to stimulate immunity was the celebrated experiment in which he established the efficacy of immunization against anthrax (Chapter 17).

A number of vaccines consisting of organisms which have been deliberately attenuated by laboratory culture are currently used in human immunization. The most important of these, ranking with diphtheria and tetanus toxoids as the most effective agents currently used for active immunization, are the yellow fever, smallpox, BCG and polio vaccines. Live vaccines have also been used on a limited scale for immunization against bubonic plague, brucellosis, mumps and measles.

From certain organisms, e.g. tubercle bacilli and the yellow fever and smallpox viruses, it has not so far been possible to prepare an effective non-living antigen. This may be because the methods used for vaccine preparation have inactivated the immunizing antigen or because the immunizing antigen is not produced in sufficient quantity, if at all, unless the organism multiplies in the tissues.

The process of attenuation as employed in the preparation of vaccine strains consists in the selection of mutants of diminished virulence. The emergence of such mutants usually requires a long period of cultivation in laboratory media or a long period of passage in laboratory animals or in tissue cultures. The selection of the avirulent 17D variant of the yellow fever virus, which is that currently used for immunization against yellow fever, is illustrative of the techniques employed (p. 470).

The attenuation of a micro-organism for the purpose of producing an effective and safe vaccine presents the microbiologist with three major problems.

1. The organism must be sufficiently attenuated to ensure safe administration. This in effect means that it should not be capable of causing a progressive infection or that the risk of its doing so should be so small compared with the risk against which it protects that it can be safely ignored.

2. The degree of attenuation should not be so great as seriously to deprive the organism of its immunizing efficiency. The difficulty of steering a course between these extremes has been well illustrated in the development of a measles vaccine (p. 507). The first attenuated strain of measles virus introduced for active immunization—the Edmonston strain—was insufficiently attenuated to be administered by itself, producing a severe febrile reaction in quite a high proportion of vaccinated individuals. Many further attenuated virulents, however, have appeared to be insufficiently immunogenic.

3. The attenuated variant should be stable, i.e. it should have no significant tendency to revert to its original virulent form. This condition has required particular attention in the development of poliomyelitis vaccines (p. 456).

On first principles, attenuated vaccines are the ideal antigens for active immunization. They most nearly simulate the conditions of natural infection, and since they have not been inactivated they are more likely to contain the major immunizing antigens. In many cases, however, the development of attenuated variants suitable for human immunization has not been possible, frequently because the antigenic diversity of the species has made this impracticable.

Killed Vaccines

Killed bacterial vaccines are used for immunization against the typhoid and paratyphoid fevers, cholera, plague and whooping cough. The degree of immunity produced by these vaccines, although considerable, is much less than that obtained either with the living attenuated vaccines, which have just been discussed, or with the toxoids. Killed vaccines are also highly effective in immunization against poliomyelitis—a viral—and typhus—a rickettsial—disease. Autogenous vaccines, i.e. vaccines made from organisms present in the patient's own flora, were at one time widely used in the treatment of conditions such as rheumatism and chronic bronchitis for which no satisfactory therapy was available. There is, however, no evidence that they have any significant prophylactic or therapeutic effect.

For the preparation of these vaccines the organisms may be killed in a variety of ways, e.g. by heat, formalin, phenol, alcohol or ultra-violet irradiation. The particular method chosen must be one that will not damage the immunizing antigen. The vaccine is preserved with an antiseptic, e.g. dilute phenol, merthiolate or alcohol.

The testing of the immunizing efficiency of killed vaccines poses problems of particular difficulty, and must be carried out in the first place by determining the capacity to protect experimental animals infected by parenteral injection. Since the route of infection is a completely unnatural one, and since the susceptibility of the animal may be quite different from that of the human subject, the results of such protection experiments may have only a very limited applicability to human immunization. This difficulty has been particularly illustrated in the case of TAB vaccine. On the basis of mouse protection tests the alcoholized TAB vaccine in which the Vi antigen of the typhoid bacillus is fully preserved (p. 304), has been found to be considerably more effective than phenolized heat-killed vaccine. The situation in man appears to be quite the reverse (p. 314). Animal experiments, however, are of considerable value in determining the capacity of a vaccine to a stimulate antibody production, and where the identity of the antigen responsible for the stimulation of protective antibody is known, as in the case of the poliomyelitis vaccine, the antigenic efficacy of the vaccine in animals can be expected to bear some relationship to its efficacy in man. Nevertheless a final assessment of the efficacy of an antigen for human immunization must be obtained as a result of controlled trials in the human population.

Toxoids

Toxoids are toxins which have been treated to deprive them of their toxicity without impairing their capacity to stimulate the production of antibodies.

Only the protein exotoxins can be converted into toxoid. For immunization purposes this is achieved by treatment with formalin; the resulting antigen is known as formol toxoid. The formol toxoids which have been most used are the diphtheria and tetanus toxoids. Since diphtheria and tetanus are almost entirely due to the action of the exotoxin they can be prevented by active immunization with toxoid. In the case of diphtheria it is possible that although the prevention of the disease requires the establishment of an antitoxic immunity, some degree of antibacterial immunity is also of value. In support of this contention is the finding that the more highly purified toxoids appear to be somewhat less effective as immunizing agents than the cruder preparations.

Administration of Prophylactics

The principal indications for active immunization may be summarized as follows:

1. Immunization of all members of the community in infancy or early life against the more serious diseases prevalent in the community. The conditions for which a programme of general immunization is required naturally vary from one community to another, and also vary in the same community from time to time. Thus when a disease which was once widely prevalent has been brought under effective control by active immunization and/or other procedures it may be possible to modify the immunization programme. This appears now to be the position in relation to tuberculosis in Scandinavian countries (p. 365) and possibly in other western European countries as well. In western Europe, diseases for which general immunization of the community is currently required are diphtheria, tetanus, whooping cough, poliomyelitis, measles, smallpox and, in most cases, tuberculosis.

2. Immunization of individuals travelling to countries where they may encounter diseases not prevalent in their own country. Important examples are yellow fever, cholera, plague and various rickettsial infections.

3. Vaccination in the face of an impending epidemic. Thus in a community in which smallpox does not occur as an endemic disease, mass vaccination may be required if the disease is introduced into the community from outside and the immediate measures to contain it have been unsuccessful.

4. Immunization under conditions of special risk. Under this heading we may include the use of influenza vaccine for elderly people and patients with cardiovascular insufficiency, the immunization against rabies of individuals believed to have been bitten by rabid animals, and immunization against tetanus of patients sustaining severe wounds (p. 390).

The occurrence following the administration of TAB vaccine of a so-called 'negative phase' in which the bactericidal power of the blood for *Salm. typhi* is considerably diminished was described by Wright in 1901. The reality of this negative phase has been the subject of considerable controversy. Recently, however, evidence has been presented by Raettig, both on epidemiological and experimental grounds, suggesting that such a phase may occur, and that immunization during the incubation period of typhoid fever, for instance, may considerably increase the severity of the disease. Because of this it would seem advisable not to vaccinate with TAB vaccine during the course of a typhoid epidemic. No such effect has been demonstrated with live vaccines; in fact there is evidence that the administration of live poliomyelitis vaccine may—by interference with the infecting strain of poliomyelitis virus—tend to abort an epidemic.

With the passage of time the immunity produced by active immunization inevitably diminishes, as does the immunity produced by natural active immunization. The rate of decline is much greater in some cases than in others. Thus immunity is very persistent following smallpox and yellow fever vaccination, or immunization with tetanus toxoid, but quite transient following immunization with TAB vaccine.

Not only does the duration of immunity vary with the antigen employed, but with the same antigen can differ considerably from one individual to another. Some individuals are good responders, others are poor responders. A waning immunity can be reinforced, however, by periodic booster injections. Where the initial immunity has been transient, as following immunization with TAB vaccine, booster inoculation would be required at frequent intervals, in the case of those who continue at risk. In respect of diseases with which an individual may periodically come in contact appreciable natural boosting of immunity will occur under natural conditions. Although insufficient to protect completely against infection, a waning immunity may nevertheless be of considerable value in preventing a serious overt attack of the disease, permitting instead a latent subclinical infection. The latter may in turn effect a considerable restimulation of the antibody-producing machinery. This natural boosting of immunity is believed to be of considerable importance in the maintenance of immunity following a single administration of BCG vaccine, one inoculation of which therefore, in a community in which tuberculosis is prevalent, may give rise to a long-lasting immunity.

Most of the preparations used in active immunization are introduced directly into the tissues, being inoculated either subcutaneously, intramuscularly or into the skin, the latter route being reserved for the BCG and smallpox vaccines. Except for live polio vaccine the oral route is not a satisfactory one for vaccine administration. With other antigens the antibody response to oral administration is capricious and cannot be relied on. The satisfactory antibody response following the oral administration of live polio vaccine is due to the fact that the virus multiplies in the cells of the intestinal tract.

The antigenicity of a number of substances can be increased by combination with a variety of compounds which have an adjuvant effect. Aluminium hydroxide and aluminium phosphate both of which are used as adsorbents for diphtheria toxoid are, however, the only adjuvants which have so far found an application in immunization in man. The potentiating effect of these substances on antigenicity may be due to their low solubility and their high capacity to adsorb the antigen; consequently they form a depot of antigen in the tissues from which the antigen is slowly released. There appears to be a definite risk that the intramuscular injection of preparations containing alum may predispose to the development of paralytic poliomyelitis in the injected limb. The use of these is, therefore, best avoided at times when poliomyelitis is prevalent except in the case of individuals who have already been immunized with polio vaccine. It has been claimed that this complication, known as provocation poliomyelitis, is also, but to a much less extent, associated with the administration of combined prophylactics incorporating pertussis vaccine. Most workers however consider that this association has not been sufficiently firmly established to justify rejection of immunization programmes employing combined prophylactics.

Combined prophylactics containing more than one immunizing agent are frequently employed. Combined immunization has the great advantage of reducing the number of injections that have to be given; in the immunization of children this is of considerable practical importance. The following combined preparations are frequently used: diphtheria-pertussis, diphtheria-tetanus, diphtheria-tetanus-pertussis and TAB—tetanus prophylactics. There is, however, the danger in combined immunization that most of the antibody response may be directed towards only one of the antigens present. This type of interference has been shown to occur in persons who have been immunized with a diphtheria toxoid preparation and are subsequently given a combined prophylactic which includes diphtheria toxoid. In such cases, most of the antibody response may be concerned with the production of diphtheria antitoxin. Another difficulty arises in the case of combinations of pertussis with polio and/or diphtheria toxoid. In order to provide protection when it is most needed pertussis vaccine should be given within the first few months of life; at this time, however, the response to polio vaccine and to diphtheria toxoid is poor and may be reduced still further by the presence of maternally transmitted passive immunity. Immunization schedules for children must, however, to some extent represent a compromise between the ideal and the expedient. They must provide a full range of protection but at the same time must not involve the giving of an unduly large number of injections. Because of this latter requirement combined vaccines, especially the triple vaccine containing diphtheria, tetanus and pertussis antigens, have in recent years come increasingly into favour. An immunization schedule in which three injections of triple vaccine are given as a primary course within the first 6 months of life has been recommended for use in the United Kingdom and has been adopted by many authorities.

When killed vaccines or toxoids are used more than one injection is required. Although appreciable potential immunity may be found after a single injection it is important that the number of injections prescribed by the makers of the vaccine and the amount indicated for each injection should be closely adhered to.

Naturally Acquired Passive Immunity

During intra-uterine development the foetus appears to be very effectively protected from antigenic stimulation. Consequently, at birth, it is normally devoid of acquired active immunity. Nevertheless, the new-born infant shows a very high resistance to a number of infections, e.g. measles, chickenpox, diphtheria and scarlet fever, to which older children are highly susceptible. This resistance is due to antibody passively acquired from the mother.

Transmission of antibody from mother to foetus may occur immediately after birth via the milk or colostrum, or before birth by direct transfer from the maternal to the foetal circulation, across the placenta or through the yolk sac. Different animal species differ in the relative importance of these two methods. In cattle, horses and pigs transfer is virtually entirely postnatal via the milk or colostrum. The colostrum secreted during the first few days after delivery is of particular importance since it contains a high concentration of antibody. The ingested antibody is absorbed through the intestinal mucosa which is highly permeable for the first few days after birth. This mechanism has been assumed to be of little importance in man but the evidence so far available is insufficient to say that it is completely without significance. Thus it has been suggested that breast feeding of infants may impede the establishment of enteroviruses in the alimentary tract. Significantly, human milk has been shown to contain all the immunoglobulins in appreciable concentration. In rabbits and guinea-pigs, transfer of maternal antibodies occurs mainly from the yolk sac, which is prominent in these animals and to which antibodies gain access from the lumen of the uterus. In man, transfer of maternal antibodies occurs mainly as an antenatal event across the placenta. This can readily occur since there are only two tissue layers between maternal and foetal circulations at term as compared with five layers in ruminants and six in pigs. The failure to acquire antibodies from the milk or colostrum after birth is presumably due to an impermeability of the intestinal epithelium. The placental route of transfer is highly selective, permitting the passage only of IgG antibodies. This selectivity is probably of considerable biological significance in man, since IgG antibodies appear to be the most efficient variety, at least in toxin neutralizing and virus neutralizing capacity. Moreover the barrier to IgM antibodies prevents transfer of iso-agglutinins which, in cases of ABO blood group incompatibility, would have a damaging effect on the foetal red cells. The capacity of IgG antibodies to cross the placenta appears to be due to the presence of a placental transfer site on the Fc moiety of the antibody molecule (p. 101). When this is removed as in pepsin digestion of diphtheria antitoxin (p. 165), placental transfer cannot occur. Infants cannot therefore be passively immunized against diphtheria by administration of commercially refined antitoxin to their mothers.

Certain antibodies, notably diphtheria antitoxin, have been shown to be present in the foetal circulation in considerably higher concentrations than in the maternal circulation. This difference in concentration would appear to be due in the first place to the fact that transfer of protein from mother to foetus seems to be mainly unidirectional. It would also be necessary, however, to assume some active transport mechanism by virtue of which the foetus could build up antibody levels against a concentration gradient.

After birth there is a progressive fall in the concentration in the infant's blood of passively transferred antibodies. This fall is due to the metabolism in the infant's circulation of the maternal gamma globulin which to the infant is virtually a foreign protein. The gamma globulin levels reach their lowest values at from 3 to 10 weeks of age, and thereafter begin to rise. Full adult levels are not usually attained, however, until between 1 and 4 years. That this rise in gamma globulin level is due to antibody synthesis is clear from the fact that it is grossly deficient in animals brought up in a germ-free environment.

Passively transferred antibody shows a logarithmic rate of decline, with a half-life (that is the time required to fall by 50 per cent) of approximately 30 days. This is shown both in the fall in the concentration of specific antibodies in normal infants, and of total gamma globulin in hypogammaglobulinaemic infants born of normal mothers. As a result of this rate of fall little if any of the transferred antibody is detectable at the age of 6 months.

Artificially Acquired Passive Immunity

Passive immunity is achieved artifically by the injection of antibodies produced in one animal into another. This procedure, known as passive immunization, is carried out both for treatment and prophylaxis.

Passive immunization differs from active immunization in the following respects: (1) Immunity is rapidly established. This technique is therefore of value as an emergency measure to protect persons who have been in contact with cases of infectious diseases. (2) The immunity produced is of short duration. In the case of the antitoxins the antibody, being a foreign protein, is rapidly eliminated; the diphtheria and tetanus antitoxins prepared in the horse having in the normal human subject a half-life of about 7 days. In some individuals an initial phase, in which the concentration of the antibody falls logarithmically, is succeeded by a phase of accelerated elimination due to the formation of antibody against the injected protein. This immune elimination may be associated with the appearance of the serum sickness syndrome (p. 177). Immune elimination is almost certain to occur if the individual has received a previous injection of horse antitoxin. The protection afforded by the injection of such persons is therefore of particularly short duration. (3) In passive immunity there is no education of the reticulo-endothelial system in the production of antibody and the individual has therefore no potential immunity. Consequently, when the immediate protection has disappeared, he is again fully susceptible to infection. In active immunity, on the other hand, the reticulo-endothelial cells have been educated and he therefore has a potential immunity which may last to a greater or lesser extent for life.

As a prophylactic measure passive immunization is of value in giving short-term and immediate protection to persons who have been in contact with an infectious case. Active immunization on the other hand is a prophylactic measure to be adopted before the risk of infection becomes imminent.

At one time crude unrefined serum was used as antibody source, but this is no longer considered justifiable and preparations consisting of immunoglobulins which have undergone a considerable degree of purification are used instead.

These preparations have the following advantages as compared with whole serum.

1. They are less dangerous. Crude animal sera, especially horse serum, may give rise to severe allergic reactions, and crude human sera may produce serum jaundice. The risk of allergic reactions is greatly reduced, and that of serum jaundice eliminated, by the use of purified globulins.

2. Purification permits a considerable degree of concentration, thus allowing the injection of a relatively large amount of antibody in a small volume of fluid.

The immunoglobulins which are of importance in this context are (a) the antitoxins, and (b) human gamma globulin. At one time antibacterial sera, prepared by the immunization of animals, were used extensively in the treatment of a variety of bacterial infections. Their use except possibly in the case of leptospirosis (p. 412) has been rendered obsolete by the introduction of chemotherapy. Antibacterial sera have no value as prophylactics.

Antitoxins

The most important of the antitoxins are the diphtheria, tetanus and gas-gangrene antitoxins and the antivenoms. These are normally prepared by the immunization of horses. Unfortunately, some people are hypersensitive to horse products and develop serious allergic reactions following the injection of horse serum. These reactions are much less severe with purified immuno-globulin preparations. In a minority of persons, however, even the latter can produce fatal anaphylactic reactions.

Human Gamma Globulin

Since most adults have been exposed to a variety of virus infections, gamma globulin prepared from large pools of adult plasma will contain a variety of antiviral antibodies. Its main use, however, has been in the prevention of measles in very young or debilitated children (p. 507). Gamma globulin should never be given by the intravenous route as it may contain aggregates of de-natured globulin capable of giving rise to fatal systemic reactions. Since gamma globulin is not a foreign protein it does not give rise to allergic reactions.

HERD IMMUNITY

Herd immunity is the immunity possessed by a population group as a whole. It varies in extent with the number of individuals comprising the population who are immune. When herd immunity is low an infectious disease capable of assuming an epidemic form may spread rapidly and is often clinically of severe type. When herd immunity is high the disease spreads less rapidly and is of relatively mild form.

Natural active immunization is the major factor in determining the extent of herd immunity. Consequently a disease is of less gravity in a population in which it occurs in endemic form than in a population into which it is introduced for the first time. Natural immunization, however, is not the only factor contributing to this situation. The population may have a low degree of susceptibility due to high basic immunity as a result of the operation of natural selection. When a disease is establishing itself in endemic form in a population it tends to eliminate all individuals in the population who are highly susceptible to it, thereby leaving a stock which is relatively resistant.

The devastating results which may follow the introduction of an organism to an unprotected population is well demonstrated by the experience of the Fiji Islands in relation to measles. Prior to 1875 no epidemic of measles had occurred in Fiji in living memory; the Islands were therefore virgin soil for the measles virus. In 1875 measles was introduced by a visiting ship. This resulted in the development of a severe epidemic which affected all age groups and caused the death of about 25 per cent of the population.

Alterations in the extent of natural immunization in a community, occurring spontaneously or as the result of the application of preventive measures, may have important epidemiological effects. Thus, in the case of poliomyelitis, modern hygienic measures have greatly diminished the chance of infection in childhood. As a result many more adults are susceptible to infection and the disease has in consequence shown a considerably increased incidence in the older age groups.

Spontaneous alterations in herd immunity play an important part in determining the periodicity of epidemic infections such as measles and influenza, which can be readily and rapidly spread. A major epidemic of these infections can begin only if there is a high proportion of susceptibles in the population. When, during the course of the epidemic, the proportion of susceptibles falls below a certain level, the epidemic begins to withdraw. The community remains immune against further serious epidemic invasion while the proportion of susceptibles remains low. This proportion ultimately rises and when it reaches a critical level the scene is set for a further epidemic.

A high level of herd immunity may be achieved against some diseases, e.g. diphtheria, by means of artificial active immunization. In such a case it is vitally important that if large-scale immunization of a population has been adopted it should be fully maintained. Immunization, by reducing the prevalence of a disease, diminishes the opportunities for natural active immunization against it. Consequently if the programme of active immunization is relaxed, the infection might be reintroduced and would then encounter a highly susceptible population with possibly disastrous results.

CHAPTER 9

HYPERSENSITIVITY

In this chapter we are concerned with a number of conditions in which the tissues show an increased capacity to react to some foreign substance. For this abnormal reactivity the terms *allergy* and *hypersensitivity* will be used synonymously.

The conditions considered here as hypersensitivities are extremely diverse in their clinical manifestations but are nevertheless believed to have a common basic mechanism—namely that they are the result of antibody–antigen reactions occurring in the tissues. The evidence for this common mechanism may be summarized as follows.

1. Hypersensitivities are elicited by substances which are either known to be antigens or which can be shown to combine with plasma or tissue proteins to form antigens.

2. The reactions are specific in a serological sense, the reactivity being directed towards the substance responsible for stimulating the allergic response, and to any closely related substance.

As was considered in Chapter 6, immune responses are of two varieties—humoral and cellular. Both types of response can form the basis of hypersensitive reactions. Humoral antibodies are the basis of the *immediate-type* hypersensitivities, and cellular responses the basis of *delayed-type* hypersensitivities. In both cases hypersensitivity may be transferred from a hypersensitive subject to a normal one. In the case of the antibody-mediated immediate hypersensitivities, passive transfer is achieved by the injection of serum or plasma containing the antibody. In the case of the cell-mediated delayed hypersensitivities, passive transfer is achieved by the injection of appropriately sensitized lymphoid cells.

The allergic reaction is the response which develops on contact with the homologous allergen in an animal previously sensitized to that allergen. In experimental allergies the sensitizing contact with the antigen can be defined precisely, since it involves the deliberate exposure of the animal—usually by inoculation—to the allergen in question. In the case of clinical allergies, however, it is not usually possible to identify the sensitizing or immunizing contact; a notable exception is the injection of horse serum, e.g. as a prophylactic against tetanus.

IMMEDIATE-TYPE HYPERSENSITIVITY

This term is applied to hypersensitive states in which an allergic reaction develops within a short period after contact with the antigen. In some cases the response may be clinically obvious within a few seconds after contact, whereas in others it may not appear for some hours. Immediate-type hypersensitivities may be divided into two varieties, (a) anaphylactic type and (b) Arthus type.

Anaphylactic Hypersensitivity

As previously indicated, immediate-type hypersensitivity is due to the reaction of antigen with humoral antibody. In contrast to the antigen–antibody reactions responsible for immunity, however, those involved in the production of immediate-type anaphylactic hypersensitivity occur in, or in association with, tissue cells. As a result the tissue cells are damaged, releasing pharmacologically active substances—the most important of which is histamine—into their immediate environment. These may be circulated by the blood to act on tissues and organs remote from the site of production. The clinical symptoms associated with anaphylactic hypersensitivity are the result of the action of these substances on susceptible tissues. The tissues principally involved are the smooth musculature of the bronchi and gastro-intestinal tract, which undergo contraction, and the blood vessels, particularly the capillaries, which show a considerable increase in permeability.

The symptoms of anaphylactic sensitivity depend in the first place on the route by which the animal makes contact with the allergen. Different animals, however, exhibit different and often quite characteristic types of allergic response. These differences depend both on the nature of the substances released and on variations in the reactivity of different animals to them. Much of our knowledge of anaphylactic hypersensitivity has been derived from study of anaphylaxis in the guinea-pig—the experimental animal of choice because of its extremely high susceptibility to anaphylactic reactions.

In experimental animals three types of anaphylactic reaction may be distinguished, depending on the way in which the hypersensitivity is demonstrated.

1. Systemic Anaphylaxis

This is a condition of acute shock, usually terminating in death, which follows the injection of antigen into a previously sensitized animal. When protein antigens are used sensitization can usually be achieved with a single dose of antigen. The amount of antigen required for sensitization—the sensitizing dose—depends on its antibody-producing capacity. Thus with horse serum, a very potent antigen, a dose of as little as 0·0001 ml may be sufficient to sensitize. Sensitivity usually appears some 10 to 21 days after the sensitizing injection. At this stage the intravenous injection of a larger amount of the same antigen will bring on the symptoms of shock. In the guinea-pig almost immediately after the shock injection the animal becomes restless, its hair bristles, its respirations become embarrassed and slowed. Death which occurs within a few minutes of the injection is due to suffocation from contraction of the smooth muscle in the walls of the small bronchioles. At post-mortem examination, the lungs are grossly distended, the bronchioles contracted, and the intestine may show active peristalsis.

In rats, circulatory collapse and increase in intestinal peristaltic activity are the main features. As a result the intestinal tract is believed to be the main shock organ. Rats, unlike guinea-pigs, are insusceptible to histamine, and anti-histamines have therefore no protective effect. On the other hand, rat smooth muscle is noticeably susceptible to the action of serotonin, and there is a marked increase in intestinal capillary permeability in relation to the serotonin-containing chromaffin cells to the intestinal tract. In the rabbit, death is associated with extreme dilatation of the right side of the heart caused apparently by pulmonary hypertension following constriction of the branches of the pulmonary artery. Both histamine and serotonin are believed to play a part in this but a mechanical factor due to the deposition in the pulmonary capillaries of antigen–antibody aggregates in platelet-leucocyte clumps appears to be of importance as well.

The guinea-pig can be passively sensitized to systemic anaphylaxis by the injection of serum from another guinea-pig already sensitized, or of human and rabbit immune sera. Certain animal sera, e.g. those of horses and rats, will not, however, passively sensitize guinea-pigs.

An animal can be shocked only with the antigen which is used for sensitization or one which is serologically closely related to it. Animals which have been sensitized with conjugated protein antigens, such as those used by Landsteiner in his studies of serological specificity, can be shocked by injection of the corresponding hapten. This appears to occur, however, only if the hapten is capable of precipitating with antibody. If the hapten is incapable of precipitation it will inhibit the production of shock by the complete antigen.

Although the most efficient method of producing shock is by intravenous inoculation it also occurs following intraperitoneal, intramuscular or subcutaneous injection. When these routes are used, however, considerably larger amounts of antigen are required.

A sensitized animal may be *desensitized*, without producing the symptoms of acute shock, by the injection of small but increasing doses of antigen over a period of some hours. By this procedure the animal becomes refractory to shock for some days, but the state of sensitivity eventually returns. Desensitization occurs because the antigen combines with the tissue-fixed antibody, thereby neutralizing it but, since this combination takes place gradually and over a long period, no serious symptoms result.

The development of anaphylactic sensitivity is delayed, if, instead of the usual sensitizing dose, the animal is given initially a large dose or a series of doses of antigen capable of stimulating the production of a large amount of circulating antibody. This refractory state is known as *anti-anaphylaxis*. The isolated organs of such animals, however, show organ anaphylaxis. The circulating antibody therefore appears to act as a barrier preventing the antigen from gaining access to the tissue-fixed antibody.

2. Local Cutaneous Anaphylaxis

By the intradermal injection of antigen into actively sensitized guinea-pigs, local wheal-and-flare reactions may be produced. Cutaneous anaphylaxis may also be induced passively, passive cutaneous anaphylaxis (PCA), by the intradermal injection of antisera capable of passively transferring systemic anaphylactic sensitization. Passive cutaneous anaphylaxis may be demonstrated some 4 to 6 hours after the injection of antibody, by intravenous injection of a mixture of the antigen with a dye, e.g. Evans blue, which is capable of combining with serum protein. At the sensitized site, combination of antigen with antibody increases capillary permeability and permits the escape of the protein-dye complex into the tissues.

3. Organ Anaphylaxis

If the uterus or a segment of the ileum or bronchus of a sensitized animal is washed and exposed to a solution of the sensitizing antigen, it will contract as a result of smooth muscle spasm. This phenomenon has been applied in the Schultz-Dale test as a highly specific and sensitive method for the demonstration and estimation of antigen. Organ anaphylaxis may also be induced passively by exposing the isolated tissue to antisera capable of passive in vivo transfer of sensitization.

Mechanism of Anaphylaxis

The participation of antibody in anaphylactic reactions in the guinea-pig is clear from: (*a*) The serological specificity of the reaction, which can be induced only by the antigen responsible for sensitization or one closely related to it. (*b*) The passive transfer of sensitivity by specific immune sera. Since it is possible to elicit reactions such as muscle contraction and histamine release from the washed tissues of a sensitized animal by exposure to antigen, it can be concluded that the antibody involved in sensitization is firmly fixed to cells present in the tissues.

Anaphylactic sensitization and histamine release from perfused guinea-pig lung can be achieved also by exposure to antigen–antibody complexes obtained in the region of antigen excess. There is some evidence, however, that the complexes may not be active per se but act as sources of antibody which dissociates and is then adsorbed to the tissue. Since it is possible passively to transfer anaphylactic sensitization by non-precipitating rabbit antibody, the reaction does not require the formation of a precipate between antibody and antigen.

In the guinea-pig and, almost certainly, in man the cell type of greatest importance in the production of anaphylactic reactions is the mast cell (see below). There is, however, no reason to believe that the mast cell is the only cell which is sensitized by antibody. It seems more likely that the antibody site which binds to mast cells will bind to other cells as well.

It can therefore be seen that the first stage in anaphylactic sensitization is the production of an antibody capable of binding to tissue cells and in particular, to mast cells. In order to do so the antibody must presumably possess a configuration permitting adsorption to the specific receptor site on the appropriate tissue cell. There is clear evidence that only certain of the antibodies which an animal produces possess the configuration enabling them to bind to the tissue cells in such a way as to induce anaphylactic sensitization. Thus in the guinea-pig this capacity has been demonstrated for the electrophoretically relatively fast-moving 7S antibody designated γ_1 but is absent from a slower moving 7S antibody designated γ_2. An analogous distinction has been made in the mouse and the rat. Moreover it would appear that the antibodies which can transfer anaphylactic hypersensitivity within a species can do so only within that species, and cannot transfer sensitivity to a different species. Sensitivity may however be transferred to a different species, if the animal produces antibodies capable of fixation to the cells of that species. Thus human IgG antibodies, which do not appear to be involved in anaphylactic hypersensitivity in man, can nevertheless transfer anaphylactic hypersensitivity to the guinea-pig. There is evidence in this case, and it is probably a general rule, that the appropriate fixation site is on the Fc fragment, and is therefore a function of the heavy chain. Similarly, anaphylactic hypersensitivity may be transferred to guinea-pigs by mouse, dog and monkey antibodies analogous to human IgG antibodies; like the latter these antibodies do not produce anaphylactic hypersensitivity within the producer species.

Whether the combination of an antigen with tissue fixed antibody causes direct damage to sensitized tissue cells is in doubt. It has been suggested, for example, that the combination of antibody with antigen may have a damaging effect on collagen. There is no doubt, however, that the major symptoms of anaphylactic hypersensitivity are due to the release of pharmacologically active substances as a result of the antigen–antibody reaction. Before a substance can be accepted as playing a role in the symptomatology of anaphylactic hypersensitivity it should fulfil the following criteria: (a) It should be released at the site of the reaction. (b) It should be capable of mimicking the symptoms of the hypersensitive state. (c) The symptoms of the hypersensitive state should be susceptible to inhibition by known antagonists of the pharmacologically active substance. Currently four substances require consideration as possible pharmacological mediators—histamine, the slow-reacting substance SRS(A), bradykinin and serotonin. All four have been found to be released by sensitized guinea-pig tissue in the course of in vivo or in vitro anaphylactic reactions.

Histamine

The main source of histamine is the mast cell, the granules of which appear to be composed of a loose complex of histamine and heparin. Histamine is a potent constrictor of both human and guinea-pig smooth muscle, including that of the bronchioles. In addition it causes a marked increase in capillary permeability and is a potent vasodilator. Considerable information on the mechanism of histamine release from sensitized mast cells in the presence of antigen, has been obtained by the use of chopped guinea-pig lung preparations. Under these conditions, as shown by Mongar and Schild, release of histamine depends on the activation of an esterase which, like $C'1$, can be inhibited by the esterase inhibitor, diisopropylfluorophosphate. The esterase involved can be differentiated from $C'1$ esterase by differences in susceptibility to various inhibitors, and by its activation by guinea-pig γ_1 but not γ_2 antibodies.

The importance of histamine in the pathogenesis of anaphylactic reactions in the guinea-pig is established by a number of lines of evidence.

1. Anaphylactic shock is associated with an increase in blood histamine levels, and histamine is readily released from perfused or chopped sensitized guinea-pig lung on exposure to antigen.

2. Guinea-pig bronchiolar tissue is highly susceptible to the action of histamine, and the symptoms of acute anaphylaxis can be mimicked by the administration of histamine.

3. Guinea-pigs can be protected from fatal anaphylactic shock by the administration of anti-histamines. Anti-histamines, however, have diverse chemical structures, and some of their recorded effects on anaphylactic syndromes could therefore be due to activities other than histamine antagonism.

Certain substances are capable of inducing a non-specific release of histamine from cells and have been found capable, on injection, of producing reactions resembling those found in anaphylactic shock. To distinguish these reactions from anaphylaxis they are known as *anaphylactoid* reactions. The resemblance to anaphylaxis is most marked in the reactions produced by peptone. In addition, trypsin, organic mercurials and serum which has been treated with various agents such as starch, agar or kaolin are capable of producing anaphylactoid reactions.

SRS(A)

This substance was shown by Kelleway and Trethewie to be released from sensitized guinea-pig lung when challenged with antigen. A pharmacologically identical substance has been obtained from human asthmatic lung. Under in vitro conditions SRS(A) has a marked capacity to contract guinea-pig ileum and human bronchiolar muscle but its action differs from that of histamine in showing a characteristically slow and prolonged contraction, and in being insensitive to anti-histamines. The precise cell of origin is unknown but it is probably not the mast cell. Unlike histamine, SRS(A) is not preformed in the tissues and is produced apparently as a result of antigen–antibody combination. SRS(A) has not yet been chemically characterized but is an acidic substance possibly an unsaturated fatty acid.

Bradykinin

This is a nonapeptide which can be produced by the action of trypsin and other proteases on a precursor—*bradykininogen*—present in the α 2 fraction of the plasma globulins. In anaphylactic reactions bradykinin is produced by the action of proteolytic enzymes released from tissue cells as a result of antibody-antigen combination. Bradykinin resembles histamine in its action on human and guinea-pig smooth muscle, and has a marked capacity for increasing capillary permeability. It is reported to have a marked vasodilator effect on the coronary vessels. Like histamine it is rapidly destroyed in the tissues. There is no known antagonist, and since its action is not antagonized by anti-histamines, it probably makes only a minor contribution to anaphylactic shock in the guinea-pig.

Serotonin (5-hydroxytryptamine)

This substance can cause bronchial and ileal smooth muscle contraction in the guinea-pig but has no effect on human bronchiolar muscle; nor does it increase capillary permeability. It appears to have a constrictor effect on the larger blood vessels. Serotonin is rapidly destroyed in vivo and is neutralized by lysergic acid. It appears to be the main mediator of anaphylactic reactions in rats and mice, in the mast cells of which it is present in considerable concentration. Although present in the chromaffin cells of the intestinal tracts of man and other animals it does not appear to play any significant role in human or guinea-pig anaphylactic syndromes.

Systemic Anaphylactic-Type Hypersensitivity in Man

Man develops systemic anaphylactic hypersensitivity much less readily than the guinea-pig. Systemic anaphylaxis has been described under the following conditions.

1. After injecting diphtheria or tetanus antitoxins. The majority of people affected have had a history of spontaneous local hypersensitivity, particularly of asthmatic type (see below), to horse dander. Less frequently, sensitization is the result of previous administration of horse serum.

2. Following the administration of drugs, penicillin—to which many people have now been rendered hypersensitive—undoubtedly being the worst offender. Many cases of fatal anaphylaxis in man, following the injection of penicillin, have occurred as a result of self-administration. In persons highly sensitive to penicillin it has been estimated that as little as 3×10^{-6} units of benzyl penicillin can give rise to a systemic reaction. The antibodies primarily involved appear to be specific for benzyl penicilloic acid, a degradation product of penicillin, which when complexed with plasma or tissue protein, constitutes the sensitizing antigen. In some cases the antibody specificity has also been directed to the carrier protein. Although in man most cases of fatal anaphylaxis due to penicillin have followed injection of the drug, some have been the result of oral administration.

3. Following insect bites, particularly bee or wasp stings. It has been estimated that from six to twelve people per year die in the British Isles in this way. Persons with an allergy to insect bites appear to acquire first a delayed hypersensitivity (p. 179), which is then followed by an immediate skin reactivity. After further bites this cutaneous hypersensitivity usually disappears but in a few individuals it may become intensified, ultimately to form the basis of a systemic anaphylactic reaction.

4. Following the injection of various prophylactics—e.g. tetanus toxoid (p. 390)—prepared from media containing components to which very exceptionally an individual may exhibit a spontaneous hypersensitivity.

5. Following intradermal injection of pollen extracts for the identification of allergens in atopic, particularly asthmatic subjects (p. 174).

6. Following miscellaneous intravenous injections, e.g. of contrast media in intravenous pyelography.

The commonest clinical pattern in acute anaphylaxis in man is that of severe repiratory distress due, as in the guinea-pig, to bronchiolar constriction, together with the signs of vascular collapse consequent on vasodilatation. Laryngeal oedema, which may itself be sufficient to cause death, is an important additional component. As in the guinea-pig, the main pharmacological mediator appears to be histamine, presumed, though not shown conclusively, to be derived from mast cells.

Local Anaphylactic Reactions in Man

Hypersensitive states in which a person reacts to substances encountered during the course of everyday life, are frequently known as *idiosyncrasies* or, collectively, as *atopy*. The most important of these conditions are hay fever and asthma, in which the symptoms are confined to the respiratory tract, and eczema and urticaria which involve the skin. Respiratory allergies are usually due to plant pollens and to various types of vegetable and animal dusts. The allergic state is normally the result of the inhalation of the allergen, but asthmatic symptoms may be caused by the ingestion of the antigen which is then carried to the respiratory tract via the blood. Eczema and urticaria are usually the result of the ingestion of an allergen in food. Children with atopic eczema are often sensitive to eggs. In adults, the food allergens of most importance are nuts and fish. Skin allergies of immediate type are also caused by a variety of drugs, mainly as a result of direct contact of the drug with the skin rather than by transmission through the blood from the intestinal tract.

In most, but not in all cases of idiosyncrasy, hypersensitivity can be passively transferred to normal persons. Passive transfer is most readily achieved by the *Prausnitz-Kuestner* technique. In this procedure serum from the sensitive person is injected into the skin of a normal one. If the allergen is subsequently injected into the same area, a local immediate-type reaction occurs. The technique was first used in the case of Kuestner, who was sensitive to a variety of cooked fish. Some of Kuestner's serum was injected into Prausnitz's skin; following introduction of a small amount of cooked fish at the same site a local reaction developed. The Prausnitz–Kuestner reaction can also be elicited when the allergen is injected first and is followed by infection of the serum.

The substances responsible for passive transfer are known as *reagins*. Reagins are non-precipitating, have a marked tendency for fixation to human skin, in which they may persist for some weeks, are heat-labile—being destroyed in half-an-hour at 60° C—and are unable to cross the placental barrier. Unlike IgG precipitating antibodies, however, they do not sensitize guinea-pigs to anaphylactic reactions. They have many of the properties of IgA antibodies with which they have for some years been identified. Recently however evidence has been presented by Ishizaka suggesting that reaginic activity is a property of a newly described immunoglobulin IgE (γE) which is distinguishable immunologically from IgA.

Most of the clinical manifestations of the idiosyncrasies can be attributed to smooth muscle contraction and increased capillary permeability—changes characteristic of histamine action. The beneficial effect of the anti-histamine drugs in treatment also supports the view that histamine release plays an important part in the production of symptoms. Anti-histamine drugs appear to be more effective in controlling the vascular than the muscular manifestations of the idiosyncrasies and there is reason to believe that, at least in the latter, factors other than histamine may be involved.

Introduction of the allergen into the skin of a patient with an idiosyncrasy is followed by an immediate wheal-and-flare type reaction. Skin tests are frequently used clinically, although often unsuccessfully, in an attempt to identify the substance responsible for a clinical allergy.

In some cases it is possible to desensitize a sensitive patient by giving a course of injections of small amounts of antigen over a period of some weeks. The injections appear to stimulate the production of a relatively heat-stable non-precipitating antibody which is capable of neutralizing the allergen and does not become fixed to the tissues. This antibody apparently blocks the action of the antigen and prevents it from combining with the tissue-fixed sensitizing antibody (reagin).

Although the idiosyncrasies are characterized by the development of local anaphylactic reactions, subjects who exhibit these syndromes nevertheless possess a general anaphylactic sensitization. This is indicated by the development of an immediate wheal-and-flare type reaction following introduction of the allergen into the skin. Skin tests are frequently used clinically, though often unsuccessfully, in an attempt to identify the substance responsible for a clinical allergy. They must be applied with considerable care, however, as they can induce serious, and occasionally fatal, systemic anaphylactic reactions.

In one type of human atopy, that of hypersensitivity to ragweed, it has been found possible to demonstrate the release of histamine from the leucocytes of sensitive persons by exposure to antigen. The kinetics of the reaction appear to be identical with that of the antigen induced liberation of histamine from sensitized guinea-pig lungs (p. 171).

It is frequently stated that there is a marked hereditary tendency in the idiosyncrasies, but the evidence for this is doubtful. It is nevertheless true that atopic persons possess an unusual capacity for allergic sensitization. This is shown by the frequent occurrence of cutaneous allergy and respiratory allergy in the same subject. It has been estimated that about 60 per cent of children with atopic eczema subsequently develop respiratory allergy. We do not know, however, why such subjects are hypersensitive to only one, or at most, a limited number of allergens, nor what determines the localization of the allergic reaction to the skin or to the upper or lower respiratory tract.

Recent work with pollen allergens has shown that the most potent of these are polypeptides of low molecular weight. It is possible that this property may be important in allowing them to traverse respiratory or intestinal mucous membranes. In this case, differences in permeability may explain the differences in localization of allergic reactions in different individuals or in the same individual at different ages.

Arthus Reaction

This name is applied to an inflammatory reaction with particular involvement of the blood vessels which may occur in the tissues of a sensitized animal as a result of local antibody–antigen reaction. The reaction was first described in the rabbit. Rabbits repeatedly injected intradermally with horse serum produce no reaction to the earlier injections. With later injections, however, an oedematous and haemorrhagic reaction, in some cases progressing to necrosis, may appear at the injection site. Arthus-type reactions have been produced in a wide range of experimental animals and in a variety of tissues but are most readily studied in the skin. As an experimental animal the rabbit is preferred to the guinea-pig as it less readily develops anaphylactic-type sensitivity. Like anaphylactic reactions the Arthus reaction is dependent on humoral antibody. In contrast to the anaphylactic reaction the antibody is not fixed to tissue cells and the antigen–antibody reaction involved takes place freely in the tissue fluids. Although it is classified as an immediate-type hypersensitivity, the Arthus reaction is much slower in development than anaphylactic reactions, the lesions attaining their maximal extent usually from between 4 and 10 hours after injection.

On histological examination the characteristic feature is an inflammatory reaction, associated with the infiltration of large numbers of polymorphonuclear leucocytes, in the walls of small blood vessels, particularly of venules. In addition to polymorphonuclear infiltration, antigen–antibody complexes and complement are demonstrable in the vessel walls, by the fluorescent antibody technique. Sensitization may be induced passively by the intravenous injection of serum from a sensitized animal. The reaction may then be elicited if the antigen is injected into the skin. The antigen is usually injected immediately after the injection of antibody, but if it is delayed the cutaneous reaction produced, particularly in the guinea-pig, may be of anaphylactic type. Arthus-type sensitivity may also be elicited if the antibody is injected into the skin and is followed by intravenous injection of the antigen. This is known as the reversed passive Arthus reaction.

Two features of passive Arthus sensitization should be noted: (1) The reaction may be elicited if the antigen is injected before or immediately after the antibody, indicating that no latent period is required for tissue fixation of the antibody, as would be required in anaphylactic reactions. (2) The typical Arthus reaction requires that either the antibody or the antigen should be present in the circulation, and the other reagent outside it. As a result antibody–antigen complexes can be formed, through diffusion of the antigen and antibody towards one another, in the walls of the blood vessels.

Arthus reactions can be produced only by antibody capable of precipitating the antigen. This is apparent in the incapability of antisera containing only non-precipitating antibodies to effect passive transfer of Arthus sensitivity. Also the capacity of different animals to undergo sensitization parallels their capacity to produce precipitating antibody. Moreover, reactions produced in different animals of a species by active sensitization vary directly with the titre of precipitating antibody produced.

There is considerable evidence that complement is essential for the development of the Arthus reaction.

1. Passive Arthus sensitization may be produced by guinea-pig γ_2 antibodies which can fix complement, but not by guinea-pig γ_1 antibodies which are incapable of doing so.

2. Arthus reactions do not occur in rabbits which are congenitally deficient in the $C'3$ component.

3. Arthus reactions do not occur in animals which have been depleted of complement by injection of aggregated gamma globulin, zymosan or carrageenin. The work of Boyden suggests that the adsorption of complement to the antigen–antibody complex on the vascular wall stimulates the release of a heat-stable leucotaxic substance from plasma.

The principal mediators of the Arthus reaction are undoubtedly the polymorphonuclear leucocytes. In animals which have been depleted of polymorphs by administration of nitrogen mustards, antigen–antibody complexes have been found to accumulate in blood vessel walls but Arthus reactions do not develop. It is probable that the polymorphs accumulating at the site of an Arthus reaction liberate hydrolytic enzymes which are responsible for degenerative changes in the walls of the blood vessels. A definitive substrate for such enzymes, however, has not yet been defined. Anti-histamines appear to be without significant effect in the prevention of Arthus reactions, and although histamine may be released as a result of tissue damage it clearly does not play an important role in the pathogenesis of the condition.

Arthus-like reactions can also be produced by the injection of soluble antigen–antibody complexes prepared in the region of antigen excess. These may be obtained by precipitating an antigen such as bovine serum albumen with antibody, washing the precipitate and redissolving the latter in excess antigen. The reactions produced by soluble complexes differ from those previously described in being slower in onset, showing maximal activity some 20 to 24 hours after injection, and in that the polymorphonuclear accumulation occurs mainly in the interstitial tissues, with little evidence of vascular involvement.

In man, Arthus-like cutaneous reactions similar to those observed in experimental animals have been observed in patients who have received several injections of antitoxic sera for the prophylaxis of tetanus or diphtheria, and in those receiving repeated injections of insulin. It is probable, however, that Arthus-type sensitivity is of much greater importance in the human subject than is indicated by these examples. There is little doubt that it plays a major role in the pathogenesis of the serum sickness syndrome, whether this is produced by the injection of serum or following drug administration. It could also be implicated in the production of rheumatic carditis, glomerulonephritis and possibly in other chronic diseases of undetermined aetiology which are believed to have an immunological component.

SERUM SICKNESS

The term serum sickness was first applied by Von Pirquet and Schick to a condition which may occur in man following the injection of horse serum. Its incidence is much less with modern refined antitoxins than with the crude horse serum at one time widely used. The symptom complex of a serum sickness has also been observed after the administration of various drugs—notably the sulphonamides, penicillin, streptomycin and the organic arsenicals. These drugs are not antigenic in themselves but form antigenic complexes by combination with plasma and tissue protein. In the case of serum sickness proper, the onset of symptoms is usually from 7 to 14 days after injection.

The first symptom is in general the appearance of an urticarial rash at the site of injection. This is followed by a general urticaria, oedema of the subcutaneous tissues, particularly of the neck with, in more severe cases, pain and swelling of the joints, glandular enlargement, particularly of the glands draining the site of injection and pyrexia.

That the condition has an immunological basis was strongly suggested by the demonstration—shortly after the onset of symptoms—of precipitins for horse serum in the sera of affected patients, and from the fact that subjects who fail to produce precipitins do not develop serum sickness. A precise examination of the relationship between antibody production and antigen elimination, to the development of symptoms, has, however, proved virtually impossible in patients injected with horse serum, because of the mutiplicity of antigens present even in purified preparations of the latter. Such a correlation has however been achieved, by Kendall, following the injection of purified bovine albumen. Three phases were distinguishable.

1. A period of rapid fall in blood antigen concentration—due to equilibration of antigen between intravascular and extravascular fluids.

2. A phase of slow logarithmic decrease in antigen concentration—due to non-immune catabolism of the antigen.

3. A phase of rapid exponential immune elimination. The onset of this phase was found to coincide with the appearance of symptoms, and only at the end of this phase was antibody demonstrable in the patient's serum; coincident with this the symptoms disappeared.

The coincidence of the appearance of symptoms with the onset of the third or immune phase of antigen elimination clearly relates the development of symptoms to the presence in the circulation of antigen–antibody complexes, formed in the region of antigen excess. As we have seen (p. 177), such complexes have been found to be highly effective in eliciting Arthus-type reactions. There is therefore good reason to believe that the inflammatory lesions found in serum sickness are due to reactions of this type. Antigen–antibody complexes capable of producing Arthus-type reactions must be formed frequently in the tissues during bacterial and other infections, and following various forms of immunization. These, however, are not associated with overt symptoms of the serum sickness syndrome. This is probably due to the fact that the complexes are present only in low concentration. Following the administration of serum or as a result of drug therapy, however, complexes are formed in sufficiently high concentrations to produce overt symptoms.

In addition to Arthus-type reactions some of the components of the serum sickness complex are clearly caused by concomitant anaphylactic-type hyper-sensitivity, viz. fever, urticaria, oedema of the eyelids and the asthma which occasionally develops. Consistently with this, reaginic-type antibodies have on occasion been demonstrated in the serum of serum sickness patients. The presence of an anaphylactic component explains why anti-histamines have some ameliorative effect in these conditions.

The pathogenesis of the serum sickness syndrome has been considerably elucidated by a study of similar syndromes in experimental animals. It has long been known that various forms of tissue damage, notably glomerulonephritis, endocarditis and arteritis could be produced in rabbits by the injection of complex, naturally occurring proteins. With the demonstration that such lesions could be produced by the injection of purified proteins, e.g. bovine albumen, and bovine gamma globulin, a more detailed analysis of the experimental disease became possible. Under these conditions the three phases of antigen elimination referred to above, and the relationship of the onset of symptoms to the initiation of the immune phase of antigen elimination, have been clearly demonstrated. Following the elimination of antigen and the appearance of excess antibody the symptoms gradually subside. From such data it is apparent that the onset of symptoms is related to the presence in the circulation of antigen--antibody complexes formed in the region of antigen excess. For bovine albumen, it has been estimated that the most damaging complexes are those formed with a ratio of three molecules of antigen to two of antibody.

The specific damaging effect of complexes produced in the region of antigen excess appears to be due to the fact that, unlike the larger complexes produced in the equivalence zone, they are not readily disposed of by the reticulo-endothelial system. Precisely in what way they initiate the lesions responsible for the condition is, however, unknown. There is little doubt that symptoms are produced as a result of damage inflicted at the site of localization of the complexes, the presence of which has been demonstrated by the fluorescent antibody technique. The basis for this tissue localization has not been explained. In the case of the glomeruli, however, it can be presumed that localization is in some way a result of their filtration function. In addition glomerular endothelium has been shown to have a phagocytic effect. These factors may also be of importance in the pathogenesis of the acute nephritis which sometimes develops in human subjects after streptococcal infection (Chapter 14).

DELAYED-TYPE HYPERSENSITIVITY

This term is applied to a group of hypersensitivities in which there is an appreciable delay between the exposure to the antigen and the development of symptoms. Delayed-type hypersensitivities are demonstrable by a cutaneous reactivity which usually attains a maximum some 24 to 48 hours after introduction of the antigen. This is in marked contrast to immediate-type hyper-sensitivities of anaphylactic type in which the cutaneous reaction occurs almost immediately. A second major difference from anaphylactic-type hypersensitivity is that the reactions are histologically of an inflammatory character with a preponderance, when fully developed, of mononuclear type cells. The cutaneous reactions are erythematous and indurated, and not of the wheal-and-flare type characteristic of anaphylactic hypersensitivity. Thirdly, delayed-type hypersensitivities show no evidence of the participation of any of the pharmacologically active mediators found in anaphylactic hypersensitivity.

In contrast to both varieties of immediate-type hypersensitivity, delayed-type hypersensitivities cannot be passively transferred by the serum of a sensitive animal. They occur in the absence of demonstrable humoral antibody, and may be present in subjects—hypogammaglobulinaemics—who are constitutionally incapable of producing such antibody. Delayed-type hypersensitivity can, however, be transferred passively to normal animals by the injection of cells taken from lymph nodes, spleen or peritoneal exudates or of leucocytes from the peripheral blood, of sensitive animals. The cell responsible for the transfer of sensitivity has been identified beyond reasonable doubt as the lymphocyte.

Although delayed-type hypersensitivity can be readily produced in experimental animals, man appears to be particularly outstanding in his capacity to develop this type of immunological reactivity. It occurs in two main clinical forms:

1. Delayed Hypersensitivity to Microbial Antigens Developing during the Course of Infection

It seems likely that delayed-type hypersensitivity to microbial components plays an important part in the pathogenesis and evolution of most, if not all, human microbial infections. This is notably so in the case of tuberculosis. The presence of delayed-type cutaneous reactivity can also be demonstrated in leprosy, brucellosis, soft sore, glanders, lymphogranuloma venereum, most fungal infections and many viral diseases. In all cases in which it has been possible to identify the antigen responsible for sensitization, it has been found to be protein.

The paradigm of delayed-type bacterial hypersensitivity is that which develops as a result of infection with the tubercle bacillus, and is demonstrable by the tuberculin reaction (p. 359). This was the first bacterial hypersensitivity to be discovered and is still the most dramatic in its clinical manifestations. The hypersensitive state is in this case directed towards the tuberculoprotein commonly known as tuberculin. Tuberculin, now usually employed in a highly purified form—PPD—will elicit a characteristic erythematous indurated cutaneous reaction on introduction into the skin of hypersensitive subjects. The cutaneous reaction normally attains a maximum between 24 and 48 hours. The reaction subsides slowly and may take several days or some weeks to disappear completely. In highly sensitive subjects there may be considerable swelling at the reaction site, and the centre of the lesion may undergo necrosis. Injection of tuberculin into experimental animals suffering from an active tuberculous infection is associated also with the development of focal reactions around the sites of infection, and with general systemic reactions which can be very severe.

Histologically, the cutaneous tuberculin reaction is characterized by an infiltration of mononuclear cells, and it has usually been assumed on the basis of morphological evidence that most of these cells are primarily lymphocytic in origin. Recent observations on cells labelled with tritiated thymidine, however, suggest that many of the cells previously identified as leucocytes are in fact histocytes or macrophages. Although delayed-type reactions can be elicited by the injection of tuberculin, the injection of tuberculin alone cannot induce sensitization. Sensitivity is readily produced, however, by a tuberculous infection, by injection of live attenuated bacilli, e.g. the BCG strain or by the injection of killed organisms, though the latter are much less effective in inducing hypersensitivity than are live organisms.

2. Contact Sensitivity

This denotes a hypersensitivity that develops from the contact of potentially sensitizing material with the skin. Spontaneous hypersensitivity of this type is quite common in man, when it is known as *contact dermatitis*. It can be produced as a result of exposure of the skin to a variety of substances; sulphonamides, organic arsenicals, antibiotics, formalin, paraphenylene-diamine (a substance used in the dyeing of furs), active agents present in poison ivy, primula and other plants, laundry marking-ink derived from the nut of the ral tree, picric acid and various ions including mercury, iodine, nickel, cobalt, zirconium and beryllium. It is clear that many of these substances are not antigens. All the available evidence, however, indicates that they become antigenic by combination with proteins found in the skin or the tissues.

In contact sensitivity, it may be possible to identify the substance responsible for the sensitivity by patch tests in which the suspected substance is applied to the skin. In such cases positive reactions may be obtained not only from the area initially sensitized, but from any part of the skin surface.

Contact sensitivity can be readily produced in the guinea-pig, and this model has been extremely useful in the study of delayed-type hypersensitivity in general. Most work has been carried out using picryl chloride, and nitro and halo substituted benzenes, e.g. 2,4-dinitrochlorobenzene and 2,4-dinitro-fluorobenzene. These compounds have been found to form complexes readily with the amino and sulphydryl groups of proteins. Some substances which are incapable of combining with protein themselves, however, give rise to degradation products which can combine with protein. Thus it is probable that penicillin hypersensitivity of anaphylactic as well as of delayed type is due to the formation of complexes of protein with benzyl penicilloic and benzyl penicillenic acid. As in the human subject, positive reactions may be elicited from any part of the skin surface. In spite of this, the skin does not itself appear to be sensitized since a skin graft from a sensitive animal to a normal non-sensitive animal does not retain the sensitivity. A skin graft from a non-sensitive animal to a sensitive animal, however, does acquire sensitivity. It is clear that the sensitivity is due to the migration of sensitized cells or, possibly, of some soluble substances capable of effecting sensitization into the skin.

Mechanisms Involved in Delayed-Type Hypersensitivity

From what has already been said, it can be seen that a great variety of antigens are capable of stimulating the production both of humoral antibodies, including those responsible for anaphylactic hypersensitivity, and of delayed-type hypersensitivity. Whether a delayed hypersensitivity is produced would appear to depend, at least among the protein antigens (there is some doubt as to whether polysaccharides can produce delayed-type hypersensitivity), on the circumstances and conditions under which the antigen makes contact with the animal body, rather than on an inherent property of the antigen itself.

1. Certain substances, notably the wax D of the tubercle bacillus, have a directive effect on the immune response so that delayed-type hypersensitivity is produced. The way in which this effect is exerted is unknown. It has recently been shown by White and his associates that the wax is capable of combining with protein, and this capacity may play an important part in its directive function. Moreover it is possible that the adjuvant material stimulates a specific mononuclear type of inflammatory response which is essential for the establishment of this type of hypersensitivity.

2. Soluble antigens, particularly those of low molecular weight, are most likely to cause delayed-type hypersensitivity when introduced into the skin. It is possible that the role of the skin in facilitating the development of delayed-type reactions may be due to its rich supply of lymphatic channels which allow ready access of the antigen to the lymph nodes. Alternatively it is possible that the skin contains substances with an adjuvant action analogous to that of the wax of the tubercle bacillus. In this context the high fatty acid content of the skin is undoubtedly of interest.

Transient delayed-type hypersensitivity to protein antigens has also been produced following the injection of very small amounts of antigen. Thus delayed-type hypersensitivity has been produced in guinea-pigs by the injection of very small amounts of egg white or horse serum—the hypersensitivity appearing on the fourth or fifth day after injection and disappearing with the appearance of humoral antibody. Similar transient reactions may be produced by antigen–antibody complexes formed in the region of antibody excess, and by the injection of proteins heavily coupled with haptenic groups.

Immunological Basis of Delayed-Type Hypersensitivity

There is no doubt that delayed-type hypersensitivity has an immunological basis. This is clearly shown in the serological specificity of the reactions. In fact they appear to be more specific than concomitant immediate-type sensitivities or in vitro reactions involving the same antigens. Thus guinea-pigs sensitized with 2,4-dinitrophenol (DNP) guinea-pig albumen complex, only show delayed-type reaction to the corresponding homologous antigen, and fail to react, for example, to 2,4-dinitrophenol bovine gamma globulin. The reaction has a specificity directed towards both the haptenic group and the carrier. On the other hand, guinea-pigs anaphylactically sensitized with DNP guinea-pig albumen produce anti-DNP precipitating antibodies which react with all conjugated proteins incorporating DNP as haptenic group. It is clear that the delayed-type reaction involves a larger antigenic determinant than is involved in classical antigen–antibody reactions. In the case of substances, such as picryl chloride, which are not in themselves antigenic but against which contact hypersensitivity may be induced, clear evidence has been obtained of an immunological specificity directed towards conjugates of the sensitizing substances and the animal's own protein.

The capacity of hypogammaglobulinaemics to develop delayed-type hypersensitivity, the failure to transfer sensitivity passively with serum, together with the ability to transfer it passively with cells derived from lymphoid tissues and with blood leucocytes, have created a strong prima facie case that delayed hypersensitivity is a manifestation of cellular rather than of humoral immunity (p. 117). It must nevertheless be considered possible that it could be due to a type of humoral antibody which might be manufactured by hypogammaglobulinaemics and might be produced by the lymphoid cells used in passive transfer experiments or their descendants or by cells which can accept specific instructions from these. Karush and Eisen have suggested that it may be due to an antibody which is present in such low concentration in the blood that passive transfer is not possible, but which at the same time has a very high affinity for antigen. No such antibody has been demonstrated, however, and in general, highly avid antibodies are produced late in immunization rather than at the early stage at which delayed hypersensitivity normally appears. An alternative suggestion is that it may be due to a *cytophilic* antibody of the type described in guinea-pig sera by Boyden. Cytophilic antibody has a high affinity for macrophages, and macrophages which have been passively sensitized with it will adsorb homologous antigens, and if these are particulate, e.g. red cells, will agglutinate them. So far, however, it has not proved possible to transfer delayed-type hypersensitivity in animals, by injection of macrophages which have been passively sensitized with macrophage cytophilic antibody.

The case against humoral antibody, and for a cellular mechanism, has been greatly strengthened in recent years by the demonstration of the dissociability of antibody producing capacity, and of the capacity to develop delayed-type hypersensitivity. This dissociation is particularly readily demonstrated in fowl, in which removal in ovo of the bursa of Fabricius in the hind gut eliminates the capacity to produce antibody without affecting the capacity to produce delayed-type hypersensitivity, and removal of the thymus eliminates the capacity to produce delayed-type hypersensitivity without affecting antibody production. In animals the latter effect has also been achieved by administration of 6-mercaptopurine, by the injection of anti-lymphocyte serum, and by the induction of tolerance in neonates, followed by the injection of antigen in Freund adjuvant, when some animals subsequently develop the capacity to produce antibody. In man, the converse of hypogammaglobulinaemia is seen in Hodgkin's disease, in which there is impairment of the capacity to develop delayed-type hypersensitivity but in which antibody production is unaffected. Evidence has been presented by Turk of an anatomical separation of antibody producing and delayed-hypersensitivity function. In animals actively producing antibody, Turk observed a marked development of germinal centres in the lymphoid follicles of lymph glands. In animals showing delayed hypersensitivity responses, no alteration in lymphoid follicles was observed but there was a marked proliferation of pyroninophilic cells in the paracortical areas of the glands.

There is evidence that macrophages also have a role of considerable importance in delayed hypersensitivity: (1) Most of the cells which infiltrate and take part in delayed-type reactions appear to be macrophages. (2) In passive transfer experiments with tritium-labelled lymphocytes the proportion of labelled cells in the lesions range only from 2 to 8 per cent. (3) In plasma clot explants of lymphoid tissue the migration of macrophages from the clot is markedly inhibited by antigen, whereas the migration of lymphocytes is little, if at all, affected. The sensitivity of the macrophage does not, however, appear to be an intrinsic property but to depend on the presence of sensitized lymphocytes. The sensitivity of macrophages from sensitized animals is lost after a relatively short period of culture, and a small population of lymphocytes has been shown to be capable of transferring sensitivity to a very much larger population —up to 50 times greater—of macrophages. The substance responsible for transfer has been shown to be released by sensitized lymphocytes, following exposure to antigen. Its precise nature has not been identified. It may be an antibody or an antibody-like substance, its release constituting in effect a secondary response, or it could be some pharmacologically active substance which has the capacity to modify the response of the macrophage.

Passive Transfer of Delayed-Type Hypersensitivity

The capacity to transfer delayed-type hypersensitivity passively by lymphoid cells and blood leucocytes of sensitive animals has played a major part in the development of the concept that the immunological specificity of these reactions depends on the surface specificity of sensitized lymphoid cells. The passive transfer of all types of delayed reactivity is readily achieved in the guinea-pig. Peritoneal exudate cells have been mostly used for this purpose. The persistence of hypersensitivity after passive transfer in the guinea-pig is of short duration since it appears to require the continued viability of the transferred cells. In man, passive transfer of tuberculin hypersensitivity and of other delayed-type bacterial hypersensitivities has been achieved by the injection of leucocytes from sensitive persons. Contact sensitivity has proved more difficult to transfer passively in man but has been achieved in hypogammaglobulinaemic subjects. Although the cell suspensions used for transfer contain a variety of cell types it is generally believed that the cell which mediates transfer is the lymphocyte.

It has been shown by Laurence that it is possible in man to transfer tuberculin hypersensitivity by leucocyte extracts obtained in various ways, e.g. by lysis in distilled water or by alternative freezing and thawing. The active agent in these extracts has been shown to be stable to desoxyribonuclease, ribonuclease and trypsin, to be diffusible and to have a molecular weight of 10,000 or less. The transferred hypersensitivity has in some subjects persisted for 1 to 2 years. As the recipient's leucocytes were also found to yield extracts capable of passive sensitization it was proposed by Laurence that the transfer factor was capable of undergoing replication in the recipient. The significance of these observations are not at the moment clear but they are obviously of the utmost importance in relation to the mechanism of delayed-type hypersensitivity. There are three main possibilities.

1. The transfer factor is in fact sensitizing antigen, associated in the cells with highly active adjuvant which allows it to establish a state of delayed-type hypersensitivity with great rapidity. In the case of passively transferred tuberculin hypersensitivity all efforts to demonstrate material in the extract showing any antigenic resemblance to tuberculin have, however, been unsuccessful.

2. The transfer factor may be an antibody sub-unit. The evidence suggesting replication of the transfer factor is, however, against this possibility. Moreover the reactions involved in delayed-type hypersensitivity differ considerably from those found in the anaphylactic- and Arthus-type antibody mediated hypersensitivities. Immuno-electrophoresis has failed to reveal any antibody globulin or globulin sub-units in active fractions.

3. The transfer factor may be a nucleic acid or a nucleic acid derivative. This appears to be the only basis by which, in the context of our present knowledge, the replication of transfer factor could be explained, but efforts to establish it have so far proved unsuccessful.

Tissue Damage in Delayed-Type Hypersensitivity

In the lungs of tuberculous patients there is extensive damage to the tissue cells, including those of the lung parenchyma. This damage is generally attributed to delayed-type hypersensitivity with which it is certainly significantly correlated. Consistent with the cellular theory of delayed-type hypersensitivity there are three main ways in which this may occur.

1. It may be caused by a direct reaction between sensitive lymphocytes or macrophages and antigen adsorbed to the tissue cells. No experimental model to test this mechanism appears to have been examined.

2. The reaction between antigen and sensitized lymphocytes may result in the liberation of a substance capable of damaging the tissue cells by direct interaction. No such substance has so far been demonstrated.

3. The reaction of antigen with sensitized leucocytes may lead to the liberation of a substance capable of causing damage to the blood vessels.

Recently, evidence has been obtained by Willoughby, Walters and Spector of the accumulation at sites of delayed-type reactions of a vascular permeability factor identified first in lymph nodes (LNPF). It is proposed that this substance may be a natural mediator of delayed-type reactions by causing an increase in vascular permeability, with resultant migration of inflammatory cells from the blood vessels. Although it has not been chemically identified, the behaviour of LNPF appears to resemble that of a highly polymerized RNA. Its precise role in delayed-type hypersensitivity has still to be determined.

There has been considerable controversy as to whether bacterial allergy of delayed type plays a part of any importance in the defence against infection. On the whole it would seem likely that, since it results in the stimulation of an inflammatory reaction, it is of value. The problem has been most studied in connexion with tuberculosis (p. 360). In the present state of our knowledge the problem cannot, however, be decided, and we cannnot say either that the allergic reaction is an important defensive mechanism or, since it results in considerable damage to the sensitized cells, that it is a harmful and undesirable concomitant of immunity.

ALLERGY TO ANTIBACTERIAL DRUGS

Allergic reactions due to the administration of antibiotics and other anti-bacterial drugs are now, because of the very extensive use of these drugs, both on a medical prescription and, as the result of self-administration, of considerable clinical importance. Virtually any type of allergic reaction may be produced. Reactions are observed more frequently in patients who have previously been treated with a drug than in those who are receiving it for the first time. Application to the skin is a particularly potent source of sensitization, and sensitization may occur in persons, such as nurses, who merely handle the drug. There is no evidence that persons of allergic disposition are unduly liable to develop drug reactions. When reactions do occur, however, they are more serious than in the normal person.

By far the worst offender in the production of allergic reactions is penicillin. It is, in fact, responsible for more of these reactions than all the other chemo-therapeutic agents together; this is presumably because it has been used much more frequently.

The reactions observed with these drugs are usually mild, those most frequently found being some degree of fever and rash. Occasionally, however, more serious reactions occur. Anaphylactic shock, although extremely rare, has been observed following the administration of penicillin, and the serum sickness syndrome has been caused by penicillin, streptomycin and the sulphonamides.

PHYSICAL ALLERGY

Certain reactions to physical reagents, e.g. to heat, cold and light, clinically resemble the reactions found in the idiosyncrasies. The mechanism of these physical allergies has not been explained. In some cases the physical agent may act by stimulating the release of histamine in the tissues; in others it may induce hypersensitivity by rendering allergenic some substance normally present in the body.

ALLERGIC DISEASES

By immunization with certain antigens it has been found possible to produce cardiovascular and renal lesions in experimental animals resembling those found in certain of the so-called collagen diseases of man, viz. rheumatic fever, rheumatoid arthritis and acute glomerulonephritis. Lesions of this type were produced in rabbits by Rich by immunization with large amounts of horse serum and by Hawn and Janeway by immunization with beef protein. The lesions were found only when antigen was still present in the circulation and resolved when the antigen was eliminated. They were consequently believed to be allergic in character. The production of these experimental lesions has given support to the view that the human diseases referred to above are also allergic in character. In the case of rheumatic fever and glomerulonephritis many of the proponents of the allergic hypothesis believe that the exciting allergen is some component or product of *Str. pyogenes*, an organism with which these conditions are epidemiologically associated. There is, however, no indication of the particular bacterial antigens which might be responsible nor has any antibody or antibody-like substance capable of producing sensitization been discovered.

More recently evidence has been adduced suggesting that these conditions might instead be manifestations of auto-immunization. If this view should prove to be correct, and at the moment there is no concrete evidence in support of it, they might be regarded as allergic reactions induced by endogenous allergens and possibly associated with a local production of antibody. The role of *Str. pyogenes* in these circumstances would presumably be that of precipitating the auto-immune process. The pathogenesis of these conditions is considered further in Chapter 14.

CORTICOIDS IN ALLERGIC STATES

Many types of allergic reaction, both of immediate and delayed types, are considerably diminished by the administration of corticoids. The effect of these compounds on delayed-type hypersensitivity is probably a result of their capacity to inhibit the inflammatory response. When employed in the control of clinical allergies they must, however, be used with caution since, by depressing the inflammatory reaction, they may permit the rapid spread of any unrecognized infection which may be present.

THE SHWARTZMAN REACTIONS

These are reactions which may be produced in various animals, but most readily in rabbits, by the endotoxins of a variety of Gram negative bacteria and by certain other macromolecular substances. Although they do not appear to have an immunological basis they exhibit a superficial resemblance to certain hypersensitivity states. Two types of reaction have been described—local and general. In the local reaction a small amount of endotoxin is injected into the abdominal skin of the rabbit and then after 24 hours a larger dose of endotoxin is injected intravenously. Within a few hours after the second injection the prepared area of skin shows the development of petechial haemorrhages which coalesce to form a large circular haemorrhagic area. In the production of the generalized reaction both injections are given intravenously. In this case in from 12 to 24 hours after the second injection many of the injected animals die exhibiting at post mortem various haemorrhagic lesions of which the most prominent is a bilateral haemorrhagic cortical necrosis of the kidneys. There is no evidence that Shwartzman-type reactions occur during the course of any bacterial infections but it has been suggested that certain of the biological effects associated with the injection of the endotoxins of the Gram negative bacteria may in fact be due to reactions of this type occurring in naturally sensitized animals.

The mechanism of the Shwartzman reactions is still in dispute. Recent evidence suggests that in the generalized reaction the first injection causes an alteration in fibrinogen so that it becomes precipitable by a substance or substances released from leucocytes by the second injection and that the precipitation of the altered fibrinogen in the small blood vessels is the immediate cause of the vascular damage observed.

CHAPTER 10

ANTIBIOTICS AND OTHER ANTI-BACTERIAL AGENTS USED IN CHEMOTHERAPY

The term chemotherapy was introduced by Ehrlich to indicate the treatment of microbial disease by the administration of a drug which has a lethal or inhibitory effect on the microbe responsible, but which in therapeutic concentrations has little or no toxic action on the tissues. He described such a drug as a 'magic bullet' which, when introduced into the body, would destroy only the bacteria at which it was aimed. This requirement is not met by the disinfectants and antiseptics which were considered in Chapter 4. These substances, although highly active against bacteria, have considerable toxic action on tissue cells.

The substances used in chemotherapy are of very diverse chemical structure. For convenience they may be divided into two categories: (1) Relatively simple compounds which were obtained in the first place by laboratory synthesis. The more important compounds of this type in general use are the sulphonamides, isoniazid (INAH) and PAS. (2) Antibiotics. The term antibiotic is applied to any substance produced by a living organism and which is active against other living organisms. Most are produced by soil actinomycetes. Their production is usually regarded as a mechanism of value to the organism in the struggle for survival. It has been suggested, however, that this view is too facile, that in fact antibiotics are produced by micro-organisms after growth has passed its maximum, and therefore not at a time when their production would have significant survival value.

The various antibacterial agents differ considerably in their range of action, that is in the number and variety of species against which they are effective. The range of action of the agents currently used is considered in some detail at the end of this chapter. As a general rule Gram positive organisms are more susceptible than Gram negatives—the only drug in current clinical use which is selectively active against Gram negatives being polymyxin. The neisseriae share the general susceptibility of the Gram positives. Of the Gram negative bacilli *Pseudomonas aeruginosa* and *Proteus* species are distinguished by their high resistance to most agents. Tubercle bacilli are also highly resistant to chemotherapeutic agents; of the drugs commonly used against other organisms they are sensitive only to streptomycin. They are, however, susceptible to the action of some drugs—e.g. PAS and INAH which have no effect on other organisms. Some antibacterial drugs are active also against chlamydiae and rickettsiae but none have any activity against viruses. The specific problems of antiviral chemotherapy are considered in Chapter 31.

In respect of the type of action they exhibit against bacteria, antibacterial agents are commonly divided into two classes—the bacteriostatic and the bactericidal. Bacteriostatic drugs are drugs which in the concentrations attainable in the body merely inhibit bacterial growth. When the growth of bacteria is inhibited, however, they eventually die and to this extent the bacteriostatic drugs may be described as having a bactericidal effect; this effect is, however, secondary to that of growth inhibition. In contrast to the bacteriostatic drugs the bactericidal drugs have a rapid lethal action. Of the drugs in more general use chloramphenicol, the sulphonamides and the tetracyclines belong to the bacteriostatic group and penicillin, polymyxin, streptomycin, novobiocin and erythromycin to the bactericidal. As a general rule bactericidal drugs are more effective chemotherapeutic agents than bacteriostatic drugs since they are able to sterilize the tissues by themselves. Because of this, and other things being equal, they are usually preferred. Bacteriostatic drugs are nevertheless very effective chemotherapeutic agents, though necessarily somewhat slower in action. Bacteria whose growth has been inhibited by them eventually die. But of greater importance is the fact that a bacterial population which has been controlled by the use of a bacteriostatic drug can be more readily disposed of by the tissue defences.

MODE OF ACTION

In recent years considerable advances have been made in our knowledge of the mode of action of antibacterial drugs. In most cases, however, it is still far from being formulated in precise chemical terms. The problem can be considered from two aspects: (1) Identification of the site of action of the drug and (2) Its precise mechanism of action.

1. With a particular drug more than one biochemical effect may frequently be demonstrated. In such cases it is difficult to determine which is the primary effect and which effects are secondary to this primary change. It may be assumed, however, that a biochemical lesion will be responsible for the death of the cell, or for growth inhibition, only if it is demonstrable in the same concentrations of drug as those which exercise an antibacterial effect. With this qualification we can distinguish the following four major loci of action.

(i) Inhibition of synthesis of the cell wall. This is the point of action of the pencillins, cephalosporins and cycloserine, and almost certainly of bacitracin, vancomycin and ristocetin. As the development of resistance to any one of these is not associated with the development of resistance to the others, they must be presumed to interfere with different stages in the synthesis.

All of these drugs have two features in common: (a) When exposed to them, sensitive bacteria accumulate Park nucleotides in the medium—these compounds were first identified by Park in cultures of Staph. aureus exposed to penicillin, and the most important and largest is a uridine muramyl pentapeptide containing D- and L-alanine, D-glutamic acid and L-lysine, in the same proportions as in the cell wall mucopeptide. The discovery of this compound was the first clear indication that penicillin interfered with the synthesis of the cell

SYNTHESIS OF CELL WALL MUCOPEPTIDE OF *Staphylococcus aureus*

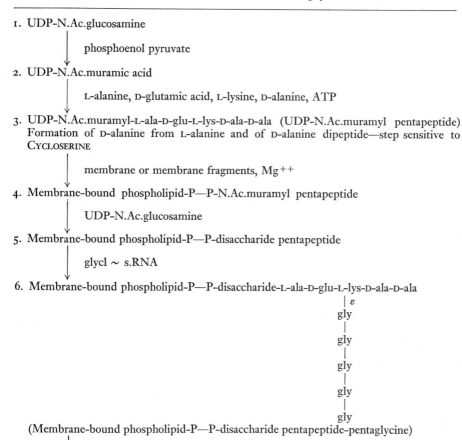

1. UDP-N.Ac.glucosamine

   phosphoenol pyruvate

2. UDP-N.Ac.muramic acid

   L-alanine, D-glutamic acid, L-lysine, D-alanine, ATP

3. UDP-N.Ac.muramyl-L-ala-D-glu-L-lys-D-ala-D-ala   (UDP-N.Ac.muramyl pentapeptide) Formation of D-alanine from L-alanine and of D-alanine dipeptide—step sensitive to CYCLOSERINE

   membrane or membrane fragments, Mg++

4. Membrane-bound phospholipid-P—P-N.Ac.muramyl pentapeptide

   UDP-N.Ac.glucosamine

5. Membrane-bound phospholipid-P—P-disaccharide pentapeptide

   glycl ~ s.RNA

6. Membrane-bound phospholipid-P—P-disaccharide-L-ala-D-glu-L-lys-D-ala-D-ala

   | ε
   gly
   |
   gly
   |
   gly
   |
   gly
   |
   gly

   (Membrane-bound phospholipid-P—P-disaccharide pentapeptide-pentaglycine)

   Mg++

7. (disaccharide-pentapeptide-pentaglycine)$_n$ = polymerization stage with release of murein from membrane. Possibly step sensitive to VANCOMYCIN, RISTOCETIN, BACITRACIN.
8. Cross-linking of terminal glycine to penultimate D-alanine on neighbouring peptide chain through peptide bond formation between free glycine NH_2 and D-alanine COOH. Terminal D-alanine eliminated. This is step sensitive to PENICILLINS and CEPHALOSPORINS.

wall. (*b*) They are inactive against L forms or, in the case of bacitracin which is active against staphylococcal L forms, active against the L form in much higher concentration than against the normal form. It might be expected that a drug which inhibited cell wall synthesis and was inactive against L forms could also be used to produce L forms. So far, however, this has only been achieved with penicillin, the cephalosporins, cycloserine and bacitracin, the latter, however, inducing formation of L forms only in streptococci. Decisive proof that a drug acts by inhibiting the synthesis of the cell wall requires a precise definition of the particular step in synthesis which it affects in an in vitro synthesizing system. This has been established beyond reasonable doubt for the penicillins (p. 201)—the cephalosporins are presumed to have a similar action—and for cycloserine (p. 216).

(ii) Damage to the permeability of the cytoplasmic membrane. Such an effect can be demonstrated with tyrocidin, gramicidin, the polymyxins and the anti-fungal polyene antibiotic nystatin.

(iii) Inhibition of protein synthesis. There is little doubt that this is the primary site of action of chloramphenicol and, probably, of streptomycin, the related antibiotics kanamycin, neomycin, viomycin, paromomycin, and, possibly, of the tetracyclines and erythromycin. Drugs which inhibit protein synthesis without affecting synthesis of nucleic acids act at the level of the ribosome. Failure of a particular synthesis, e.g. that of certain bacterial polypeptide antibiotics, to be inhibited by such drugs can therefore be taken as evidence that the synthesis is non-ribosomal.

(iv) Inhibition of nucleic acid synthesis. A number of antibiotics appear to act by inhibiting the synthesis of nucleic acids. Although of considerable theoretical interest, none of these are of importance in chemotherapy. From the chemotherapeutic standpoint, the most important group of compounds inhibiting nucleic acid synthesis are the sulphonamides.

2. So far as the mechanism of action of chemotherapeutic agents is concerned, the most clearly defined is that generally known as *nutritional antagonism*. This denotes the interference of a drug with the utilization of an essential bacterial metabolite or intermediate resembling it in chemical structure. Because of this resemblance the drug can compete with the metabolite in some essential reaction involving the latter, but is nevertheless incapable of fulfilling the function of the metabolite in the cell.

The classic model of nutritional antagonism is the action of the sulphonamides, shown by Woods, in 1940, to interfere competitively with the utilization of para-aminobenzoic acid (PABA), of which they are structural analogues. Woods demonstrated that the relationship between PABA and sulphonamide is a competitive one, the inhibitory action of the sulphonamide being reversible by the addition of PABA. It was subsequently shown that, together with glutamate and pteridine residues, PABA is an essential component of the molecule of folic acid. The synthesis of folic acid from its components, and the inhibition of this synthesis by sulphonamide have been clearly demonstrated in bacterial extracts. It is of interest, however, that while preventing the incorporation of PABA into the corresponding pteroic acid, the sulphonamide is incorporated into a similar but non-functional product. The role of folic acid in the cell has been established as that of providing derivatives which can function as carriers of one-carbon units in the synthesis of various compounds—particularly purine bases, thymine and the amino acids serine and methionine. As might be expected, these end products, as well as folic acid, are able to inhibit sulphonamide activity non-competitively.

A second analogue of para-aminobenzoic acid with appreciable antibacterial properties is para-aminosalicylic acid (PAS). This compound presumably acts in the same way as the sulphonamides but its spectrum of action is surprisingly different, being active only against the tubercle bacillus. Conversely, the growth of tubercle bacilli is not inhibited by sulphonamides. The precise basis for these differences remains unexplained but, presumably, the configuration of the enzyme of the tubercle bacillus responsible for PABA incorporation is such that it combines with PAS and not with the sulphonamides. Per contra, organisms whose growth is inhibited by sulphonamide presumably possess enzymes whose configuration does not permit combination with PAS. On this basis it seems possible that the insusceptibility of many bacteria to sulphonamides is due to a lack of affinity of the homologous enzyme for sulphonamide.

The lack of toxicity of sulphonamides for tissue cells is due to the fact that tissue cells require preformed folic acid, the utilization of which—unlike the incorporation of PABA—is not sulphonamide sensitive. Appreciable amounts of folic acid and folic acid derivatives are present in animal tissues. These compounds cannot however be used directly by the great majority of pathogenic bacterial species. They will not substitute for the PABA requirement of the latter, and therefore will not antagonize sulphonamide action.

Attempts have been made to develop other chemotherapeutic agents on the sulphonamide model, which would antagonize the action of various essential growth factors because of structural resemblance to them. A number of these growth factor analogues, e.g. pantoyl taurine and pyridine-3-sulphonic acid, have considerable in vitro antibacterial activity, but none so far has proved to be of any value as a therapeutic agent. In some cases at least this appears to be due to the fact that the antagonized growth factors have been essential factors for the host's cells as well as for the bacteria. The analogues are therefore competitively inihibited by growth factor present in the tissues and if this inhibition is overcome interfere with the metabolism of the host's cells.

Because of this the search for new chemotherapeutic agents has consisted largely of the routine screening of diverse compounds, both of synthetic and natural origin, for antibacterial activity. A rational chemotherapy based on tailor-made nutritional antagonists has not, at least so far as the bacteria are concerned, proved possible. Nevertheless, a number of naturally occurring compounds with antibacterial activity have been discovered, and have been shown to owe their activity to a structural analogy with some essential metabolite. The most interesting of these are *azaserine* and 6-diazo-5-oxo-L-norleucine, both of which are glutamine analogues and both have been found to inhibit the transfer of amide groups from glutamine, to formyl glycinamide ribonucleotide—a key intermediary in the biosynthesis of purine. Other compounds or analogues of particular biochemical interest are *psicofuranine*, an analogue of adenosine capable of inhibiting the synthesis of guanine, and *hadacidin*, which is an analogue of L-aspartic acid and interferes with purine synthesis by blocking the conversion of inosinic to adenylosuccinic acid. The only antibiotic of chemotherapeutic value whose action has been decisively shown to be due to nutritional antagonism is cycloserine, a structural analogue of D-alanine. Cycloserine inhibits both the formation of D-alanine from L-alanine, and of the alanine dipeptide required in mucopeptide synthesis. It has been suggested that penicillin may possess sufficient structural resemblance to some part of the cell wall mucopeptide as to explain its inhibitory effect on mucopeptide synthesis (p. 208), but the evidence for this is inconclusive.

STRUCTURAL RESEMBLANCE BETWEEN D-ALANINE
AND CYCLOSERINE

$$H_3C\text{——}CH.NH_2 \qquad\qquad H_2C\text{——}CH.NH_2$$

D-Alanine   Cycloserine

A particularly interesting type of nutritional antagonism is that shown by the antibiotic *puromycin*, which is produced by *Streptomyces alboniger*. Puromycin is a potent inhibitor of protein synthesis, a property which it owes to the fact that it is a structural analogue of the adenosyl end of amino acyl RNA, and therefore competes at ribosomal level. Puromycin apparently forms peptide bonds with the carboxyl groups of the terminal amino acids of peptide chains in process of synthesis, thereby blocking the incorporation of further amino acids carried by the soluble or transfer RNA. This results in the release of incomplete peptides from the ribosome. Consistent with this explanation is the finding that

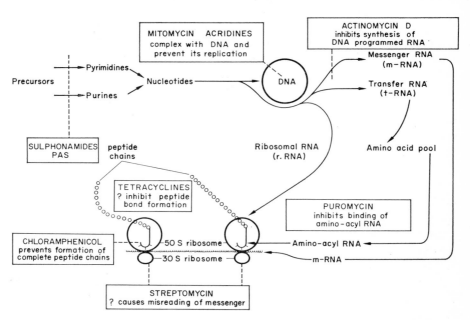

FIG. 13. ACTION OF ANTIBACTERIAL DRUGS ON PROTEIN AND NUCLEIC ACID SYNTHESIS

the released peptides each contain a single molecule of puromycin. Puromycin is an inhibitor of protein synthesis in mammalian, as well as bacterial cells, and has sufficient nephrotoxicity to prevent its application as a chemotherapeutic agent. It has, however, been of considerable value, through its specific effect on protein synthesis, in elucidating the mechanisms involved in the replication of viral nucleic acids.

ACQUIRED RESISTANCE

There are two main ways in which bacteria initially sensitive to a chemotherapeutic agent may become resistant; these are (*a*) by mutation and (*b*) by infective transfer.

Mutation

Resistant mutants are readily selected in the laboratory from initially sensitive strains by growing them in progressively increasing but subinhibitory concentrations of drug. This may be achieved as follows: a series of dilutions of the drug are made in broth, and inoculated with a sensitive organism. After incubation subcultures are made from the tube containing the highest concentration of drug permitting growth into a second similar series of tubes. A subculture is

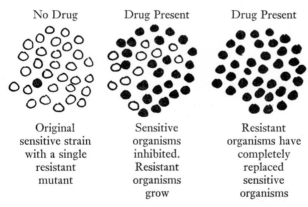

No Drug	Drug Present	Drug Present
Original sensitive strain with a single resistant mutant	Sensitive organisms inhibited. Resistant organisms grow	Resistant organisms have completely replaced sensitive organisms

FIG. 14. SCHEMATIC REPRESENTATION OF THE ACTION OF AN ANTIBACTERIAL DRUG IN SELECTING DRUG-RESISTANT MUTANTS

then made from the highest subinhibitory concentration of this series into a further series of tubes and so on.

When the technique described above is used, two contrasting patterns in the development of resistance are observed. (1) A high level of resistance may suddenly develop at any stage in subculture; it may even appear at the first subculture. This pattern is characteristic of the development of resistance to streptomycin and, in the case of tubercle bacilli, to INAH. (2) With penicillin, chloramphenicol, the tetracyclines and the sulphonamides, on the other hand, resistance develops slowly and a high level of resistance can be achieved only by a considerable series of transfers in progressively increasing concentrations of drug. This type of resistance appears to develop in a stepwise fashion by a small increment each time. A pattern of resistance development intermediate between these two types is shown by erythromycin and novobiocin.

There is little doubt that, in such cases, the development of drug resistance is due to mutation. These mutations occur spontaneously in cultures and independently of the presence of drug at a frequency of about one in 10^7 to 10^{10} cell divisions. The mutants have a relatively low survival value which is less than that of the parent sensitive strain; they are therefore unable to replace the parent sensitive organisms in cultures not exposed to drug. If the drug is present, however, the parent sensitive is inhibited and the drug-resistant mutants can grow out. The action of the drug is therefore not to stimulate the development of drug-resistant forms but to select them. On prolonged growth in the absence of drug, strains that have been made resistant by selection in the laboratory normally revert to drug sensitivity. This change is due to the occurrence of back-mutations. As a general rule reversion, when it occurs, is incomplete—the organism rarely, if ever, regaining its original sensitivity. Different variants show considerable differences in their capacity to revert, some in fact failing to do so under prolonged observation.

There is so far little precise information as to the mechanisms responsible for drug resistance acquired by mutation. The following types of mechanism could be involved: (1) Acquisition by the organism of a capacity to destroy the drug. Some instances have been described of coliform bacteria possessing initially a low level of penicillinase activity acquiring by mutation a high level of activity. No instance has been described, however, of an organism acquiring by mutation the capacity to destroy a drug when it had initially lacked the capacity to do so. (2) Decreased permeability to the drug. There is some evidence that acquired resistance to chloramphenicol and the tetracyclines may be of this type. (3) Diminished affinity of the drug-sensitive site. This probably operates in some cases of laboratory-acquired resistance to streptomycin and penicillin. (4) Increased production of a drug inhibitor. Some organisms resistant to the sulphonamides have been described as having an increased capacity to synthesize PABA; this, however, is not a general mechanism of sulphonamide resistance. (5) The acquisition by the organism of an altered metabolism in which the drug-sensitive reaction is by-passed. No clear example of this mechanism has been observed.

In the past there has been some controversy as to whether resistance could not develop also by a mechanism of *adaptation*, i.e. a change occurring uniformly throughout the organisms of the culture, and produced directly by exposure to the drug. As we shall see, this mechanism does operate to create full resistance in penicillinase-producing staphylococci, and there may well be other instances in which the presence of the drug in environment can induce the synthesis of a hydrolytic enzyme capable of inactivating it. As a mechanism, however, by which initially sensitive bacteria become resistant, adaptation, although in the past receiving considerable mathematical support from Hinshelwood, has now been largely discarded.

Organisms may also be isolated which are not only resistant to a drug but which are dependent upon it and which will therefore grow only in its presence; such dependence has been observed in relation to the sulphonamides and streptomycin. As might be expected the growth of sulphonamide-dependent organisms is inhibited by PABA.

Infective Transfer

This mechanism was first postulated in 1957, by Akiba in Japan, to explain the considerable increase in the numbers of strains of shigellae and of coliform bacteria possessing multiple resistance to chloramphenicol, streptomycin, tetracycline and the sulphonamides. The resistance exhibited by these organisms to chloramphenicol, tetracycline and sulphonamides was in each case considerably greater than that which could be expected as a result of mutation. Akiba and Watanabe subsequently showed that the increase was due to the infective transmission from resistant to sensitive strains of a genetic determinant for resistance known as a *resistance* or R *factor*. Like sex factors (p. 26) and certain colicinogeny determinants (p. 567), R factors can be transmitted by growing a resistant strain possessing them, with a sensitive recipient. Resistance is transferred much more efficiently by strains that have recently been infected with an R factor than by strains in which an R factor has been firmly established. As in bacterial conjugation and colicinogeny transfer the factor is not demonstrable in the cell-free state and can only be transferred by a conjugation-like mechanism involving cell to cell contact.

The first instances of the infective transfer of resistance were of the simultaneous transfer of resistance to a number of drugs. It therefore seemed possible that a common mechanism bringing about an overall decrease in cell permeability was involved. It was subsequently found, however, that resistance to antibacterial agents could occur in any combination, and that the resistance to individual agents could be segregated in conjugation and transduction experiments. Resistance to each drug is therefore specific. In most cases it appears to involve a decrease in the permeability of the organism to the particular drug, but a more precise biochemical definition is not at the moment possible. In addition to the drugs initially incriminated, infective transfer has since been demonstrated in relation to kanamycin, neomycin, the penicillins and the cephalosporins. Resistance to penicillins and cephalosporins has been found to be associated with the transfer of penicillinase and/or cephalosporinase activities. So far, R factors have been demonstrated only in the enterobacteriaceae, *Serratia marcescens*, *V. cholerae* and *Past. pestis*.

There is now clear evidence, on the basis of direct analysis of nucleic acid content, that R factors consist of DNA, and show many points of resemblance to the F factor and to the colicinogeny determinants. They can be transduced by various bacteriophages, and in the case of *E. coli* strains, can function as sex factors capable of determining transfer of the bacterial chromosome from an F^- strain. The resemblance to the F factor is also shown in the demonstration by Datta and Meynell that certain R^+ strains, rendered resistant by infection with an R factor, are capable of synthesizing a specialized pilus, identical with that synthesized by F+ strains, and like the latter, capable of adsorbing F+ bacteriophage. This pilus is presumed to constitute the conjugation tube through which the transfer factor is transferred to a recipient strain. Such R factors, if introduced into an F+ strain, interfere with the function of the F factor, lowering its capacity to produce specialized pili, and as a result, its capacity to mediate chromosomal transfer. This interference appears to be due to the production, by the R factor, of a repressor substance which acts on both R and F factors. Its action on the R factor is manifested in the low frequency of transfer in established R+ cultures. Production of the repressor is minimal in freshly infected strains, a phenomenon which explains the relative ease of transfer of R factors from such strains. R factors depressing the function of F are known as fi+, those which do not as fi−. More recently it has been shown that cells possessing fi− R factors also synthesize specialized pili, but are distinguishable from those determined by fi+ R factors in electron microscopic morphology and in their capacity to absorb a specific fi− bacteriophage. Similar pili are also produced by strains carrying certain colicinogeny determinants.

A strain which owes its resistance to an R factor may lose its capacity to transfer resistance, while itself remaining resistant. In this case its capacity for infective transmission can be restored by growth with other R+ strains. A strain may also lose its resistance to one or more of the agents to which it was initially resistant. These findings indicate that the R factor is in fact a complex of resistance determinants, together with a transfer factor (RTF), which determines the capacity of the strain to transfer resistance. This complex of transfer factors and resistance factors exists in the cell as a single genetic unit, which may on occasion, however, lose one or more of its components.

There seems little doubt that the transfer factor component must be regarded as a sex factor, but one which has in some way acquired the genetic determinants which control resistance to antibacterial agents. So far, the presence in transfer factors of genes other than those responsible for drug resistance has not been demonstrated. The origin of the resistance determinants of R factors is in doubt, but the most reasonable supposition is that they are chromosomal genes which have become integrated into the transfer factor in precisely the same way as has been shown for integrated F factors (p. 28). The possible ultimate chromosomal origin of the R factors is suggested by base composition analysis of their DNA, using the buoyant density procedure. Thus an R factor determining chloramphenicol resistance in *Proteus* has a guanine plus cytosine content of 56 per cent, which is in fact the combined guanine plus cytosine content of the DNA of the *Klebsiella* genus. Other R factors in *Proteus* have been reported to have a guanine plus cytosine content of 50 per cent, which is that of the DNA of *E. coli*. By contrast, *Proteus* DNA has a guanine plus cytosine content of 39 per cent. These findings suggest that chloramphenicol resistance factors are derived from the *Klebsiella* chromosome, and resistance factors for other agents from the *E. coli* chromosome. A serious difficulty in this hypothesis is that of explaining why the mechanisms involved in infective resistance should be different from those of strains which have been selected by deliberate exposure to the drug. A further problem is that of explaining why a single transfer factor should be associated with a number of different resistance determinants. Possibly, the reason is that the transfer factor picks up the appropriate gene in passage from one strain to another, natural selection operating to favour survival of the R factor with multiple resistance determinants. As against this explanation, however, R factors determining multiple resistance were the first to be identified, not, as might be expected on this hypothesis, appearing at a later stage. An alternative possibility is that R factors carrying multiple resistance determinants are the result of recombination between R factors carrying individual determinants. This raises the possibility that the individual resistance determinants may not have been of chromosomal origin, but may be derived by spontaneous mutations of the transfer factors themselves.

It is obvious that the existence of R factors is of the greatest importance for the future of chemotherapy. Even though they have been encountered most frequently in commensal coliform bacteria, they are capable of being transferred to highly pathogenic organisms such as the salmonellae and shigellae. Their occurrence in coliform bacteria, however, is not to be dismissed lightly. Coliform bacteria are of great importance as causes of urinary tract infections, hospital wound infection and infantile gastro-enteritis.

The dissemination of bacterial strains carrying R factors is obviously favoured by the large-scale clinical use of antibacterial agents. In this connexion, the recovery by Anderson of strains of *Salm. typhimurium* carrying R factors from calves and pigs, is of the greatest importance. Control of the dissemination of these agents must therefore involve not only close attention to drug policy in respect of the human population, but also for domestic animals which constitute a reservoir of such agents, extremely difficult, if not impossible, to control.

The Persister State

The name *persister* was originally applied by Bigger to staphylococci which had temporarily acquired resistance to penicillin. It was found that if staphylococci were mixed with high concentrations of penicillin most of the organisms were killed within 24 hours, but a few survived; when the penicillin present was destroyed by penicillinase the survivors sooner or later multiplied. Persisters are believed to be organisms in a dormant or non-metabolizing state in which they are insusceptible to the killing action of the drug. This state of dormancy may be the result of the bacteriostatic action of penicillin. Alternatively, a small proportion of any penicillin-sensitive bacterial population may, at any given time, be in the persister state. The duration of the period of dormancy varies greatly from one organism to another. In some it may last only a few hours, in others for days, in a few for more than a week. As soon as a dormant form resumes activity it becomes sensitive to penicillin and is killed. Penicillin in relation to persisters acts in the same way as a trained police dog in relation to a fugitive. So long as he remains quiet he is not attacked, if he displays any activity it attacks him. Persisters are probably of greatest importance in the chemotherapy of tuberculosis (p. 365).

Drug Resistance as a Clinical Phenomenon

Since drug resistance can be produced in the test tube, it is to be expected that it will occur also in the bodies of patients who are under treatment. As might be expected it occurs very readily in relation to streptomycin and INAH. In patients under treatment with these drugs organisms may rapidly become completely resistant, due to the selection by the drug of mutants having a high level of resistance. As in the laboratory, resistance may develop regardless of the amount of drug used. With penicillin, and other drugs exhibiting the multistep resistance pattern, however, resistance rarely appears to develop during the course of treatment in organisms originally sensitive provided that adequate amounts of drug are administered. This probably applies also to other drugs showing the same type of in vitro resistance pattern.

It is probable that many cases in which resistance appears to develop during the course of chemotherapy, particularly with drugs showing the multi-step resistance pattern, are due not to the acquisition of resistance by an originally sensitive organism but to replacement or substitution infection. This is a process in which the sensitive organisms initially responsible for the infection are inhibited but the lesion becomes reinfected by resistant organisms present in the environment. It is most likely to occur with surface lesions such as wounds and burns which are directly exposed to environmental organisms. The risk is greatest with patients treated in a hospital environment where resistant organisms are lurking in abundance.

When a patient is treated with an antibacterial drug the drug acts not only on the organisms responsible for his infection but also on the normal flora of his respiratory and intestinal tracts. If this action is sufficient to cause a substantial reduction in the normal flora a bacteriological vacuum is created which tends to become populated with drug-resistant strains. Usually this is without serious consequence for the patient although it may render him a danger to others since he becomes a focus from which resistant organisms may be spread. Occasionally, however, resistant organisms with pathogenic propensities may become established and may initiate an infection. This process is known as superinfection. The most serious infection of this type is the acute enterocolitis which may complicate treatment with the wide-spectrum antibiotics. This is not a common complication of antibiotic therapy but is an extremely grave one. It is most frequently caused by *Staph. aureus*, but *Proteus*, *Pseudomonas* and other Gram negative bacilli are sometimes involved. The organisms responsible are frequently resistant not only to the drug being administered but also to a number of other antibacterial drugs as well. In many but not in all cases this complication has followed abdominal operation.

Another type of superinfection that has assumed clinical importance is that due to overgrowth of *Candida albicans*—a yeast-like fungus which is a normal inhabitant of the respiratory and alimentary tracts. Following the administration of wide-spectrum antibiotics, especially the tetracyclines, extensive overgrowth of *C. albicans* has on occasion been found to occur in the intestinal, respiratory and urogenital tracts. In exceptional cases the fungus invades the blood stream with the development of metastatic abscesses in the kidney, liver and brain. This complication has also been reported following the administration of penicillin, a drug which appears in fact to have a direct stimulating effect on the growth of *Candida*.

Since antibacterial agents can transform sensitive strains into resistant ones, and can select for resistant strains, however produced, it is not surprising that, when a drug has been used in a community for some time, the relative proportion of organisms resistant to it should increase. This has occurred in relation to all the agents now in common use, but not to the extent that was at first feared— the increased prevalence of resistant strains having fortunately affected only a few species. The problem is greatest with *Staph. aureus*, many strains of which are now resistant to penicillin, streptomycin and the tetracyclines—the antibiotics which have been most used—and with the coliform bacteria, almost certainly as a result of the spread of R factors. Many strains of *Pseudomonas* and *Proteus* species now isolated from clinical material are also highly resistant, but since these species have considerable natural resistance to antibiotics the relative increase is not so marked. It is reported that a small proportion of tubercle bacilli isolated from fresh cases of tuberculosis are by laboratory tests appreciably resistant to streptomycin or INAH, and clinical evidence suggests that there has been some increase in the resistance of viridans streptococci and of gonococci to penicillin. There is no evidence of any significant increase in the resistance of other pathogenic species. The fact that the pathogenic staphylococci, organisms which are frequently present in the upper respiratory tracts of healthy individuals, and coliform bacteria, which are intestinal commensals, are the main offenders in this respect suggests that exposure of the respiratory and intestinal flora to drug, an exposure which occurs to some extent every time an antibiotic is administered, is of special importance as a factor in the emergence of resistant strains.

The Control of Drug Resistance

In the control of drug resistance three distinct problems have to be considered. (1) The prevention of the development of resistance in initially sensitive organisms. (2) The prevention of replacement infection with resistant strains present in the patient's environment. (3) The reduction of the apparently inevitable increases in the prevalence in the population as a whole of resistant strains of *Staph. aureus* and coliform bacteria.

In order to prevent the development of resistance in organisms originally sensitive the first principle of chemotherapy is to ensure that an adequate amount of drug is administered. No procedure is more calculated to favour the development of resistance, particularly of the multistep penicillin type, than half-hearted inadequate treatment. Although the maintenance of an adequate drug concentration in the tissues may be expected to minimize the chance of resistance developing to drugs showing the multistep resistance it will not do so in the case of drugs showing the single step resistance pattern especially if treatment with these drugs is prolonged. With these compounds, however, the development of resistance may be diminished by the use of combined therapy. The rationale of combined therapy is that if any organisms are to survive combined treatment they must become resistant to both drugs employed and the probability that they would do so is very much less than the probability that they would become resistant to either drug if given alone. Theoretically the probability of the development of resistance to two drugs given at the same time should be the product of the independent probabilities for each of them. The value of combined therapy in preventing the development of resistance has been clearly shown in the treatment of tuberculosis, in which resistance develops much less frequently if patients are given a combination of two antituberculous agents, e.g. streptomycin and INAH, than if they are given either alone.

The problem of preventing replacement infection in surface lesions, e.g. wounds and burns, is essentially that of the control of cross-infection in general. In cases, e.g. urinary tract infection, in which there is an underlying lesion—stone, congenital defect, prostatic obstruction—which predisposes to infection, this lesion must be dealt with. If this is not done, when one organism has been eliminated by chemotherapy the patient may simply become reinfected with another organism resistant to the drug previously used.

Ultimately the most important of the problems in connexion with bacterial resistance is the more general one of preventing increases in the prevalence of resistant strains. Since the prevalence of resistant strains is a direct result of the widespread use of antibacterial drugs, this can be achieved only by ensuring that antibiotic and chemotherapeutic agents are used as little as possible. They should not be given for trivial infections from which the patient would certainly recover. They should not be casually administered as prophylactics (p. 91). They should not, except in emergency, be prescribed blindly in the absence of a bacteriological diagnosis or of a reasonable expectation that the organisms are sensitive. Surface lesions should be treated, if possible, by topical application of drugs not normally used systemically, e.g. bacitracin and neomycin, and only in severe surface infections should systemic treatment be employed.

ANTAGONISM AND SYNERGISM

Antibacterial drugs are frequently given to patients in various combinations not only with the object of preventing the development of resistance, as in the treatment of tuberculosis, but also to achieve a synergistic effect, that is, an effect greater than that which could be achieved with either drug alone.

It is generally agreed that the use of combined therapy is indicated in the circumstances mentioned below. (1) In the case of infections due to organisms of relatively low susceptibility to any of the available antibiotics, e.g. the treatment of infections due to *Str. faecalis* with a combination of penicillin and streptomycin or of *Ps. aeruginosa* infections with a combination of polymyxin and a tetracycline. In these circumstances combined therapy should be undertaken only when its potential value is indicated by laboratory sensitivity tests. (2) In mixed infections due to organisms of differing sensitivities, e.g. in combined infection with a streptococcus and a Gram negative bacillus. (3) In grave undiagnosed infection where combined therapy may be necessary as a life saving measure. (4) In certain empirically determined conditions in which it has been shown that the combined therapy gives the most satisfactory therapeutic result, e.g. in the treatment of subacute bacterial endocarditis due to viridans streptococci (Chapter 14), or of brucellosis (p. 351). (5) To prevent the development of resistance when antibiotics showing the single step high level resistance pattern are employed.

Under in vitro conditions, however, it has been found that certain antibiotics may antagonize the actions of others, and this has naturally given rise to the fear that a similar antagonism might occur during the course of treatment. The antagonisms observed in vitro have, however, been of limited nature. Thus the mainly bacteriostatic drugs, in particular chloramphenicol and the tetracyclines, have been found to inhibit the bactericidal action of penicillin and streptomycin. This antagonism has been found only against organisms highly sensitive to the bactericidal drug and only with certain drug concentrations. The mainly bacteriostatic drugs do not inhibit each other, nor do they affect the bacteriostatic action of penicillin and streptomycin. Penicillin and streptomycin have not been found to antagonize each other and may in fact show synergism. The antagonism of bactericidal by bacteriostatic drugs has been observed not only in the test tube but also in the treatment of certain experimental infections in animals. There is, however, insufficient evidence to indicate to what extent antagonism occurs as a result of combined therapy under clinical conditions.

SENSITIVITY TESTS

These are tests in which the bacteriologist attempts to determine whether an organism is sufficiently sensitive to an antimicrobial drug to permit the use of that drug in treatment. In the tests normally used for this purpose it is the bacteriostatic effect of the drug which is investigated. We determine the extent to which the growth of the organism is inhibited by the drug and on the result of this examination we base an opinion as to whether the drug can be effectively used in treatment.

Although sensitivity tests are of great value in the control of treatment the decision as to which drug or drugs to use should be based in the first place on clinical diagnosis supplemented, where possible, by simple diagnostic laboratory tests. In most types of infection the establishment of a bacteriological diagnosis immediately indicates the appropriate chemotherapeutic agent to use, and sensitivity tests on the causative organism are not normally required. However, in pyogenic infections due to species, viz. *Staph. aureus*, coliforms, etc., which are not uniformly sensitive, sensitivity tests are essential—although treatment should normally be begun without waiting for the result of these tests.

For clinical purposes sensitivity tests are usually carried out by the agar plate diffusion technique. When carried out on organisms already isolated in pure culture the following technique may be used. The surface of a blood agar plate is flooded with a broth culture or with a suspension in broth of the organism (or with a dilution of these). The excess fluid is pipetted off and the surface of the medium allowed to dry. Discs or tablets impregnated with antibiotic are then placed on it and the plates incubated with the lid uppermost. After incubation the diameter of the zones of inhibition surrounding the discs or tablets is measured. By determining the size of the zones obtained with known sensitive organisms the bacteriologist can fix standards by reference to which the sensitivity of any organism can be graded. The data obtained do not sufficiently closely parallel clinical results to warrant attaching any great significance to relatively small differences in zone diameter, and a comparatively simple grading of organisms as into 'sensitive', 'moderately resistant' and 'resistant' is all that is required. The diameter of the inhibition zone depends not only on the sensitivity of the organism but also on the concentration of antibiotic in the disc or tablet used and on its rate of diffusion. It is consequently not permissible to base any opinion on the relative efficacy of different drugs against a particular organism on differences in zone size except in so far as these

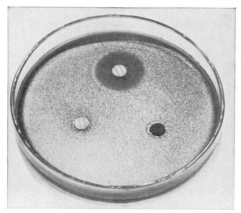

FIG. 15. ANTIBIOTIC SENSITIVITY TEST USING
IMPREGNATED TABLETS
Sensitivity is indicated by a zone of inhibition
around the tablet

permit a sensitivity grading such as that indicated above. When organisms are reported as being within an apparently sensitive range the clinical choice of drug should be made on other grounds.

Sensitivity tests on organisms that have first been isolated in pure culture may not, however, give a completely reliable picture of the sensitivity of the organisms in the original material. This is because the culture tested is obtained by random picking of a single colony from the isolation plate, and this colony may differ in sensitivity from the majority of the organisms present. In addition indirect tests are slow, since they require prior isolation of the organism. More rapid and therefore clinically more useful results are obtained if the tests are carried out directly, i.e. using the clinical material (e.g. pus) as an inoculum. Direct tests also give a more reliable picture of the sensitivity of the organisms present, since sampling errors are avoided; they have the disadvantage, however, that they are appreciably less accurate.

The sensitivity of tubercle bacilli to streptomycin, INAH and PAS may be determined by inoculation on to slopes of Löwenstein medium containing various concentrations of drug. The sensitivity is commonly expressed as a ratio of the concentration inhibiting growth to that inhibiting growth of a known sensitive strain, e.g. H37Rv.

If the bacteriologist is required to investigate the possible antagonistic action of one drug on another in relation to a particular organism, tests indicating bactericidal rather than bacteriostatic activity must be employed. In one type of test used for this purpose dilutions of the drugs under test, singly and in various combinations, are made in broth and inoculated with the organism. After overnight incubation subcultures are made on to blood agar from each of the tubes inoculated to determine whether the organisms introduced into it have been killed. If one of the drugs has an antagonistic effect on the other, their combination should be less efficient in killing the organism than the more actively bactericidal of the drugs by itself. Tests of this type are cumbersome and ideally require the testing of a large number of antibiotic concentrations. Whether the information gained is of significant clinical value is doubtful.

Some indication of the existence of synergism between two antibiotics can be obtained by the use of comparatively simple plate tests. For this purpose discs containing the antibiotics are placed on the surface of a seeded plate at a distance apart approximately equal to that of the sum of the diameters of the zones of inhibition produced by each antibiotic independently. If one of the antibiotics potentiates the action of the other the zone of inhibition produced by the latter will be increased. Antagonistic effects are much less readily demonstrable by this technique.

ASSAY OF ANTIBIOTICS

Methods similar to those that have been described for sensitivity testing can be used for assay of the concentration of an antibacterial drug present in various clinical fluids: blood, cerebrospinal fluid, urine, etc. As in sensitivity testing, plate diffusion techniques, although less precise than broth dilution techniques, are technically simpler. The filter-paper disc technique may be used but the 'cup' method is more frequently employed. In this the dilutions of the antibiotic and of the fluid being tested are pipetted into shallow glass or porcelain cylinders placed on the surface of a plate which has been seeded with a known sensitive organism. In a simple but quite satisfactory modification of this technique the dilutions of fluid and antibiotic are pipetted into small holes cut out of the surface of the agar with a cork borer. From the inhibition zones obtained with the known antibiotic dilutions a curve, which relates inhibition zone diameter to antibiotic concentration, can be drawn. If the inhibition zone produced by one of the dilutions of the fluid being examined falls on this curve, the antibiotic concentration present in that dilution can be read off immediately.

LABORATORY USES OF ANTIBIOTICS

Antibiotics have been used in the laboratory for a variety of purposes. Of these the undermentioned are the most important for diagnostic medical bacteriology.

1. They may be incorporated as selective agents in culture media. Thus penicillin may be used to facilitate the isolation of *H. influenzae* from material taken from the upper respiratory tract since it inhibits most of the Gram positive organisms and the neisseriae present. Neomycin, as in Willis and Hobbs's medium, is of value for the isolation of clostridia, particularly of *Cl. perfringens*, from material, e.g. faeces or food, contaminated with other organisms.

2. Antibiotics are universally employed for the control of bacterial contamination in tissue cultures used for virus isolation. The antibiotics normally used are penicillin and streptomycin for the control of bacterial contamination and nystatin for the control of fungal contamination.

3. The pattern of sensitivity of an organism to a battery of antibiotics constitutes a simple method of typing which has been found to be of considerable epidemiological value. It may, for example, be used as a preliminary to phage typing in the investigation of epidemics of staphylococcal infection. The strain isolated from the putative source of the infection should have the same antibiotic sensitivity pattern as that isolated from the infection. The pattern of sensitivity of an organism to different antibiotics is sometimes known as an *antibiogram*.

ANTIBIOTICS IN CURRENT USE

Antibiotics may be conveniently classified on the basis of the range of bacteria against which they are active.

1. Antibiotics mainly or exclusively active against Gram positive organisms. The antibiotics falling into this group are penicillin G and V, methicillin, cloxacillin, erythromycin, novobiocin, vanomycin, bacitracin and fucidin. Except for vancomycin these compounds are also highly active against the pathogenic neisseriae—the gonococcus and meningococcus and, to a lesser extent, *H. influenzae* and *Bordetella pertussis*. Of the Gram positive group the enterococci are the most resistant, particularly to the less active penicillins—methicillin and cloxacillin.

2. Antibiotics mainly or exclusively active against Gram negative organisms. The important compounds in this group are streptomycin, neomycin and polymyxin.

3. Antibiotics which are highly active against both Gram positive and Gram negative organisms. This group includes the so-called 'wide-spectrum' antibiotics—the tetracyclines, chloramphenicol, ampicillin and the cephalosporins —cephaloridine and cephalothin.

4. Antibiotics active against fungi. Those currently available are nystatin, griseofulvin and amphotericin B (p. 572).

The Penicillins

The penicillins constitute a family of antibiotics, the first member of which was discovered by Fleming in 1929. It was not at that time possible, however, to obtain it in a sufficiently concentrated and purified form for clinical use. This was subsequently achieved by Chain, Florey and their associates in 1941.

Penicillins consist of a nucleus of 6-aminopenicillanic acid (6 APA) to which are attached various side-chains in amide linkage. Penicillin G and penicillin V are produced entirely by fermentation processes using a mutant strain of *Penicillium chrysogenum* which is capable of producing large amounts of penicillin in submerged culture. At an early stage it was found that the *Penicillium* mould was capable of incorporating a variety of substituted acetic acids into

THE PENICILLINS

$$R—CO—NH—CH———HC \overset{S}{\diagup} \overset{CH_3}{\underset{CH_3}{C}}$$

β lactam ring   thia-zolidine ring

$$CO———N———CH—COOH$$

peptide bond hydrolysed by *penicillin amidase (acylase)* to yield 6-aminopenicillanic acid (6-APA) which has little anti-bacterial effect.

Penicillin amidase, produced by some Gram negative bacteria, is used in preparation of semi-synthetic penicillins. It plays little if any part in bacterial resistance to penicillin.

peptide bond hydrolysed by *penicillinase* to yield penicilloic acid. Susceptibility depends on nature of side group. Penicillinase is basis of penicillin resistance in *Staph. aureus* and many Gram negative bacilli.

the side-chains of the penicillin molecule. The addition of such compounds therefore became standard practice in penicillin production, penicillin G being produced in large amounts following addition of phenylacetic acid and phenoxymethyl penicillin in the presence of phenoxyacetic acid. The next major advance was the discovery by Chain, Bachelor et al. that the penicillin nucleus, 6-APA, was produced in appreciable amounts in fermentation media in the absence of added precursor. From this it was but a short step to the semi-synthetic penicillins—methicillin, ampicillin and the isoxazolyl penicillins—in which various side-groups are incorporated by chemical manipulation. In the production of these, however, it has been found more convenient to obtain the parent compound, 6-APA, by treating benzyl penicillin with penicillin amidases (or acylases) of bacterial origin.

Penicillin G fulfils many of the requirements of an ideal chemotherapeutic agent. Active against sensitive organisms in extremely low concentration, it is bactericidal and appears to be without toxicity in the highest concentrations attainable in the tissues. Its defects are its limited range of action, its lability to acid so that it cannot be administered orally, its high susceptibility to bacterial penicillinases, and its capacity to induce allergic sensitization. It is these defects that the more recent penicillin derivatives have attempted to rectify. Two of the newer penicillins, methicillin and cloxacillin, are resistant to staphylococcal

SOME IMPORTANT PENICILLINS

Name	Side chain (R)	Acid stability	Resistance to staphylococcal penicillinase	Active against Gram negative bacilli
Benzyl penicillin (Penicillin G)	—CH₂— (benzyl)	−	−	−
Methicillin (Celbenin)	OCH₃ … OCH₃	−	+	−
Ampicillin (Penbritin)	—CH— | NH₂	+	−	+
Cloxacillin (Orbenin)	Cl … —C=C—CH₃ (isoxazolyl)	+	+	−
Carbenicillin (Pyopen)	—CH— | COO Na	−	−	+ Active against Pseudomonas

penicillinase. Ampicillin and cloxacillin are acid-resistant, and can therefore be administered orally, and ampicillin and carbenicillin exhibit a wide spectrum of activity embracing many Gram negative bacteria. Of the five compounds shown above, benzyl penicillin and ampicillin possess much the same order of activity against Gram positive organisms. Methicillin and cloxacillin are appreciably less active but have the enormous advantage that they can be used against penicillinase-producing staphylococci.

Early work suggested that penicillin specifically inhibited the incorporation of the muramyl pentapeptide from the Park nucleotide, viz. UDP-N-acetyl muramyl pentapeptide, into the cell wall, possibly because of a three-dimensional structural resemblance of penicillin to muramic acid. This interpretation, however, has not been supported by later work. More recently Wise and Park have presented evidence that the immediate effect of penicillin is to prevent cross-linking of the mucopeptide peptide side-chains. In *Staph. aureus*, cross-linking is due to a pentaglycine bridge between lysine on one peptide chain and D-alanine on an adjacent chain. Wise and Park propose that penicillin inhibits the formation of the peptide bond between glycine and D-alanine. They suggest that it does so because of a structural resemblance to the L-alanine D-glutamic region of the mucopeptide, as a result of which it combines with the enzyme involved in transpeptidation, preventing binding of the latter to the mucopeptide. How this interference leads to the accumulation of Park nucleotide has still to be clarified. It is possible that continued synthesis of the mucopeptide can only occur if cross-linking proceeds normally. This co-ordination might be achieved through the operation of some, as yet unidentified, bio-chemical control mechanism.

Penicillinase

Penicillin is broken down by two types of bacterial enzyme: (*a*) penicillinase, or more correctly β-lactamase, and (*b*) penicillin amidase or acylase. The action of these enzymes on penicillin is shown on p. 207.

Penicillinases are produced by naturally resistant strains of *Staph. aureus*, by certain *Bacillus* species and by a variety of enterobacteriaceae, particularly of the coliform and *Proteus* groups. It is usually demonstrated by a biological assay procedure which determines the capacity of a bacterial culture to destroy the inhibitory activity of penicillin against a known sensitive organism, e.g. the Oxford staphylococcus. As normally carried out, such bioassays usually reflect β-lactamase activity but decisive proof that the agent responsible is a β-lactamase rather than a penicillin amidase requires the demonstration of penicilloic acid production, e.g. by chromatography or by the iodometric technique of Perret.

From the clinical point of view the most important of the β-lactamases is that produced by *Staph. aureus*. It is produced by all naturally resistant strains of *Staph. aureus*, and is responsible for their resistance. Without penicillinase such strains are intrinsically sensitive to penicillin. This may be demonstrated in sensitivity tests with dilute inocula, when the sensitivity of penicillinase-producing strains approximates that of non-penicillinase-producing strains. When, however, large inocula are employed the organisms appear resistant because of the presence of larger amounts of penicillinase sufficient to destroy the penicillin present.

Staphylococcal penicillinase is inducible, normal wild-type resistant strains producing it in significant amounts only in the presence of penicillin. Non-inducible mutants have however been isolated in the laboratory, and these produce considerable amounts of the enzyme constitutively. Induction of the enzyme is currently explained on the Jacob-Monod hypothesis (p. 31). Inducing capacity is a property of 6-APA and all its known derivatives, includ-ing compounds such as methicillin and the isoxazolyl penicillins, which are highly resistant to penicillinase action. It seems very unlikely therefore that it would be possible to develop a penicillin derivative with high antibacterial activity but having little capacity to induce penicillinase.

As previously indicated, the genes controlling penicillinase production in *Staph. aureus* are carried on extrachromosomal genetic elements or plasmids (p. 250). These may be transduced by bacteriophages from one cell to another, but differ from the resistance transfer factors of the enterobacteriaceae in not being capable of spontaneous transfer. A penicillinase-producing staphylococcus may lose its plasmid, becoming as a result fully sensititive to penicillin. It does not seem possible, however, for a non-penicillinase-producing strain to gain a plasmid spontaneously. Consequently, penicillin-resistant mutants selected in the laboratory are non-penicillinase producers.

The penicillinases of the Gram negative bacteria are a diverse group of enzymes which have not so far been fully investigated. Those of the coliform bacteria differ from staphylococcal penicillinase in being non-inducible, and in having a more specifically intracellular location. They differ amongst themselves in their activity towards different penicillins, most having much the same order of activity against both penicillin and ampicillin, some being more active against penicillin than against ampicillin, and others—especially in *Klebsiella* strains— being more active against ampicillin than against penicillin. The genetic basis of these penicillinases has not been fully explored. It is clear, however, that ampicillin resistance determined by R factors is the result of a penicillinase active against ampicillin and genetically controlled by the R factor.

Since on the whole penicillin- and cephalosporin-producing fungi and penicillinase-producing bacteria share the same natural environments, it is reasonable to presume that the capacity to produce penicillinase has evolved in penicillin sensitive bacteria as a form of protection against penicillins and cephalosporins produced in their environment. That this evolution has not been a recent event is indicated by the observation of Pollock that spores of *Bacillus licheniformis* which had remained dormant on dried plants held in the British Museum since 1689 germinated into vegetative organisms which were active producers of penicillinase. Pollock found also that the penicillinase they produced showed biochemical and immunological properties identical with those of penicillinase produced by *Bacillus* species of the present day. He suggests that penicillinase production may have arisen by a mutation affecting some enzyme involved in the synthesis of the cell wall (p. 191) whose activity is inhibited by penicillin.

Penicillin Resistance of Gram Negative Bacteria

Although possessing a mucopeptide component in their cell walls, Gram negative bacilli are intrinsically much less susceptible to benzyl penicillin than are Gram positive bacteria. This could be due to a diminished affinity of the transpeptidation enzyme (p. 191) for penicillin, or to interference by lipid and/or other non-mucopeptide cell wall components with access of penicillin to the enzyme site. A possible role for the lipid is suggested by the finding that the sensitivity of various Gram positive bacteria is decreased under conditions leading to accumulation of lipids. The introduction of an amino group into benzyl penicillin, to yield ampicillin, results in considerably increased activity against Gram negatives. In the case of non-penicillinase producers this increase must presumably be achieved by an increase in the capacity of the drug to reach or to adsorb to the transpeptidation enzyme. Many coliform bacteria and other enterobacteriaceae, however, are resistant to ampicillin. In most cases this appears to be associated with a β-lactamase active against ampicillin. But there is also evidence that certain Gram negative bacteria may have an intrinsically high level of ampicillin resistance, quite apart from penicillinase production. The role of penicillin amidase in the resistance of Gram negatives to the penicillins is in doubt. Some Gram negatives produce this enzyme, which does not, however, appear to make a significant contribution to resistance, under normal growth conditions.

The Cephalosporins

The first member of this family of antibiotics, which possess the β-lactam ring structure of the penicillins and which apparently have an identical mode of action, cephalosporin C, was identified by Newton and Abraham in 1953 as one of a number of antibiotics produced by the mould *Cephalosporium acremonium.* This mould had been originally isolated by Brotzu from a sewage outfall in Sardinia in 1945, in a deliberate attempt to isolate an organism producing an antibiotic active against the typhoid bacillus. In addition to cephalosporin C, the mould produces two other compounds of interest—cephalosporin P, an acidic steroid structurally related to fucidin (p. 217), and cephalosporin N. Cephalosporin N is in fact a penicillin with an α-amino-adipic acid side-chain. It shows appreciable activity against various Gram negative bacteria but is considerably less active than ampicillin. Cephalosporin C consists of a nucleus of 7-amino-cephalosporanic acid (7ACA), which consists of fused β-lactam and dihydrothiazine rings, and an α-amino-adipic acid side-chain. Its potential value was indicated by its resistance to staphylococcal penicillinase and its activity against various Gram negative organisms, but its antibacterial action was in general much less than that of other penicillins.

$$H_2N.CH—HC \overset{S}{\diagup} CH_2$$
$$CO——N \diagdown_C \diagup C.CH_2.O.CO.CH_3$$

7-amino-cephalosporanic acid

Clinical interest has centred mainly on various derivatives of 7-amino-cephalosporanic acid, which have been prepared by chemical manipulation. Of these, *cephalothin* and *cephaloridine* are the two currently of therapeutic importance. Both are highly resistant to staphylococcal penicillinase but susceptible to the penicillinases of most Gram negative bacteria—though apparently much less sensitive to some than benzyl pencillin. On the other hand, certain *Proteus* and *Klebsiella* strains have been found to produce β-lactamases which are highly specific for the cephalosporins. Whether β-lactamase and cephalosporinase activity is, however, the function of distinct enzymes, is not at the moment clear.

The cephalosporins have a broader range of action against Gram negative bacteria—particularly against *Proteus* and *Klebsiella* strains—than does ampicillin, and are more effective against penicillinase-producing staphylococci than either methicillin or cloxacillin. Of the two, cephaloridine appears to be distinctly the more active against Gram positive organisms. Their activity against Gram negative bacteria appears to be about the same but cephalothin is reported to be somewhat more active against *H. influenzae* and the neisseriae.

A particularly valuable feature of the cephalosporins is that they can be used safely in cases of allergy to penicillin. Whether they can themselves induce sensitization comparable with that produced by penicillin remains to be seen.

Streptomycin and Related Antibiotics

Streptomycin produced by *Streptomyces griseus* was discovered by Waksman in 1944 as a result of an intensive search, prompted by the discovery of penicillin, for chemotherapeutic agents of fungal origin. It is a highly basic compound consisting of the base streptidine, an unusual sugar, streptose and N-methyl-L-glucosamine.

Streptomycin is highly active against the common Gram negative bacillary pathogens with the exception of *Proteus* species and *Ps. aeruginosa*—organisms which possess a high natural resistance to all the major antibiotics active against Gram negative bacilli. It is also active against *Staph. aureus*, *B. anthracis*, *A. israelii* and the neisseriae. It has little or no activity against streptococci, pneumococci, clostridia, spirochaetes, rickettsiae or chlamydiae. Undoubtedly the most important and most valuable feature of streptomycin is its high degree of activity against the tubercle bacillus. Streptomycin is not adsorbed from the alimentary tract. It has little power of penetration into the cerebrospinal fluid; its capacity to penetrate into serous cavities is about the same as that of penicillin.

A major difficulty in the use of streptomycin is the readiness with which organisms become resistant to it during the course of treatment. The more prolonged the treatment the greater is this risk. Consequently when streptomycin is used in the treatment of tuberculosis, for which treatment is necessarily prolonged, it must be combined with some other antituberculous drug. The development of resistance may not be a serious difficulty in the treatment of acute coccal and bacillary infections if the course of treatment is of short duration. A further disadvantage in the use of streptomycin is its toxic effect on the eighth nerve.

The action of streptomycin has been variously attributed to an effect on respiration, on oxidative phosphorylation, on the cytoplasmic membrane, and on protein synthesis. There seems little doubt, however, that the interference which has been described, both on respiration and on oxidative phosphorylation, are secondary to an inhibition of protein synthesis which is now generally considered to be the main action of the drug. In an in vitro synthesizing system using C^{14}-labelled polyuridylic acid as messenger, streptomycin was found to inhibit the formation of polyphenylalanine—the polypeptide coded for by polyuridylic acid. When 70S ribosomes prepared by aggregation of 30S and 50S ribosomes derived from both streptomycin-sensitive and streptomycin-resistant strains were examined, inhibition was found only when the 30S component was derived from a sensitive strain. No inhibition was observed when the 30S component was derived from a resistant strain.

The precise way in which streptomycin affects the ribosomes is unknown. The failure of the drug to bind to ribosomes already associated with messenger RNA suggests that it may in some way interfere with the association of messenger RNA and the 30S ribosome. An alternative hypothesis proposed by Gorini et al. is that streptomycin affects the association of messenger RNA with the ribosome, by altering the conformation of ribosomal RNA in such a way that the messenger code is misread. Thus, in the presence of polyuridylic acid as messenger, streptomycin was found to inhibit the incorporation of phenylalanine, while at the same time stimulating the incorporation of isoleucine, serine and leucine. This hypothesis might provide a simple explanation of streptomycin dependence; in this case dependence could be due to the correction at messenger level of what would otherwise be a lethal mutation.

The major difficulty with the hypothesis that the antibacterial action of streptomycin is due to an inhibition of protein synthesis is the demonstration of an early effect of the drug on the cytoplasmic membrane. The first demonstrable effect of streptomycin is in fact a loss of potassium ions from the cell, a loss which apparently does not occur in streptomycin-resistant organisms. In addition there is evidence of a secondary uptake of streptomycin, following an initial rapid adsorption similar to that occurring in cells whose membranes have been damaged by treatment with toluene. An action on the cytoplasmic membrane might moreover provide a more satisfactory basis for the marked bactericidal effect of streptomycin. Although this effect is most readily demonstrable with growing organisms it can be shown to occur, though to a lesser extent, with resting suspensions. It is possible that an effect on protein synthesis may be coupled with damage to the cytoplasmic membrane—as a result of combination of the drug with ribosomes closely associated with the membrane. At present, however, a precise definition of the relationship between these two phenomena is not possible.

Three other basic antibiotics incorporating amino sugar components, and also produced by various species of *Streptomyces*, show considerable structural resemblance to streptomycin. These are *neomycin, kanamycin* and *paromomycin*. They have a similar spectrum of action to streptomycin and have a toxic effect on the eighth nerve. They are, however, appreciably more toxic than streptomycin on the kidney. Among themselves they exhibit complete cross-resistance but show a unidirectional cross-resistance with streptomycin. Strains with acquired resistance to neomycin, kanamycin and paromomycin are resistant also to streptomycin, but strains resistant to streptomycin are not resistant to neomycin, kanamycin or paromomycin. Because of their toxicity they are mainly used for local application and for the pre-operative sterilization of the intestinal flora, for which they are highly effective since they are not absorbed from the intestinal tract. Of the three, only kanamycin possesses sufficient marginal safety for systemic use.

Neomycin, as commercially available, is a mixture of two chemically similar compounds, neomycin B and neomycin C. Neomycin B is also known as *framycetin*. Neomycin, kanamycin and paromomycin appear to be somewhat more active against the *Pseudomonas* group than streptomycin. In addition, resistance against them appears in general to be much less readily developed. Like streptomycin, they are more active at an alkaline than at an acid pH, presumably due to a greater ionization of bacterial acid groups.

Some relationship to this group is also shown by *viomycin*, a drug which appears to have a polypeptide structure. Viomycin-resistant strains are usually resistant also to streptomycin and kanamycin, while strains resistant to the latter drugs are often sensitive to viomycin. Viomycin has been used as a second-line drug in the treatment of tuberculosis (p. 366).

Chloramphenicol

This compound, first isolated by Ehrlich and his associates—from an actino-mycete, *Streptomyces venzuelae*—in 1947, when it was known as chloromycetin, is now produced by laboratory synthesis. A number of derivatives have been prepared by chemical manipulation but none has shown any improvement in antibacterial action or has remedied the main defect of chloramphenicol, its toxicity to haemopoietic tissues. Chloramphenicol has a wide spectrum of action against both Gram positive and Gram negative bacterial species, although it appears to be somewhat less active against Gram positives than the tetra-cyclines. Its use as a chemotherapeutic agent has been considerably restricted because of its capacity to cause aplastic anaemia—a complication which has nevertheless been observed only in a small number of cases. As a result of this, it is generally recommended only for the treatment of typhoid fever and *H. influenzae* meningitis, conditions for which it is currently accepted as the drug of choice. Toxicity apart, chloramphenicol possesses many of the properties of an ideal chemotherapeutic agent, and it is readily absorbed from the intestinal tract. Although some coliform bacteria possess an enzyme *nitroreductase* which reduces the nitro group, this alteration does not appear to affect the antibacterial action. The drug readily crosses tissue barriers, and gains easy access to the cerebrospinal fluid. In addition it penetrates tissue cells, a factor which must play a considerable part in determining its efficacy in the treatment of typhoid fever. Because of the hazard of aplastic anaemia it is doubtful if chloramphenicol should ever be given when an acceptable alternative is available. When its use is unavoidable, administration should be controlled by repeated blood examina-tion—a fall in reticulocyte count apparently being demonstrable at a stage at which the damage caused by the drug is still reversible.

Chloramphenicol unquestionably acts at ribosomal level. As shown by Gale and Folkes in 1953, it causes an immediate interruption in protein synthe-sis while stimulating the synthesis of RNA. The synthesis of DNA is not affected.

When taken up by bacteria, as shown by Vazquez, chloramphenicol binds to 50S component of 70S ribosomes. It is suggested that this combination causes a slight deformation of the structure of the ribosome, thereby affecting the proper association of the amino-acyl transfer RNA complex attached to the 30S ribosome with messenger RNA attached to the 50S ribosome. As a result the progressive addition of amino acyl s-RNA complexes is inhibited, and protein synthesis stops. The partially completed peptides are not released, however, messenger RNA remaining attached to the ribosome. Because of this continued association it is protected from normal decay. As messenger RNA synthesis is not interrupted, this would explain the apparently stimulatory effect of chlor-amphenicol on RNA production.

The Tetracyclines

The tetracyclines are a family of antibiotics produced by various species of *Streptomyces*. The important members of the group are tetracycline, chlortetracycline, oxytetracycline and demethylchlortetracycline. After the penicillins the tetracyclines are undoubtedly the most widely used antibiotics. This may

THE TETRACYCLINES

	R	R$_1$	R$_2$
Tetracycline	H	CH$_3$	H
Chlortetracycline	Cl	CH$_3$	H
Oxytetracycline	H	CH$_3$	OH
Demethylchlortetracycline	Cl	H	H

be attributed to their wide antibacterial spectrum, their virtual absence of toxicity except in very high doses, their ease of administration—they are readily absorbed from the intestinal tract—and their very low tendency to induce allergic sensitization. Like chloramphenicol, their action is primarily bacteriostatic; because of this they should preferably not be given in combination with penicillin unless laboratory confirmation of the value of the combination has been obtained. Being amphoteric compounds the tetracyclines are used mainly as the hydrochlorides. Their action is optimal at an acid pH.

The only significant toxic effect of the tetracyclines is on the liver, and then only when very large doses have been given by the intravenous route. In practice the most serious complication of tetracycline therapy is that, by creating a bacteriological vacuum in the alimentary tract, intestinal superinfection by *C. albicans, Proteus, Pseudomonas* and most seriously of all, by resistant strains of *Staph. aureus* may develop (p. 200).

Again, like chloramphenicol, the tetracyclines have been found to have an inhibitory effect on protein synthesis—an effect which has been demonstrated in cell-free protein synthesizing systems. Tetracyclines also act as chelating agents, however, and this function may be of importance in their antibacterial effect.

The Erythromycins

The erythromycins constitute a group of antibiotics consisting of a macrocyclic lactone ring, linked glycosidically to various sugars, because of which they are referred to as *macrolides*. They are basic in character and are most active under alkaline conditions. A number of individual members, differing mainly in their sugar residues, have been described: erythromycin, oleandomycin, carbomycin and spiramycin, of which erythromycin appears to be generally the most effective. The range of action of erythromycin is very similar to that of penicillin but its action is mainly bacteriostatic. For a time, erythromycin was used extensively in the treatment of infections due to penicillinase-producing staphylococci but has now been largely replaced by the newer penicillins and cephalosporins. The drug may, however, still be of value for the treatment of streptococcal and pneumococcal infections, in patients exhibiting penicillin hypersensitivity. The mode of action of erythromycin is unknown, but there is some evidence that it inhibits protein synthesis without affecting synthesis of nucleic acids. Its action may therefore be very similar to that of chloramphenicol.

Novobiocin

Novobiocin is an acidic antibiotic consisting of a phenolic residue—a substituted coumarin which confers on it a resemblance to dicoumarin—and an unusual sugar, noviose. It is active against most Gram positive organisms, *H. influenzae*, the neisseriae and, somewhat surprisingly, some strains of *Proteus*, and it is well absorbed from the intestinal tract.

It has been suggested that novobiocin interferes with the synthesis of the cell wall, since staphylococci exposed to it accumulate UDP-muramyl peptides. This would not, however, explain the inhibitory effect which has been demonstrated on staphylococcal and streptococcal L forms. Novobiocin binds magnesium ions, and it is possible therefore that this may play some part in its antibacterial action.

Resistance to novobiocin develops rapidly, and though of low toxicity, the drug has a considerable tendency to produce allergic sensitization. Currently it has only a limited place in chemotherapy.

Vancomycin and Ristocetin

These compounds—possessing appreciable toxicity—no longer have a place in therapy, but they are of considerable theoretical interest. They lead to the accumulation of UDP-muramyl peptides and have been found, in in vitro synthesizing systems, to inhibit a late stage in cell wall synthesis involving the incorporation of the glucosaminyl-muramyl pentapeptide into cell wall mucopeptide.

Cycloserine

Cycloserine is a relatively weak antibiotic active against the tubercle bacillus and a wide range of Gram positive and Gram negative organisms. It is of considerable value in the treatment of tuberculosis resistant to the major antituberculous agents and is claimed to be of special value in lesions of chronic type. Cycloserine has considerable neurotoxicity and has given rise to convulsions in a number of patients. It acts by inhibiting cell wall synthesis (p. 194).

Fucidin

This steroid antibiotic produced by *Fusidium coccinium* is the sodium salt of fusidic acid. Fucidin has a limited range of action, being highly active against staphylococci, neisseriae, corynebacteria and clostridia, but of low activity against streptococci. Resistance develops rapidly in vitro and combination with other antibiotics is therefore advised if prolonged administration is required. For this purpose erythromycin and novobiocin have been recommended. Fucidin is readily adsorbed from the intestinal tract. It possesses little if any toxicity.

Lincomycin

This antibiotic shows an antibacterial spectrum very similar to that of erythromycin with which it may show some cross resistance. Resistance however develops much less readily to lincomycin. It does not possess a macrolide structure. Lincomycin is readily absorbed from the intestinal tract. It may play a minor role in the therapy of resistant staphylococcal infections.

Gentamycin

This new antibiotic from *Micromonosporium purpurea* is a mixture of two components—gentamycin C_1 and C_2—of closely similar structure. Both contain a deoxystreptamine component and are chemically related to the streptomycin group. Gentamycin is a bactericidal antibiotic with a wide range of action against both Gram positive and Gram negative organisms. Perhaps the most interesting feature of its action is its activity against *Pseudomonas aeruginosa*. Unfortunately it has a high degree of toxicity for the 8th nerve. Although an appreciable degree of cross resistance has been shown between gentamycin, neomycin, kanamycin and streptomycin in mutants selected in the laboratory, strains of *Staphylococcus aureus* resistant to neomycin and kanamycin which have been isolated from patients have been found to be fully susceptible to gentamycin. The antibiotic may have some value in the treatment of *Pseudomonas* infections not amenable to other drugs and, by local application, in the treatment of nasal carriers of *Staphylococcus aureus* resistant to other antibiotics.

Polypeptide Antibiotics of Bacterial Origin

A number of highly potent bactericidal antibiotics have been isolated from members of the *Bacillus* genus. They include *gramicidin* and *tyrocidin* which were isolated by Dubos from a soil bacillus—*Bacillus brevis*—and are of historical interest as the first antibiotics discovered as a result of a planned search for such agents; because of their toxicity, however, they are suitable only for local application. *Bacitracin* produced by *B. subtilis*, is also too toxic for systemic use but is of theoretical interest since it appears to act by blocking some stage in cell wall synthesis.

The Polymyxins

These are the only polypeptide antibiotics with a place in current therapy. Five polymyxins—A, B, C, D, and E—have been identified. The commercially available compounds are polymyxin B, and colistin or polymyxin E, both supplied as the sulphate or sulphomethyl derivatives. Polymyxins A, C and D are too nephrotoxic for clinical use. Polymyxins B and E are, however, relatively non-toxic, and are undoubtedly the antibiotics of choice in the treatment of infections due to *Ps. aeruginosa*. Resistance to the polymixins is acquired only with difficulty in the laboratory, and resistant strains of coliform bacteria and *Pseudomonas* in clinical material are very rare. There is considerable evidence that the polymyxins act by damaging the cytoplasmic membrane. Initially, a rapid leakage of low molecular weight constituents occurs from the cell, and if the membrane damage becomes more intense the cell undergoes autolysis. Unlike penicillin lysis, the lysis produced by polymyxin is not dependent on cell growth, and can be produced in protoplasts.

SYNTHETIC CHEMOTHERAPEUTIC AGENTS

The Sulphonamides

Prontosil (sulphonamido-crysoidin), introduced by Domagk in 1935, was the first chemotherapeutic agent active against bacteria. In spite of its therapeutic

NH$_2$	NH$_2$	NH$_2$
COOH	SO$_2$.NHR	HO / COOH
p-aminobenzoic acid	Sulphonamides	p-aminosalicylic acid
(PABA)		(PAS)

effectiveness, however, it had no in vitro antibacterial activity. Its in vivo activity was shown, by Tréfouel, to be due to the fact that in the tissues it is broken down to yield sulphanilamide or para-amino benzene sulphonamide— the parent drug of the sulphonamide series and from which all the currently used sulphonamides have been derived by substitution for one of the hydrogen atoms of the sulphonamide—SO$_2$NH$_2$—group. The most active sulphonamides are those in which the substituent is a heterocyclic ring. In most cases substitution of the para-amino group has led to loss of activity, as a result of loss of structural resemblance to PABA (p. 192). One such compound, however, para-aminomethyl benzene sulphonamide—Marfanil—has appreciable antibacterial activity. This activity is not of sulphonamide type as it fails to be neutralized by PABA.

To a considerable extent, the antibacterial action of the sulphonamides can be correlated with the electronegativity of the SO$_2$ group. At pH 7 the electronegativity of this group and, as a result, the degree of dissociation of the compound may be increased by introducing substituent groups of increased electron-attracting power. This process can reach a limit, however, the maximum increase in activity being achieved with sulphadiazine which is about 70 per cent dissociated at pH 7. The failure of the more highly dissociated compounds to exert a greater antibacterial effect—one which might be expected from the virtually complete dissociation of PABA—is a result of the diminishing similarity between the electronic structure of the sulphonamide molecule and PABA as substitution progresses.

The sulphonamides have a comparatively limited range of action. They are active against the neisseriae—although many strains of gonococci are now resistant—and against *Str. pyogenes*, pneumococci, *B. anthracis* and the gas-gangrene clostridia. They are sufficiently active against *H. ducreyi*, *H. influenzae*, *Past. pestis* and the shigellae to be of therapeutic value in infections caused by these organisms. They are also of value in the treatment of coliform infections of the urinary tract because, although not highly active against the coliform group, they are excreted in effective concentration in the urine. The sulphonamides penetrate readily into the cerebrospinal fluid and are therefore of considerable value in the treatment of meningitis, particularly that due to the meningococcus.

Nalidixic acid (Negram)

This compound, one of a series of naphthyridine derivatives, is active against a variety of Gram negative bacteria but is without effect against staphylococci, streptococci or pneumococci. It is well absorbed from the gastro-intestinal tract and is excreted mainly in the urine. There is some evidence that the drug is concentrated in renal tissues. Excellent results have been reported for nalidixic acid in the treatment of urinary infections due to the coliform and *Proteus* groups.

Nitrofurantoin (Furadantin)

This compound, a nitrofuran derivative, has been used extensively by the oral route for Gram negative bacillary infections of the urinary tract. It has in addition appreciable activity against *Streptococcus faecalis*. It is most active at an acid pH.

Para-aminosalicylic Acid (PAS)

As previously considered, para-aminosalicylic acid is a PABA antagonist but is distinguished from the sulphonamides by the fact that its action is exclusively demonstrable against the tubercle bacillus. As an antituberculous agent it is merely bacteriostatic, and as a result, is much less effective than either streptomycin or INAH. As PAS is rapidly excreted it must be administered in high doses, in which, however, it causes gastro-intestinal disturbance. No modification of the drug so far achieved has resulted in any improvement in its antibacterial efficacy or in its capacity to persist in the tissues.

Isoniazid (INAH)

Although discovered in 1912, isoniazid was first reported to have activity against the tubercle bacillus in 1952. The β-isomeric form of the drug is inactive, suggesting that it acts as a competitive antagonist. The most obvious metabolite which it might antagonize is nicotinamide. However, the drug is without inhibitory effect on NAD-requiring dehydrogenases, nor is its inhibitory action overcome by nicotinic acid or nicotinamide. It is clear therefore that INAH does not act by nutritional antagonism of nicotinamide. An observation which may have some relevance to its mode of action is the fact that tubercle bacilli rendered resistant to it, lose the power to synthesize catalase and peroxidase. It has therefore been suggested that peroxidase may convert the drug into an

Isoniazid (INAH)   Pyrazinamide   Ethionamide

active form. However, the fact that atypical mycobacteria have normal catalase and peroxidase activity but show considerable resistance to INAH, makes this possibility less likely. INAH is an active chelating agent but there is no evidence for a correspondence between chelating activity of this and similar compounds, and their antitubercular action. Recent evidence tends to implicate INAH as having an inhibitory role in the synthesis of lipid. In this way it could cause damage to the cytoplasmic membrane and to intracellular lipid-associated enzyme systems.

INAH is well absorbed from the intestinal tract, and has marked powers of penetration across membranes and into cells. It has little, if any, toxic effect much of which appears to be reduced by concomitant administration of pyridoxine. Considerable differences have been shown between different individuals in the rapidity with which they metabolize INAH. In some, inactivation of the drug is slow, in others rapid, and there is evidence that these differences are genetically controlled. They are not of significance in chemotherapy provided that adequate doses of drug are administered.

Pyrazinamide

The discovery by Chlorine, in 1945, that nicotinamide possessed some activity against the tubercle bacillus—an activity not possessed by nicotinic acid—prompted the examination of other pyridine derivatives for similar activity. This led to the introduction of the amide, pyrazinamide, which, though not as active an antituberculous agent as INAH is appreciably more active than PAS. Unfortunately, it has a marked toxic effect on the liver, and is therefore not an acceptable alternative to PAS in the standard tuberculosis therapeutic regimen. Nevertheless it is of considerable value as a second-line drug which can be used in cases showing resistance to the primary drugs—streptomycin, INAH and PAS (p. 365).

Thiosemicarbazones

The thiosemicarbazones have been used extensively in Germany for the chemotherapy of tuberculosis. They are active only against mycobacteria. The most completely investigated member of the group—para-acetamidobenzyl thiosemicarbazone, or thiacetazone, has considerable activity against the tubercle bacillus but is, unfortunately, highly toxic. Its degree of toxicity makes it unacceptable except when other antituberculous drugs have proved ineffective.

Ethionamide (α-ethyl thio-isonicotinamide)

This pyridine derivative, because of its possession of the S:C.NH-group, shows a structural resemblance to the thiosemicarbazones. Because of this relationship there is complete cross-resistance between ethionamide and thiacetazone—the most important of the thiosemicarbazones.

Ethionamide is readily absorbed from the intestinal tract. It is now regarded by many authorities as the first choice when resistance to one or other of the major chemotherapeutic agents has developed.

Isoxyl (Iso-amyl oxythiocarbanilide)

This is another compound which has some resemblance to the thiosemicarbazones in possessing the S:C.NH-group. Isoxyl is not adsorbed from the intestinal tract. Recent evidence suggests that it may have a role in the treatment of tuberculosis, in combination with other active drugs, and that its toxicity is slight. Not surprisingly, in view of its structure, there appears to be some cross-resistance with the thiosemicarbazones.

The sulphones

These drugs, the most important of which is diaminodiphenylsulphone (DDS), are analogues of PABA. They are of historical interest in that they were the first chemotherapeutic agents shown to be effective in the experimental treatment of tuberculosis. They have appreciable toxicity but are nevertheless the drugs of choice in the treatment of leprosy against which, even though the disease is caused by a mycobacterium, INAH is quite ineffective.

CHAPTER 11

DIAGNOSTIC BACTERIOLOGY

The primary object of diagnostic bacteriology is to establish that the causative organism of a disease is present in the body of the patient. This may be attempted in one or both of two ways: (1) *Directly* by microscopy and cultural isolation. (2) *Indirectly* by the demonstration that the patient has developed an antibody response to the organism.

Collection of Material for Bacteriological Examination

The first step in the demonstration and/or isolation of a pathogenic organism is the collection of a satisfactory specimen from the patient. This should be taken with full aseptic precautions to prevent contamination by adventitious bacteria. It should be adequate in amount and be transmitted to the laboratory in an appropriate sterile container, clearly labelled and accompanied by a statement of the patient's main symptoms and of the possible clinical diagnosis. This statement is of considerable value to the bacteriologist in providing a guide to the type of laboratory examination required. Since delay may cause the death of delicate organisms the specimen should be transmitted to the laboratory as rapidly as possible. In the case of particularly delicate organisms, e.g. *Neisseria, Haemophilus* and *Bordetella*, cultures should be inoculated directly from the patient.

Fluid specimens should be transmitted to the laboratory in screw cap containers or bottles. Waxed disposable cardboard cartons are suitable for sputum. They must not however be sent through the post. Faeces are best collected in special glass or plastic containers carrying a collecting spoon attached to the cork or cap of the container. Blood for blood culture should be transported in a special blood culture bottle (p. 225). Cotton wool swabs wound on wooden or wire holders are used for the sampling of pus and exudate from wounds, discharging ears etc., and for obtaining specimens from the nose, throat, nasopharynx, larynx, urethra, cervix uteri and rectum. If the swabs cannot be sent to the laboratory immediately they should be immersed in a suitable transport medium. For the transport of swabs from urethral exudates for the isolation of gonococci Stuart's medium is recommended; for other organisms a simple agar medium is satisfactory.

Inspection

Before any specific bacteriological examination is undertaken the specimen

222

should be carefully inspected. Direct visual examination may reveal, for example, the presence in pus of the granules of *Actinomyces israeli* or of pus and mucus in a dysenteric stool. The colour of pus may suggest infection with *Pseudomonas aeruginosa* or its putrid smell the presence of certain anaerobic bacteria.

Microscopy

Unstained wet preparations which will reveal pus cells or red cells are important in the examination of urine and cerebrospinal fluid. For the demonstration of bacteria, however, wet preparations are of limited value, their most important use being in the demonstration of *Treponema pallidum* in primary syphilitic lesions by dark ground examination.

In the examination of some material (faeces, for example, for the presence of bacilli of the enteric or dysentery groups) the examination of the bacteria in stained films does not yield any information of value; but in the great majority of cases films should be prepared as a routine and stained by Gram's method. These will not only be of value in establishing the diagnosis but will frequently indicate the use of a particular cultural method, and will often help materially in the selection of suitable chemotherapy. Although the Gram stain may indicate the general nature of the organism responsible for the infection it will only rarely permit a completely definite immediate diagnosis. It is most valuable in doing so in infections due to organisms with a characteristic morphology, e.g. in gonorrhoea in the male, in Vincent's angina and in meningococcal meningitis.

For the demonstration of tubercle bacilli, films are stained by the Ziehl–Neelsen method. This should be used routinely for pus, sputum and serous fluids. It must be remembered, however, that acid alcohol-fast organisms are not necessarily tubercle bacilli. A particular danger lies in the use of the Ziehl–Neelsen method for demonstration of tubercle bacilli in urine which has not been taken by catheter. In these specimens *Myco. smegmatis* may be present and may be confused with the tubercle bacillus. In some cases special staining methods, such as that to demonstrate capsules, may be employed on films made from the material under examination.

In recent years the fluorescent antibody technique has been increasingly used for the direct demonstration of organisms in clinical material. It has been particularly valuable as a diagnostic procedure in conditions in which specific identification would not have been possible by the use of conventional microscopic techniques. In such cases the method has permitted a much more rapid diagnosis than cultural examination. Currently, the procedure is used, with appropriately absorbed sera—so as to eliminate nonspecific reactions—for the identification of group A streptococci in throat swabs, of enteropathogenic strains of *E. coli* in faecal smears and of gonococci in urethral exudates. The method also appears to be of some value in the demonstration of *Bordetella pertussis* in nasopharyngeal swabs and in the examination of the cerebrospinal fluid from cases of acute pyogenic meningitis due to *Haemophilus influenzae*,

Neisseria meningitidis and the pneumococcus. Other applications under investigation are the demonstration of typhoid bacilli and dysentery bacilli in faecal material and of diphtheria bacilli in throat swabs. There is little doubt that in the near future the range of usefulness of this technique will be considerably increased.

Cultural Examination

In some cases (e.g. tuberculosis, gonorrhoea, Vincent's angina) these preliminary examinations will suffice for the identification of the organism for purposes of diagnosis. In general, however, cultures are essential. Isolation by culture not only permits precise identification based on a study of the characteristics of the organism in pure culture, but is also a more sensitive technique than microscopic examination for the detection of bacteria. It is, furthermore, the only way in which it is possible to recognize the presence of most pathogens in sites, e.g. throat and intestinal tract, with a normal mixed flora.

As a routine medium for the cultivation of many of the organisms causing disease in man, blood agar is used. Where, however, the clinical history of the case, the source of the material, or the preliminary examination points to a certain organism or group of organisms, media appropriate for these must be employed.

If the specimen is fluid it should be centrifuged and cultures and films prepared from the centrifuged deposit. In the case of urine it is now a common practice to prepare cultures from the uncentrifuged fluid in such a way as to provide an estimate of the number of organisms present. Such an estimate can be simply obtained by inoculating plates with a single standardized loopful of the urine. In the cultivation of sputum the culture should be prepared from any purulent material present. The chances of isolating a pathogen, particularly *H. influenzae*, from sputum are improved if the sputum is homogenized, e.g. by shaking with glass beads, prior to culture. The procedures employed in the isolation of tubercle bacilli are considered in detail in Chapter 26.

Plates are incubated aerobically as a routine in all cases. When, however, the presence of anaerobic organisms is suspected anaerobic cultures are obligatory. They are desirable though not essential in the routine cultivation of material, e.g. pus and other exudates, from which aerobic bacteria are usually isolated but in which anaerobes, notably anaerobic streptococci, are occasionally present. A convenient method of anaerobic culture used for this purpose by many bacteriologists is to inoculate an iron strip broth or Robertson's meat medium along with the primary aerobic plate. If the latter is sterile the broth or meat is subcultured to blood agar plates which are incubated both aerobically and anaerobically. Aerobic subcultures prepared in this way not infrequently show the presence of aerobic pathogens when the primary aerobic plates are sterile. This is because many facultatively anaerobic bacteria grow best from small inocula when the pH of the medium is low. In cases of suspected *Neisseria* or *Brucella* infection a plate should also be incubated in an atmosphere of 5 to 10 per cent carbon dioxide.

Blood Culture

Isolation of bacteria from the blood is an important method of diagnosis in a number of conditions, in particular the coccal septicaemias, subacute bacterial endocarditis, brucellosis and typhoid fever.

A special blood-culture bottle is generally employed. This is an 8-oz bottle with perforated screw cap fitted with a rubber washer and containing approximately 50 ml of medium. For most purposes nutrient broth is a satisfactory medium, but for the isolation of streptococci some bacteriologists prefer a 1 per cent glucose broth. If the patient has been under treatment with a sulphonamide, a broth containing 5 mg per cent *p*-aminobenzoic acid should be used. Penicillinase may be added to the medium when cultures are being carried out on patients under treatment with penicillin. Broth containing liquoid (sodium polyanethyl sulphonate) in a concentration of 0·05 per cent is used in many laboratories. Liquoid is an anticoagulant and also inhibits the bactericidal power of the blood. Consequently when it is used a large volume of medium is not necessary—10 ml giving satisfactory results. This volume can be issued in a universal container.

In the taking of blood for culture great care must be exercised to avoid contamination of the blood by organisms present in the air or on the patient's skin. The blood culture bottle is inoculated at the bedside and should be warmed to body temperature before use. Since bacteria may be present in the blood only in small numbers a large volume of blood—5 to 10 ml—should be used as inoculum.

After inoculation the bottle is incubated overnight and then subcultured on to blood agar. At the same time films are made from the broth and stained by Gram's method. Subcultures should be made every 48 hours for a week, and at intervals up to at least 3 weeks from receipt. This long period of incubation is necessary because some organisms—viridans streptococci and brucellae—may grow very slowly. When the bottles are removed from the incubator they should not be allowed to cool before subculture.

For the isolation of brucellae a special liver extract broth should be used; after incubation this is subcultured on to liver extract agar. Both bottles and plates are incubated in an atmosphere of 10 per cent carbon dioxide. Before incubation, the screw cap should be removed from the bottle and replaced with a cotton wool plug.

It is frequently possible to isolate enteric organisms from blood clots sent for agglutination tests in cases of suspected enteric fever. The clot should be placed in a wide test tube and covered with broth. If there is any reason to believe that the blood was not taken aseptically, the clot may be cultured in lactose bile salt broth. Some workers add streptokinase to the culture medium used for clot culture. This breaks down the clot and may possibly facilitate the release of organisms trapped in it.

Species Identification

This may require the investigation of a considerable number of bacterial characteristics for which subcultures will be required. For this purpose a pure culture of the suspected pathogen is prepared by picking off a single colony from the isolation medium and inoculating it onto or into an appropriate subculture medium, e.g. agar slope, broth or blood agar plate. In the isolation of non-lactose fermenters from faeces it is desirable to subculture a single colony from the selective isolation medium onto a MacConkey plate, all further investigation being carried out with cultures derived from a single colony on the latter.

Microscopy

Gram's method is used as a routine and will show whether the organisms under examination are cocci or bacilli, whether they exhibit any characteristic arrangement and whether they are Gram positive or Gram negative. When necessary stains for capsules, spores and metachromatic granules are employed. Motility may be determined by the examination of wet preparations from fluid cultures (p. 34) or by the demonstration of a swarming or spreading growth on semi-solid agar.

Colonial Appearance

The colour, size, shape, outline and surface of the colony of the organism is of considerable value in its identification. If blood agar is employed it should be noted whether the colonies are surrounded by a clear zone of haemolysis—β haemolysis, in which the blood is not only lysed but digested, or, as occurs with the pneumococci and viridans streptococci, by a zone of greenish discoloration—α haemolysis.

Growth Requirements

Growth requirements are of value in some cases. Thus in the identification of *H. influenzae* it may be necessary to determine the organism's requirements for haematin and cozymase. The demonstration of a requirement for carbon dioxide is of value in the recognition of *Br. abortus*. If an acid-fast organism grows freely on blood agar it can be identified as a saprophytic mycobacterium —not a tubercle bacillus. It frequently is possible to show that an organism is a saprophytic contaminant, because it grows better at a low temperature, e.g. $25°$ C, than at $37°$ C. The capacity to utilize citrate as sole source of carbon and to grow in the presence of KCN is important in the identification of the enterobacteriaceae.

Biochemical Reactions

Many species have specific biochemical characteristics which are of value in identification. The biochemical characteristics most commonly examined are: (*a*) the presence of particular enzymes in bacterial cultures; (*b*) the presence in cultures of certain compounds as metabolic end products. These are, of course, produced as a result of enzyme action but are for convenience classified separately.

PLATE II

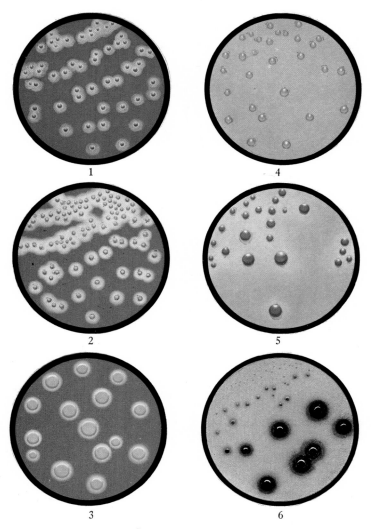

1

4

2

5

3

6

COLONIES OF BACTERIA

1. Streptococci on blood agar showing α haemolysis
2. Streptococci on blood agar showing β haemolysis
3. *Staphylococcus pyogenes* on blood agar
4. *Salm. typhi* on MacConkey's medium
5. *E. coli* on MacConkey's medium
6. *Salm. typhi* on Wilson and Blair's medium

[*To face p.* 226

The enzymes most frequently looked for specifically are *gelatinase, urease, oxidase, coagulase, lecithinase* and *catalase.*

For the detection of gelatinase a tube of gelatin is inoculated with a straight wire and incubated at 22° C. In the case of the anthrax bacillus a characteristic type of gelatin liquefaction occurs having the appearance of an inverted fir tree. Urease is detected by growing the organism in a urea-containing medium such as Christensen's. If the urea is decomposed, ammonia is liberated and the indicator changes to a purple-pink colour.

Catalase may be detected by adding a few drops of hydrogen peroxide (20 volumes) to a broth culture of the organism or to the growth on a solid medium. If the organism produces catalase there will be a vigorous evolution of bubbles of oxygen due to decomposition of the peroxide.

The demonstration of oxidase, coagulase and lecithinase are of importance in the recognition of the gonococcus, *Staph. aureus* and *Cl. perfringens* respectively; the tests used are considered in the appropriate sections.

The most important tests in which metabolic end products are demonstrated are the sugar fermentation reactions (p. 45). They are of value in the identification of many species.

For the differentiation of the enterobacteriaceae a great variety of biochemical tests may be employed. The most important of these are the following:

1. The production of indole in 24-hour broth or peptone water culture prepared from a peptone rich in the amino acid tryptophane. The presence of indole may be detected by layering a small amount of Ehrlich's reagent—para-dimethylaminobenzaldehyde—on the surface of the medium. A red ring develops if indole is present. Kovac's reagent which contains amyl alcohol in addition to para-dimethylaminobenzaldehyde is more sensitive than Ehrlich's reagent since the amyl alcohol extracts the indole from the culture. Organisms such as the cholera vibrio which in addition to producing indole reduce nitrate to nitrite give the cholera red reaction. This is the development of a red colour—due to the nitroso-indole reaction—on the addition of sulphuric acid to the culture.

2. The production of acetyl methylcarbinol (acetoin) in buffered glucose broth cultures is known as the Voges Proskauer (V.P.) reaction. Cultures are incubated at 37° C or preferably 30° C for 48 hours. Acetoin may be detected by O'Meara's or by Barritt's methods. In the former an equal volume of 40 per cent sodium hydroxide and a knife point of creatine are added to the culture which is then vigorously shaken. If acetoin is present a red colour develops usually within 2 to 5 minutes. In Barritt's method 0·6 ml of a 5 per cent solution of alpha naphthol in alcohol and 0·2 ml of a 40 per cent solution of potassium hydroxide are added to 1 ml of culture. A positive reaction is indicated by the development within 2 to 5 minutes of a pink colour which deepens to crimson or magenta in the course of the next hour.

3. The methyl-red test. This depends on the final reaction of the medium after glucose fermentation. Buffered glucose broth is inoculated with the organism and incubated for 4 days. A few drops of methyl-red solution are added and the resulting colour noted. If red (showing high and persisting acidity), the test is positive; if yellow (indicating low or transient acidity), it is negative.

4. Production of phenylalanine deaminase. The organisms are grown on agar slopes containing phenylalanine and a few drops of 10 per cent solution of ferric chloride allowed to run over the surface of the slope. Deamination of phenylalanine to phenylpyruvic acid is shown by the development of a green colour. Alternatively a low concentration of ferric ammonium citrate may be incorporated in the medium, the green colour in this case developing in the agar on incubation.

Antigenic Structure

In many cases specific identification requires the use of serological methods. Serological identification is usually carried out by the agglutination technique. In the ordinary diagnostic laboratory agglutination tests are mainly required for the identification of *Salmonella* and *Shigella* species. Diagnostic antisera specific for the more important of these are available commercially. For bacterial identification agglutination tests are carried out in the first place by the slide method using living suspensions. Positive results are then confirmed by the tube technique (Chapter 7). The most important application of the precipitin reaction is in the identification of the different varieties of haemolytic streptococci (Chapter 14).

Pathogenicity Tests

Many of the bacteria pathogenic for man are pathogenic also for laboratory animals. In such cases virulence tests in animals may be of considerable value in species identification. They have been used most for the identification of tubercle bacilli, anthrax bacilli, diphtheria bacilli, pasteurellae and clostridia. In the case of exotoxin-producing organisms, viz. diphtheria bacilli and the clostridia, the identity of the organisms can be completely established by showing that their lethal effect on laboratory animals is neutralized by the appropriate antitoxin. Virulence tests are now less frequently used than formerly, more reliance being placed on in vitro characteristics, but in particular instances they may still be necessary.

In some bacterial infections, notably tuberculosis and brucellosis, animal inoculation is used as a method of isolation. Animal inoculation is also employed in the isolation of viruses, rickettsiae and certain spirochaetes.

Differentiation of Types

Many bacterial species can be subdivided into types, and on occasion the bacteriologist may have to determine not only the species but the type within a species to which a particular organism belongs.

The criteria on which type differentiation is made vary with different species. In some, e.g. *Str. pyogenes* and the pneumococci, it is possible to distinguish a number of serologic types which differ from one another by the possession of type-specific antigens. *Staph. aureus* and some of the salmonellae, notably *Salm. typhi*, may be divided into types on the basis of their susceptibility to various bacterial viruses—bacteriophages—which are capable of lysing them

(Chapter 41). The diphtheria bacilli are divided into three types—*gravis*, *intermedius* and *mitis*—on the basis of morphology and cultural properties. In a few species type differentiation may be based on biochemical properties; this method, however, is not as valuable as those indicated above. When a species can be subdivided into types by different criteria the types are usually quite independent of each other.

Typing by serologic methods and by bacteriophage has been found to be of considerable value in epidemiological investigations. By the use of these methods it may be possible to trace the source of an infection or to follow the spread of an organism in the community with a degree of certainty which could not be achieved by a mere species identification.

SEROLOGICAL DIAGNOSIS

In certain conditions, it may be difficult or impossible to demonstrate the organism responsible by either microscopic or cultural methods. In these circumstances, serological methods, if available, may be employed. In these, attempts are made to demonstrate the presence of antibodies to a suspected organism in the patient's serum, and from the presence of antibody, or from the presence of a large amount of antibody, we infer that the patient is infected with that organism. Ideally, a rising antibody titre should be demonstrated, because only in this way is there any certainty that the antibody demonstrable has developed in response to the current infection. For this purpose two specimens of serum must be examined, one taken at an early stage of the disease and the second a week or ten days later. In many cases, however, this is not feasible and the diagnosis must, if possible, be made on the results of a single serological examination. The interpretation of single tests will depend on the normal level of antibody in the population, the stage in the disease at which the specimen is taken and on whether the patient has been previously immunized by a vaccine which stimulates production of the antibody in question (p. 312).

Antibodies may be demonstrated by a variety of serological techniques (Chapter 7). The most important of these for diagnostic bacteriology are the complement fixation test, which is of particular value in the diagnosis of syphilis and of viral infections, and the agglutination reaction, which is the most generally useful technique for the demonstration of antibody responses in bacterial infections. Agglutination tests are most frequently carried out in the ordinary clinical laboratory for the diagnosis of enteric infection and in this context are known collectively as the Widal test. They are also of considerable value in the diagnosis of brucellosis (p. 350) of various rickettsial diseases and, using the MG streptococcus as test antigen, of primary atypical pneumonia (p. 380).

Agglutination Techniques

Two types of techniques are used—the Dreyer and the Felix. The Dreyer method is used for the estimation of both H and O agglutinins, the Felix method only for O and Vi agglunins. The bacterial suspensions required for the Widal test in any particular area depend on the *Salmonella* pathogens prevalent in that area. In Britain it is customary to employ the following: *Salm. typhi* H and O; *Salm. paratyphi* B, H and O; non-specific *Salmonella* H; and since brucellosis is a not uncommon cause of undiagnosed pyrexia in Britain a *Br. abortus* suspension is also normally included. Standard agglutinable suspensions for use in these tests can be obtained commercially. The titres obtained in different laboratories using standard suspensions are directly comparable.

These techniques are also used with known antisera to confirm the results of slide agglutination tests in the identification of unknown organisms. For this purpose appropriate killed suspensions of the organisms under investigation are required. H suspensions may be prepared from motile organisms by the addition of formalin to a final concentration of 0·1 per cent to suspensions of the organisms prepared from broth or agar cultures. O suspensions may be prepared by boiling for half an hour. Alternatively the suspension may be mixed with twenty times its volume of absolute alcohol and heated at 40 to 50° C for half an hour. In all cases the density of the suspension to be used for the test is standardized nephelometrically to correspond to that of an accepted standard agglutinable suspension.

Dreyer Technique

The tests are carried out in special narrow agglutination tubes of $\frac{1}{5}$ to $\frac{1}{6}$ in. internal diameter. Reagents are conveniently measured in drops, with a standardized dropping pipette, following the schema shown in the accompanying table. When required a further series of dilutions may be set up using a 1 in 200 initial dilution of the serum. Alternatively serial halving dilutions of the serum

Tube No.	1	2	3	4	5
Saline	0	5	8	9	10
1 in 10 serum	10	5	2	1	0
Suspension	15	15	15	15	15
so yielding Final dilution of serum	1:25	1:50	1:125	1:250	0

Figures indicate the number of drops used.

may be made, usually starting from a 1 in 10 or 1 in 20 dilution in $3 \times \frac{1}{2}$ in. test tubes, and an appropriate volume of agglutinable suspension added, the mixture then being transferred to the small agglutination tubes. In the estimation of H agglutinins the results are read after incubation for 2 hours at 52 or 37° C. H agglutination is shown by the development of loose floccular clumps, due to the adherence of the flagella, which sediment to form a fluffy mass at the bottom of the tube. In the estimation of O agglutinins the tubes are incubated for 4 hours at 37° C when a preliminary reading may be made. The final reading should be made after the tubes have been allowed to stand overnight at 4° C. In O agglutination the agglutinated cells form a fine compact deposit in the bottom of the tube.

Felix Technique

Serial doubling dilutions of the serum are made in saline, starting from a 1/10 dilution, in 3 × ½ in. test tubes (Kahn tubes), so as to leave 1 ml of serum dilution in each tube. One drop of a concentrated agglutinable suspension is then added to each tube. The tubes are thoroughly mixed, incubated at 37° C for 2 hours and allowed to stand in the cold room overnight. Agglutination is shown by the accumulation on the bottom of the tube of a carpet of agglutinated cells. This frequently presents a wrinkled margin at the junction of the side and bottom of the tube. Unagglutinated cells collect in the centre of the bottom of the tube as a small circular button or spot. The sediment is conveniently examined by observation of its magnified reflection in a concave mirror.

The sedimented cells in the Felix technique can be used for the performance of the antiglobulin test for the detection of non-agglutinating antibody. In this case the tubes are centrifuged, the cells washed three times in saline and resuspended in an appropriate dilution of antihuman globulin serum. Alternatively antiglobulin tests may be carried out with cells recovered after an incubation period of 2 hours, from a parallel series of tubes set up independently at the time of performance of the direct agglutination test. Antiglobulin tests are of particular value in the diagnosis of *Brucella* infections; they have also been used for the estimation of non-agglutinating antibody to *Salmonella* antigens.

Complement Fixation Tests

As previously indicated complement adsorbs specifically to antigen–antibody complexes. Consequently fixation of complement can be used as an indicator that an antigen–antibody combination has occurred. The fixation of complement may be shown by demonstrating that, when added to the test system under suitable conditions, it is not available to cause immune haemolysis (p. 135) or conglutination (p. 137). Tests of this type are known as complement fixation tests. They are mostly used to demonstrate the presence of antibodies in a patient's serum but may also be used under appropriate conditions for the detection of antigen.

A typical haemolytic complement fixation test is divided into two stages. In the first stage the patient's serum, which has been heated to 56° C for half an hour to destroy any complement present, antigen and complement are mixed and allowed to remain in contact sufficiently long to allow the complement to become fixed. In the second stage, sheep red cells sensitized with immune body are added. The mixtures are then incubated, and the results read. If the patient's serum does not contain antibody, complement is not fixed in the first stage of the test and is therefore available to cause lysis of the sensitized sheep red cells added in the second stage. If, on the other hand, the patient's serum does contain antibody, the complement is fixed to the antigen–antibody complex in the first stage and lysis of the sensitized red cells added in the second stage cannot occur. Haemolysis therefore indicates a negative result and the absence of haemolysis a positive result.

The reagents employed in complement fixation tests must be carefully standardized. This applies particularly to the complement since there is a quantitative relationship between the amount of antibody present in the patient's serum and the amount of complement which can be fixed. If a large excess of complement is present, sufficient may be left over in spite of fixation to cause haemolysis, so giving a false negative result. The amount of immune body is not so critical, since it is only in low concentrations of immune body that its concentration affects the amount of complement required for lysis. In this range, increase of the concentration of immune body reduces the amount of complement required. To minimize the effects of variation in haemolysin concentration the tests are carried out using concentrations of immune body that lie appreciably above this range.

The unit of immune body and complement normally employed is the *minimum haemolytic dose* or MHD. This is the smallest amount of either reagent which under the conditions of the test will cause complete haemolysis. In the standardization of complement the minimum haemolytic dose of immune body is first determined. This is carried out in the presence of excess complement (5 MHD), since under these conditions the minimum haemolytic dose of immune body is not affected by the amount of complement used. The minimum haemolytic dose of complement is then determined by titrating the complement in the presence of excess immune body (5 MHD).

Usually two or three concentrations of complement falling within the range of from 2 to 6 minimal haemolytic doses are used in complement fixation tests. The inclusion of two different concentrations of complement permits a semi-quantitative estimate of the amount of antibody present, since the amount of complement fixed depends on the amount of antigen–antibody complex formed, and this with a constant concentration of antigen on the amount of antibody present in the patient's serum. Thus if 3 and 5 MHDs of complement are used, a serum that can fix 5 MHDs of complement must contain more antibody than one that can fix merely 3 MHDs of complement. A more complete estimate of the amount of antibody present in a serum can be determined by testing serial dilutions of the serum in the presence of a fixed quantity, e.g. 3 MHD of complement. The results are expressed, as in agglutination tests, as a titre; this is the highest dilution of the serum which in the presence of the antigen will fix all the complement employed in the test.

Complement may also be non-specifically fixed by a variety of materials—yeast, some bacteria, high concentrations of serum, tissue extracts, and inert particles such as kaolin and quartz. This non-specific fixation, i.e. fixation occurring in the absence of antigen–antibody reaction, is known as an *anticomplementary effect*. The dilutions of serum normally employed in complement fixation tests rarely show non-specific fixation. The test should, however, include a control to exclude the possibility of such fixation. This is provided for by including a tube which contains the dilution of serum used but to which antigen has not been added. The possibility of non-specific complement fixation is much less with serum that has been heated to 56° C than with unheated serum. Viral antigens derived from infected tissues are very liable to give non-specific complement fixation, and with these particular care has to be taken to ensure that they are not anticomplementary in the concentrations used in the test and that appropriate controls are included.

CHAPTER 12

THE CLASSIFICATION OF BACTERIA

In Chapter 1 bacteria were subdivided on purely morphological grounds into a number of large groups. Such a classification is, however, inadequate for practical purposes for which a greater degree of subdivision is needed. There is general agreement that bacteria should be classified as far as possible in the same way as plants and animals. On this basis each distinct kind of bacterium is designated as a species, and species with a number of common characters are grouped into genera.

Each species receives two Latin or Latinized names, e.g. *Staphylococcus aureus*—both of which should be italicized. The first name is the genus name. It is a noun in the singular and is always written with a capital initial letter. The second name is the species name. It is usually either a noun in the genitive qualifying the genus name, e.g. *Salmonella typhi*, or an adjective agreeing with the latter in gender, e.g. *Proteus vulgaris*. The species name is always written with a small initial letter.

The genus name may be used in the plural for descriptive purposes; in this case it is written with a small initial letter and is not italicized. We may for example describe the properties of the clostridia or of the neisseriae.

For practical purposes many species are subdivided into *types*; these are not regarded as being sufficiently distinct from each other as to warrant being given species rank. Subdivision into types is usually based on antigenic differences but occasionally other criteria are employed (Chapter 11). The term *group* is also used to indicate a subdivision of a species, but loosely and without any generally agreed application. It is usually employed for a number of types with sufficient resemblance to each other to justify their being grouped together. The ultimate unit in descriptive bacteriology is the *strain*. The term is applied to all the descendants derived by single colony isolation from a single source.

The application to bacteria of a system of classification similar to that employed for plants and animals, however, raises two major problems.

1. The concept of species is a concept based on sexuality—a species being a group of organisms that regularly interbreeds. This concept cannot however be applied directly to bacterial taxonomy since bacteria are normally asexual, and sexual equivalents in bacteria are of too restricted a distribution to constitute a basis for a comprehensive classification. Consequently species in bacteria must be defined on the basis of other criteria. For this purpose a variety of properties are used, viz. structure—both at the anatomical and antigenic level—staining

reactions, cultural characteristics and biochemical capabilities. In the application of these criteria to taxonomic definition two approaches are possible: (*a*) Certain characters may be regarded as being of particular importance, e.g. coagulase production for the definition of *Staphylococcus aureus* or the production of the Lancefield Group A hapten for the definition of *Streptococcus pyogenes*. In this way species are defined on the basis of a limited number of 'important' properties. This is the conventional and traditional approach, and for the day-to-day identification of individual bacteria the only feasible one. Its main disadvantage is that the importance of particular characters may be determined by a variety of adventitious factors—the techniques available, the fashions of the day and the particular interests of the taxonomist. The selection of differential criteria must therefore, to some considerable degree, be arbitrary. (*b*) The second approach involves the abandonment of the weighting of characteristics and the acceptance of all characteristics as of equal importance. This is the basis of modern numerical or neo-Adansonian taxonomy. The data obtained are fed into a computer which provides association indices, on the basis of which taxonomic groups or 'clusters' of individual organisms may be defined. Apart from its impracticability for bacterial identification, many bacteriologists have rejected numerical taxonomy from the conviction that some characteristics are more important than others in defining phylogenetic relationships. Nevertheless, numerical taxonomy has provided information of considerable value and can, at the least, assist the conventional taxonomist in the selection of the more important differential criteria.

Although sexual equivalents do not provide a practicable basis for bacterial classification, the concept of sexuality has in recent years been reintroduced at a biochemical level in the determination of DNA base composition. Wide differences in base composition, as shown by guanine-plus-cytosine content, have been found amongst bacteria. So far, data available for several hundred bacterial species have shown on the whole very substantial consistency within individual species, which are clearly defined by current procedures. Thus strains of *Staph. aureus* have a guanine-plus-cytosine content of 30 to 40 per cent, while tubercle bacilli have a guanine-plus-cytosine content of 60 to 70 per cent. Such findings clearly indicate that DNA base composition must in future be taken into account in species definition. Although the data available so far have provided substantial confirmation of current taxonomic definition at species level, they have, however, indicated considerable heterogeneity at the generic level.

2. The second problem is that of classification of species and genera into higher groups. Bergey's *Manual of Determinative Bacteriology* which is, for the bacteriologist, probably the most widely accepted system of bacterial classification, at least in its general outline, classifies genera into families, families into tribes, tribes into orders and orders into classes. Many bacteriologists feel, however, that such a rigid hierarchical structure is not justified, as it stresses too firmly phylogenetic relationships which must be a great deal more speculative than the relationships believed to be defined at species and genus level. To numerical taxonomists such a scheme is virtually meaningless. Nevertheless a

classification of this type is of great convenience for the description of bacteria, provided that it is not given an evolutionary significance or allowed to obscure the fact that bacteria constitute a spectrum of closely interrelated organisms.

As presented in the 7th edition of Bergey's manual, bacteria are assigned to the class *Schizomycetes* of the division *Protophyta*. The class Schizomycetes is subdivided into ten orders, only five of which are of medical importance. The main characteristics of each order and of the medically important families in each will be briefly described.

Order I. Pseudomonadales

Rigid Gram negative non-sporing rod-shaped or spiral forms. Usually motile by means of polar flagella. Polar flagellation is in fact the primary characteristic on the basis of which organisms are assigned to this order. Aerobic.

Families

Pseudomonadaceae. Rod-shaped forms. Many produce water-soluble pigments.

Spirillaceae. Curved or spiral organisms.

Order IV. Eubacteriales

Rigid cells—coccal or rod-shaped—which may be motile. Motility is due to peritrichous flagella. Aerobic and anaerobic.

Families

Achromobacteriaceae. Gram negative non-sporing rods. Rarely ferment glucose. Usually saprophytic in soil and water. Aerobic and facultatively anaerobic.

Enterobacteriaceae. Gram negative non-sporing rods. Ferment glucose and sometimes lactose, frequently producing gas (CO_2 and H_2). Many species parasitic in alimentary tracts of animals. Aerobic and facultatively anaerobic.

Brucellaceae. Very small Gram negative non-sporing rods. Usually have exacting nutritional requirements needing body fluids for growth. Restricted fermentative ability. Obligate parasites. Aerobic.

Bacteroidaceae. Usually anaerobic Gram negative non-sporing rods. Some show a rudimentary branching.

Micrococcaceae. Spherical usually Gram positive non-sporing organisms. Cells occur in masses, tetrads—groups of four arranged in one plane or in cubical packets of eight cells.

Neisseriaceae. Gram negative cocci usually occurring in pairs. Non-motile. Non-sporing. Many grow poorly without body fluids.

Lactobacillaceae. Gram positive non-sporing cocci and rods which usually form chains. Produce lactic acid in sugar fermentation. Growth stimulated by carbohydrate.

Corynebacteriaceae. Gram positive non-sporing rods frequently club-shaped.

Tend to stain irregularly. Some species show marked metachromatic granule formation.

Bacillaceae. Gram positive sporing rods.

Order V. Actinomycetales

Rigid cells. Frequently branching with the formation of a mycelium-like structure. In some species aerial hyphae give the colony a mould-like appearance.

Families

Mycobacteriaceae. Gram positive non-sporing organisms. Mycelium rudimentary or absent.

Actinomycetaceae. Branching cells with the formation of a true mycelium.

Order IX. Spirochaetales

Non-rigid unbranched cells of spiral shape. Only one family of medical importance—*Treponemataceae*: spiral cells 4 to 16μ in length. Motile by rotation round long axis and by lashing and uncurling movements. Non-flagellated.

Order X. Mycoplasmatales

This order comprises a group of highly pleomorphic organisms which are usually referred to as the pleuropneumonia group. Their relationship to other bacteria is in doubt.

CLASS SCHIZOMYCETES

Order	Family	Genus
Pseudomonadales	Pseudomonadaceae	Pseudomonas
	Spirillaceae	Vibrio
		Spirillum
Eubacteriales	Achromobacteraceae	Alcaligenes
	Enterobacteriaceae	Escherichia
		Klebsiella
		Proteus
		Salmonella
		Shigella
	Brucellaceae	Pasteurella
		Bordetella
		Brucella
		Haemophilus
		Actinobacillus
		Moraxella
	Bacteroidaceae	Bacteroides
		Fusobacterium
		Sphaerophorus
		Streptobacillus
	Micrococcaceae	Staphylococcus
	Neisseriaceae	Neisseria

Order	Family	Genus
	Lactobacillaceae	Diplococcus
		Streptococcus
		Lactobacillus
	Corynebacteriaceae	Corynebacterium
		Listeria
		Erysipelothrix
	Bacillaceae	Bacillus
		Clostridium
Actinomycetales	Mycobacteriaceae	Mycobacterium
	Actinomycetaceae	Nocardia
		Actinomyces
Spirochaetales	Treponemataceae	Borrelia
		Treponema
		Leptospira

CHAPTER 13

THE STAPHYLOCOCCI

Staphylococci are Gram positive, non-capsulated, non-sporing cocci which occur characteristically in irregular grape-like clusters. This arrangement is due to the way in which the organisms divide, successive divisions tending to occur in different planes. Their average size is from 0·7 to 1μ. Staphylococci are facultative anaerobes but grow best under aerobic conditions. Although their growth is improved by the presence of blood, they grow readily on any of the common laboratory media. The optimum temperature of growth is 37° C, but growth will occur from about 12° C up to 43° C. As defined by Bergey the genus *Staphylococcus* contains two species, the pathogenic *Staphylococcus aureus* and the non-pathogenic *Staphylococcus epidermidis*.

Staphylococcus aureus (*Staphylococcus pyogenes*)

Staphylococcus aureus produces a readily recognizable colony on blood agar, which is the medium most frequently used for its isolation; after overnight incubation the colony measures about 2 mm in diameter, has a smooth, highly refractile surface and an entire edge.

The colonies of most strains have a characteristic golden-yellow colour which, on longer incubation or on standing, becomes more intense. Pigmentation only develops in the presence of oxygen, and is due to the carotenoids—δ carotene and rubizanthene. On blood agar the colonies are usually surrounded by a narrow zone of haemolysis. *Staph. aureus* is highly tolerant of salt, and media containing a high concentration of salt are therefore of value for isolation from contaminated sources.

Most strains produce gelatinase and ferment a variety of sugars—of which mannitol is of some differential importance—to give acid but no gas. All strains are strongly catalase positive.

Antigenic Structure

A species-specific antigen demonstrable by precipitation tests has been identified in the cell wall, from which it can be readily extracted. The antigen appears to be a ribitol teichoic acid which owes its serological specificity to N-acetyl glucosamine residues. A non-species-specific red cell sensitizing antigen is demonstrable in cell extracts and culture supernatants. A similar antigen is produced by a variety of Gram positive organisms, and appears to be a glycerol teichoic acid.

By the use of agglutination tests with boiled suspensions the majority of strains may be classified, as first shown by Cowan, into three groups which show a minor degree of antigenic overlap. This classification has, however, been of only limited epidemiological value. A method of typing which appears to have greater potential value for epidemiological purposes has been described by Oeding. Using slide agglutination tests with living 5-hour cultures Oeding has been able to distinguish eight major antigenic components which participate in agglutination reactions. These antigens occur in different combinations in different strains and on the basis of their distribution it is possible to define a large number of agglutination types. The main limitation of this method as an epidemiological tool is that the majority of strains normally encountered appear to belong to a limited number of the possible types.

Bacteriophage Types

On the basis of their susceptibility to a series of symbiotic bacteriophages *Staph. aureus* strains may be classified into a number of types (p. 565). Most

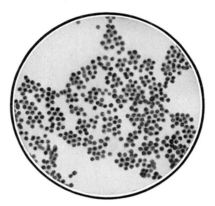

FIG. 16. *Staphylococcus aureus* FROM
AGAR CULTURE (× 950)

strains are susceptible to lysis by more than one typing phage. In such cases the type of the strain is defined by its pattern of susceptibility to different phages. With the currently standard set of 22 typing phages, several hundred bacteriophage types or patterns can be distinguished. The majority of strains isolated from human sources are susceptible to one or other of the typing phages, but a minority are untypable. The types fall into four broad groups—I to IV—the strains within each group being as a rule susceptible only to phages active within that group. The majority of typable strains from human sources belong to groups I, II and III, those found in hospitals being usually either group I or group III. The groups show a general, but not detailed correspondence with the serological groups determined by agglutination tests. The strains of the different groups also produce antigenically distinct coagulases, and show certain differences in pathogenicity and in the capacity to develop antibiotic resistance.

Many of the bacteriophages used in typing staphylococci have been derived from a limited number of symbiotic phages, which were subsequently adapted to different strains. This adaptation has, as in the case of *Salm. typhi*, involved changes in specificity due either to host range mutations or phenotypic host controlled modification. As for *Salm. typhi* (p. 561), the bacteriophage type of a particular strain may be modified by infecting it with a different symbiotic bacteriophage. Thus strains showing the pattern 80, 81, 52, 52A can be derived in the laboratory from 80, 81 strains by infection of the latter with certain bacteriophages belonging to serological group A. This transformation is believed to have occurred under natural conditions and to have been responsible for the emergence of the 80, 81, 52, 52A type. As most, if not all staphylococci are lysogenic, it would seem possible that the type specificity of lysogenic strains might depend on the nature of the symbiotic phage they carry. Evidence has not been obtained, however, to support this hypothesis as a general explanation of type specificity.

Phage typing has been of particular value in epidemiological investigations, especially in the investigation of sources of infection in outbreaks of bacterial food poisoning, and in tracing the spread of staphylococcal cross infection in hospital. Because of the larger number of types it reveals—several hundreds have now been encountered—phage typing is potentially a more useful epidemiological tool than serological typing.

Pathogenicity

At least three antigenically distinct haemolysins, α, β and δ, are found in cell-free filtrates. The α and δ haemolysins are produced by the great majority of strains irrespective of source. The β haemolysin is produced mainly by strains from animal sources.

Of the three haemolysins the α haemolysin is undoubtedly the most important in pathogenicity. Under in vitro conditions it is produced only in the presence of oxygen, and its production is enhanced by a high CO_2 concentration. Its haemolytic range is narrow, being lytic for rabbit, to a lesser extent for sheep and only slightly for human red cells, but it is toxic for a variety of cells in tissue culture. It has a rapidly lethal effect on experimental animals, following intravenous inoculation, and produces necrosis of the skin on intradermal injection. The toxin has been obtained in a highly purified form as a protein with a molecular weight of about 44,000. It shows a peculiar behaviour towards heat, crude preparations being inactivated rapidly at 60° C. Their activity is to some extent restored if they are subsequently heated at temperatures between 80 and 100° C. This paradoxical behaviour has been attributed to combination of the toxin with a heat-labile inhibitor at 60° C, at higher temperatures the inhibitor being destroyed and the toxin released. On further heating, however, the toxin is inactivated.

The β-haemolysin is lytic for sheep but not for human or rabbit red cells. The haemolytic process, initiated by incubation of cells with the haemolysin at 37° C may also be completed by exposure to a variety of substances—glycerol, low concentrations of δ-lysin, supernatants of cultures of *Streptococcus agalactiae*

(p. 260) and of various other organisms. The β-lysin has not been obtained in purified form but appears to be a phospholipase, hydrolysing various sphingomyelins, the distribution of which would explain the specificity of the lysin for the red cells of different animal species. It is produced under anaerobic as well as aerobic conditions, and does not require an increased CO_2 tension for optimal production.

The δ lysin is lytic for sheep, and less so for human and rabbit cells. It has been isolated as a crystalline protein with a molecular weight of about 70,000. Like the β haemolysin, it is much less toxic for experimental animals than is the α lysin.

Staphylococcal filtrates have considerable toxic action on human white cells. The substance responsible, known as *leucocidin*, is a complex of two serologically distinct components. These components will adsorb to red cells treated with tannic acid. Antibody to each of them can consequently be estimated independently by passive haemagglutination tests (p. 129).

In addition to their haemolytic action, filtrates of *Staph. aureus* have a rapidly lethal effect on experimental animals on intravenous injection and produce necrosis of the skin on intradermal injection. There seems little doubt, though this has not been formally proved, that these effects are due to the action of the α lysin.

Some strains of *Staph. aureus* produce an enterotoxin which is responsible for a variety of bacterial food poisoning. The enterotoxin is heat stable and can withstand boiling for 30 minutes. Consequently it may be present in food which has been heated sufficiently to kill all the staphylococci present. The existence of the toxin was first recognized by feeding experiments in human volunteers and in monkeys, and unfortunately these are still the only satisfactory test animals. The enterotoxin has been purified by Dack who has found it to be a trypsin-resistant protein. Three distinct antigenic types of enterotoxin A, B and C—of which A and B are the most important—have been identified. The toxin may be demonstrated by the Outcherlony agar gel diffusion technique, using antisera prepared against purified toxins. The mode of action of the toxin is unknown but since it produces vomiting in monkeys following intravenous administration, it is more likely to act on the central nervous system than on the gastric mucosa. Animals which have been exposed to enterotoxin become refractory to enterotoxin of the same antigenic type for some days. Most enterotoxin-producing strains belong to phage group III or to type 42D.

All strains of *Staph. aureus* have the property of clotting human and rabbit plasma by inducing the transformation of fibrinogen into fibrin. This is due to the secretion by the staphylococcus of a substance known as coagulase. Coagulase, however, is not itself the active agent of clotting but reacts with a second substance, variously referred to as *coagulase reacting factor* or *coagulase activator*, present in plasma and in tissue fluids, to produce the active agent; the latter has properties very similar to those of thrombin, both splitting off identical peptides from fibrinogen, and both being inhibited by the esterase inhibitor di-isopropylfluorophosphate (DFP) and by heparin. Because of this resemblance it is referred to as coagulase-thrombin. The plasmas of certain animal species, e.g.

the guinea-pig, are deficient in coagulase reacting factor. Because of this, these plasmas are not clotted by staphylocoagulase, even though their fibrinogen is fully susceptible to coagulase-thrombin.

Coagulase is antigenic; immune sera can be prepared against it in animals, and antibodies to it are demonstrable in the sera of patients suffering from chronic staphylococcal infections. Seven distinct antigenic varieties of coagulase have now been described. The majority of human strains of *Staph. aureus* produce coagulase A.

Coagulase is an extremely important component of the offensive armoury of *Staph. aureus*. By laying down a fibrin barrier which is impermeable to leuco-cytes in the immediate vicinity and on the surface of the organism, it gives the latter considerable protection from phagocytosis. Since under in vitro condi-tions coagulase is produced in the lag phase and in the early log phase, it can be presumed to protect the organism from phagocytosis at a time when such protection is most needed, i.e. during the early stages of infection. In addition there is evidence that coagulase protects the staphylococcus against bactericidal substances present in the tissue fluids. How this is achieved is not known.

For the demonstration of coagulase 0·1 ml of an overnight broth culture of the organism and 0·9 ml of a 1 in 10 dilution of human or rabbit plasma are pipetted into a Kahn tube. The mixture is incubated at 37° C and the result read after 2 hours. If the organism produces coagulase, the plasma will form a clot which is usually sufficiently firm to remain adherent to the sides of the tube when the latter is inverted. It is important that incubation should not be prolonged for more than 2 hours, since on prolonged incubation some organisms are capable of utilizing the citrate employed as anticoagulant and, as a result, spontaneous clotting of the plasma may occur.

When staphylococci are mixed on a slide with the plasma of certain animal species the staphylococci are rapidly clumped or agglutinated. It was first assumed that this agglutination was due to coagulase activity. It was shown by Duthie, however, that this was not the case, the clumping being due to the combination of fibrinogen in the plasma with a receptor, known in this context as *clumping factor*, present on the surface of the organism. Clumping does not require the co-operation of the coagulase reacting factor and the fibrinogen is not transformed into fibrin. From the evidence presented by Duthie it is appa-rent that the staphylococcal component involved in the clumping phenomenon is distinct from coagulase:

1. It is an integral component of the cell wall, and unlike coagulase, is not secreted into the medium except on autolysis of the cell.

2. Though resembling coagulase in being a protein it is markedly heat-stable, while coagulase is heat-labile.

3. Coagulase and clumping factor are serologically distinguishable, only one antigenic type of the latter having been described.

4. Clumping is produced only by the fibrinogens of certain animal species. Coagulase thrombin, on the other hand, is active against all fibrinogens, regardless of source.

Staphylococcus aureus also shows some fibrinolytic activity, but not as actively as *Str. pyogenes*. Fibrinolysin is produced by the action of a staphylococcal product, *staphylokinase*, on plasminogen—a protease precursor which is a normal component of plasma. Staphylokinase is produced only during the later stages of growth, and its contribution to staphylococcal pathogenicity is therefore in doubt. It may, however, play a part in the production of staphylococcal septicaemia, by dislodging infected intravascular thrombi. Most strains of *Staph. aureus* also produce hyaluronidase and desoxyribonuclease.

Staphylococci have been shown to produce a number of lipolytic enzymes at least one of which, described by Alder and Gillespie, can produce opacity in egg yolk media, and may have some relation to pathogenicity. Its substrate appears to be the lipoprotein, *lipovitellin*. This enzyme is produced by most strains isolated from boils and carbuncles, and is thought to play a part in the invasion of staphylococci through the intact skin.

Staphylococcal Infections

The nose is the natural home of *Staph. aureus,* and the organism can be isolated from the anterior nares of about 50 per cent of normal persons. In many of these the carrier state is of short duration, but in some it is more persistent. The nasal carriage rate is considerably higher in hospital patients than in the general population. From 5 to 10 per cent of people are skin carriers— probably in many cases as a result of contamination from the nose. Staphylococci are also frequently present in the intestinal tract and may be isolated from the faeces of about 20 per cent of normal persons. The perineum, particularly in infants, is also an important carrier site.

Staphylococcus aureus is probably the most frequent cause of acute pyogenic infections in man. The lesions produced are characteristically localized, and septicaemia, though it occasionally occurs, is infrequent. In this respect staphylococcal lesions contrast sharply with those produced by *Str. pyogenes*.

Staphylococcus aureus has a marked predilection for the skin. It produces pustules, boils and carbuncles—the organisms responsible in many cases being derived from the nose—and is a frequent cause of sepsis in wounds and burns. About 10 per cent of people with cutaneous staphylococcal lesions are subject to recurrent infections, which are particularly frequent in persons infected with so-called hospital staphylococci (p. 246). The capacity to produce boils and other cutaneous staphylococcal infections is apparently not possessed equally by all strains of *Staph. aureus*. Many strains capable of causing hospital wound sepsis do not, apparently, cause boils. *Staph. aureus* appears to be the causative organism of most cases of *impetigo contagiosa*, a condition which may also be caused by *Str. pyogenes* (p. 258). Most of the strains of *Staph. aureus* isolated from cases of impetigo belong to a single bacteriophage type, type 71, and are strong producers of hyaluronidase. The latter property may explain the epidermal character of the lesion in impetigo, which contrasts with the subepidermal type of infection found in boils and carbuncles. A closely similar condition in babies, *pemphigus neonatorum*, is also caused by the staphylococcus.

Staphylococcus aureus is the causative agent in about 90 per cent of cases of acute osteomyelitis. This condition, which occurs mostly in children, is the result of haematogenous spread from a superficial site of infection such as a boil or furuncle. Staphylococcal osteomyelitis may also occur as a result of infection of a compound fracture.

Staphylococcus aureus is frequently isolated from infections of the air sinuses and is responsible for a relatively uncommon but severe type of pneumonia. As a primary infection staphylococcal pneumonia appears to occur most frequently in the neonatal period. In the adult it is usually secondary to some other infection of the respiratory tract and is particularly important as a complication of influenza. The pulmonary lesions in staphylococcal pneumonia are of bronchopneumonic distribution and frequently progress to abscess formation.

On rare occasions the staphylococcus may give rise to septicaemia. This is, fortunately, an uncommon complication of staphylococcal infection. Currently, however, about 50 per cent of cases of septicaemia are due to the staphylococcus, the remainder being caused by miscellaneous Gram negative bacilli, particularly of the coliform group. In septicaemia, the patient is gravely ill and multiple foci of metastatic infection appear. Less extensive blood invasion may result in isolated metastatic lesions such as meningitis, renal and perinephric abscesses and liver abscess.

Reference has already been made to the severe enterocolitis which may complicate treatment with antibiotics, especially the tetracyclines, which are highly active against the normal Gram negative flora of the intestinal tract. This condition is most frequently caused by *Staph. aureus*. As a rule it occurs sporadically but epidemics have been described. It is thought that only certain strains of staphylococci have the capacity to produce enterocolitis.

Staphylococcus aureus is an important cause of bacterial food poisoning. This condition is an intoxication and not an infection. It is due to the ingestion of enterotoxin formed as a result of multiplication of the organisms in food. The foods responsible are usually made up meat dishes and foods containing a high concentration of milk or cream. Food poisoning is most likely to occur if the food has been held under warm conditions for some time prior to eating, thereby permitting bacterial multiplication. The food is usually infected in the course of preparation by a nasal carrier or by an individual with a superficial staphylococcal lesion, e.g. furuncle, boil or impetigo.

Staphylococcal food poisoning is usually rapid in onset, the symptoms, the most prominent of which are vomiting and abdominal pain, appearing within 4 to 6 hours of ingestion of the food. It is of short duration usually resolving in a further 24 hours, has a negligible mortality, and is a much less serious condition than salmonella food poisoning. The lack of fever and the prominence of vomiting as a symptom help to differentiate it clinically from the latter condition.

Hospital Infections

In recent years considerable attention has been directed to the problem of the infection, in hospital, of clean surgical wounds by pyogenic organisms. *Staph. aureus* is the single most important cause of such infections. Thus in a survey of wound sepsis carried out by the Public Health Laboratory Service staphylococci were isolated alone in 45 per cent of cases and in association with coliform bacteria in a further 15 per cent. There is a widespread belief that these infections have increased in frequency. Reliable evidence on this point has, however, been difficult to obtain, since, not only is the incidence of sepsis different in different hospitals but it is also different in different types of operation. As a rule wound infection merely results in a delay in healing, though this, by prolonging the patient's stay in hospital is of considerable economic importance. Occasionally, however, it may be the starting point of a septicaemia which not infrequently leads to the death of the patient.

Though in some cases wound infection is due to a strain of staphylococcus which the patient was carrying on his admission to hospital it is much more frequently due to organisms which he has acquired from the hospital environment—the so-called hospital staphylococci. The application of the phage-typing technique has shown that the majority of strains of staphylococci responsible for hospital infections belong to a quite limited number of bacteriophage types. This finding has created the concept of epidemic or hospital strains of enhanced virulence and infectivity. The existence of such strains—although earlier suggested by paediatricians as being involved in neonatal infections—was first clearly demonstrated by the identification of the notorious phage type 80 as being responsible for a high proportion of epidemics of hospital sepsis in Australia in 1953 to 1954, and, shortly afterwards, as an important cause of hospital cross infection in other parts of the world. In 1957 strains giving the pattern 52, 52A, 80, 81 started to appear. This pattern was shown to be the result of lysogenization, with type determining phages, of 80/81 strains. The phages 52, 52A, 80 and 81 appear in fact to determine a closely interrelated complex of strains which may give all possible combinations of reactions with these typing phages. From 1957 onwards group III strains of type 83A, which is quite unrelated to the important 80/81 complex appeared as important causes of epidemics.

In view of the wide use of antibiotics in the hospital environment, it is not surprising that hospital strains should show a high level of antibiotic resistance. They are invariably resistant to penicillin and usually to the tetracyclines as well. In addition they have been shown by Moore to have frequently a high level of resistance to mercury salts. It is not immediately clear how this property could confer a selective advantage on a strain possessing it, since mercurial disinfectants are now little used in hospital practice.

The properties of epidemic staphylococci which are ultimately responsible for their high infectivity and their capacity to persist in the hospital environment are not known. There is some evidence that they may have a higher degree of viability outside the body than non-epidemic strains. There is, in addition, evidence that they not only possess a higher infectivity than non-epidemic strains but are also more pathogenic. Thus Barber found that highly drug-resistant strains more frequently give rise to generalized, as opposed to localized, infections than drug-sensitive strains. Moreover, carriers of epidemic strains more frequently develop infections caused by the carried strains than do carriers of non-epidemic strains.

Although they may be isolated from floors, hangings and other inanimate objects, the great reservoirs of staphylococci in the hospital environment are patients and members of the hospital staff who are carriers or who are suffering from staphylococcal infections. As sources of staphylococcal infection *people* are much more important than *things*, and patients suffering from overt infections— of which the most dangerous in this context are exposed skin lesions, enterocolitis and pneumonia, from which the environment is readily contaminated— are much more important than carriers. At one time it was thought that staphylococcal carriers disseminated staphylococci into their environment by direct droplet contamination. There is little evidence that this mode of spread is of any great importance. More important is spread by hands and contaminated handkerchiefs to the clothing and bedding, from which in turn the organisms are disseminated mainly by frictional movements and by shaking.

When patients are first admitted to hospital their anterior nares rapidly become colonized by the resident hospital strains. Many such patients develop wound infections in which the staphylococci are of the same phage type as those carried in the nose. Such infections are therefore presumably auto-infections. At the same time, control of the nasal carrier state in such patients by the application of antiseptic creams to the anterior nares does not, however, appear to reduce significantly their chances of acquiring a wound infection. This makes it possible that the wound or the nose, or perhaps both, are infected from the same source. There is, however, considerable reason to believe that auto-infection plays an important role in the pathogenesis of cutaneous staphylococcal infection acquired outside hospital.

Infection of wounds may occur at any time from their infliction until they are completely healed but is most likely to be acquired at the time of operation or during dressing of the wound.

Infection in the operating theatre is probably most frequently due to contamination of the air. On occasion this has been shown to be caused by the use of an exhaust ventilation system sucking in unfiltered contaminated air from wards and corridors. More important sources of infection are bed-clothes brought in with patients from the wards; individuals entering the theatre—other than members of the operating team—without being required to change their clothes; patients with staphylococcal sepsis, and members of the operating theatre staff who may be carriers or who may be suffering from superficial staphylococcal infections. A clear relationship has been established between the total bacterial content of the air of the theatre, as measured by slit sampler, its staphylococcal content and the frequency of wound sepsis. If the theatre is used for a number of consecutive operations it is inevitable that the air contamination will increase. Consistent with this is the finding that the lower the patient is in the operation order the greater the likelihood of his developing wound sepsis. The extent of air contamination also depends on the amount of movement permitted in the theatre.

Wounds may also be infected by direct contact, e.g. by improperly sterilized instruments and sutures, and through punctures in rubber gloves, by organisms derived from the surgeon's hands, and as a result of improper sterilization of the patient's skin prior to operation. Operative technique is also important; if the tissues are roughly handled, thereby lowering their resistance to infection, or if haemostasis is incomplete, allowing the formation of haematomata in the depths of which bacteria can grow, the chances of infection are greatly increased.

Occasionally a hospital experiences a sharp increase in the incidence of staphylococcal wound infection. The more serious epidemics appear in most cases to be produced by strains of staphylococci, e.g. the notorious phage type 80, with an exceptional capacity to spread and to produce superficial cutaneous lesions. Epidemics may on occasion be due to a breakdown at some point in the sterilizing, operative or wound dressing procedures or to a nurse or surgeon who has a superficial staphylococcal lesion or who is a persistent nasal carrier.

A high incidence of staphylococcal infection has also been reported in newborn infants in maternity wards. Cutaneous lesions and blepharitis are of frequent occurrence and staphylococcal pneumonia is not uncommon. Infants are particularly susceptible to colonization with *Staph. aureus* and within a short period after birth from 80 to 100 per cent of those born in hospital become first skin and then nasal carriers. The organisms responsible appear in the majority of cases to be derived from other children in the ward rather than from the nursing staff. Other frequent sites of colonization are the umbilical stump and the perineum. There is now considerable evidence that the incidence of neonatal sepsis due to the staphylococcus can be greatly reduced by measures designed to prevent the colonization of these major carrier sites. Newborn infants frequently transmit the staphylococci they acquire in hospital to their mothers during breast feeding. This often results in the production in the mother of a staphylococcal mastitis which may not become clinically apparent until after she leaves hospital.

Diagnosis

Colonies of *Staph. aureus* are usually readily recognizable on blood agar, although occasional strains of the organism are encountered which do not produce the characteristic golden pigment. For normal diagnostic purposes the identity of the organism is confirmed by coagulase tests.

In the isolation of staphylococci from heavily contaminated material such as food, vomit or faeces, the specimen should be plated on one of the selective media, viz. blood agar containing 7 per cent sodium chloride or Ludlam's medium. Phenolphthalein phosphate agar is sometimes used, and after incubation the plate is exposed to ammonia vapour. Colonies of *Staph. aureus* turn pink as a result of the liberation of phenolphthalein.

In recent years considerable interest has been taken in the possibility of using serological tests for the diagnosis of staphylococcal infections. In most cases serological tests are quite unnecessary, but in certain occult infections, e.g. osteomylitis of the spine and hip, a reliable serological test would be of considerable value. Relatively simple techniques have been developed for the estimation of antibodies to α haemolysin, leucocidin, coagulases and staphylokinase. Of these, the tests for anti-leucocidin—carried out by the haemagglutination technique—appears to be the most generally useful.

Treatment

Of all bacterial species *Staph. aureus* has shown the greatest tendency to develop resistance to antibiotics to which, when first introduced, the species as a whole appeared uniformly sensitive. Because of this, the choice of antibiotic in any particular case should, where possible, be based on the results of sensitivity tests. Antibiotic-resistant strains of staphylococci are much more numerous in the hospital environment than in the general population. Nevertheless, the number of resistant strains isolated from sources outside hospital has, though to a much lesser extent, increased as well.

Many of these strains are resistant to other commonly used antibiotics, particularly to the tetracyclines and streptomycin. In general the number of strains resistant to a particular antibiotic in any environment depends on the frequency with which that antibiotic has been used in the environment. If the antibiotic is discontinued or its use curtailed the frequency with which strains resistant to it are isolated immediately falls.

Penicillinase-producing staphylococci are resistant to ampicillin, as well as to benzyl penicillin, but are sensitive to the semi-synthetic penicillins—methicillin and the isoxazolyl penicillins—and to the cephalosporins as well as a variety of other antibiotics outside the penicillin group. Some strains have been described which have been resistant to methicillin. The resistance of some of these strains examined by Barber, was only partial, requiring for its full expression growth on hypertonic media. Systemic antibiotic therapy should not be used for mild cutaneous staphylococcal infections which can be effectively treated by topical applications of various antimicrobials which are not suitable for systemic administration, e.g. bacitracin, neomycin, chlorhexidine, framycetin and gramicidin, given singly or in various combinations.

Penicillinase Plasmids

Naturally occurring penicillin-resistant strains of *Staph. aureus* owe their resistance to the production of penicillinase (p. 209). Staphylococcal penicillinase is inducible and is excreted by the organism into the medium. The amount excreted, however, varies considerably in different strains. By analysis of mutants obtained in the laboratory it has been possible to identify two genes controlling penicillinase production, a gene p, which determines the structure of the enzyme, and a gene i, which controls its inducibility. It is generally accepted, though not formally proved, that inducibility is dependent on the production of a cytoplasmic repressor (p. 31). Three antigenic varieties of penicillinase have been distinguished: A, B and C. Type B only occurs in phage group II strains, and types A and C in strains of groups I and III. The type B enzyme is much less active, and has a lower substrate affinity than types A and C. This may explain the lower frequency as causes of human infections of phage group II strains compared with strains of groups I and III.

Penicillinase production is controlled by extrachromosomal genetic determinants known as *plasmids* (p. 24). These resemble R factors but are not spontaneously transmissible. They may, however, be transferred from one strain to another by transduction, for which phage 80 has been most frequently used.

The plasmids may be spontaneously lost and in some cases the rate of loss is higher than 1 in 1000 cell divisions—a frequency much greater than that of spontaneous mutations. Loss of plasmid is accelerated by exposure of the cell to acridine dyes. In addition to penicillinase production, penicillinase plasmids have been found to carry determinants for other bacterial characters, viz. resistance to mercuric chloride and to erythromycin, and a colonial morphology marker. They may be divided into two groups, *pla* I and *pla* II, depending on their compatibility in the same cell. On transduction of a plasmid of one compatibility group into a cell already possessing a plasmid of another compatibility

PENICILLINASE PLASMIDS IN *Staphylococcus aureus*

Plasmid type	α	β	γ	δ	ε	ζ
Phage groups of carrier strains	I/III	I/III	I/III	II	I/III	I/III
Erythromycin resistance	−	−	+	−	−	−
Penicillinase type*	A	C	A	B	A	C
Resistance to HgCl₂	+	+	+	+	−	−
Compatibility group†						
pla I	+	−	+	?	+	+
pla II	−	+	−	?	−	−

From: M. H. Richmond (1965), 'Penicillinase plasmids in *Staphylococcus aureus*'. In *Recent Research in Molecular Biology* (Ed. R. C. Clowes). *Brit. med. Bull.*, *21*, 260.

* Types differ serologically. B is less active against penicillin than A and C.
† Plasmids in same compatibility group cannot coexist in one cell as separate components, but may undergo recombination.

group, both plasmids can coexist in the cell as separate entities, and each may be lost from the cell independently. This coexistence is referred to as the *poly-plasmid* state. If, however, a plasmid of one compatibility group is transduced into a strain already harbouring a member of this group, the polyplasmid state is not produced but recombination between the plasmids may occur. On the basis of their compatibility group, the antigenic type of penicillinase produced, and the non-penicillinase markers they carry, ten types of plasmid have so far been distinguished. The properties of the first six plasmids to have been described are shown in the accompanying table.

There is some evidence that staphylococcal antitoxin may be a useful adjunct to chemotherapy in the treatment of acute staphylococcal infections in which there is marked toxaemia.

Prophylaxis

The control of hospital infections is now a problem of such magnitude as to require planning at the administrative level. The general principles which should be adopted are: (1) The elimination of all reservoirs of infection. This involves the institution of measures designed to reduce dust, the sterilization of bed clothes, the control of nasal carriers for which topical application of anti-septic creams or sprays has been favourably reported on and the exclusion of all persons with superficial septic lesions from contact with the patient, either in the operating theatre or in the ward. (2) The employment of a fully aseptic technique in the operating theatre and during the dressing of wounds. (3) The recording and investigation of all cases of wound sepsis. Phage typing should be employed in the investigation of all major outbreaks of infection. If several phage types are found the presumption is that the outbreak is due to a breakdown at some point in aseptic technique. The isolation of a single phage type from the majority of cases would indicate on the other hand the likelihood of infection from a single source or the wide dissemination of a rapidly spreading epidemic type.

Staphylococcal vaccines have been extensively used both in the treatment and prophylaxis of recurrent cutaneous staphylococcal infections, and occasionally have been found to be of value. Better results have been claimed in these conditions with a staphylococcal toxoid, prepared by treatment of a filtrate containing the α toxin with formalin. The immunity produced by the toxoid is of short duration and frequent boosting doses are required. The toxoid is sometimes of value in aborting a superficial staphylococcal infection such as a boil if given at the first sign of development of the lesion.

Staphylococcus epidermidis

This species occurs as a normal inhabitant of the skin. It is coagulase-negative, and produces a porcelain-white colony because of which it is sometimes referred to as *Staphylococcus albus*. It is of low pathogenicity but is occasionally responsible for such relatively minor lesions as stitch abscesses and blepharitis.

CHAPTER 14

THE STREPTOCOCCI

Cocci which occur in chains are known as streptococci. The chains are due to the fact that the successive divisions of cocci occur in the same plane and that after division the organisms tend to adhere together. Chains are produced best in fluid media. On solid media, long chains are rarely found, the organisms usually occurring in short chains of 3 or 4, in pairs or as single cocci. Streptococci are Gram positive, non-motile and do not form spores. They grow poorly on simple media but growth is greatly enhanced by the addition of fermentable carbohydrate, e.g. glucose, or of serum or blood. Most are facultative anaerobes which, since they lack cytochrome components possess an essentially anaerobic metabolism. Consequently, as a rule they grow as well under anaerobic as under aerobic conditions. Except for group D streptococci which will grow at 45° C, the growth of most human parasitic strains is restricted to the neighbourhood of 37° C.

Classification of the Streptococci

Most of the streptococci from human sources are aerobic and facultatively anaerobic. The classification of the aerobic streptococci has, however, given rise to considerable difficulty. The criterion which has so far been of most value in classification is the presence of polysaccharide haptens which can be extracted from the organisms by a variety of methods and which are demonstrable by precipitin tests. On the basis of these haptens 17 groups of streptococci (A, B, C, D, E, F, G, H, K, L, M, N, O, P, Q, R and S) may be distinguished, all the strains in a particular group possessing an antigenically identical polysaccharide. Since they were first recognized by Lancefield these divisions are known as Lancefield groups.

In the majority of the Lancefield groups the group polysaccharide appears to be bound firmly to the cell wall mucopeptide, presumably through covalent bonds but not in sufficiently superficial a location as to be demonstrable by agglutination tests. In groups D and N, however, the polysaccharide appears to be much less firmly attached, being removable from the cell by comparatively simple washing procedures. It has been suggested that in these groups the polysaccharide may form a layer between the cell wall and the protoplast membrane. There is, however, no direct evidence for this view, and the experimental data can be otherwise explained.

Most of the organisms which possess Lancefield group haptens produce a wide zone of haemolysis on blood agar which is usually referred to as β haemolysis. This is an area of complete clearing of from 2 to 5 mm in diameter surrounding the colony. Since the Lancefield group haptens were first recognized amongst the β haemolytic strains, organisms possessing them are frequently referred to as haemolytic streptococci. The term is a convenient one but it should be noted that it is by no means a correct description of the group since many are non-haemolytic or may produce the viridans change.

In addition to being classified into groups on the basis of their possession of Lancefield haptens many streptococci have been assigned species rank. In some instances, e.g. groups A, B and N, the species is co-terminous with a Lancefield group. In some, e.g. groups C and D, the group is subdivided into species distinguished by various physiological characteristics. In others, species are defined by physiological characteristics only, without reference to serological properties, e.g. *Streptococcus sanguis* and *Streptococcus salivarius*. Many streptococci, however, including all those of groups E, L, M, O, P, Q, R, S, are classified simply by serological group and have not been given a species designation.

Other criteria that have been suggested as a basis of classification, but whose ultimate value for this purpose has still to be determined, are the chemical composition of the cell wall, particularly the presence or absence of rhamnose as a cell wall component, and the production of various red cell sensitizing antigens which are secreted by the organism into its environment but which would nevertheless appear to have a close association with the cell wall.

Streptococcus pyogenes

The most important of the haemolytic streptococci as causes of human infection are those of Lancefield group A. Group A streptococci form a homogeneous group which has received species rank as *Streptococcus pyogenes*.

Morphology

The individual cocci vary from 0·5 to 1·0µ in diameter. In shape they are spherical, but frequently, adjacent cocci in a chain are slightly flattened. *Str. pyogenes* is capsulated—the capsules consisting of hyaluronic acid. Capsules are demonstrable, however, only in young cultures examined after 2 to 3 hours incubation. In the later stages of growth the capsular hyaluronic acid is secreted into the medium, and in some cases broken down by the action of hyaluronidase.

Cultural Properties

On blood agar *Str. pyogenes* produces small colonies about 1 mm in diameter which have a finely granular or matt surface. The colonies are surrounded by an area of clear β haemolysis which may be as much as 5 mm in diameter. The haemolysis on aerobic plates is due to the oxygen-stable haemolysin. A small number of strains are deficient in this haemolysin and show haemolysis only on anaerobic or deep culture. Occasionally strains are encountered which synthesize large amounts of hyaluronic acid, and which give rise to large mucoid colonies measuring about 4 to 5 mm in diameter. On subculture in the laboratory, avirulent variants producing either glossy or rough irregular colonies may arise. Both these types of variants have shown to be deficient in the M or type-specific proteins (see below).

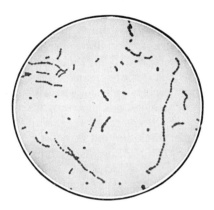

Fig. 17. *Streptococcus pyogenes* FROM
BROTH CULTURE (× 950)

Antigenic Structure

The species may be subdivided, as first shown by Griffith, using the slide-agglutination technique, into a number of distinct antigenic types. Type specificity depends in most cases on a group of antigenic trypsin-sensitive alcohol-soluble proteins—M proteins which are also, because of their anti-phagocytic properties, essential for virulence. The M proteins may be extracted from the cells with hot acid, and typing is now normally carried out by precipitin tests, using antigen extracted in this way. Since acid extracts also contain the group antigen the type-specific antisera employed must be absorbed so that the group antibody is removed.

In addition to the M antigen most strains of *Str. pyogenes* possess a second antigenic protein known as the T antigen. Many of the serologic types possess a T antigen specific for the type, but the correlation is not by any means complete. The T antigens differ from the M antigens in being trypsin resistant and in playing no part in the determination of virulence. Since they are acid labile they are not present in the acid extracts used for typing and grouping. T antigens may be extracted from the cell by digestion with proteolytic enzymes but are usually demonstrated by agglutination tests.

Certain M serotypes—2, 28 and 48—also possess a common antigenic protein known as the R antigen which may cause difficulties in type identification. Neither the R nor the T antigens are of importance in determining virulence.

The hyaluronic acid of the capsule is non-antigenic, presumably because of its structural similarity to the hyaluronic acid of animal tissues.

Pathogenicity

Streptococcus pyogenes produces a number of substances which play a part in pathogenicity. The most important of these are the *O* and *S haemolysins*, *streptokinase, desoxyribonuclease* and the *erythrogenic* or *Dick* toxin.

The O haemolysin is an oxygen-labile exotoxin which readily undergoes oxidation to an inactive form. It may be obtained in an active state by growing the organism in broth containing a reducing agent such as sodium hydrosulphite. The O lysin is lethal on injection into animals and has in particular a highly toxic effect on the heart. It is strongly antigenic, and antibody to it is found in the sera of many persons during the course of, or during convalescence from, streptococcal infection. This antibody—antistreptolysin O—may be demonstrated in vitro by its capacity to inhibit the haemolytic action of the toxin. Streptolysin O is strongly inhibited by cholesterol to which it is apparently adsorbed. Although normal serum contains appreciable amounts of cholesterol it is not present in a form capable of inhibiting the streptolysin, but in old or contaminated sera the cholesterol may be released in an active form. Such sera, therefore, may show considerable inhibitory properties for streptolysin O. In its pharmacologic properties streptolysin O closely resembles the oxygen-labile haemolysins produced by *Cl. perfringens*, *Cl. tetani* and the pneumococcus. These haemolysins are also similar antigenically, but each is neutralized most effectively by its homologous antitoxin.

In contrast to streptolysin O, streptolysin S is oxygen stable. It is more closely bound to the cell than streptolysin O but active cell-free preparations of it can be obtained by growing the organisms in serum broth or by suspending them in ribonucleic acid. These substances act by stimulating the release of the lysin. Streptolysin S appears to be a protein but is non-antigenic. Its haemolytic action is antagonized by a lipoprotein present in normal serum. The concentration of this inhibitor is diminished in the course of streptococcal infection. Streptolysin S has been shown to be capable of producing necrosis of the convoluted tubules of the kidneys of mice when implanted intraperitoneally. Its role in the pathogenesis of human lesions, however, appears to be less well established than that of streptolysin O.

The *erythrogenic toxin* is so called because it produces a local erythema when injected into the skin. If large amounts of it are injected subcutaneously into susceptible persons, it produces a skin rash which is identical with that of scarlet fever. Although it has not yet been obtained in purified form its susceptibility to trypsin indicates that it is a protein. It is relatively heat stable, but is destroyed by boiling for 1 hour. The Dick toxin is produced by only certain strains of *Str. pyogenes*, and it is only these strains which can cause scarlet fever. Its mode of action is unknown. At least two different antigenic types of Dick toxin have been identified; only one of the types is commonly found, being that produced by about 80 per cent of toxin-producing strains. Recent evidence suggests that, as in the case of the diphtheria bacillus, the capacity of *Str. pyogenes* to produce erythrogenic toxin may depend on lysogenization by a specific temperate bacteriophage. Toxin production only occurs when the phage is induced (p. 558) to give rise to mature phage particles.

Culture filtrates of *Str. pyogenes* are actively fibrinolytic for human fibrin. As in the case of the staphylococci the fibrinolytic agent is a plasma protease (plasmin) produced by activation of plasminogen. There is some evidence that the immediate activator of plasminogen is a plasma kinase which is formed from a plasma precursor by the action of the streptococcal agent—*streptokinase*. Streptokinase almost certainly plays a part in the pathogenicity of *Str. pyogenes* by breaking down the fibrin barrier formed by the tissues in response to infection. In contrast to staphylokinase it is produced maximally in the early stages of growth, and therefore can be presumed to be produced at an early stage of streptococcal infection. Streptokinase is antigenic and increase in the antistreptokinase activity of serum is frequently found in the course of streptococcal infections. Antistreptokinase, however, is not as valuable an indicator of streptococcal infection as antistreptolysin O.

Four antigenically distinct desoxyribonucleases (streptodornases)—A, B, C and D—have been described; of these B is the most antigenic in man. One or more of these is produced by all strains of *Str. pyogenes*. Since DNA may be present in considerable concentration in inflammatory exudates, and accounts for much of their viscosity, these enzymes are probably the substances mainly responsible for the serous character of streptococcal pus. Mixtures of streptokinase and streptodornase have been used therapeutically for breaking down blood clots and fibrinous exudates in closed spaces such as the joints or pleural cavity. Like streptokinase, desoxyribonuclease is produced in the early stages of streptococcal growth. It seems likely therefore that together they may contribute appreciably to the spreading character of streptococcal infection.

Some strains produce *hyaluronidase*, an enzyme which breaks down the hyaluronic acid of the tissues. In most cases the amount of hyaluronidase produced is small and can be detected only by very sensitive in vitro tests. In the course of streptococcal infection, however, most patients develop antibody against hyaluronidase suggesting that the enzyme, though produced only in small amounts in laboratory cultures, may be produced in larger amounts in the tissues. Hyaluronidase also breaks down the hyaluronic acid of the streptococcal capsule; consequently strains which produce a large amount of hyaluronidase produce little hyaluronic acid. Hyaluronidase might be expected to play a part in the virulence of *Str. pyogenes* by facilitating its spread through the tissues, but whether, or to what extent, this effect is counterbalanced by its capacity to break down the hyaluronic acid capsule is not clear.

Another substance of dubious significance in pathogenicity is a protease, produced in cultures grown at 37° C, but not at 32° C, which is capable of breaking down the M type specific protein. Streptococcal protease also inhibits the production of streptokinase. Since it is produced only at an acid pH it may not be present during the early stages of infection. It may possibly be produced in areas of inflammation in the tissues and, by destroying the M protein, on which the virulence of the organism depends, might contribute to the patient's recovery.

Many strains of *Str. pyogenes* produce an enzyme—diphosphopyridine nucleotidase which releases nicotinamide from diphosphopyridine nucleotides. The distribution of this enzyme is reported to be correlated with the capacity of the organism to kill leucocytes, a property which was previously attributed to the O lysin.

Many strains produce an amylase but whether this enzyme plays any role in pathogenicity has not been determined.

Recently it has been shown that, in the rabbit, the intradermal injection of the group polysaccharide may lead to the appearance of multiple skin nodules, as a result of some toxic action on the dermal connective tissue. The possible significance of this effect in relation to human infection is not clear.

Infections due to *Streptococcus pyogenes*

Streptococcus pyogenes is intrinsically a much more dangerous organism than *Staph. aureus*, and has a much greater tendency to spread in the tissues, therefore being more likely to give rise to septicaemia—the most serious complication of pyogenic infection. The last few decades, however, have seen a considerable fall in the incidence of streptococcal infection, as well as a marked diminution in its severity.

The main site of streptococcal infection is the throat, where a purulent tonsillitis is the most typical lesion. This condition is found characteristically in older children and in adults. In younger children the infection is more diffuse— a pharyngitis rather than a tonsillitis—and less acute in character. The more acute localized lesion of the older person is believed to depend on a previously acquired allergy.

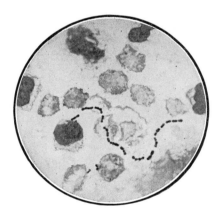

FIG. 18. *Streptococcus pyogenes* IN PUS
(× 950)

When a throat infection is caused by a strain which produces the erythrogenic toxin the resultant symptom complex is known as scarlet fever. During the course of outbreaks of scarlet fever many people develop a sore throat but without the appearance of a skin rash. This is because they are immune to the erythrogenic toxin owing to antitoxin in their blood, developed as a result of a previous infection with a toxin-producing strain of *Str. pyogenes* of a different serotype from that responsible for the present infection. Though immune to scarlet fever they can nevertheless develop a streptococcal throat infection because their blood does not contain type specific antibody for the currently infecting strain.

From the throat the infection may spread locally, particularly to the neighbouring lymphatic glands and to the middle ear. Occasionally a peritonsillar or retropharyngeal abscess is produced and, infrequently, a diffuse cellulitis of the floor of the mouth known as Ludwig's angina. From the throat the organism may also invade the lungs, causing a pneumonia of severe type. Streptococcal pneumonia occurs infrequently as a primary condition and is usually a complication of other infections involving the respiratory tract such as influenza.

Streptococcus pyogenes is an important cause of superficial infections. Infections of wounds, abrasions and burns are of frequent occurrence. In recent years, however, the staphylococcus has completely ousted *Str. pyogenes* as the primary cause of wound infection in hospitals. Local extensions of the infection to subcutaneous tissues may give rise to cellulitis. The lymph vessels may be involved with the production of lymphangitis and of lymphadenitis in the local lymphatic glands. If the infection is not checked at this stage, invasion of the blood with septicaemia may occur. Streptococcal septicaemia is usually accompanied by endocarditis and frequently shows purulent joint involvement. It may result from any streptococcal lesion, but most frequently is a complication of wound infection. The wound responsible may be quite trivial.

Erysipelas is a diffuse streptococcal skin infection involving the superficial lymphatic vessels. The skin is swollen with a brawny induration and the area of inflammation shows a characteristic sharp edge. The condition may progress to pus formation. *Str. pyogenes* also appears to be responsible for some cases of impetigo. The strains of *Str. pyogenes* isolated from cases of impetigo have been found to belong to only a limited number of serological types, most frequently to types 4 and 25.

Streptococcus pyogenes is the most important cause of puerperal sepsis; in this condition the organisms are almost invariably derived from attendant nurses or doctors or from contaminated instruments. In the pre-antibiotic era puerperal sepsis progressing to septicaemia was a major cause of maternal mortality.

Meningitis may occur, though rarely, as a result of spread from infection of the middle ear.

A small proportion of normal individuals carry *Str. pyogenes* in their throats. The carrier state appears to be most frequent during the winter and spring. Some persons are nasal carriers. Both types, but particularly the nasal carrier, are of great importance in the spread of streptococcal infection, the mechanism of environmental contamination being essentially the same as that already considered for the staphylococcus.

Sequelae of Streptococcal Infection

There is a considerable body of evidence that *Str. pyogenes* is in some way the cause of acute rheumatism and of most cases of acute glomerulonephritis in man. These conditions differ, however, from the streptococcal infections we have so far considered in that they only appear between the first and third week after the acute stage of the precipitating infection. Many cases are not preceded by overt streptococcal infection but in many of these, high titres of antibodies to streptococcal extracellular antigens, particularly to streptolysin O, are frequently demonstrable. Streptococci are not directly demonstrable in the lesions in either condition, and it is clear that they are not due to direct invasion of the tissues by the organism. Apart from the differences in the organs involved there are certain differences in the mode of occurrence of these conditions which must be taken into account in any proposed explanation of their pathogenesis. (a) When streptococcal in origin, acute glomerulonephritis is usually associated with infection due to particular serotypes of Str. pyogenes, particularly type 12. No specific serological types have so far been associated with acute rheumatism. Since streptococcal immunity is type specific these findings presumably explain the fact that acute nephritis is a non-recurrent condition whereas acute rheumatism recurs with each subsequent streptococcal infection. (b) There is some evidence that susceptibility to acute rheumatism but not to acute nephritis is genetically determined. It appears to occur most frequently in non-secretors of blood groups other than O. In addition, persons who suffer from rheumatic fever develop higher antibody responses to streptococcal antigen, and appear to have a higher susceptibility to recurrent streptococcal infection than the normal subject. There are two main theories to explain the role of the streptococcus in producing these conditions.

1. They may be due to the direct toxic action of some streptococcal product. The association of acute nephritis with only a few serological types of Str. pyogenes suggests that these strains may in fact produce some substance that is toxic to the kidneys. Claims to this effect have not, however, been adequately documented. In the case of acute rheumatism the presumed toxic component would have to be produced by all the serological types of streptococci. The most likely substance would appear to be streptolysin O but the susceptibility of the rheumatic subject to recurrent attacks of acute rheumatism in the presence of a high titre of antistreptolysin O renders this hypothesis unlikely.

2. They may have an immunological basis. This could be an allergy to some streptococcal component—the allergic reaction occurring in the tissues giving rise to tissue damage—or it could be an auto-immune process resulting in the development of antibody reacting with a normal tissue antigen. An immunological basis could provide a satisfactory explanation for the delay in the development of the lesions.

The evidence for an immunological basis is clearer in acute nephritis than in rheumatic fever. Glomerular lesions resembling those occurring in acute nephritis in man have been produced in rabbits by the injection of protein antigens. When a single large dose of protein was injected the nephritis was transient. When the protein was injected in a series of small doses the renal lesions were progressive and permanent. Nephritis may also be produced in rabbits by the injection of antigen–antibody complexes. It is possible therefore that in man acute nephritis may be due to the production of Arthus-type reactions in the glomeruli, as a result of the formation or retention of antigen–antibody complexes. The most likely antigen would in this case be the M protein. This possibility is consistent with the demonstration by the fluorescent antibody technique, of the presence of gamma globulin and complement in glomeruli from cases of acute nephritis, and with the lowering of serum complement levels found in the condition. The possibility of an auto-immune reaction is suggested by the development of kidney lesions in rabbits—as first shown by Masugi—following inoculation with anti-rabbit kidney antiserum, and the production of renal lesions in rats and sheep injected with kidney tissue suspended in Freund adjuvant. The reports on the development of renal auto-antibodies in human nephritis, however, are conflicting, and all attempts to elute such antibodies from affected kidneys have been unsuccessful. The gamma globulin demonstrable in the glomeruli, therefore, presumably does not possess anti-kidney specificity.

Cardiac lesions have been produced in rabbits as a component of the serum sickness syndrome, following the injection of large amounts of protein. The lesions found, however, have consisted primarily of a peri-arteritis, and were quite different from the lesions observed in acute rheumatism in man. Lesions more closely resembling those of rheumatic carditis were observed—by Murphy—in rabbits, following a series of intradermal injections of streptococci of different serological types. In man the presence of gamma globulin adsorbed to heart muscle cells has been described, and also the presence in the blood of antibodies to human heart tissue.

The latter have been found, however, in conditions other than rheumatic fever, and may be a result rather than the cause of the disease. The occurrence in streptococci of an antigen which will stimulate the development of antibodies which react with heart muscle cells and which can be absorbed out with streptococcal cell walls has been reported. It is conceivable that antibody to this antigen might be responsible for the cardiac lesions in acute rheumatism. An alternative possibility is that a streptococcal product might confer antigenicity on an antigen present in the heart, thereby allowing it to by-pass the tolerance mechanism (p. 125).

Erythema nodosum is also in some cases associated with streptococcal infection and is believed to have a similar allergic aetiology. A number of cases of this condition, however, are undoubtedly associated with tuberculosis, and are assumed to be an allergic response to the tubercle bacillus.

Other Haemolytic Streptococci

Streptococci of Lancefield group B constitute the species *Str. agalactiae*. This organism is the main cause of bovine mastitis and is only very slightly if at all pathogenic for man. It may occur as a commensal in the nose, throat and vagina. Its differentiation from *Str. pyogenes* in milk is of some epidemiological importance since *Str. pyogenes* may cause mastitis, and when present in milk it can cause infections in consumers of the milk while *Str. agalactiae* cannot. *Str. agalactiae* produces a substance—CAMP factor—which causes lysis of sheep cells which have been exposed to the β lysin of *Staph. aureus*. *Str. agalactiae* is capsulated and is subdivided into types on the basis of capsular polysaccharide composition.

Streptococci of groups C and G can produce lesions very similar to but less severe than those of *Str. pyogenes*. Many strains of groups C and G produce streptokinase and streptolysin O and a number also produce erythrogenic toxin. Other points of resemblance between groups A, C and G are the findings that strains of all three groups are lysed by an enzyme produced when group C streptococci are infected with a specific bacteriophage and that strains of groups C and G possess an R antigen serologically identical with that found in group A. Group G streptococci occur not infrequently as throat commensals. Group C streptococci are primarily animal pathogens being responsible for mastitis in cows and for strangles and contagious bronchopneumonia in horses. On the basis of their biochemical characteristics they have been subdivided into four species—the species responsible for human infections being sometimes known as *Streptococcus equisimilis*.

Group D strains rank next in importance to group A strains as causes of human infection. Since their natural home appears to be the intestinal tract of man and other animals group D streptococci have been grouped together as 'enterococci'. Two species of enterococci occur as human commensals, *Streptococcus faecalis* and *Str. faecium*. *Str. faecalis*, which is the species most frequently encountered, may be distinguished by its capacity to grow on media containing 0·05 per cent potassium tellurite, by its fermentation of sorbitol and by its failure to prevent arabinose. *Str. faecalis* and most strains of *Str. faecium* grow and ferment mannitol in mannitol bile salt broth—a property which is of some value in distinguishing them from other streptococci. Some strains of both species are haemolytic on blood agar, but most are completely non-haemolytic (*Str. faecalis*) or produce the viridans change (*Str. faecium*).

Although normally non-pathogenic, enterococci may invade the tissues and produce pyogenic lesions. The lesions most frequently caused are urinary infections and wound sepsis. The enterococci are second only to coliform bacilli as a cause of acute pyelitis, and are occasional causes of puerperal sepsis and of subacute bacterial endocarditis, usually of severe type. Many of these infections have occurred after genito-urinary manipulation.

Streptococcus faecalis is of considerable value as an indicator organism in the bacteriological examination of water. Its presence in a water sample is presumptive evidence of faecal contamination, and since it dies fairly quickly in water is an indication of recent contamination.

Strains of groups F, H and O occur as commensals in the throat. They may be either β haemolytic or of viridans type. Amongst the viridans strains of group F, are a group of strains which have been assigned species rank as *Streptococcus MG*. They form a serologically homogeneous group, and produce colonies which fluoresce in UV light. Their importance can be attributed to the fact that antibody to them, demonstrable by the agglutination test, is present in the sera of cases of primary atypical pneumonia, a condition with which, however, the streptococcus has no causal relationship (p. 380).

For some strains of group H, which have the distinctive property of producing, when grown in sucrose broth, a dextran precipitated by antiserum to the capsular polysaccharide of the type 2 pneumococcus, the species *Streptococcus sanguis* has been proposed. Many strains of *Str. sanguis* lack the group H hapten, however, and the species, as currently defined, is clearly heterogeneous. *Str. sanguis* strains appear to be of importance as causes of subacute bacterial endocarditis.

Streptococci of other Lancefield groups are primarily of animal origin. Though some have occasionally been isolated from human lesions their pathogenicity for man is doubtful.

The Viridans Streptococci

Many streptococci isolated from human sources do not possess Lancefield polysaccharide haptens. Most of these produce a greenish discoloration of the blood in the immediate vicinity of the colony—the greenish zone being frequently surrounded by a very narrow rim of almost complete haemolysis. This type of change is usually referred to as α haemolysis. It is to these organisms that the designation viridans streptococci is primarily applied by bacteriologists. The term is, however, a confusing one since many viridans-type streptococci isolated from human sources possess identifiable Lancefield group haptens. The majority, however, do not. They are a heterogeneous group, and their classification presents particular difficulties because of the paucity of criteria which will permit satisfactory species definition. Because of this the species designations *Streptococcus viridans* and *Streptococcus mitis*, which are sometimes applied to them, cannot be considered justified. Viridans streptococci occur as commensals of the upper respiratory tract. They are of particular importance as causes of subacute bacterial endocarditis.

Subacute Bacterial Endocarditis

Although viridans streptococci are responsible for the great majority of cases, subacute bacterial endocarditis is occasionally due to *H. influenzae* and *Haemophilus parainfluenzae* (p. 338), and, very rarely, to *Coxiella burneti* (p. 548).

It occurs usually in valves which have been damaged by a previous rheumatic endocarditis or which are the seat of a congenital defect. Bicuspid aortic valves are particularly prone to involvement. The organisms gain entrance to the valves from the blood stream. Other important precipitating causes are tonsillectomy and manipulation of the cervix uteri. In the case of group D streptococci, the infection frequently occurs after genito-urinary manipulation. In group D infections, previous cardiac damage does not appear to be so essential a predisposing condition as in viridans infections.

Anaerobic Streptococci

These organisms are found as normal inhabitants of mucous membranes, but can occasionally invade the tissues, producing pyogenic lesions. They can cause infection in any organ but are most commonly found as invaders of wounds, particularly those that have been extensively damaged or contused. They are of special importance as causes of a severe type of puerperal sepsis. They have marked proteolytic properties and usually produce large amounts of hydrogen sulphide from sulphur-containing amino acids. Because of this, pus from anaerobic streptococcal lesions has an unpleasant putrefactive smell. Anaerobic streptococci are assigned by Bergey to a separate genus, *Peptostreptococcus*, in which a number of species are defined. Characterization of these organisms, however, is at present incomplete. The most clearly differentiated species has been designated *Peptostreptococcus putridus*—the chief distinguishing characteristic of which is the production of large amounts of gas from certain sugars in the presence of sulphur-containing compounds.

Diagnosis of Streptococcal Infections

Streptococci are usually isolated from clinical material by aerobic culture on blood agar. For the isolation of *Str. pyogenes*, however, anaerobic cultures give more satisfactory results particularly for the recognition of the occasional strain which is deficient in the S lysin and which does not therefore produce haemolysis on surface aerobic culture. Pike's medium has been favourably reported on as an enrichment medium prior to plate culture. Gentian violet is of considerable value as a selective agent in the isolation of *Str. pyogenes* from sites, e.g. the throat, with a normal mixed flora. The dye may be incorporated in blood agar to give a concentration of 1/300,000 to 1/500,000.

When a haemolytic streptococcus has been isolated on culture its Lancefield group should be determined. For this purpose the group hapten is extracted and its identity determined by a tube precipitin test (p. 131) with appropriate grouping sera. A variety of methods may be used for antigen preparation. In most the starting point is the deposit obtained by centrifugation of digest or glucose broth cultures. The antigen may be extracted by Lancefield's method with N/20 HCl at 100° C, by Fuller's method with formamide at 160° C or by Rantz's method by autoclaving at 10 to 15 lb/in² in saline. Alternatively, Maxted's method, which has the advantage that it can be applied to primary plate cultures, may be used. In this, some of the growth is emulsified in a small volume of filtrate from a culture of *Streptomyces albus*—which contains enzymes capable of breaking down streptococcal cell walls—and the mixture incubated at 50° C until it becomes clear. The method is only effective with streptococci of Lancefield groups A, C or G.

An alternative method of grouping which has been used increasingly in recent years and which does not require prior extraction of the antigen is by the fluorescent antibody technique. It is highly specific but occasionally gives false positive reactions with some strains of group C. The bacitracin sensitivity test, which has been recommended as a substitute for grouping in the identification of group A strains, has a low degree of specificity and is not reliable.

The diagnosis of subacute bacterial endocarditis is made by isolating the organism from the blood. If the patient is under treatment with penicillin, penicillinase should be incorporated in the broth used for culture. Since many of the streptococci responsible grow slowly, blood culture bottles should not be discarded as negative for at least 4 weeks.

Estimation of antistreptolysin O titres is sometimes carried out for the diagnosis of infection with *Str. pyogenes*, and particularly to indicate recent episodes of infection in children suffering from juvenile rheumatism. The average levels of antistreptolysin titres in persons who are suffering from, or who have recently had, an acute streptococcal infection are higher than in normal ones. The titre level obtained at a single examination is, however, difficult to assess, since a number of normal persons give high titres, and a significant number of these who have recently been infected give low titres. An increase in antistreptolysin titre is more important as evidence of streptococcal infection than a high titre obtained at a single examination.

It should be noted that antistreptolysin titres when significant are indicative only of streptococcal infection and are not specifically diagnostic of rheumatic fever. It is claimed that rheumatic fever subjects show an unusual response to streptolysin O—the antibody appearing later than in uncomplicated streptococcal infection, but attaining higher levels and persisting for much longer.

Treatment

Streptococcal throat infections should be energetically treated with penicillin, and the drug is usually continued for some time after the disappearance of symptoms in order to minimize the risk of the development of acute rheumatism as a sequela. Penicillin has given excellent results in the treatment of subacute bacterial endocarditis due to viridans streptococci, although some viridans strains are reported to have appreciable resistance to penicillin. In such cases, and in enterococcal infections, combined therapy with penicillin and streptomycin has proved satisfactory. Relapses of subacute bacterial endocarditis, even after intensive antibiotic therapy, are frequent. There is some reason to believe that these relapses may be due to reinfection from infected teeth, and the complete removal of the teeth has been recommended for all patients apparently recovered from the condition. This, however, must be done while the antibiotic is being administered. Penicillin appears to be the drug of choice for most infections due to the anaerobic streptococci.

In severely toxic cases of scarlet fever the administration of scarlet fever antitoxin is of considerable value. These cases are now fortunately very uncommon.

Penicillin and the sulphonamides have both been used successfully in the prophylaxis of streptococcal infection in persons who have at one time suffered from acute rheumatism. Penicillin, because of its capacity to sterilize the tissues, has now been accepted as the agent of choice for this purpose. In the case of children it is recommended that prophylaxis should be continued at least until adult life. Penicillin has also been used as a prophylactic for children living in closed communities in the face of an epidemic of streptococcal throat infection but is not generally used for this purpose because of the dangers of sensitization and because it interferes too much with natural active immunization.

CHAPTER 15

PNEUMOCOCCI

Diplococcus pneumoniae (Pneumococcus)

The pneumococcus has much in common with the streptococci but is assigned to a distinct genus *Diplococcus* of which it is the only member.

Morphology

The pneumococcus is a non-motile, non-sporing Gram positive coccus. In material taken from the body it occurs characteristically in pairs of flame-shaped cocci about 1μ in length, the rounded ends of the cocci being adjacent to each other. This typical morphology is not often seen in laboratory cultures where the appearance and arrangement is similar to that of the streptococci. The pneumococcus is capsulated, the capsule being best seen in material taken directly from the tissues.

Cultural Properties

Very poor growth is obtained on unenriched media. On blood agar normally capsulated strains produce a highly characteristic, smooth, flat colony frequently showing umbilication and resembling a draught-board piece in appearance. Growth is improved in the presence of 5 to 10 per cent CO_2. Like *Str. pyogenes*, it grows well under both aerobic and anaerobic conditions. Many of the strains found as normal inhabitants of the nasopharynx are non-capsulated on primary isolation, and as a result give rise to rough colonies. The colony on blood agar is surrounded by a zone of greenish discoloration of the medium and often by an outer zone of haemolysis—the changes being similar to those associated with the viridans streptococci. Type 3 pneumococci produce large, highly mucoid colonies of characteristic appearance.

Pneumococci readily undergo autolysis in culture, the flat appearance of the colony in fact being due to these autolytic changes. The enzyme system responsible for autolysis may be activated by a number of agents such as bile salts, saponin, soap and alkali. This is the basis of the bile solubility test, which is of considerable value in the differentiation of pneumococci from viridans streptococci. It can be carried out by adding 0·1 ml of a 10 per cent solution of sodium desoxycholate to 1 to 5 ml of a digest broth culture. The latter must not be more acid than pH 6·8 as, in more acid solutions, the desoxycholate is precipitated. Solution may take place almost at once or after a few minutes' heating to 37° C.

Pneumococci are highly sensitive to ethylhydrocuprein (Optochin); a property which is also valuable in differentiating them from viridans streptococci.

Antigenic Structure

In their antigenic composition pneumococci resemble the streptococci. They possess a species-specific polysaccharide hapten, which is chemically, although not serologically, similar to the Lancefield group haptens. The most important of the pneumococcal antigens are the capsular polysaccharides on the basis of which the species is subdivided into serologic types, some 75 of which have so far been described. Serologic typing may be carried out by the capsule-swelling or by the agglutination reaction. The purified polysaccharides, although fully antigenic for man, are non-antigenic in the rabbit. Pneumococci also possess type-specific M proteins whose distribution closely parallels that of the capsular polysaccharides. The reactivity of the type-specific proteins is masked by the presence of the capsule.

Rough pneumococci derived from capsulated organisms of one type can be permanently transformed into capsulated organisms of a different type by treatment with DNA derived from the latter (p. 29). This transformation is of considerable historical interest, since its discovery by Griffith was the first indication that properties could be transferred from one micro-organism to another. The extent to which this type of change occurs under natural conditions is unknown, but it is likely to be infrequent since the in vitro transformation requires special conditions and occurs at a low rate.

Immunity to pneumococcal infection depends on the presence of antibody to the capsular polysaccharides and is, therefore, type-specific. Consequently an individual can undergo a number of infections, each infection being due to an organism of different serologic type.

Pathogenicity

The pneumococcus produces an oxygen-labile haemolysin resembling streptolysin O. Pneumococcal cultures which have undergone autolysis also contain a substance which can produce purpuric lesions in experimental animals. Neither of the substances referred to above, however, appears to play any significant part in pathogenicity. Consequently it has been suggested that the severe toxaemia which is so characteristic a feature of pneumococcal pneumonia is due to the fact that the organisms growing in the lung deprive the tissue cells of adequate nutriment. It is significant in this connexion that the dramatic improvement in cases of lobar pneumonia, known clinically as the crisis, coincides with an outpouring of antibody and cessation of growth of the organism. The improvement in the patient at the time of the crisis is certainly not the result of any marked change in the lesion in the tissues, which remains histologically precisely the same for some time after the crisis; it may therefore well be the result of the mere inhibition of bacterial growth.

Like many viridans streptococci, pneumococci produce large amounts of an enzyme resembling the receptor-destroying enzyme of the influenza virus. No role has so far been assigned to this enzyme in pathogenicity.

The capsule of the pneumococcus is essential for virulence—its role being to protect the organism from phagocytosis. This protective function is lost on combination with specific antiserum. The role of the capsule in virulence is clearly shown in an interesting experiment carried out by Dubos. Dubos found that it was possible to remove the capsule from type 3 organisms without affecting their viability by exposing them to the action of a polysaccharide-splitting enzyme which he had isolated from a soil bacillus. The decapsulated organisms were avirulent. Further evidence of the importance of the capsule in determining virulence is provided by the finding that immunization with purified capsular polysaccharide will protect against pneumococcal infection.

Pneumococcal Infections

Pneumococci are widely distributed as commensals of the upper respiratory tract. Many of the commensal pneumococci are, however, non-capsulated and avirulent. Capsulated and potentially virulent pneumococci may also occur as commensals but the capsular types normally found as commensals are of relatively low pathogenicity and are only infrequently responsible for disease. The majority of pneumococcal infections are due to a limited number of capsular types the most important of which are types 1, 2 and 3. These appear to be much more invasive than the usual commensal types; in addition they are more likely to show epidemic spread in closed communities where the conditions are such as to facilitate the spread of respiratory pathogens.

Pneumonia is the most important disease caused by the pneumococcus. Although occurring as a primary condition pneumococcal pneumonia is more frequently secondary to some damage to the respiratory tract, especially that caused by virus infections, e.g. influenza, which render the lungs more liable to bacterial invasion.

Pneumococcal pneumonia occurs clinically in two forms—bronchopneumonia and lobar pneumonia, classified according to the distribution of the area of consolidation in the lung. The two types of pneumonia show important differences in incidence and pathogenesis. Bronchopneumonia is characteristically a disease of young children and of the older adult, i.e. over 50 years. It is essentially a sporadic infection and is usually due to one of the less commonly pathogenic types which occur as commensals in the upper respiratory tract. In contrast lobar pneumonia is almost exclusively a disease of the age group 10 to 50 years. The majority of cases are caused by a limited number of the more virulent capsular types; types 1, 2 and 3 are particularly important, being responsible for over half the cases. The pneumonia caused by the type 3 pneumococcus is considerably more severe than that caused by types 1 and 2. The latter types, however, are more invasive and as a result more frequently gain access to the bloodstream with the production of secondary foci of infection. These occur particularly in the meninges, peritoneum, joints and the endocardium. Lobar pneumonia occurs both as a sporadic and as an epidemic disease. Epidemics of the disease occur almost exclusively in closed communities, e.g. barracks and asylums. In such communities an epidemic type when once introduced spreads rapidly. If such spread should occur at a time when other respiratory infections, and particularly influenza, are prevalent, there is a considerable risk that a number of individuals carrying the epidemic type will develop lobar pneumonia. It has been suggested that the typical lobar distribution of pneumococcal pneumonia in the adult may be the result of a previously acquired allergy. In the allergic individual contact with the organism might lead to an outpouring of fluid by which invading organisms are swept throughout an entire lobe.

The pneumococcus is occasionally responsible for acute episodes of infection in individuals suffering from chronic bronchitis but is of less importance in this respect than *H. influenzae*. It is probably the organism most frequently found in pyogenic infections of the air sinuses. It is a frequent cause of otitis media and is occasionally responsible for a primary peritonitis occurring in young girls.

The pneumococcus is one of the major causes of acute pyogenic meningitis. This condition is commonest in children in whom it frequently occurs as a complication of otitis media. It may also develop as a sequel to fractures of the skull. Occasionally pneumococcal meningitis assumes a very acute and rapidly fatal form. In these cases the appearance of the cerebrospinal fluid is highly characteristic showing the presence of large numbers of pneumococci with comparatively few pus cells.

Diagnosis

The diagnosis of pneumococcal meningitis can usually be made with reasonable certainty from the examination of Gram stained films of a centrifuged deposit from the cerebrospinal fluids. For the diagnosis of pneumococcal pneumonia, however, culture is essential. It should be noted that although the majority of lobar pneumonias are caused by the pneumococcus, a few are due to *Klebsiella pneumoniae*. Since the latter carry an extremely grave prognosis if treatment is at all delayed, it is essential that they should be identified at the earliest possible moment. This can usually be readily achieved by the examination of Gram stained films.

When Gram positive cocci of typical colonial morphology are found on blood agar they can usually be safely identified as pneumococci. The typical colony appearance is, however, not always observed, and the organisms may then be indistinguishable from viridans streptococci. Their differentiation from the latter can be made either by the bile solubility test or by determining their susceptibility to ethylhydrocuprein. For the latter test a subculture is made to a blood agar plate from a suspicious colony and on the inoculum is placed a filter paper disc impregnated with 1/1000 ethylhydrocuprein. If the organism is a pneumococcus, an appreciable area of inhibition of growth will appear round the disc. Viridans streptococci are not inhibited, or are so only slightly.

Treatment

Pneumococci are sensitive to sulphonamides, penicillin and the wide-spectrum antibiotics. Penicillin is the agent of choice; in the treatment of meningitis it is claimed to give best results when combined with a sulphonamide, and should be given by the intrathecal, as well as by the intramuscular route.

CHAPTER 16

THE NEISSERIAE

The neisseriae are aerobic Gram negative cocci which characteristically occur in pairs. The cocci have a highly distinctive bean or kidney shape. In the diplococcal form they are arranged with their long axes parallel and with their flattened sides adjacent to each other. They are non-motile and non-sporing, and are devoid of morphological capsules. All the neisseriae give strong positive oxidase (i.e. indophenol oxidase) reactions. This reaction is of particular value for the recognition of the pathogenic species in mixed cultures. They are catalase positive and are strict aerobes, because of which they grow very poorly in fluid media.

The genus comprises both pathogenic and non-pathogenic members. A number of species of non-pathogenic neisseriae have been described, all of which, however, are clearly parasites. Of these, the most important is *Neisseria catarrhalis*, which occurs as a commensal of the human upper respiratory tract. *N. catarrhalis* is easily distinguished from the pathogenic species by the fact that it grows readily on ordinary media such as unenriched nutrient agar. It frequently occurs in a rough colony form, the organisms of which are spontaneously agglutinable in saline.

The pathogenic members of the genus *Neisseria meningitidis* and *Neisseria gonorrhoeae* are extremely delicate organisms and are among the more difficult to grow in the laboratory. They die out rapidly outside the body and, in the laboratory, if not preserved in the dry state must be frequently subcultured. Though Gram negative their antibiotic susceptibility pattern is very similar to that of the streptococci. They are strictly human parasites and on inoculation possess a very low pathogenicity for experimental animals. Neither produces exotoxins but both possess endotoxins, the nature of which has not been fully investigated.

They will not grow on ordinary media but grow in media to which blood or serum has been added. It is thought that blood and serum permit growth not because they supply essential growth factors but because they neutralize toxic substances, particularly long-chain fatty acids, normally present in agar media. The growth of both species especially on primary isolation is considerably improved by incubation in an atmosphere containing from 10 to 20 per cent carbon dioxide.

In agglutination, precipitin and complement fixation tests, both species appear to be antigenically heterogeneous and show in addition considerable antigenic overlap with *Neisseria catarrhalis* and other non-pathogenic neisseriae.

Neisseria meningitidis (Meningococcus)

The diplococcal form of *N. meningitidis* is most readily seen in films prepared from the cerebrospinal fluid from cases of meningococcal meningitis. In the cerebrospinal fluid the cocci are found chiefly within the polymorphonuclear leucocytes though in the early stages of very acute cases many may be seen lying free of the cells which may be few in number. In films prepared from cultures the diplococcal form is less regularly found, and the organisms may show considerable irregularity in size and staining due to the occurrence of autolytic changes. Capsules are not demonstrable by ordinary microscopic techniques; they have, however, been demonstrated by the use of the capsule swelling reaction with immune serum.

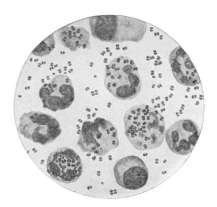

FIG. 19. MENINGOCOCCI IN PURULENT
CEREBROSPINAL FLUID

On blood agar the meningococcus produces, after about 24 hours' growth, a smooth, translucent and rather viscid colony of from 1 to 2 mm in diameter, with a shining surface and an entire edge. It is non-haemolytic. The meningococcus ferments glucose and maltose without gas production and has no action on saccharose. Fermentation tests are best carried out on agar media containing added rabbit serum.

The species has been divided into four serologic groups—A, B, C and D—by the agglutination test. The groups, however, are by no means homogeneous, and the differentiation between them is not clear-cut. They are of no diagnostic importance.

Meningococcal Infections

Meningococci are present in the nasopharynx of from 2 to 5 per cent of normal people. These commensal strains are most frequently of group B. Group

A strains which are those mainly responsible for epidemics rarely occur as commensals.

The meningococcus is the most important cause of acute pyogenic meningitis. Meningococcal meningitis occurs most commonly, although not exclusively, in children. Mortality from the condition is maximal at the extremes of life. Meningitis, however, is the final and most dramatic phase of meningococcal infection—the evolution of which can be divided into three stages. In the first stage the organism appears in the nasopharynx, where it may cause a pharyngitis. In the second stage the blood is invaded. The characteristic lesion of this stage is the development of petechial skin lesions, due to foci of infection in the capillaries. In the third stage the organism localizes in the meninges producing an acute pyogenic meningitis. The infection may abort at either of the earlier stages without the production of meningitis.

In some cases of meningococcal infection bacteraemia may become a chronic condition without evidence of meningeal localization. In a small proportion of cases the bacteraemic stage appears as a fulminating septicaemia which may be fatal in a few hours. In this condition, known as the *Waterhouse-Friderichsen* syndrome, the patient dies in a state of severe shock; at post-mortem examination diffuse haemorrhagic infiltration of the adrenals is invariably found.

Meningococcal meningitis may occur either as a sporadic or as an epidemic infection. The development of epidemics is favoured by conditions of overcrowding and they are particularly liable to occur in institutions with a susceptible young population, e.g. schools and barracks. Under such conditions the organisms can be isolated from the nasopharynx of a high proportion of individuals in whom there may be no evidence of infection and in whom the condition does not develop beyond the stage of nasopharyngitis. Most epidemics are due to organisms of serological group A while most sporadic infections are due to groups B and C.

Metastatic meningococcal lesions also sometimes occur in the heart, where they give rise to endocarditis, or in the joints where they cause a purulent arthritis.

Diagnosis

In meningitis the organisms may be demonstrable in Gram films prepared from the centrifuged deposit of the cerebrospinal fluid. In some cases, however, even when there is a considerable amount of pus, they may be so few in number that this is not possible. Since the meningococcus dies rapidly outside the body, it is imperative that cultures should be made as soon as possible, blood agar being normally used. The plates are best incubated in an atmosphere containing 5 to 10 per cent CO_2. The cerebrospinal fluid should also be incubated directly or better still with the addition of an equal volume of glucose broth, and, after incubation, subcultures made onto blood agar. This procedure may yield a growth of the organism when immediate plating has been negative. A precipitin reaction using the ring technique for the demonstration of meningococcal antigens in the cerebrospinal fluid is employed by some workers as a rapid diagnostic method; it has been of particular value when organisms cannot be demonstrated in stained films. In early cases it may be possible to isolate the organism from the blood. The blood should be inoculated into a blood culture bottle and should also be spread directly onto a blood agar plate.

The identification of *N. meningitidis* in the cerebrospinal fluid presents no difficulty. In cultures taken from the nasopharynx, considerable trouble is experienced, for a number of other Gram negative diplococci are frequently found in that situation. The chief one of these likely to cause confusion is *N. catarrhalis*, which may be distinguished from the meningococcus by its capacity to grow on nutrient agar at room temperature, by its lack of fermentative actions on sugars, by its colonies which are larger and whiter and by the fact that it is usually spontaneously agglutinable in saline.

Treatment

The sulphonamides are the drugs of choice in the treatment of meningococcal meningitis.

Neisseria gonorrhoeae (Gonococcus)

Neisseria gonorrhoeae resembles *N. meningitidis* very closely in microscopic appearance. In stained films of the pus obtained from the urethra in acute gonorrhoea, the great majority of the cocci are seen to lie within leucocytes. As many as one hundred cocci may occasionally be seen within a single pus cell. In the very early stages of gonorrhoea, when the discharge is mucoid rather than purulent, very many gonococci may be seen outside pus cells, and a similar picture may be obtained in an old standing case of gleet, except that in this condition the cocci may be very scanty. The microscopic appearance of gono-cocci in culture resembles that seen in direct films, but there is much greater irregularity in size, swollen and badly staining degenerated cocci being present.

The gonococcus is even more difficult to grow than the meningococcus. A satisfactory medium contains 20 per cent of citrated blood with an agar con-centration sufficiently low to produce a distinctly soft medium. The colonies, which usually appear within 24 hours, very closely resemble those of the meningococcus. The gonococcus ferments glucose with the production of acid only. It does not ferment maltose or saccharose.

Gonococci are serologically very heterogeneous and do not show a clear differentiation into distinct antigenic types.

Gonococcal Infections

Man is the only animal naturally infected by gonococci. Infection is, on account of the delicacy of the organism, almost always direct from individual to individual and almost exclusively by venereal contact.

The gonococcus attacks chiefly the urethra both in the male and female, producing an acute urethritis. From the urethra the disease, if untreated, tends to spread locally. In the male spread occurs to the prostate, testes, seminal vesicles, epididymis and sometimes into the peri-urethral tissues. In the female the cervix uteri is invaded early; later the infection may spread to Bartholin's glands, to the uterus—producing an endometritis—and to the Fallopian tubes, ovaries and pelvic peritoneum. In adult women the vagina usually escapes because of the acid pH of the vaginal secretions but a severe vulvovaginitis can occur in young girls. Outbreaks of the latter condition were at one time not uncommon in children's hospitals and schools, the organism apparently being spread indirectly by the use of contaminated utensils and clothes. Occasionally in either sex, but more frequently in the female, the mucous membrane of the rectum and anus may be involved. Arthritis is an unusual complication of gonorrhoea which tends to occur in old standing rather than in acute cases; this suggests that an allergic factor may be involved in its aetiology.

Gonococcal conjunctivitis occurring in the newborn is now a very uncommon condition because of the universal practice of instilling sulphonamide or silver nitrate into the new-born infant's eyes immediately after delivery. The condition is due to infection of the child's eyes during delivery from gonococci present in the genital tract of the mother.

Diagnosis

In the male a diagnosis of gonorrhoea can usually be made in the acute stage by the demonstration of typical intracellular Gram negative diplococci. In chronic cases, and in the female, a microscopic diagnosis is rarely possible and isolation of the organism is essential. Where possible cultures should be made directly from the patient onto the medium. Where this is not feasible swabs should be transmitted to the laboratory in one of the special transport media, e.g. Stuart's medium.

The oxidase reaction is of considerable value for the recognition of colonies of the gonococcus on primary plates. The test is carried out by flooding the plate with a fresh 1 per cent solution of tetramethyl-para-phenylenediamine hydrochloride, when the gonococcal colonies rapidly develop a purple colour. Subcultures can be obtained from oxidase positive colonies if made within a few minutes after the performance of the test. The reaction is not specific for the gonococcus—strong reactions being given by other neisseriae, and weak reactions by miscellaneous other organisms. The test, however, is of very great value as a screening procedure to indicate colonies which require further investigation.

If typical colonies of Gram negative cocci giving a positive oxidase reaction are isolated from a case of urethritis in the male, they can be safely accepted as gonococci. For more precise identification, and this is particularly necessary in infections in the female, fermentation reactions would be decisive. Recent work indicates that equally reliable, and considerably more rapid identification can be achieved by the use of the fluorescent antibody technique.

In chronic cases, in which microscopic and cultural examination may be equivocal, and in late complication of the disease—such as arthritis—the gonococcal complement fixation test is of considerable value. Because of the antigenic heterogeneity of the species, however, a polyvalent antigen prepared from a number of strains is essential. Positive results are rarely obtained in the test until at least 2 weeks after infection, and are most frequently given by cases in which the infection has spread from the anterior urethra.

Treatment

The treatment of gonorrhoea was revolutionized by the introduction of the sulphonamides, but unfortunately after a few years' use of these drugs a high proportion of strains isolated were found to be sulphonamide-resistant.

Penicillin has for many years been the treatment of choice. Recent reports, however, show an increasing number of strains with a substantial resistance to penicillin. Fortunately, gonococci are still highly sensitive to various other antibiotics, of which the tetracyclines and erythromycin appear to be the most generally useful. Gonococci appear also to have regained, to a very considerable extent, their original sensitivity to sulphonamides.

Gonorrhoeal patients not infrequently have a coexistent syphilitic infection contracted at the same time. The administration of penicillin or any other antibiotic active against *Treponema pallidum* to such patients may delay or in some cases completely inhibit the development of the primary syphilitic lesion. It is therefore important to carry out serologic tests for syphilis over a period of some months after such treatment. It is stated that if chills and fever are found during the course of penicillin treatment of gonorrhoea, there is a considerable possibility of coexistent syphilis.

Non-specific Urethritis

Not all cases of urethritis are due to the gonococcus. A more chronic form which is generally known as non-specific urethritis appears to have been increasing in frequency in recent years. This condition is apparently not of gonococcal origin but its precise cause has not been determined. It has been suggested that it may be due to a *Mycoplasma* (Chapter 28). Suggestive but not conclusive evidence has been obtained for this identification in certain cases. It is possible that the disease may have a multiple aetiology. Successful results have been claimed for a variety of therapeutic regimens—sulphonamides, penicillin, tetracycline, chloramphenicol, streptomycin—but without precise information as to aetiology, treatment must be entirely empirical. Non-specific urethritis is occasionally a component of a more serious generalized disease of undetermined aetiology, known as Reiter's disease, in which lesions are also found in the joints and the conjunctiva.

CHAPTER 17

BACILLUS

Organisms of the *Bacillus* genus are aerobic Gram positive sporing rods. Only one species, *Bacillus anthracis*, is pathogenic for man.

Bacillus anthracis

Morphology

Bacillus anthracis is a large non-motile bacillus measuring 5 to 10μ by 1 to 2μ. In the tissues it is found singly, in pairs and in short chains and is surrounded by a capsule which is continuous over the whole chain. In culture long chains of bacilli may be found.

As in other capsulated pathogenic species the capsule is essential for virulence. Chemically, it is composed of a polymer of D-glutamic acid. Similar glutamyl polypeptides are found in other members of the *Bacillus* genus. The capsule therefore is not the sole determinant of virulence. Normal virulent bacilli do not produce capsules on nutrient agar under normal atmospheric conditions. Capsulation may be induced, however, by incubation in an atmosphere containing a high concentration of CO_2, or by the addition of bicarbonate to the medium, or, in physiological CO_2 concentrations, by growth in the presence of albumen, serum, charcoal or starch. From the work of Meynell and Meynell, it would appear that the role of high CO_2 concentrations is to secure an adequate concentration of bicarbonate ion in the medium. This, in turn, may be the natural inducer of the enzymes involved in the synthesis of the glutamyl polypeptide. Serum, albumen, charcoal and starch appear to act by neutralizing an inhibitor—possibly oleic acid—present in ordinary media. When the inhibitor is neutralized, capsulation occurs in the presence of normal physiological concentrations of CO_2. The mechanism by which the inhibitor acts is unknown. Certain non-virulent strains of anthrax bacilli are capsulated when grown on nutrient agar under ordinary atmospheric conditions; there is evidence that these strains have lost their sensitivity to the inhibitor. Other non-virulent strains are non-capsulated under all conditions of growth.

Spores are produced only in the presence of oxygen. Consequently they are found in culture only when the organism is grown under aerobic conditions; they are never seen in material taken directly from the tissues. Characteristically the spores are centrally situated, of the same width as the bacillus, and oval in shape.

Cultural Properties

The anthrax bacillus is aerobic and facultatively anaerobic. The organism grows well on all ordinary media at temperatures between 19° C and 40° C. Growth is not improved by the presence of blood. After overnight incubation the colonies on agar are highly characteristic. They are of a greyish-white or cream colour, opaque, with an uneven surface and an irregular wavy edge,

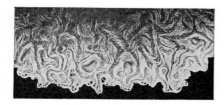

FIG. 20. EDGE OF A COLONY OF *B. anthracis* ON AGAR (× 75)

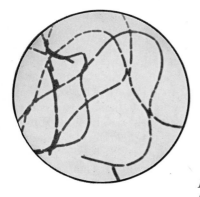

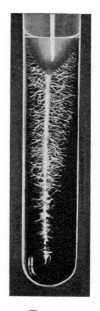

FIG. 22.
B. anthracis FROM AN AGAR CULTURE (× 750)

FIG. 21
B. anthracis IN GELATIN (× ½)

showing the so-called Medusa head or 'barrister's wig' appearance. On microscopic examination the edge of the colony can be seen to consist of long, interlacing strands comprising parallel chains of bacilli. When grown under conditions which favour capsule development, e.g. on serum agar or in the presence of a high concentration of CO_2, the colony has a smooth, mucoid character. Normally the organism is non-haemolytic on blood agar, but a few strains may show a narrow zone of haemolysis.

In gelatin stab-culture *B. anthracis* produces a highly characteristic type of liquefaction in which lines of growth radiate from a central stem—the whole resembling an inverted fir tree with delicate filamentous branches.

Antigenic Structure

The main component of the capsule is a polypeptide of D-glutamic acid. Similar glutamyl polypeptides are found in other *Bacillus* species. Although essential for virulence there is some doubt as to whether the polypeptide is antigenic. A polysaccharide which cross-reacts serologically with the type 14 pneumococcal capsular polysaccharide is the principal antigenic component of the cell wall. Antibody to this antigen nevertheless plays no part in protection against infection. An antigen which stimulates the production of protective antibody is demonstrable, however, in the oedema fluid produced in response to the inoculation of living anthrax bacilli. This antigen is not produced in the conventional type of laboratory culture but is produced when the organism is grown in the presence of a high concentration of bicarbonate. Without bicarbonate the antigen appears to accumulate intracellularly but with bicarbonate it is released into the medium, possibly as a result of some alteration in the permeability of the cell membrane. The antigen is a heat-labile protein, and has been identified as one of the components of the anthrax toxin (see below).

Pathogenicity

The anthrax bacillus produces a specific toxin which is lethal and oedema-producing on injection into experimental animals. The toxin, which is not demonstrable under ordinary cultural conditions, was first identified in the plasma of animals dying of anthrax infection. It was subsequently found in very young cultures of the organism growing in heparinized or defibrinated guinea-pig blood. As shown by Smith, the toxin is a complex of the three protein components I, II and III, each of which by itself is non-toxic. Component II is identical with the protective antigen referred to above. It is the only component which is antigenic per se. A mixture of components I and II has marked oedema-producing capacity but relatively low lethality. The addition of component III considerably enhances lethality while reducing oedema-producing capacity. The lethal effect of the toxin appears to be the result of shock but the precise nature of the biochemical lesion involved is not known.

Most mammals are to a greater or lesser extent susceptible to experimental anthrax infection. For diagnostic purposes mice and guinea-pigs are most used. Following subcutaneous injection of fully virulent strains guinea-pigs die within two days of inoculation. At post mortem there is a marked inflammatory lesion at the site of inoculation with a surrounding gelatinous oedema. Large numbers of bacilli are present in the blood and may also be seen in various internal organs, particularly in the spleen.

Anthrax

The natural disease affects herbivora—chiefly sheep and cattle—in which the mortality may be as high as 80 per cent. Horses, goats and pigs are less commonly attacked. In animals, anthrax is a septicaemic disease which may be acute or subacute in type. The most marked post-mortem finding is the great enlargement of the spleen, from which fact the name 'splenic fever' has been given to the disease.

There is little doubt that infection in animals is chiefly by the ingestion of spores present in their food. Since, however, laboratory animals can only rarely be infected by feeding, it is probable that some damage to the mucous membranes, such as might be inflicted by thorns, is essential. Infected animals excrete large numbers of anthrax bacilli in discharges from the mouth, nose and rectum and in this way contaminate their pasturage where the spores may survive for years and constitute a source of infection for other animals.

The disease is uncommon in animals in Britain—most infections being caused by spores present in imported foods. Consequently the majority of cases occur in winter when imported foodstuffs are generally used. In countries in which it is enzootic the disease occurs most frequently during the late summer and autumn.

Anthrax is not a common disease in man. In countries where the disease is prevalent in animals infection occurs mainly in persons whose work brings them into close contact with animals, viz. veterinary surgeons, butchers and farmers. In others it is found mainly as an industrial disease, infection occurring almost entirely in workers whose occupation involves the handling of imported hair, hides or wool. Infection of members of the general population may occur through the use of shaving brushes, the bristles of which have come from infected animals.

In man the disease assumes three clinical forms, cutaneous, respiratory and intestinal. In the cutaneous form, which is the commonest variety of the disease, the spores or bacilli gain entrance through cuts or abrasions or possibly by way of the hair follicles. The face and neck, hands, arms or back are the usual sites for the characteristic lesion, which is known as the 'malignant pustule'. From 1 to 3 days after infection a small papule, usually painful, occurs. This soon becomes vesicular, the contained fluid being clear or blood-stained. The centre becomes necrotic and black in colour and around it a ring of vesicles forms: the whole area is congested and oedematous. The cutaneous lesion usually resolves spontaneously but in a minority of cases, if untreated, the blood stream is invaded, and the outcome is, invariably, fatal.

The respiratory form of anthrax, known as 'woolsorter's disease', occurs almost exclusively in the wool industry, as a result of the inhalation of dust from infected wool. Respiratory anthrax has a high mortality rate, and the organisms appear to multiply mainly in the mediastinal glands from which the blood stream is rapidly invaded. Though it is the normal route of infection in animals, infection by the intestinal tract is rare in man. As in the respiratory form the condition carries a grave prognosis.

Diagnosis

In the early stages of cutaneous anthrax the organisms are usually readily demonstrable in the skin lesions; in the later stages, however, this may not be possible. Whatever the source of the material examined, the organism should be isolated on culture. Since the anthrax bacillus does not spore in the body the material should not be heated prior to culture. For routine purposes blood agar is a satisfactory medium for isolation.

If anthrax bacilli are sought in material which is heavily contaminated with other organisms, a portion of the material should be heated at 70° C for 10 minutes as a preliminary to culture or animal inoculation. Pearce and Powell's medium, which contains haemin, lysozyme, peptone and agar, may be used for cultures from heavily contaminated material.

The cultural features distinguishing the anthrax bacillus from other sporing bacilli are: the characteristic colony, absence of haemolysis on sheep blood agar, absence of motility, typical fir-tree growth in gelatin, susceptibility to specific bacteriophages, sensitivity to penicillin and production of morphological capsules on serum or bicarbonate agar.

Post-mortem examination should never be carried out for the diagnosis of anthrax in animals since spores develop readily when the organisms are exposed to the air and might be responsible for further spread of the disease. Instead an ear should be removed and an attempt made to demonstrate the bacillus in blood from the ear vein.

Ascoli's test has been widely used for the recognition of anthrax in the tissues of dead animals. In this test extracts are made of the infected tissue by boiling for 5 minutes with normal saline containing 1/1000 acetic acid and tested by the ring-precipitin technique with immune serum. The test is not completely specific.

Treatment

Penicillin is the treatment of choice. Although very effective in treatment, penicillin does not modify the evolution of the skin lesion since it has no effect on the anthrax toxin. In severely toxaemic cases the administration of an antiserum, sometimes known as Sclavo's serum, prepared by immunization of asses, may be combined with chemotherapy. The treatment of respiratory and intestinal anthrax is, however, unsatisfactory.

Prophylaxis

A considerable degree of immunity can be produced against anthrax in animals by the inoculation of vaccines prepared from living attenuated strains. This was first demonstrated by Pasteur in his classic experiment at Pouilly-le-Fort in 1881. Pasteur inoculated 24 sheep, 1 goat and 6 cows with living cultures of an anthrax bacillus whose virulence had been attenuated by prolonged growth at 42° C. The animals were given two injections with 12 days' interval between; 2 weeks later the inoculated animals and a similar number of controls were injected with a fully virulent culture. All the control animals died of anthrax, whereas all of the inoculated animals, except one sheep, survived. The latter did not die of anthrax. Following this dramatic proof of its value vaccination was widely adopted. The results generally obtained with it, however, did not fully realize the initial expectations. It did not give complete protection, but of more serious consequence was the fact that it killed about 1 per cent of animals inoculated. This, however, was preferable to the very high mortality from the natural disease, which was then widespread throughout France.

Because of the difficulty of ensuring the stability of the attenuated strains prepared by Pasteur's method his method of vaccine preparation has been abandoned. The most satisfactory of the vaccines now in use for immunization of animals appears to be that of Mazzuchi. This consists of a spore suspension of the stable attenuated Carbazoo strain in 2 per cent saponin. The immunity produced by any form of anthrax vaccine is of short duration and animals require annual reinoculation. Vaccines are not used for human immunization but preparations of the protective antigen may be valuable for persons exposed through their occupation.

Prophylaxis, so far as man is concerned, is chiefly a matter of industrial hygiene, viz. adequate exhaust ventilation to remove dust and the sterilization of wool, hides and hair. In Britain the control of industrial anthrax has been greatly facilitated by restricting the importation of potentially infected hides and hair to a single port—Liverpool. Since most infections occur through the skin, the hands of the workers should be protected as much as possible. Abrasions should immediately be treated with iodine.

Other Bacilli

Non-pathogenic aerobic sporing bacilli are widely distributed in nature. Some may resemble the anthrax bacillus sufficiently closely to cause confusion in identification. These non-pathogenic species usually show one or more of the following characters: motility, haemolysis, diffuse growth in broth and gelatin liquefaction of a diffuse type. In any case of doubt a pathogenicity test should be carried out. The following species are of special interest.

Bacillus subtilis. Some strains of this organism produce an extracellular penicillinase. Since the penicillinase produced by *B. subtilis* is an adaptive enzyme, it is produced in appreciable amount only by growing the organism in the presence of penicillin. *B. subtilis* is a particularly troublesome organism to the bacteriologist since if introduced into a laboratory its spores are very persistent and may cause contamination of media.

Bacillus mesentericus. This organism is responsible for the condition of ropiness occasionally found in bread.

Bacillus polymyxa is important as the source of the antibiotic polymyxin.

CHAPTER 18

THE CORYNEBACTERIA

The corynebacteria are irregularly staining Gram positive non-sporing, non-motile and non-capsulated rods. They frequently show club-shaped swellings, a characteristic which is responsible for the name of the genus. Only one species—*Corynebacterium diphtheriae* is pathogenic for man. Other species—*Corynebacterium ovis*, *Corynebacterium pyogenes* and *Corynebacterium equi*—are important animal pathogens.

Corynebacterium diphtheriae

Morphology

Diphtheria bacilli vary considerably in morphology. This is to a considerable extent correlated with cultural type (p. 283), but even within the same type they may show considerable strain variation. Morphology also depends on the precise cultural conditions employed. The bacilli may appear as short, more or less uniformly stained organisms, but more often, as long (5 × 0·4μ) slender, slightly curved, irregularly stained bacilli. They are rarely of uniform diameter throughout their length, swellings at one or both ends, producing the characteristic 'club' appearance, being common. The most striking morphological feature of diphtheria bacilli are the metachromatic granules—intensely staining round or oval bodies usually located at the ends of the bacilli—which consist of highly polymerized metaphosphate. In films made from cultures, diphtheria bacilli, particularly the longer forms, tend to be grouped in pairs with the individual organisms lying at an acute angle. The pairs frequently occur in groups, giving rise to the so-called 'Chinese letter' appearance.

Cultural Properties

The diphtheria bacillus grows best aerobically; under anaerobic conditions growth is poor. It will grow on nutrient agar but growth is better on media containing blood or serum. For isolation, Loeffler's serum medium, on which, though not a particularly good medium, diphtheria bacilli will grow more rapidly than do other bacteria likely to be found in the nose and throat, and media containing potassium tellurite, which are highly selective for the diphtheria bacillus and on which it produces a black colony, are the media of choice.

Three cultural types of diphtheria bacillus, distinguished by their colonial morphology on a special blood tellurite medium, were described by McLeod.

PLATE III

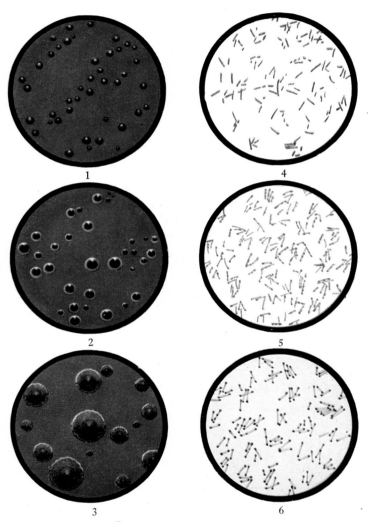

1

4

2

5

3

6

CORYNEBACTERIUM DIPHTHERIAE

1. *Intermedius* type on McLeod's medium
2. *Mitis* type on McLeod's medium
3. *Gravis* type on McLeod's medium

4. Film stained by Gram's method
5. Film stained with methylene blue
6. Film stained by Neisser's method

[*To face p.* 283

These types are known as *gravis*, *intermedius* and *mitis*, the names indicating the severity of clinical disease with which each type is most frequently associated. This classification, however, is not exhaustive and many strains cannot be assigned to any of the three types. There is some evidence that the types are not completely stable, organisms initially of one type being capable of mutation to another type.

The *gravis* variety, on McLeod's medium, produces large, grey or grey-black, daisy head colonies: in broth it produces a heavy pellicle and granular deposit with the bulk of the fluid clear. Most strains ferment starch. *Gravis* strains are haemolytic for rabbit blood but not for ox blood. They are shorter than the strains of the other types and rarely show the presence of metachromatic granules. The *intermedius* variety, on McLeod's medium produces very small, flat, black, granular colonies with central papillae: in broth it causes a fine, dust-like deposit without clouding or surface growth; it does not ferment starch and is never haemolytic. The bacilli are almost entirely of an irregularly barred form with poor development of metachromatic granules. The *mitis* variety, on McLeod's medium, grows in colonies which are black, glistening and smoothly convex; in broth it produces a uniform turbidity with or without a fine pellicle; it does not ferment starch and is haemolytic for ox and rabbit cells. Most *mitis* strains show well-marked metachromatic granule formation on serum media.

Diphtheria bacilli ferment glucose and maltose, producing acid, but no gas. Except for a few very rare strains they do not ferment saccharose.

A large number of serologic types have been defined by agglutination tests. Serological typing is of some epidemiological value but, though the antigens responsible appear to be restricted to diphtheria bacilli, is not carried out as a routine procedure.

Pathogenicity

The diphtheria bacillus produces a potent exotoxin which, by diffusing from the site of multiplication in the tissues, plays the key role in the disease picture of diphtheria. The toxin, which is a protein, has been isolated in crystalline form. It is extremely potent, 0.0001 mg of a purified preparation constituting a lethal dose for a 250-g guinea-pig. Toxin is produced by all *gravis* and *intermedius* strains, but about 20 per cent of *mitis* strains are nontoxigenic. The toxins produced by different strains are antigenically identical, and can all be neutralized by a single antitoxin. Examination by the Ouchterlony plate technique has however shown three or four distinct antigens in the most highly purified preparations so far available.

Toxin production is closely dependent on the iron concentration of the medium, being optimal with concentrations of iron just sufficient to permit growth. During growth the toxin begins to accumulate only when the exogenous supply of iron is exhausted. Evidence has been presented by Pappenheimer in support of the view that the toxin is the protein part of a bacterial cytochrome —cytochrome b_1, a respiratory pigment which contains iron, porphyrin and protein. In concentrations of iron greater than those required for optimal toxin production, the entire cytochrome molecule would be synthesized. With low concentrations of iron the organisms could synthesize the protein and the porphyrin but could not form the complete cytrochrome molecule. The protein would therefore be free, and be excreted into the medium. Considerable, but not decisive, evidence has been obtained in support of this theory.

As shown by the production of a cytopathogenic effect in a wide range of tissue cultures, the diphtheria toxin appears to have a toxic effect on most tissue cells. The subcutaneous inoculation of a guinea-pig with a sufficient amount of a virulent culture of bacilli produces death in 36 to 72 hours. The local lesion is a small greyish area of necrosis surrounded by a zone of gelatinous oedema. A pathognomonic feature is the appearance of the adrenals which are usually markedly congested and often haemorrhagic. These effects are due entirely to the toxin and there is little or no invasion of the animal's body by the organism.

The capacity of the diphtheria bacillus to produce toxin depends on the presence in the organism of a symbiotic bacteriophage known as β phage. The phage appears to act as a genetic determinant controlling toxin production. By infecting them with β phage or with one of its variants non-toxigenic bacilli can usually, though not invariably, be converted into toxigenic bacilli. This transformation is known as phage conversion (p. 559). The phages responsible for conversion may be derived from non-toxigenic as well as from toxigenic strains. Bacilli which have been rendered toxigenic by phage infection will remain toxigenic only as long as they remain lysogenic (Chapter 42). Thus by growth in the presence of antiphage serum it is possible to cure them of the phage infection; concomitantly with the loss of the phage the bacilli become non-toxigenic. There is no evidence that the release of toxin depends on lysis of the cells by phage.

Diphtheria

The natural disease in man affects chiefly the upper part of the respiratory tract, especially the fauces, the toxin of the organism producing necrotic changes in the mucous membrane of the affected area. This stimulates a local inflammatory reaction as a result of which a 'false membrane' composed of laminae of fibrin, in which are entangled leucocytes, red cells, epithelial cells and, in the more superficial layers, diphtheria bacilli, is formed. The membrane is most conspicuous in the tonsillar area but, as the condition progresses, spreads over the palate around the pharyngeal wall and into the larynx. In the latter situation it can cause respiratory obstruction leading, unless relieved by tracheotomy, to the death of the patient. In addition to membrane formation there occurs a general toxaemia as a result of spread of toxin in the blood stream from the local lesion. This produces remote toxic effects, particularly on the adrenals, which cause a fall in blood pressure; on the heart muscle, which may be sufficient to produce cardiac failure, and on the kidneys, leading to albuminuria. The acute stage of the infection is not infrequently followed by a peripheral neuritis, usually of a transient character. This condition is possibly due to allergic sensitization, rather than to the direct action of the toxin. In some cases, particularly in young children, the nasopharynx is mainly involved. A false membrane may be found in other parts of the body, such as the ear, conjunctiva, vulva and vagina, but much more rarely than in the respiratory tract. Infection of wounds or abrasions with the production of an indolent ulcer is not uncommon in the tropics but is rare in temperate zones. This type of infection is associated with relatively little systemic disturbance.

As previously indicated, the severity of diphtheria depends on the type of bacillus (p. 283) causing the infection. Thus in McLeod's original series the mortality from the *gravis* type was 8·1 per cent, from the *intermedius* type 7·2 per cent, while that from the *mitis* type was 2·6 per cent. *Gravis* and *intermedius* cases also frequently show an extensive oedema of the tissues of the neck which may spread down to the chest and give rise to the appearance known clinically as 'bull-neck'. These differences in mortality can be attributed to the fact that toxaemia is much more marked in *gravis* and *intermedius* than in *mitis* infections. In addition to these differences there is some evidence that *gravis* and *intermedius* strains have a greater potential for epidemic spread. *Mitis* strains, on the other hand, have a greater capacity to persist in artificially immunized populations.

The relatively greater severity of infection due to the *gravis* type has not been adequately explained. The classical toxins produced by *gravis* and *mitis* strains appear to be identical both pharmacologically and antigenically. It has been suggested that recently isolated *gravis* strains produce in addition to the classical toxin a substance which facilitates spread of the toxin through the tissues and which also interferes with the avidity of antitoxin. A second view which has received some support proposes that *gravis* strains are more active toxin producers than *mitis* strains in the environment of the tissues. It has been suggested that this may be due to a more active growth rate as a result of which they would more rapidly deplete the local tissue concentration of iron which would otherwise have a limiting effect on toxin production.

Diagnosis

In no condition is it more important to achieve an early diagnosis than in diphtheria. Films made from the lesion are quite unsuitable for a microscopic diagnosis and culture is therefore essential.

A throat swab is charged from the area involved, care being taken to include a portion of any membrane present. The swab is inoculated onto a Löffler slope and onto a blood tellurite plate. The swab should also be inoculated onto blood agar for the detection of *Str. pyogenes*.

After overnight incubation, smears are made from the serum slope and from any grey or black colonies present on the tellurite medium and stained with one of the special stains used for diphtheria bacilli. The appearance of the colonies on tellurite is of considerable diagnostic value; they should be examined under magnification, preferably with a colony microscope. The experienced observer can usually make a reliable presumptive diagnosis at this stage and can also indicate the type of diphtheria bacillus present. Any suspicious colonies appearing on tellurite should be subcultured to serum. The serum slope cultures are used for a further morphological examination and for fermentation reactions and virulence tests when these are considered necessary. A full examination should be undertaken on all strains obtained from carriers, from isolated cases at non-epidemic times, or in any case of doubt.

Virulence tests may be carried out by injecting the growth from a young serum culture subcutaneously into each of two guinea-pigs, one of which has been protected by 250 units of antitoxin, injected the previous day. If the organism is a diphtheria bacillus the unprotected animal will die, usually within 5 days, showing at post mortem the characteristic signs of diphtheritic toxaemia while the protected animal will survive. Some non-toxigenic strains stimulate a local pyogenic reaction in guinea-pigs. This reaction is, however, readily distinguishable from the local reaction produced in response to the diphtheria bacillus and is not neutralized by diphtheria antitoxin. An intradermal method which permits the testing of a number of strains on a single guinea-pig can also be used. In this case the presence of toxin is indicated by the development of an erythematous reaction, progressing to necrosis, in the animal's skin. A control protected animal shows no skin lesion.

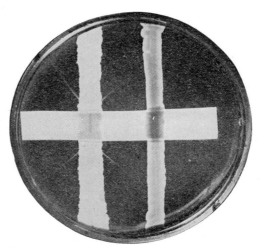

FIG. 23. PLATE VIRULENCE TEST FOR *C. diphtheriae*

Two strains of *C. diphtheriae* have been streaked vertically and a strip of filter paper laid horizontally across the plate. The strain on left had yielded 4 lines of toxin–antitoxin precipitate and is therefore toxigenic. The strain on right is non-toxigenic

The performance of virulence tests has been made very much simpler by the plate technique introduced by Elek. In this method a strip of filter paper soaked in antitoxin is laid across a plate of serum agar. The strains to be tested are streaked at right angles to the strip and the plate incubated. If the strain is toxigenic, a line of precipitate is observed in the angle between the streak of growth and the filter paper strip. The test has been found to give very good correlation with in vivo toxigenicity tests.

Treatment

Since the efficacy of antitoxin depends on the stage of the disease at which it is given, it is of the utmost importance that the antitoxin should be given as early as possible—*without waiting for the bacteriologist's report*. A dose of 5000 to 100,000 units of antitoxin is recommended, depending on the severity of the case and the stage at which it is seen. In severe cases, and in cases seen at a late stage, antitoxin should be administered by the intravenous route. In other cases the intramuscular route is to be preferred to the subcutaneous. When serum is administered intramuscularly it reaches its maximum concentration in the blood in 24 hours, whereas, by the subcutaneous route, maximum concentration in the blood is attained in 72 hours.

The diphtheria bacillus is sensitive to penicillin, and penicillin has been found to be a useful adjunct in treatment. Although it does not affect the toxaemia it assists in the sterilization of the tissues, thereby shortening the course of the disease and preventing the development of a convalescent carrier state. In addition it will assist in the control of concomitant streptococcal and staphylococcal infection which is sometimes present, particularly in *gravis* and *intermedius* infections. Erythromycin also appears to be of some value but has been less used than penicillin. It should be noted that chemotherapy is no substitute for the administration of antitoxin.

Following recovery from the clinical manifestations of diphtheria, the patient may continue to carry the organism in the nose or throat for some time, and is therefore capable of spreading the disease to others. Consequently, patients should not be discharged until it is reasonably certain that they no longer carry the organism. Nasal carriers constitute a considerable proportion of the convalescent carriers of diphtheria bacilli, the organism apparently disappearing more slowly from the nose than from the throat. They are particularly dangerous as sources of infection since they shed more organisms into their environment than do throat carriers. The carrier state may on occasion develop without an antecedent attack of diphtheria.

Immunity

Immunity against diphtheria can be produced both by an attack of the disease and by a subclinical infection, as well as by artificial immunization and is due to antitoxin in the blood of the immune person. This can be detected by the Schick test, in which a small amount of toxin in a total volume of 0·2 ml is injected into the skin of one forearm, and a similar amount of heated toxin—which acts as a control—into the other. Readings should be made twice, the first at 48 hours, the second from 5 to 7 days after the test. A positive reaction is shown by the development in 24 to 48 hours at the site of injection of the toxin, of a red flush, from 1 to 5 cm in diameter. The colour usually begins to fade after about a week, to be succeeded by a brownish discoloration which, in exceptional cases, may persist for some months. The occurrence of this reaction indicates that there is insufficient antitoxin present in the subject's blood to neutralize the test dose of toxin. If the patient's blood contains enough antitoxin to neutralize the test dose of toxin this reaction does not occur. The blood antitoxin concentration required to give a negative reaction with the test concentrations of toxin usually employed is on an average $\frac{1}{200}$ unit per ml. This is usually but not always sufficient to protect against diphtheria. Since some subjects may give non-specific allergic reactions to components of the toxic filtrate other than the toxin it is necessary, in order to detect these 'pseudo'-reactions, to carry out a control test by injecting into the other arm the same amount of toxic filtrate which has been heated sufficiently to destroy its toxin. Such reactions consist of a transient erythema which develops as a rule within 24 hours and usually disappears completely in from 5 to 6 days, at which time the reaction to the unheated toxin is still present. Pseudo-reactions are commonest in older children and adults. The combination of positive and pseudo-reactions normally indicates susceptibility. When, however, the pseudo-reaction is very intense it has been found to be associated with the presence of an appreciable amount of antitoxin in the blood, and therefore indicates immunity.

Prophylaxis

Contacts may be passively immunized by the injection of antitoxin, 500 units being the dose normally used. The immunity produced is of short duration lasting at most for a few weeks. Passive immunization is therefore only an emergency measure but, since it is rapidly established, is a very effective one. To be effective, antitoxin must be given as soon as possible after exposure and preferably within 24 hours. Antitoxin may be combined with active immunization for children who have not been previously immunized, but it appears to interfere to some extent with the efficacy of active immunization.

For the production of active immunity the following preparations are used.

1. Formol toxoid (FT). This preparation consists of toxin which has been treated with formalin to deprive it of its toxicity. It may be used by itself or, more frequently, in combination with various other antigens, e.g. tetanus toxoid and pertussis vaccine. By itself, formol toxoid is a relatively poor antigen but in combination with pertussis vaccine its antigenicity is considerably enhanced. Pertussis-containing vaccines are suitable only for the vaccination of young children (p. 344).

2. Adjuvant vaccines (APT and PTAP). The antigenicity of formol toxoid can be greatly enhanced, as in APT and PTAP by combination with adjuvants. APT is a suspension of the precipitate formed by the addition of aluminium hydroxide to formol toxoid. PTAP is prepared by the adsorption of a purified toxoid onto aluminium phosphate. The enhanced antigenicity of these two preparations appears to be due to two circumstances: (a) They form a depot in the tissues from which the toxoid is only slowly released. (b) They stimulate the development of local granulomatous reactions in which a substantial amount of antibody may be produced. Although highly efficient as prophylactics, adjuvant preparations have the disadvantage that they give rise to a higher proportion of reactions—particularly in older children and adults—than formol toxoid. Consequently they are only recommended for immunization of children of less than 10 years of age. There is some evidence that administration of adjuvant prophylactics may predispose to the development of paralytic poliomyelitis

in the injected limb if given at a time of poliomyelitis epidemic prevalence. Because of this they are now rarely used in Britain.

3. Toxoid antitoxin floccules (TAF). This prophylactic is a suspension of the precipitate formed by the addition of antitoxin to toxin in optimal proportions. It is the purest of all the diphtheria prophylactics and appears to give the least reactions on injection. It has about the same immunizing potency as formol toxoid. It has, however, the disadvantage that, since it contains a small amount of horse serum, it may, though rarely, produce serum hypersensitivity. It has been used mainly for the immunization of older children and adults in whom the alum-containing preparations would be more liable to produce reactions. Three injections each of 0·5 ml, with an interval of at least four weeks between each injection, are usually given.

It can be safely assumed that all children under the age of 10 years are susceptible to diphtheria and therefore require immunization. With children of this age group it is therefore unnecessary to carry out a Schick test. With children over the age of 10 years a Schick test is, however, essential. In addition to indicating which children should be immunized it will also identify those who might react severely to diphtheria prophylactics. These are persons who give strong pseudo-reactions (p. 288). In those who are presumed to have some immunity the test dose of toxin probably provides an adequate booster stimulus.

Ideally, a primary course of immunization should be completed during the first year of life. For this purpose the triple vaccine—DTP—is the prophylactic of choice. A booster dose should be given at the age of 18 months, and another at 4 to 5 years, just prior to school entry. Children with a history of asthma or other allergic state constitute a special problem since they are those most likely to develop serious reactions of an anaphylactic type following immunization. When such a child is to be immunized it is advisable to give a trial dose of 0·1 ml of the prophylactic. If this causes no reaction the full dose can then be given safely.

Since the introduction of active immunization, and the resulting enormous reduction in the incidence of diphtheria, there appears to have been a concomitant reduction in the number of healthy carriers. Thus in the 1920's carrier rates of 2·5 to 5 per cent were reported for London elementary school children. In 1943, three years after the introduction of immunization the rate had fallen to 0·19 per cent.

Other Corynebacteria

The term 'diphtheroid' is loosely applied to other species of corynebacteria. Some of these resemble the diphtheria bacillus closely in appearance and may cause difficulty in identification. Non-pathogenic corynebacteria are frequently found as commensals in the upper respiratory tract and are fairly constantly present in the nose. They can usually be differentiated from C. diphtheriae by their fermentation reactions—most strains either failing to ferment glucose or fermenting saccharose.

The named species most frequently found as commensals are *Corynebacterium pseudodiphtheriticum* (Hofmann's bacillus), which is often present in the nose and less frequently in the throat, and *Corynebacterium xerosis*, which is sometimes found in the conjunctiva. *C. pseudodiphtheriticum* is readily distinguishable morphologically from the diphtheria bacillus. It is shorter, does not possess metachromatic granules and usually exhibits an unstained central bar. It does not ferment any sugars and is not pathogenic for guinea-pigs. *C. xerosis* is morphologically similar to the *mitis* type of diphtheria bacillus but ferments saccharose and is non-pathogenic for guinea-pigs.

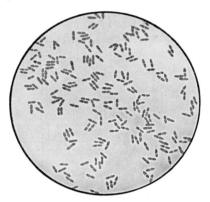

FIG. 24. *C. pseudodiphtheriticum* FROM CULTURE ON SERUM (× 800)

CHAPTER 19

COMMENSAL INTESTINAL BACTERIA

In the next three chapters we shall be concerned with organisms of the family enterobacteriaceae, so called because their normal habitat is the intestinal tract of man and other animals. The enterobacteriaceae are Gram negative non-sporing bacilli which grow readily on ordinary laboratory media under both aerobic and anaerobic conditions. All ferment glucose and most ferment a variety of other sugars as well. The enterobacteriaceae have been extremely difficult to classify precisely since they include a large number of complexly interrelated bacterial types. This difficulty is particularly acute in the classification of the coliform group. Consequently the definition of genera has in many cases been quite arbitrary, and has tended to change with the acceptance of new criteria for taxonomic characterization. From the medical point of view, for which their pathogenic potential is of a primary importance, they may be subdivided into two large groups. (*a*) Organisms occurring primarily, or exclusively, as intestinal pathogens. This group comprises the genera *Salmonella*, *Shigella* and *Arizona* which will be considered separately in subsequent chapters. (*b*) Organisms occurring primarily as intestinal commensals. These fall into two groups: the *coliform* group and the *Proteus* group.

For the differentiation of the enterobacteriaceae the capacity to ferment lactose, though not accepted as a primary taxonomic criterion, is of considerable practical importance. Lactose is fermented with the production of acid and gas by most of the eschericheae. It is not fermented by any of the salmonellae, shigellae—with the exception of *Shigella sonnei* which is a late lactose fermenter —or by the proteae.

THE COLIFORM GROUP

In this group five genera may be distinguished: *Escherichia*, *Klebsiella*, *Citrobacter*, *Cloaca* and *Hafnia*. Of these, *Escherichia* and *Klebsiella* are the most important, and are the only genera with an established pathogenic potential.

Escherichia is represented by a single species, *E. coli* and *Klebsiella* by three species—*Kl. pneumoniae*, *Kl. rhinoscleromatis*, *Kl. ozaenae*. The features distinguishing *E. coli* and the typical, and most important, *Klebsiella* species, *Kl. pneumoniae*, are shown in the following table.

Typical Reactions of *Escherichia coli* and *Klebsiella pneumoniae*

	E. coli	Kl. pneumoniae
Indole	+	−
Methyl red	+	−
Voges Proskauer	−	+
Growth in citrate as sole carbon source	−	+
Adonitol and inositol fermentation	−	+
Decomposition of urea[1]	−	+

1 This reaction occurs slowly taking as a rule 3 or 4 days to be detectable. Decomposition of urea by *Proteus* is much more rapid being detectable within 24 hours.

Escherichia coli

Escherichia coli is the typical coliform organism of the intestinal tract and is present in large numbers in the faeces of man and other animals. It is non-capsulated and usually motile, although in some cases motility may be extremely difficult to detect. It usually occurs as a short rod—0.5μ by 2 to 5μ in size—but short coccobacillary and long filamentous forms are occasionally observed, the latter particularly in urine. It exhibits no special arrangement. On solid media it produces relatively large colonies which are usually smooth and glistening. Variants are, however, occasionally isolated from pyogenic infections which give rise to very minute colonies. These small colony variants produce the normal type of colony if they are grown on media to which various organic sulphur compounds, e.g. cystine, have been added. On blood agar *E. coli* is usually non-haemolytic but haemolytic strains are occasionally encountered.

The great majority of *E. coli* strains ferment lactose promptly, i.e. within 24 hours, with the production of acid and gas. Glucose, maltose and mannitol are also fermented usually with gas production. Fermentation of dulcitol and saccharose is variable. Occasional strains have atypical fermentation reactions either failing to ferment lactose or fermenting it late, i.e. after several days' incubation or failing to produce gas from sugars. The latter, which are known as anaerogenic strains, include the *alkalescens-dispar* group previously classified as paracolon bacilli. (This nomenclature is now abandoned.) *E. coli* does not liquefy gelatin or produce hydrogen sulphide and will not grow in media containing potassium cyanide.

Because of its invariable occurrence in faeces *E. coli* is of considerable value as an indicator organism in the bacteriological examination of water supplies since if it is present it can be presumed that the water has been contaminated from a faecal source.

Klebsiella pneumoniae

In contrast to *E. coli*, *Kl. pneumoniae* is capsulated and non-motile. The capsule is large and conspicuous and is often several times the size of the bacillus. *Kl. pneumoniae* is usually shorter and plumper in appearance than *E. coli* and when present in the body frequently occurs as a coccobacillus—0·5 to 1·5μ by 1 to 2μ—which may be mistaken for a coccus. On solid media it produces a large white highly mucoid colony which is very characteristic.

Klebsiella pneumoniae ferments lactose, glucose, maltose, mannitol, saccharose, adonitol and inositol. Dulcitol may or may not be fermented. From sugars other than glucose *Kl. pneumoniae* is a less active gas producer than *E. coli*. Gelatin is not liquefied and hydrogen sulphide not produced.

Klebsiella pneumoniae occurs in smaller numbers in the intestinal tract than *E. coli*. Certain serotypes—these are the strains previously known as *Bact. pneumoniae* or colloquially as Friedländer's bacilli—are not infrequently found both as commensals and as pathogens in the respiratory tract. In spite of its name, *Kl. pneumoniae*, like *E. coli*, may cause a variety of pyogenic lesions throughout the body and is frequently isolated from infections of the urinary tract. Strains with identical properties are also widely distributed in nature being found on grasses, grains and decaying vegetation and in soil and water. These strains, which were formerly known as *Bact. aerogenes*, are included by Kaufmann in the species *Kl. pneumoniae* but are assigned by Bergey to a separate genus *Aerobacter* as *Aerobacter aerogenes*.

Also included in the genus *Klebsiella* are 2 atypical species—*Kl. rhinoscleromatis* and *Kl. ozaenae* isolated from cases of rhinoscleroma and ozaena respectively. These species are capsulated and non-motile, do not produce acetyl methyl carbinol and are of more restricted fermentative capacity than *Kl. pneumoniae*.

Citrobacter

Organisms of this genus show considerable resemblance to *E. coli*, because of which they are classified by Bergey as *Escherichia freundii*. They differ from *E. coli* in failing to produce indole, in producing hydrogen sulphide, in growing in citrate as sole source of carbon and in growing in media containing potassium cyanide. The genus as now defined includes the late lactose-fermenting Bethesda-ballerup strains formerly classified as paracolon bacilli. *Citrobacter* strains occur as intestinal commensals, and are commonly isolated from water when they are classified by water bacteriologists as intermediates. They have not so far been shown to be pathogenic.

Cloaca and Hafnia

These two genera occur as intestinal commensals but have not so far been shown to be pathogenic. They resemble *Kl. pneumoniae* in biochemical properties but are motile and, except in the case of some *Cloaca* strains, non-capsulated. *Hafnia* strains differ from other coliforms in being non-lactose fermenters and in that their motility and their typical biochemical reactions are demonstrable only when grown at 22° C. A useful distinguishing feature is their capacity to grow in media containing potassium cyanide. A distinctive feature of *Cloaca* strains is their capacity to liquefy gelatin.

Antigenic Structure of the Coliform Bacteria

Four distinct types of antigen are found in the coliform group.

1. Thermostable somatic antigens chemically resembling those of the salmonellae.

2. H or flagellar antigens.

3. K or surface antigens. These are surface antigens which, when present, mask the agglutinability of the organism by O antiserum. In *E. coli* strains most of the K antigens are non-capsular, surface antigens and are relatively heat labile; in these respects they resemble the Vi antigens of the salmonellae. They are divided by Kaufmann on the basis of their physical properties into L and B antigens; L antigens are totally destroyed—both in respect of agglutinability and capacity to combine with antibody—by exposure to 100° C for one hour. The agglutinability of the B antigens is also destroyed by this degree of heat treatment but their capacity to combine with antibody is not. Individual strains possess at the most one K antigen. In *Kl. pneumoniae* strains the K antigens are true capsular antigens; they are stable at 100° C but their agglutinability is usually destroyed by some hours exposure to 120° C. They are referred to by Kaufmann as A antigens.

4. Fimbrial antigens; these are heat labile being destroyed in 1 hour at 100° C. Fimbrial antigens are not usually found in cultures grown on solid media (p. 11). They are not of any importance in classification.

On the basis of their antigenic composition both *E. coli* and *Kl. pneumoniae* can be subdivided into a large number of serological types. In *E. coli* strains 140 serologically distinct O antigens, 75 K antigens and 40 H antigens have so far been described. These antigens may occur in various combinations and consequently permit the differentiation of a very large number of distinct serotypes. Pathogenic strains of *E. coli* usually possess heat-labile K antigens and usually belong to a limited number of serological types. Strains commensal in the intestinal tract belong to a larger number of serotypes and a higher proportion of such strains lack K antigens.

In *Kl. pneumoniae* strains 72 distinct capsular antigens have been described. Because of the technical difficulties of examining the *Klebsiella* O antigens antigenic typing of *Klebsiella* strains is based entirely on capsular antigen composition. Of the capsular antigenic types, types 1, 2 and 3 are those formerly known as Friedländer's bacilli or *Bact. pneumoniae*. *Kl. rhinoscleromatis* possesses the capsular antigen 3; capsular antigens 4, 5 and 6 have been identified in strains of *Kl. ozaenae*.

Infections due to Coliform Bacteria

While confined to the intestinal tract the coliform bacteria lead a saprophytic existence and may, in fact, by the synthesis of certain vitamins contribute to the nutrition of the host. In certain circumstances, however, they gain access to the tissues and give rise to pyogenic lesions.

Coliform bacteria are the most frequent causes of urinary infections. These infections are usually associated with some underlying predisposing factor in the urinary tract, such as the presence of stone, congenital defect, urinary retention or tuberculosis. Such underlying conditions must therefore always be sought in acute urinary tract infections, particularly if these are of a recurrent character. Infection may also follow interference with the genito-urinary tract, e.g. by catheterization—an indwelling catheter being particularly hazardous— or operations on the prostate and bladder. Infections of the latter type are serious since they frequently lead to the death of the patient from septicaemia or from bacteraemic shock due to the release of large amounts of endotoxin into the circulation. *E. coli* is an important cause of postoperative wound infection though its role in this condition ranks second to that of *Staph. aureus* (p. 245). *E. coli* has also been frequently isolated from the lesions of cholecystitis, appendicitis and peritonitis, but in these conditions other organisms are usually also present, and the precise contribution made by *E. coli* to the disease picture is difficult to assess. It is possible that it may simply play the part of a secondary invader.

Recent work has shown that certain serological types of *E. coli* are responsible for some epidemics of infantile gastro-enteritis. So far 10 distinct antigenic types, distinguished by their somatic antigen composition, have been implicated in this condition. The pathogenicity of a number of these serotypes has been confirmed by feeding experiments in both animals and children. Not all strains of the enteropathogenic serotypes, however, appear capable of causing gastro-enteritis. The properties of a strain which confer enteropathogenicity are not at present known. In many ways infantile gastro-enteritis resembles cholera; there is the same exhausting diarrhoea with associated dehydration, the same absence of invasion of the tissues and of significant inflammatory or degenerative changes in the intestinal mucosa. A striking feature of gastro-enteritis, however, is the fact that the enteropathogenic strain is found throughout the entire length of the intestinal tract, and can be readily recovered from the duodenum both of naturally infected cases and of volunteers.

The condition is much more common in bottle-fed than in breast-fed infants, possibly because with bottle feeding there is a greater opportunity for the child to become infected. Since enteropathogenic strains are common in children's hospitals, the introduction into hospital of children in the susceptible age group, i.e. up to 2 years of age, must therefore be regarded as a hazardous procedure, and one which should be avoided if at all possible. Infants are not only more susceptible to overt infection than are older children but much more frequently become carriers. Infants with gastro-enteritis cause heavy contamination of their environment. This derives not only from the faeces which may be a virtually pure culture of *E. coli* but also from the vomit in which the organisms are usually present in considerable numbers.

Klebsiella pneumoniae type strains are responsible for about 1 per cent of bacterial pneumonias. The pneumonia produced closely resembles in its early stages that 'produced by the pneumococcus; at a later stage a considerable amount of destruction of lung tissue is found, frequently with the formation of multiple abscesses.

Since coliform bacteria show considerable heterogeneity in antibiotic sensitivity, effective therapy requires the performance of sensitivity tests. Many strains of *E. coli* show appreciable sensitivity to the sulphonamide drugs which, because they are excreted in a high concentration in the urine, are of particular value in the treatment of urinary tract infections.

Diagnosis

For the diagnosis of urinary tract infections, stained and unstained preparations of the centrifuged deposit should be examined. Acute infections usually show a considerable number of leucocytes in the urine; this, however, is not always the case. At the same time a loopful of the uncentrifuged and well-mixed urine should be inoculated onto blood agar and MacConkey plates. The number and variety of organisms growing on culture should be noted. If a standard 5 mm loop has been employed, the presence of 50 coliform bacteria per plate can be accepted as presumptive evidence of infection, even in the absence of clinical symptoms or of excess leucocytes in the urine. A quantitative estimate of this type is of value in distinguishing between an actual infection and contamination occurring during the taking of the urine. Such a distinction could also be made by the examination of a catheter specimen. In the case of children, however, for whom urinary examination is most frequently required, catheterization is not now considered justified.

In the identification of enteropathogenic *E. coli* from cases of gastro-enteritis the identity of the strain as an enteropathogenic type must be confirmed serologically. Since these strains do not differ colonially from commensal *E. coli* at least ten colonies from the primary plate should be examined by the slide agglutination technique with polyvalent sera. If positive they should be tested with appropriate type-specific sera, their final identification being confirmed by tube agglutination tests with heat-killed suspensions.

Bacteriological Examination of Water

An estimation of the number of coliform bacteria present in water is the test most frequently carried out on water for the purpose of indicating possible faecal pollution. The procedure used is known as the presumptive coliform count. One 50-ml, five 10-ml and five 1-ml volumes of the water are inoculated into tubes of MacConkey's lactose bile-salt broth and incubated for 48 hours. From the number of samples producing acid and gas the presumptive number of coliform organisms in the water can be determined by the use of probability tables.

The presumptive coliform count does not, however, distinguish between *E. coli* and other coliforms which may be present in water. To achieve this differentiation use may be made of the capacity of *E. coli* to ferment lactose in MacConkey's bile-salt broth and to produce indole in peptone water, when grown at 44° C. *Klebsiella* strains and other coliforms do not possess these properties. For these tests the tubes in the presumptive coliform count which show acid and gas at 37° C are subcultured into a further series of tubes of lactose bile broth and of peptone water for incubation at 44° C; this will give a differential *E. coli* count.

Waters destined for human consumption should be tested at frequent intervals. In general a satisfactory non-chlorinated water should contain no faecal *E. coli* in 100 ml and should have a coliform count of less than 4 per 100 ml. Chlorinated waters should contain no *E. coli* or other coliforms in 100 ml.

Water is also sometimes examined for the presence of *Str. faecalis* and *Cl. perfringens*. *Str. faecalis* appears to survive poorly in water, and its presence is usually regarded as evidence of recent faecal contamination. *Cl. perfringens* on the other hand survives for longer periods than either *Str. faecalis* or *E. coli*, and its presence is of special value in indicating intermittent contamination and as an indicator in water which can only be examined at infrequent intervals.

Colony counts to determine the total number of organisms present in a sample of water are also sometimes performed. Dilutions of the water are incorporated in agar and the plates incubated at 22° C and at 37° C. The organisms capable of growing at 22° C are free-living saprophytes and are in themselves of little or no significance in relation to possible faecal pollution. The significant finding is the ratio of the count at 22° C to that at 37° C. In polluted waters the ratio of the 22° C to the 37° C count is usually less than 10 to 1. This finding is of significance only in non-chlorinated water, since in chlorinated waters the ratio is usually low.

THE PROTEUS GROUP

This group comprises two genera—*Proteus* and *Providencia*.

Proteus

These are actively motile, non-capsulated, non-lactose-fermenting enterobacteriaceae. They are highly pleomorphic, varying in length from short coccobacillary forms to long filaments which are frequently slightly curved. They differ from other enterobacteriaceae in their capacity to break down phenylalanine to phenylpyruvic acid—the PPA reaction—and in their active urease production. The most immediately recognizable property of *Proteus* strains is their capacity to swarm on solid media. If inoculated in the centre of an agar plate the growth spreads rapidly over the surface of the medium, frequently in concentric rings and forming a thin transparent layer which may be easily overlooked. Since this swarming growth may result from the presence of a single organism on a plate, *Proteus* may be erroneously regarded as the causative organism of a pyogenic lesion.

As first shown by Dienes some strains of *Proteus*, when inoculated at different points on an agar plate, produce a mixed swarming growth while with others no mixing occurs, a line of demarcation showing no growth appearing between the strains. The failure to mix appears to occur when the strains differ in antigenic structure and particularly when they differ in their H antigens.

The genus comprises four species—*Proteus vulgaris*, *Proteus mirabilis*, *Proteus morganii* and *Proteus rettgeri* differentiated by their biochemical characteristics. Of these *Pr. mirabilis* is that most frequently encountered in diagnostic material. With the exception of some strains of *Pr. rettgeri* all species produce gas in fermentation reactions.

Antigenic Structure

Proteus strains are antigenically heterogeneous. Three varieties known as *Proteus OX19*, *OX2* and *OXK* are of importance since they may be agglutinated by the sera of patients suffering from certain rickettsial infections. These three types are differentiated by their O antigen composition. In their biochemical properties *OX19* and *OX2* strains resemble *Pr. vulgaris* and *OXK* strains resemble *Pr. mirabilis*. So far on the basis of their H and O antigen composition 119 distinct serotypes have been described in *Pr. vulgaris* and *Pr. mirabilis* strains.

Pathogenicity

Proteus is of low primary pathogenicity. In recent years, however, because of their high antibiotic resistance the frequency with which *Proteus* strains have been isolated as causes of cross infection in hospitals, particularly of operation wounds and of the urinary tract, has considerably increased. Though the species as a whole has a high natural resistance to antibiotics sensitivity tests will in many cases reveal an antibiotic to which a particular strain is susceptible.

Providencia

This group of strains closely resembles *Proteus* biochemically and is classified by Bergey as *Proteus inconstans*. Like *Proteus* they give a positive PPA reaction. Providence strains, however, do not swarm and rarely decompose urea. To date at least 125 serotypes based on O and H antigen composition have been described. Strains of this type have been isolated from urinary tract infections and may be present as commensals in the intestinal tract.

LACTOBACILLI

Bacteria of the genus *Lactobacillus* are mostly long, slender rods which are Gram positive, non-motile, non-capsulated and non-sporing. They are, for the most part, micro-aerophilic or anaerobic. Although they grow best in media of neutral reaction, they are aciduric, that is, they are capable of growing in media, e.g. broth containing 0·5 per cent glacial acetic acid, sufficiently acid to inhibit the growth of other organisms.

Lactobacilli are the major organisms present in the faeces of breast-fed infants; they are also found in the faeces of adults, but in much smaller numbers. The species usually encountered are *Lactobacillus acidophilus* and *Lactobacillus bifidus*. The strains of lactobacilli occurring in the adult vagina, known as Döderlein's bacilli, closely resemble *L. acidophilus* and may, in fact, belong to this species.

Some workers believe that the lactobacilli of the mouth, *Lactobacillus odontolyticus*, may play a part in the aetiology of dental caries. It is supposed that the lactobacilli break down food residues with the production of lactic acid which dissolves out the calcium phosphate of the enamel. As a result of this initial breach, the dentine is exposed and is then disintegrated by miscellaneous proteolytic organisms. There is suggestive but not conclusive evidence in support of this view. Other workers believe that the first stage in the breakdown of the enamel may be the action of proteolytic organisms on its protein consti-tuents. It has also been suggested that bacterial invasion of the dentine may occur through fissures naturally present in the enamel.

ANAEROBIC GRAM NEGATIVE BACILLI
(Bacteroidaceae)

A considerable number of species of non-sporing anaerobic or micro-aerophilic Gram negative bacilli have been identified as normal parasites of the alimentary tract. In the lower intestinal tract organisms of this type appear in fact to be much more numerous than *E. coli*. They are obviously a very hetero-geneous group and have been very difficult to classify. A number of them are undoubtedly pathogenic and have been found in association with inflammatory lesions of the intestinal tract such as appendicitis and cholecystitis and in gangrenous lesions both in the intestinal tract and elsewhere in the body. Many have a characteristic tapered cigar shape because of which they are frequently known as fusiform bacilli. Organisms with this appearance are very common in the mouth. One group which has received species rank *Fusobacterium fusiforme* is particularly associated with Vincent's angina (Chapter 30). This organism is a strict anaerobe, but is extremely difficult to isolate in pure culture.

Other anaerobic Gram negative bacilli which may be isolated from human or animal sources are classified by Bergey in the genera *Sphaerophorus* and and *Bacteroides*. The species *Sphaerophorus necrophorus* appears to be of some importance as a human pathogen. This organism is primarily responsible for necrotic lesions in various animals. Individuals whose work brings them into contact with animals occasionally become infected with the development of localized necrotic lesions in the skin and subcutaneous tissues.

CHAPTER 20

THE SALMONELLAE

Salmonellae are Gram negative, motile, non-sporing, non-capsulated bacilli morphologically indistinguishable from *E. coli*. They do not produce indole, do not liquefy gelatin and do not hydrolyse urea. They are non-lactose fermenters but ferment glucose and various other sugars, most species producing acid and gas. Salmonellae exist in nature primarily as parasites of the intestinal tract of man and other animals.

The nomenclature of the salmonellae has undergone several changes. Some of the species earlier described were named after the disease with which they were associated and these names, such as *Salm. choleraesuis*, *Salm. typhi*, *Salm. paratyphi* and *Salm. enteritidis*, have, for the most part, been retained. A few species have been called after the persons who discovered or worked with them (e.g. *Salm. schottmuelleri*) or of the patient from whose body they were isolated (e.g. *Salm. thompson*). Many have been named after the locality in which they were first isolated, e.g. *Salm. dublin*, *Salm. london*, *Salm. poona*, *Salm. aberdeen*, *Salm. minnesota*, etc. Since the number of species recognized is steadily increasing—over 1000 have now been described—the practice of giving a separate name to each new species has been abolished and new species are now designated by their antigenic formulae. This is a more rational procedure since the great majority of species differ only in antigenic composition.

On the basis of their pathogenicity the salmonellae may be divided into two groups: (1) The enteric fever group. This group comprises the organisms capable of causing the enteric fevers in man, viz. *Salm. typhi* and the paratyphoid bacilli. These species are found only in the intestinal tract of man for whom they have a high degree of pathogenicity and in whom they frequently cause invasive disease. (2) The food poisoning group. These are essentially parasites of animals from whom man is occasionally infected. Their pathogenicity for man is relatively low, the usual result of infection being the production of a gastroenteritis. In contrast to the enteric group they are not normally invasive and will infect man only when ingested in large numbers.

Cultural Properties

Growth occurs readily on unenriched nutrient agar over a wide temperature range, although optimally at 37° C. Growth under anaerobic conditions is poor. Colonies of freshly isolated strains are almost invariably circular in outline with a smooth, glossy surface, and may be difficult to distinguish from those of

E. coli. They are, however, more translucent and have a more delicate texture.

For the isolation of the salmonellae, various selective media are employed, the most important being MacConkey's agar, desoxycholate citrate agar and Wilson and Blair's bismuth sulphite agar. On desoxycholate citrate and MacConkey's agar, salmonellae produce translucent, colourless non-lactose-fermenting colonies. On Wilson and Blair's medium, which is the most selective of the three, *Salm. typhi* and *Salm. paratyphi B* produce black colonies surrounded—particularly in the case of *Salm. typhi*—by a gun-metal sheen. The typical appearance is only seen when the colonies are well separated. Other salmonellae grow well on Wilson and Blair's medium but do not produce black colonies.

With the exception of *Salm. typhi* the salmonellae ferment maltose, glucose, mannitol and usually dulcitol producing acid and gas. None ferment lactose or saccharose. In the case of the commonly isolated aerogenic species, the amount of gas produced is often small and naturally occurring variant strains which produce no trace of gas have been described. *Salm. typhi* ferments maltose, glucose and mannitol-producing acid but not gas. Some species can be sub-divided, on the basis of certain fermentation reactions, into biochemical types which tend to show a characteristic geographical distribution.

Antigenic Structure

The antigenic structure of the salmonellae is complex. The antigens of importance in identification are the H or flagellar antigens, the O or somatic antigens and the Vi antigens.

H Antigens

These are protein in nature and are destroyed by heat, viz. by boiling for a few minutes, and by exposure to alcohol. They are not destroyed by formalin, and H suspensions may therefore be prepared by the addition of formalin to broth cultures. Agglutination of H suspensions by H antiserum occurs rapidly, the organisms aggregating into characteristic loose, open floccules. Both in rabbits and man the H antigens are much more highly antigenic than the O antigens. About 70 distinct H antigens are known; these are considered below under diphasic flagellar variation.

O Antigens

These are phospholipid protein polysaccharide complexes, the antigenic specificity of which resides in the polysaccharide component. They are stable to heat, withstanding a temperature of 100° C for several hours, and are unaffected by exposure to alcohol. O suspensions may therefore be obtained from motile organisms by heat or by alcohol treatment, both of which procedures destroy the H antigens. The O antigens are much less strongly antigenic than the H antigens.

About 60 serologically distinct O antigens have been recognized. Most species possess more than one O antigen, consequently many species share the same O antigens. On the basis of their O antigen composition the species can be classified into some 40 serological groups, each group being characterized by the possession of an O antigen not present in other groups. Thus the antigen 2 is characteristic of group A, the antigen 9 of group D, and so on. The organisms most commonly encountered fall into the first five of these A, B, C, D and E. Classification into O groups greatly facilitates the serological identification of a *Salmonella*; when it is shown that an unidentified organism belongs to a particular group the choice of possible species is considerably narrowed.

ANTIGENIC STRUCTURE OF CERTAIN SALMONELLAE

Group	Species	Phase variation	O antigens	H antigens Phase 1	Phase 2
A	*Salm. paratyphi A*	Monophasic	(1) 2, 12	a	
B { *Salm. paratyphi B*	Diphasic	(1) 4, (5) 12	b	$\longleftrightarrow$ 1, 2
{ *Salm. typhimurium*	Diphasic	(1) 4, (5) 12	i	$\longleftrightarrow$ 1, 2, 3
C { *Salm. paratyphi C*	Diphasic	6, 7 (Vi)	c	$\longleftrightarrow$ 1, 5
{ *Salm. oslo*	Diphasic	6, 7	a	$\longleftrightarrow$ e, n, x
{ *Salm. newport*	Diphasic	6, 8	e, h	$\longleftrightarrow$ 1, 2, 3
{ *Salm. tennessee*	Monophasic	6, 7	z_{29}	
D { *Salm. typhi*	Monophasic	9, 12 (Vi)	d	
{ *Salm. enteritidis*	Monophasic	(1) 9, 12	g, m	
{ *Salm. dublin*	Monophasic	1, 9, 12	g, p	

( ) Indicates the antigens may not be present.
$\longleftrightarrow$ Indicates phase variation.

The complete O antigen, which may be extracted from the cell by treatment with trichloracetic acid—as first shown by Boivin—has a molecular weight of several million, the precise value varying in different preparations, suggesting that the antigen is in fact a complex of smaller units. It is fully antigenic for rabbits and fully toxic. The protein moiety may be split off by treatment with phenol, yielding a lipopolysaccharide complex which is non-antigenic but still toxic. Treatment with alkali removes most of the lipid to leave the polysaccharide and a minor lipid component known as lipid A, consisting of glucosamine, phosphoric acid and β hydroxymyristic acid which is non-antigenic and non-toxic. In the complete antigen, lipid A exists in an acetylated form but is deacylated by alkali treatment. The alkali-treated polysaccharide has a high affinity for red cells, which are then agglutinable by a specific antiserum. Treatment with acetic acid removes lipid A, and gives the pure polysaccharide.

The chemistry of the polysaccharide has been considerably clarified in recent years by the work of Westphal and his associates. Its general structure is shown below. It possesses a backbone of heptose and 2-keto-3-deoxyoctonic acid. Anatomically, the backbone is the innermost layer of the polysaccharide, and in the complete antigen is complexed with the lipid and/or protein components. To the backbone are attached side-chains which may be divided into (a) a core section of N-acetyl glucosamine, glucose and galactose common to all *Salmonella* O antigens and (b) repeat units which carry the O

STRUCTURE OF SALMONELLA SOMATIC ANTIGENS

Each *Salmonella* species possesses a number of O antigenic specificities each of which is described as a separate O antigen and designated by an arabic numeral. The different O antigens are not, however, different molecules but *different determinants* on the *same* molecule

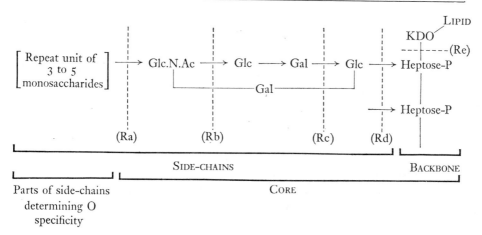

Parts of side-chains
  determining O
  specificity

Rough (R) mutants arise by failure to synthesize the entire polysaccharide. Different mutants are distinguishable by the sites at which the synthetic block occurs. These are indicated on the above structure by interrupted lines and the designation of the R mutant—(Ra), (Rb) etc.

Typical repeat units

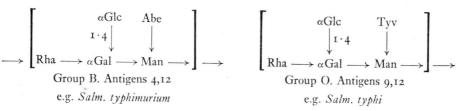

Antigen 5 by O-acetylation of galactose

Abe—abequose	Man—mannose
Gal—galactose	P—phosphate
Glc—glucose	Rha—rhamnose
Glc N.Ac—N-acetyl glucosamine	Tyv—tyvelose
KDO—2-keto-3-deoxyoctonic acid	

serological specificity. The structure of the repeat units of antigens, 4,12 and 9,12 is shown above. It will be seen that the sugars tyvelose and abequose which are 3,6-dideoxyhexoses, are the components determining group specificity. Thus tyvelose determines the specificity of group antigen 9 and abequose the specificity of the group antigen 4. 12 specificity is determined by the remaining sugars of the repeat unit. Other important dideoxyhexoses are paratose, which carries group antigen 2 specificity, and colitose, which is shared by some less common salmonellae and certain coliform bacteria.

Vi Antigens

Recently isolated strains of *Salm. typhi* possess an additional surface antigen which is assumed to be present in a layer, covering or masking the O antigen since it prevents the agglutination of the organism by O antiserum. Because of its presumed association with virulence it is known as the Vi antigen, and may be regarded as being analogous to the non-capsular K antigens of the coliform group. The agglutinability of suspensions of *Salm. typhi* by Vi antiserum is markedly heat-labile, being lost after exposure to 60° C for 1 hour. It is believed, however, that this is not due to a destruction of the antigen but to its release, on heating, into the surrounding fluid. The serological specificity of the antigen appears to depend on the presence of aminohexuronic acid residues. Vi antigens serologically similar to those of *Salm. typhi* are found in *Salm. paratyphi C* and in certain coliform bacteria, but in these species the antigens do not render the organisms O inagglutinable, presumably because they are present in much lower concentrations on the cell surface.

Antigenic Variation

A number of types of antigenic variation occur in the salmonellae. A knowledge of these is essential for the understanding of the antigenic structure of the genus.

1. H → O Variation

This is a loss of flagellar antigens due to a loss of flagella; as a consequence of this flagellar loss, the organisms are non-motile. In many non-motile cultures the flagellar loss is not complete and organisms possessing flagella are still present in the cultures, although in small numbers. In such cases the motile organisms may usually be recovered by inoculation into one side of a U-tube containing soft (0·2 per cent) agar. Any motile organisms present will grow through the agar, and after overnight incubation may be recovered from the other limb of the tube. It is not always possible to obtain motile organisms by this technique, the cultures then being described as *permanently non-motile*.

2. S → R Variation

As a result of mutation the organism may lose, to a greater or lesser extent, the capacity to synthesize the polysaccharide of the somatic antigen. Types of variant have been recognized, differing in the extent to which this capacity has been lost. These antigenic mutants are in fact biochemical mutants, lacking the capacity to synthesize the appropriate sugar or sugar nucleotide required in transfer reactions, or deficient in specific transferases. The most extreme defect is that in which there is a failure to assemble the polysaccharide backbone because of an inability to synthesize the heptose component. The commonest is that involving failure to synthesize the repeat units of the side-chains. In this case antigenic specificity is dictated by the core of the side-chain, particularly by the terminal N-acetyl glucosamine residues. Since the core is common to all *Salmonella* antigens, organisms in which this form of variation has occurred are antigenically indistinguishable. The loss is associated with a change in colony appearance from smooth to rough, because of which it is known as S → R variation. Rough organisms are also spontaneously agglutinable in saline— apparently because of a loss of hydrophilic properties conferred by the specific portion of the side-chains—and are avirulent.

S → R variation occurs infrequently under natural conditions but more frequently in strains which are maintained for long periods in laboratory cultures, and particularly when the medium contains a considerable amount of carbohydrate. The occurrence of S → R variation in stock cultures is less frequent if the organisms are maintained on Dorset egg medium and the cultures kept in the cold. The most satisfactory way to preserve the organisms so as to prevent S → R variation is, however, by freeze drying. S → R variation resembling that occurring in the salmonellae is widely encountered amongst all the Gram negative bacilli.

3. Diphasic Flagellar Variation

Many *Salmonella* species are *diphasic* in relation to their flagellar antigens. By this is meant that the organism may have one or other of two sets of flagellar antigens; these sets are known as phase 1 and phase 2 antigens. Although a particular bacterium can have flagellar antigens only in one phase, it can give rise to descendants with flagellar antigens in the second phase. In a mass culture of diphasic species one or other of the two phases is usually predominant so that the culture is agglutinated by only one of the phase antisera. In most cases the predominant phase is phase 1. Some *Salmonella* species, e.g. *Salm. typhi*, are *monophasic*, i.e. the flagellar antigens can exist in only one phase.

The first phase 1 antigens identified were designated by small letters a, b, c, etc., but, as more and more were discovered, the alphabet was soon exhausted and later antigens were therefore designated by z with a suffix number. At present at least 60 phase 1 antigens are recognized, the majority of *Salmonella* species possessing only one such antigen. Phase 1 antigens are therefore much more specific than O antigens. Phase 2 antigens, on the other hand, are less specific than either phase 1 H or O antigens. The majority of *Salmonella* species possess phase 2 antigens belonging to a series designated by Arabic numerals 1, etc. to 7. When the phase 2 antigens of an organism belong to this series the antigen 1 is always present, usually with at least one other antigen of the series. None of this series of phase 2 antigens has so far been recognized as phase 1 antigens in any species. A number of species, however, possess, as phase 2 antigens, antigens which occur as phase 1 antigens of other species. The most important of these are e, n, x and z_{15}.

4. V → W Variation

This is a variation involving loss of the Vi antigen. Loss of Vi antigen by *Salm. typhi* may be partial and the organism is then agglutinable by both O and

Vi antisera. These intermediate variants are referred to as VW forms. Partial or complete loss of the Vi antigen renders *Salm. typhi* insusceptible to the action of the Vi bacteriophages used in bacteriophage typing.

Serological Identification

If it is suspected that an unknown organism may be a *Salmonella*, the first step in its serological identification is to test it for agglutination with a polyvalent *Salmonella* O antiserum. If this confirms its preliminary identification as a *Salmonella*, it is then tested with O antisera corresponding to the main O groups. Sera for groups A to D being normally sufficient. When the O group to which it belongs has been identified the organism is tested with the phase 1 H antisera for the commonly occurring organisms of that group. If the organism is mono-phasic or is a diphasic organism in the 1 phase, these tests should serve to identify it. If no agglutination occurs with 1 phase sera, the organism may be in the 2 phase. This may be confirmed by testing it with a polyvalent 2 phase serum. If the organism is in the 2 phase, its identification requires the recovery of phase 1 organisms. This may be sometimes achieved by plating out the culture to obtain isolated colonies when some of the colonies may be found to be in the 1 phase. If this is not successful, the organism should be grown in the presence of 2 phase antiserum. This may be attempted by Craigie's method in which a plain test tube containing soft agar incorporating 2 phase antiserum with a small length of glass tubing open at both ends inserted vertically into the agar is used. The organism is inoculated into the agar inside the glass tubing; after incubation phase 1 organisms may be recovered from the agar outside the tubing. An alternative method is to subculture the organisms in broth con-taining 2 phase antiserum until it is no longer agglutinable by the serum. If, however, the organism is not agglutinated by 2 phase serum, it is probably an unusual *Salmonella* species. This can be confirmed by testing it with a poly-valent H antiserum. This is a composite serum containing antibodies to all the *Salmonella* phase 1 and phase 2 H antigens. If a positive result is obtained with this serum, it may be concluded that the organism possesses a phase 1 antigen of unusual type. The identification of rare salmonellae is beyond the scope of the ordinary clinical laboratory and such organisms are best referred to a *Salmonella* reference centre.

The tests described are carried out in the first place by the slide agglutination method. False positive results may, however, occasionally be encountered in slide agglutination tests, due to residual unabsorbed non-specific agglutinins in the serum or to a partial roughness in the organisms, not detectable in the saline control, but capable of giving rise to non-specific agglutination in the presence of serum. Positive slide results should therefore be confirmed by tube tests. For these, killed H and O suspensions are prepared and should be agglutinated to the full titre of the diagnostic serum. Freshly isolated strains of *Salm. typhi* containing the full complement of Vi antigen are not agglutinated by O antiserum and therefore cannot be grouped directly. They are agglutinated by Vi antiserum and will agglutinate with O antiserum when boiled suspen-sions are used.

Fimbrial antigens are not important in serological classification but may cause difficulty in identification, if the diagnostic antisera employed possess fimbrial antibodies. As a rule, however, fimbrial antigens are not present in laboratory cultures which have been propagated on solid media. The reaction between fimbrial antigens and their homologous antibodies results in a very loose floccular type of agglutination resembling H agglutination. In cases of doubt it may be distinguished from H agglutination by the fact that it occurs in suspensions which have been exposed to 50 per cent ethanol or to 0·005/N HCl.

Bacteriophage Types

A number of *Salmonella* species can be subdivided into types on the basis of their susceptibility to bacteriophage. These are considered in detail in Chapter 42. Phage typing is of most importance in relation to *Salm. typhi* in which a total of 72 types and subtypes have been defined. The phages used for *Salm. typhi* are specific for the Vi form and are active only against organisms possessing their full quota of Vi antigen. Since the types exhibit a high degree of stability under natural conditions, phage typing is of considerable value in epidemiological investigations, and it has been widely and successfully used to trace the source of outbreaks of typhoid fever. Thus, if a carrier is responsible for an epidemic, he should harbour the phage type found in that epidemic; if he does so a prima facie case for his responsibility is established.

Pathogenicity

The toxicity of the salmonellae is due to the somatic antigen complex. The basis of the toxicity for the somatic antigen has not been completely determined but clearly depends on the presence of lipid A—a minor phospholipid component of the complete antigen (p. 302). The smallest toxic molecule is a lipopolysaccharide obtained by phenol extraction, and containing the somatic polysaccharide and an intact lipid A component. When the latter is modified by deacylation the phospholipid loses its toxicity. The evidence suggests that lipid A is the major determinant of toxicity but it is not at the moment possible to say that it is the exclusive determinant. The participation of lipid A in toxicity provides an explanation for the failure of antibody to the somatic polysaccharide to neutralize toxicity completely. Its capacity to do so at all can be attributed to a steric effect, by virtue of which it interferes either with the fixation or activity of lipid A.

The injection of small amounts of purified somatic antigen intravenously into man and other animals gives rise to pyrexia, and leucopenia followed by leucocytosis. The pyrexia appears to be mainly due to the action of endogenous pyrogens, liberated from leucocytes as a result of the action of the endotoxin. When injected intravenously in large doses the endotoxin produces a condition of shock resembling traumatic shock. On injection into the skin it gives rise to oedema and erythema which may be followed by necrosis. On injection intraperitoneally into mice it produces diarrhoea and intestinal congestion. Other effects which endotoxin will produce in animals are abortion, the production of necrosis in certain tumours and, when appropriately administered, both local and generalized Shwartzman reactions (p. 187). The endotoxin also has a marked stimulatory effect on the reticulo-endothelial system as shown by enhanced disappearance of carbon particles from the blood following endotoxin injection. Possibly because of this it has a marked adjuvant effect on the immune response to protein antigens.

Following injection of endotoxin into animals a tolerance to further injections, which lasts for some days, is induced. This tolerance extends also to the chemically related antigens of the shigellae and other Gram negative bacilli; since it shows no serologic specificity it is not due to antibody production. It is possible that this non-specific tolerance may play a part in recovery from *Salmonella* infection, but there is no evidence on this point.

The somatic antigens of the salmonellae undoubtedly play an important part in determining virulence, since in the course of S → R variation the virulence of the organism is invariably lost, even though the variant rough form is still endotoxic. In *Salm. typhi* the Vi antigen, which is almost invariably present in freshly isolated strains, is believed to be of particular importance. It seems probable that by virtue of a strongly acidic character it may confer on the surface of the organism marked anti-phagocytic properties. Because of this, and its relatively low antigenicity—antibody to it being produced slowly and only in small amounts—it could contribute substantially to rendering Vi-containing cells much less susceptible to the humoral defence mechanisms of the host than non-Vi forms. This in turn would explain why typhoid bacilli are infective for man in much smaller numbers than are other salmonellae.

Salmonella Infections

The salmonellae are strict pathogens and have no habitat other than the human or animal body. The source of human infection is, therefore, a human or animal case or carrier, the organisms being excreted in the faeces or urine and transmitted by food or water which is ingested by another subject. The portal of entry of the organisms is always the mouth, irrespective of the subsequent sequence of events. Three types of clinical disease are associated with *Salmonella* infection: enteric fever, bacterial food poisoning and *Salmonella* septicaemia.

Enteric Fever

The term 'enteric fever' should be used to indicate the *clinical* type of disease about to be described, irrespective of the causative *Salmonella* species. The terms 'typhoid fever' and 'paratyphoid fever', often used synonymously with 'enteric fever', imply a bacteriological diagnosis (of infection with *Salm. typhi* or *Salm. paratyphi A, B* or *C* respectively) and should be used only when this has been established. Enteric fever is characterized by fever of continuous type, enlargement of the spleen, usually a 'rose-spot' rash and leucopenia. Headache and constipation are common in the early stages of the disease but diarrhoea with 'pea soup' stools is usual later when ulceration of the bowel occurs. The causative organism can be isolated by blood culture, especially in the early stages of the disease, and later from the faeces and, sometimes, from the urine. The fatality rate of enteric fever normally lies between 10 and 20 per cent.

Enteric fever is most commonly caused, throughout the world, by *Salm. typhi*. Other *Salmonella* species, and especially *Salm. paratyphi A* and *B*, may, however, be responsible both for sporadic cases and for epidemics. In Western Europe and North America, *Salm. paratyphi B* infection is common while *Salm. paratyphi A* or *C* is seldom, if ever, isolated. In India and in South America, on the other hand, *Salm. paratyphi A* is a common cause of enteric fever and *Salm. paratyphi B* a very rare one. During the last war, the isolation of a variety of *Salm. enteritidis* from cases of enteric fever in India was by no means uncommon although invasive disease due to this species is extremely rare in Europe. In Guyana *Salm. paratyphi C* is the dominant species.

The source of infection is a human case or carrier who excretes the organism either in the faeces or, less commonly, in the urine. In order that the disease may be spread, the organisms must be conveyed thence in sufficient numbers to the alimentary tracts of other people. There are two main ways in which this may occur: (1) By contaminated water. This epidemiological variety is most likely to occur in communities with inadequate systems of sanitation. It is unlikely to be found in communities with satisfactory methods of sewage disposal and water purification, unless there is some breakdown in these systems due, for example, to lack of adequate control, as in the 1962 Zermatt outbreak. Epidemics of enteric fever due to a contaminated water supply are characteristically explosive in onset and affect a large number of people. An uncommon mode of infection is the consumption of shellfish taken from the estuary of a river contaminated by sewage. A number of milk-borne epidemics have occurred in which the infection was traced to the use of contaminated water for the washing of bottles and other utensils. Canned foods may be infected if the cans are not completely watertight and if, after sterilization, they are cooled and washed in infected water. This appears to have been the mode of infection in the 1963 Aberdeen outbreak. (2) By food which has been handled by carriers. Outbreaks of this type are much less extensive than water-borne epidemics, affecting only the persons who have ingested the contaminated foods.

Enteric fever, despite its name, is not primarily a disease of the alimentary tract, but is rather a generalized infection in which the gall-bladder and the lymph follicles of the small intestine are typically involved. The sequence of events following ingestion of *Salm. typhi* has been traced by examination of material taken from various parts of the body throughout the course of the disease and after death. Corroborative findings have been obtained indirectly by experiments on mice infected by feeding with cultures of *Salm. typhimurium* which produces in these animals a disease similar to enteric fever in man.

It is probable that the bacteria which have entered the body by the mouth and have survived the acidity of the gastric juice do not at first proliferate in the small intestine but leave it by way of the lymph follicles. From there the organisms pass to the mesenteric lymph nodes and thence to the blood stream by way of the thoracic duct. A transitory bacteraemia follows, but the organisms are rapidly removed by the reticulo-endothelial cells and especially by those of the spleen, liver and bone-marrow which form the principal foci of infection. In them, and in the mesenteric lymph glands, the organisms multiply and produce a secondary bacteraemia which is of greater severity than the first and which marks the onset of the actual disease. At this stage, the bacteria are widely distributed throughout the tissues of the body and may readily be isolated by blood culture.

A feature of enteric fever which distinguishes it from *Salmonella* septicaemia is the increasing numbers of salmonellae which appear in the faeces from about the end of the first week. The organisms reach a maximum during the third week and then gradually decline during convalescence. Reinvasion of the bowel occurs through two channels. The first of these is the infected Peyer's patches and solitary lymph follicles of the small intestine which discharge salmonellae into the bowel and which may later become the sites of ulceration, haemorrhage and perforation. The main reservoir from which salmonellae reach the lumen of the gut is the gall-bladder which is constantly infected. This explains the finding of the organisms in almost pure culture in the duodenal fluid. Infection of the gall-bladder may persist long after recovery from the disease and this, as we shall see, is a factor of great importance in the spread of enteric fever.

In about 25 per cent of cases of typhoid fever, *Salm. typhi* may be found in the urine after the third week. Since the urine is free from pus there is probably no actual infection of the urinary tract. In contrast to this, when localization of infection in the renal system occurs in *Salmonella* septicaemia, the condition is always a purulent one.

Carriers

Following an attack of typhoid fever, the great majority of cases cease to excrete *Salm. typhi* during convalescence. About 5 per cent of cases continue to excrete the organism during 6 months after the attack, while some 3 per cent are still excretors at the end of a year. The majority, if not all, of those who are still excreting typhoid bacilli a year after convalescence become permanent carriers and continue to excrete the organism indefinitely. Less information is available concerning the duration of the carrier state in enteric fever due to other *Salmonella* species, but permanent carriers of *Salm. paratyphi B* are known to occur and their incidence in relation to infected persons is probably of the same order as is found in typhoid fever.

The risk of a typhoid patient becoming a carrier increases with age. Thus in an investigation, reported by Ames and Robbins, in New York State, 10 per cent of patients in the 50- to 60-year age group became carriers, as against 2·9 per cent at all ages. The risk appears to be appreciably greater in the female than in the male, particularly in the fifth decade. Since the seat of residual infection in faecal carriers is in the gall-bladder, it can be reasonably presumed that the higher carrier rate in women is associated with their greater proneness to gall-bladder disease. Urinary carriers are much less common than faecal ones, and it is possible that urinary carriage only develops when there is some concomitant renal lesion. Thus, a high incidence of urinary carriage reported from Egypt appears to have been significantly associated with the occurrence of urinary schistosomiasis.

The importance of the carrier as a source of infection is underlined by the finding that carriers frequently excrete at least 10^6 typhoid bacilli per g faeces. Urinary carriers appear to be somewhat less intermittent in their excretion of typhoid bacilli than faecal carriers. There is no reliable information on the number of organisms they excrete but the male habit of indiscriminate micturition undoubtedly renders the urinary excreter a less controllable and, probably, more dangerous source of infection than the faecal carrier.

Diagnosis

A bacteriological diagnosis of *Salmonella* infection can be made with certainty only by isolation and identification of the causative organism.

Blood Culture

In enteric fever, isolation by blood culture is the method of choice. The earlier it is performed the greater is the chance of success. During the first week, *Salm. typhi* can be isolated from the blood of 90 per cent of cases of typhoid fever, falling to about 40 per cent in the fourth week.

Isolation from Faeces or Urine

The chances of isolation from the faeces increase from about 50 per cent in the first week to about 80 per cent in the third week. Thereafter, the chances of isolation fall off rather sharply.

Cultures of faeces should be made by inoculating a tube of tetrathionate broth or one of selenite broth, and by plating on both Wilson and Blair's medium and desoxycholate citrate medium. If possible, two plates of Wilson and Blair's medium should be inoculated—one heavily, and one lightly. In addition, since dysentery, too, presents diarrhoeal symptoms, one of the less selective intestinal media (p. 43), MacConkey's agar or EMB agar, should be inoculated in order to detect dysentery bacilli, which may fail to grow on desoxycholate citrate medium. After overnight incubation, a loopful of the enrichment broth is plated on MacConkey's or desoxycholate citrate agar. The following day, all the plates are examined and suspicious colonies plated on MacConkey's agar from which, after overnight incubation, non-lactose-fermenting colonies are picked for further examination.

When other methods have failed it may be possible to isolate the organism from the urine. This can rarely be achieved before the end of the third week.

The Widal Test

In the course of the enteric fevers, the patient usually develops a high titre of agglutinins for the causative organism. The detection and estimation of these antibodies is carried out by the Widal reaction. Since the diagnostic level of the antibodies to the various antigenic components H, O and Vi is different, antibody to each must be determined independently. For this purpose H, O and Vi suspensions must be used—standardized in respect of bacterial content so that the results obtained in different laboratories are comparable. If possible two specimens of serum, the second taken about 10 days after the first, should be examined to demonstrate a rising antibody titre. If this is not feasible a diagnosis may have to be made on the results of a single serum examination. In either case it is rarely possible to obtain serological evidence establishing or supporting a diagnosis of enteric fever before the beginning of the third week, when typhoid will usually show an H titre of 1/250 or higher, and an O titre by the Felix technique of 1/1280 or higher. In some cases, however, the patient fails to develop demonstrable H agglutinins, while in others the titre of O agglutinins does not develop above the normal level. Consequently, the absence of a diagnostic titre must not be taken as excluding the possibility of infection.

In interpreting the results of the Widal reaction, the following considerations must be borne in mind.

1. The titre of antibodies to be expected depends on the stage of the illness at which the blood is taken. Thus low or negative titres are normal in the early stages of the disease but if found in the third or fourth week are presumptive, though not conclusive, evidence against infection.

2. Because of the sharing of O antigens by different salmonellae, and their occasional presence in other Gram negative bacilli—most normal sera possess an appreciable content of O antibody—titres of up to 1 in 320 against *Salm. typhi* O being occasionally found, using the Felix method. Because of this H titres are in general of greater diagnostic value than O titres. In countries in which enteric fever is prevalent appreciable H titres may be found in the absence of overt infection. Where typhoid is relatively uncommon, as in Britain, a titre of 1/25 is unusual in an uninoculated subject and should be regarded with suspicion, and a titre of 1/50 is almost diagnostic. If, however, the patient has previously been inoculated with TAB vaccine his serum may contain an appreciable amount of antibody which has persisted from the inoculation. Since H antibodies persist after immunization for a longer time than O antibodies, H titres must be interpreted with particular caution in previously immunized persons.

The Identification of Carriers

When large numbers of people are to be examined for the carrier state, a full bacteriological examination, although the ideal, is often impracticable. Under these circumstances examination of the patient's serum for antibody is of considerable value as a screening procedure. It has been generally accepted that the Vi antibody titre is of particular value for this purpose, and that Vi antibodies are unlikely to be found in significant amount unless typhoid bacilli are still present in the body. There is some evidence that the antiglobulin technique for the detection of non-agglutinating O antibodies may also be of value, but the method has not been sufficiently used for an adequate appraisal of its utility.

To establish a diagnosis of the carrier state the organism must be isolated, and, since excretion may be very intermittent, this should if necessary be attempted on a number of occasions. If repeated examination of faeces and urine is unsuccessful it may be possible to isolate the bacillus from samples of duodenal contents obtained by intubation. When a carrier has been identified it is essential, in order to establish a presumptive link between the carrier and an epidemic, to show that the phage type of the organism which he carries is the same as that responsible for the epidemic.

Considerable success in tracing carriers has been achieved by the use of the sewage-swab technique devised by Moore. The 'swabs' used are really small pads made by folding strips of gauze; they are left in position in sewers, drains and lavatories and subsequently cultured using selenite enrichment. By using these swabs it is frequently possible to identify a group of buildings or a particular house which harbours a carrier.

Treatment

Chloramphenicol is the antibiotic of choice in the treatment of typhoid fever. It has a marked effect in diminishing the duration of the disease and in lowering the fatality rate. It is most effective in the early stages of the infection. Unfortunately, relapses are of frequent occurrence even after intensive treatment with chloramphenicol, and it does not prevent the development of the carrier state. In severe infections the death of large numbers of organisms which follows the administration of the antibiotic, by releasing large amounts of endotoxin, may produce a severe and possibly fatal toxic reaction. In order to prevent relapses some workers give TAB vaccine to patients who are being treated with chloramphenicol. As a justification for this procedure they claim that the vaccine stimulates antibacterial immunity which develops poorly in cases treated with antibiotic alone. Relapses normally respond well to a further course of treatment. Ampicillin, though active against the typhoid bacillus in vitro, does not appear to be as effective in the treatment of the clinical disease as chloramphenicol.

Prophylaxis

The methods used for the prevention of enteric fever fall into two categories. The first and more important aims at preventing the spread of the organism. This is a public health problem—the essential measures being the provision of a good water supply and of satisfactory methods for the disposal of excreta, the isolation of cases, and the control of carriers. In modern urban communities epidemics of water-borne enteric fever are very rare, and when they occur are invariably due to a breakdown in the system of water protection. Practically all cases of typhoid now occurring in such communities are due to the contamination of food or milk by chronic carriers. This danger can be eliminated only by ensuring the hygienic preparation and manipulation of food, particular attention being directed to the exclusion of carriers from any contact with it during the course of preparation.

Chloramphenicol, which has been so effective in the treatment of the clinical disease, is unfortunately of no value in the treatment of the carrier. Good results have recently been claimed for ampicillin. This drug in fact appears to be more effective in the treatment of the carrier than of the established disease but it appears to be necessary to prolong the treatment for some months.

The carrier state can undoubtedly be cured by cholecystectomy. Cholecystectomy is, however, a somewhat drastic measure even in the interests of public health.

The second method, introduced by Almroth Wright at the end of the last century, is that of specific prophylaxis and aims at protecting the individual by active immunization. TAB vaccine is a suspension of killed *Salm. typhi* and *Salm. paratyphi A* and *B. Salm. paratyphi C* is sometimes included and the name TABC vaccine employed. TAB vaccine has been subjected to extensive trials under field conditions during two World Wars, when conditions have been especially favourable for the spread of enteric fever, and there can be little doubt that its use has resulted in a marked lowering in the incidence of the disease among populations exposed to the risk of infection. At best this protection is of the order of 75 per cent. There is reason to believe that the success of vaccination depends, other things being equal, on the number of organisms to which the subject is subsequently exposed. Thus vaccination may protect completely against a small infecting dose, as may be ingested from a contaminated water supply, but might be quite ineffective if the infecting dose is large, as from food contaminated by a carrier, and in which the bacilli have subsequently been able to grow. Experience gained during World War II, however, strongly suggests that the severity and fatality rate of the disease among those who do contract it in spite of inoculation are no lower than among uninoculated people.

Immunization is normally considered necessary only for those who are exposed to a special risk of infection. It is used for service personnel, for people travelling to countries where sanitary arrangements are not satisfactory and for persons such as laboratory workers and staffs of infectious disease hospitals who are particularly exposed by virtue of their occupation. Vaccination is not necessary for children under 2 years of age, since they are relatively insusceptible to infection. Because of the reactions it produces, TAB inoculation should not be given to women in the later stages of pregnancy or to any one who is in any way debilitated.

The strains selected for the preparation of vaccine are carefully chosen so that they have a full complement of Vi antigen and at the same time do not give rise to undue reactions on injection. Two methods of vaccine preparation are generally used. In the first and older method the organisms are killed by heating to 60° C for half an hour and preserved in 0·5 per cent phenol. In the second method, which was introduced by Felix, the organisms are killed by exposing them to 75 per cent alcohol and the vaccine is preserved in 25 per cent alcohol. Felix maintained that with this method the Vi antigen was more effectively preserved (but see p. 304), and that because of this the vaccine was a better prophylactic than heat-killed vaccine. This claim for its superiority is supported by the results of mouse protection experiments. In a recent trial carried out under the auspices of the World Health Organization in Yugoslavia, however, alcoholized vaccine was found to be considerably less effective in the protection of man than phenolized vaccine. More recently, in a trial carried out in children in Guyana, an acetone-killed vaccine in which the Vi antigen is also effectively preserved, was found to give superior results to a heat-killed phenolized vaccine. Acetone-killed vaccine is not commercially available, however, and at any rate requires much fuller investigation, particularly in adult populations.

TAB vaccine is usually given by subcutaneous injection; two injections with an interval of 2 to 4 weeks between them constitutes the primary course. Reactions following vaccination are common. These may consist simply of some swelling, pain and redness, at the site of the inoculation, appearing within 2 to 3 hours after injection. Not infrequently there are constitutional symptoms rather resembling an attack of influenza. These reactions usually disappear within 36 hours.

In America, in order to minimize the possibility of reactions, boosting doses of the vaccine are frequently given by intradermal injection. In the Dutch army the intradermal route is adopted for primary immunization, a combined vaccine containing tetanus toxoid—TABT—being normally employed. Unfortunately there has not so far been a controlled trial of the effectiveness of intradermal immunization.

The immunity resulting from TAB inoculation is of relatively short duration and for those who continue to be exposed to infection after inoculation, boosting doses are required. These should be given at least at yearly, and preferably at six-monthly intervals. Not long after his introduction of TAB vaccination, Wright postulated the occurrence of a negative phase of increased susceptibility to infection, developing immediately after inoculation and lasting for at most a few weeks. There has been a considerable reluctance on the part of epidemiologists, however, to accept the existence of such a negative phase. Nevertheless sufficient evidence is available from experimental infection in laboratory animals to justify regarding the negative phase as a distinct possibility. Because of this, it is considered unwise to undertake primary vaccination in the course of an epidemic. It would at any rate be unlikely that under these circumstances the vaccine would have sufficient time to exert a significant protective effect.

Salmonella Septicaemia

The next clinical type of infection to be considered is *Salmonella* septicaemia. This resembles a septicaemia due to the pyogenic cocci, with a spiky temperature of intermittent or remittent type. The disease may run an uncomplicated course of from 10 days to several weeks or, after a varying period of simple pyrexia, localization with pus formation in the urinary system, serous cavities or subcutaneous tissues may supervene. Occasionally there is an antecedent history of diarrhoea, but this is by no means constant. The causative organism can usually be isolated from the blood during the course of the disease. This is the type of disease most frequently caused by *Salm. paratyphi C* and *Salm. choleraesuis*, but it may be due to any species except *Salm. typhi*. The fatality rate is probably from 5 to 10 per cent.

Salmonella Food Poisoning

In Great Britain the salmonellae are the most important single cause of bacterial food poisoning. In America, however, the salmonellae, though important, appear to take second place to *Staph. aureus* as causes of this condition. In general, *Salm. typhimurium* is the species most frequently encountered. Thus in the U.K., in the quinquennium 1956/1960, it constituted approximately 70 per cent of all *Salmonella* isolates. Some 20 *Salmonella* species were isolated, the others of most importance being *Salm. enteritidis*, *Salm. thompson*, *Salm. newport* and *Salm. heidelberg*. The epidemiological behaviour of *Salm. heidelberg* is of particular interest. This organism was quite unknown as a cause of bacterial food poisoning prior to 1951 but since then has been isolated with increasing frequency; other European countries appear to have had a similar experience.

Infection is the result of ingestion of contaminated food, the food most frequently responsible being meat, usually in the form of made-up or reheated dishes. Eggs are an important but less frequent source of infection, and several outbreaks have been traced to the consumption of milk and sweets. The risk of *Salmonella* infection is greatest with foods which have been inadequately cooked and with food which has been kept warm after cooking, thus permitting bacterial growth. Meat may be infected because it has been derived from an infected animal or it may be infected at any time after slaughter. Cattle, sheep and pigs are frequently carriers of salmonellae. Occasionally the carrier state develops into invasive disease during transit from farm to abattoir. After slaughter meat may be infected in storage, while displayed for sale or in the course of preparation. This type of infection is frequently due to rodents, particularly mice which may infect the food directly if they have access to it, or the food may be indirectly contaminated from their droppings by flies or hands. A number of outbreaks have been traced to *Salmonella* 'virus' preparations, which were at one time popular for the eradication of mice. Cats and dogs may also be infected and might on occasion infect food. Infection may also occasionally occur from human carriers, but this mode of infection is probably not very frequent. Fowls and ducks are frequently infected and may infect their eggs. Infection of the egg may occur either in the oviduct or after laying; the latter is likely to occur if the egg is deposited in a moist environment which damages the surface waxy film, thereby permitting bacteria to pass through the shell. When eggs are pooled as in the preparation of custards, baking powders and spray-dried egg a few infected eggs may contaminate an entire batch. This may result in large-scale epidemics such as occurred following the introduction of American spray-dried egg in Great Britain in World War II.

Salmonella food poisoning is a gastro-enteritis; only the alimentary tract is involved and general invasion of the body does not occur. Following ingestion of the contaminated food there is commonly an incubation period of about 24 hours, representing the time necessary for multiplication of the organisms in the intestine. In addition to vomiting and diarrhoea, which may be severe and prolonged over several days, there is usually pyrexia. The organism can frequently be isolated from the stools and vomit as well as from the infected food.

It has been generally accepted that salmonellae can also give rise to a toxic form of food poisoning by producing enterotoxic substances in the food which remain active even after cooking sufficient to kill any organisms present. There is no conclusive evidence to support this view.

Salmonella food poisoning is usually a self-limited disease. If chemotherapy is necessary, chloramphenicol appears to be the most effective agent.

Other Types of Bacterial Food Poisoning

Bacterial food poisoning may also be caused by the following organisms:

1. Shigellae (Chapter 21).
2. Strains of *Staph. aureus* which produce enterotoxin (Chapter 13).
3. *Cl. perfringens* (Chapter 29).

There is strong evidence that food in which there has been excessive growth of almost any organism may give rise to the symptoms of bacterial food poisoning, but precisely how it does so is not known. In some of these cases there may be an active infection with the organisms present in the food, while in others the condition may be due to the local action on the intestinal tract of irritative metabolites which have accumulated in the food as a result of bacterial growth. The latter possibility recalls the theory at one time widely held that food poisoning resulted from the ingestion of ptomaines, i.e. amines produced by bacterial decomposition of food protein. Although it has been clearly established that a concentration of amines sufficient to cause toxic symptoms could hardly be present in food that could be eaten, it is nevertheless possible that other, as yet unidentified, products of bacterial growth could be responsible.

Botulism is also a variety of food poisoning, but the condition affects the central nervous system and not, as in the varieties considered above, the intestinal tract (Chapter 29).

Diagnosis

In the diagnosis of bacterial food poisoning, the patient's faeces should be examined and also, if available, a specimen of vomit and some of the incriminated food. A direct film stained by Gram's method may be valuable in revealing gross contamination of the food. The following cultural examinations may be attempted: Inoculation on to Leifson's medium and into selenite broth for isolation of salmonellae and shigellae; on to salt agar for isolation of *Staph. aureus*; into heated and unheated Robertson's meat medium and on to an anaerobic blood agar plate for the isolation of clostridia. Serological tests are of little value in the diagnosis of bacterial food poisoning due to *Salmonella* species, since the condition is of such short duration. They may, however, permit a retrospective diagnosis although the antibody response observed is usually poor.

Arizona

Only one species is defined—*Arizona arizonae*. These are lactose-fermenting enterobacteriaceae which were first isolated from reptiles in Arizona. They appear to be capable of causing intestinal infections in man and other animals similar to those produced by the salmonellae. They are rarely found as intestinal commensals. Like the salmonellae the Arizona Group are divisible into a large number of serotypes on the basis of O and H antigen composition.

CHAPTER 21

THE SHIGELLAE

The shigellae are non-motile, non-capsulated, Gram negative rods with the general properties of the enterobacteriaceae. Except for *Shigella sonnei*, which is a late lactose fermenter (p. 291), they are non-lactose fermenters. Like the salmonellae, the shigellae must be finally identified by their serological reactions. They differ from the other enterobacteriaceae so far considered in that they occur exclusively as human pathogens.

Shigella dysenteriae. These are non-mannitol-fermenting shigellae and comprise eight serotypes of which the classical *Shigella shigae* is type 1. Some of the types show characteristic biochemical reactions. All ferment glucose producing acid but not gas.

Shigella flexneri. This species is subdivided into six antigenic types, each of the types possessing an antigen specific for the type. In addition, the different types possess group antigens which occur in each type either singly or in various combinations. On the basis of the group antigens present types 1, 2 and 4 can each be divided into two and type 3 into three subtypes. In laboratory culture the organisms may show a gradual loss of the type antigens. This change, which resembles S → R variation amongst the salmonellae but without the development of spontaneous agglutinability in saline, may on occasion be found to have occurred in freshly isolated strains. The variants are sometimes referred to as X and Y types according to their residual group antigen composition. The majority of strains of *Sh. flexneri* ferment mannitol but a few—especially of type 6—comprising the so-called Newcastle variety, do not.

Shigella boydii. These strains biochemically resemble *Sh. flexneri*, but differ from it serologically. They possess type-specific antigens distinct from those of the *flexneri* group and do not possess group antigens. On the basis of their type-specific antigens they have been subdivided into 15 serological types.

Shigella sonnei. This organism differs in a number of respects from *Sh. flexneri*. It is a late lactose and saccharose fermenter. Late fermentation of these sugars is due to the appearance of variants in culture. If the organism is plated on to MacConkey's medium, the variants appear after some days' incubation as pink-coloured papillae in the centre of otherwise colourless colonies. Indole is not produced.

Shigella sonnei rapidly undergoes S → R variation. On primary isolation on MacConkey's medium colonies are frequently encountered which are partially rough and partially smooth—the rough organisms being present in a fan-shaped segment, the edge of which extends beyond the margin of the colony; this appearance is said to resemble that of a bomb crater. The colonies of other strains may at first appear smooth, but when incubation is prolonged they become rough on the surface with irregularly crenated edges. The smooth (phase 1) and rough (phase 2) forms are antigenically distinct. Phase 2 organisms do not grow on desoxycholate citrate agar.

On the basis of their capacity to produce various colicines *Sh. sonnei* strains have been assigned to sixteen types each type being characterized by the production of a specific colicine. This procedure has been applied with some success as a method of epidemiological typing.

Pathogenicity

The shigellae are endotoxic, the endotoxins, like those of the salmonellae, being associated with the somatic antigens. Though they cause diarrhoea and intestinal inflammation on injection into animals, it is by no means certain that the endotoxins are the sole agents responsible for the intestinal dysenteric lesions found in man.

Shigella dysenteriae, type 1, is unusual in producing an extremely potent heat-labile protein toxin which, because of its marked effect on the central nervous system of the rabbit, is usually described as a neurotoxin. This description, however, is probably incorrect, since the primary action of the toxin appears to be on the blood vessels. Purified preparations of the toxin have a potency of the same order as the tetanus and botulinum toxins (p. 392). Although it has the properties of a typical exotoxin, it does not appear to be secreted by the organism but is liberated by autolysis. In spite of the extreme potency of the toxin only a small amount of it is produced during growth and the toxicity of cultures is therefore low.

Bacillary Dysentery

Dysentery is an inflammatory condition of the intestine, mainly of the large intestine, characterized by necrosis, sloughing and ulceration of extensive areas of the mucosa with blood and mucus in the faeces. It may be divided into two main types, amoebic due to *Entamoeba histolytica* and bacillary, due to the shigellae. In countries in which these conditions are endemic mixed amoebic and bacillary infections are, however, occasionally found.

Cases of bacillary dysentery differ considerably in severity. In some, there is only a mild diarrhoea and, as indicated in the previous chapter, the dysentery bacilli may on occasion give rise to the symptoms of bacterial food poisoning. The most severe type of dysentery is that caused by *Sh. dysenteriae*, type 1. In this there is usually considerable toxaemia, sometimes with an effusion into the joints or evidence of myocarditis. Dysentery bacilli are normally confined to the intestine and the intestinal mucosa, and only in very rare cases is there evidence of a general invasion of the body.

Following an attack of dysentery, the organisms usually disappear from the stools in a matter of a week or so. The development of a persistent carrier state is infrequent and is most likely following *Sh. dysenteriae* infection. Carriers of *Sh. dysenteriae* are usually chronically ill and are liable to relapses of the acute condition. Relapses tend to be precipitated by dietary indiscretions and in some cases by return to work.

Dysentery occurs both as an epidemic and as an endemic infection. Epidemics of major proportions occur mainly in tropical communities and particularly in those with low standards of sanitation. In such communities the prevalence of dysentery shows a marked seasonal incidence, epidemics occurring at times of maximal density of the fly population. This relationship emphasizes the importance of flies, which act as mechanical vectors, in transferring infection from faeces to food. Epidemics of dysentery occurring under tropical or sub-tropical conditions are usually due to more than one species of dysentery bacillus; in general *Sh. flexneri* is most frequently found, with *Sh. dysenteriae*, type 1, next in frequency, but more often associated with severe disease.

In temperate zones dysentery exists primarily as an endemic infection but with a maximal incidence in the late winter and early spring. In European countries and in America, in spite of their advanced standards of sanitation and hygiene, endemic dysentery appears, in the last few decades, to have shown a marked increase in prevalence. In contrast to tropical and subtropical dysentery *Sh. sonnei* is the main organism responsible, with *Sh. flexneri* next in frequency. Both of these species have considerable tendency to establish a symptomless, but transient, carrier state. In the British Isles endemic dysentery is primarily an infection of urban communities with a maximum incidence in young children, the main foci of infection being communal nurseries, children's homes and primary schools. From such foci, once they have become established, dysentery bacilli can only be eradicated with the greatest difficulty. Dysentery is also wide-spread in mental institutions; this epidemiological variety, which is known as asylum dysentery, is usually associated with a more severe clinical disease than is the usual endemic type. In the maintenance of endemic dysentery flies are of minor importance—though they must of course be kept under control. The disease is mainly transmitted as a result of the casual contamination by cases and carriers of objects in their environment. The organisms are then transferred from contaminated objects by the hand of the recipient to the mouth. Communally used lavatories appear to be of particular importance in the spread of dysentery under these conditions.

Diagnosis

In the early stages of the disease microscopic examination may be of value in differentiating bacillary dysentery from amoebic dysentery. In bacillary dysentery 90 per cent of the cells in the stools are of polymorphonuclear type while these cells are in a minority in amoebic dysentery. In the latter condition microscopic examination should reveal the presence of *Ent. histolytica*.

Rectal swabs may be used for isolation and, when large numbers of specimens must be examined, are very convenient. They do not, however, give as high a proportion of isolations as faeces. Since shigellae die out rapidly in faeces, culture should be attempted as soon as possible. Failing this, the specimen may be preserved for a few days in buffered glycerol saline. If mucus is present it should be used as an inoculum.

Cultures should be made on both MacConkey's agar and desoxycholate citrate agar. Wilson and Blair's medium, tetrathionate broth and selenite broth are not of value as they suppress the growth of dysentery bacteria. After incubation, colourless colonies are subcultured and examined by the usual cultural methods. As with the salmonellae the final identification of a *Shigella* species is achieved by agglutination tests. Polyvalent *Sh. flexneri* and *Sh. boydii* sera and a *Sh. sonnei* serum containing antibody to both phase 1 and phase 2 antigens are available for preliminary testing.

The serum of a patient in the later stages of the disease frequently agglutinates the causative organism but, since the titre is not usually high and, since normal serum may also cause agglutination, agglutination tests are of little diagnostic value.

Treatment

The sulphonamides were for many years the drugs of choice in the treatment of dysentery. Unfortunately, many strains of dysentery bacilli are now sulphonamide resistant. In cases resistant to sulphonamides, therapy with the tetracyclines is usually successful. The drug susceptibility of the shigellae must be considerably modified, however, by the spread of R factors (p. 197) which were first recognized in the *Shigella* genus. Good results have been claimed for the use of antitoxin in severe infections with *Sh. dysenteriae* type 1 but satisfactory evidence of its value has not been presented.

Prophylaxis

The prevention of dysentery depends on the same principles as does that of the enteric fevers. Specific prophylaxis by vaccination has not been found to be feasible.

CHAPTER 22

VIBRIO, SPIRILLUM, PSEUDOMONAS

The three genera to be considered in this chapter are assigned by Bergey to the order Pseudomonadales which are distinguished from the Eubacteriales by their polar flagellation.

Vibrio cholerae (Vibrio comma)

The genus *Vibrio* comprises a group of non-sporing, non-capsulated, motile, Gram negative rods with a curved shape and a characteristic 'darting' mobility. They grow readily on ordinary laboratory media. Some are pathogenic for various animals, and only two—*Vibrio cholerae* and the *Vibrio El Tor*, which very closely resemble one another—are pathogenic for man. Most species are free-living organisms occurring naturally in soil and water.

Morphology

The cholera vibrio measures from 1.5μ to 3.0μ by about 0.5μ. As seen, usually in enormous numbers, in the dejecta from cases of cholera, it is definitely curved, and, from its resemblance to a comma, the name 'comma bacillus' was given to it. The curve, however, is not flat, but is in two planes. Frequently the organisms occur in pairs, giving either a C or, more commonly, S shape. In the stools the majority of the vibrios appear to lie with their long axes parallel, this appearance being described as resembling 'fish in a stream'. In cultures—particularly of old laboratory strains—the curved shape may be almost or completely lost, and the organism then is indistinguishable from a coliform bacillus. Involution forms develop readily.

Cultural Properties

Growth is best under slightly alkaline conditions—pH 7·6 to 8—and will occur at a pH of 9 to 9·5, sufficiently high to inhibit the growth of most other pathogenic bacteria. On agar the colonies of freshly isolated strains are usually thin and very transparent but a number of variant types have been described. In peptone water and in broth *V. cholerae* grows rapidly. In fluid media some strains produce a surface pellicle which tends to grow up the wall of the tube. Why they should do so is not known.

Indole is produced and nitrates are reduced to nitrites. The 'cholera red

323

reaction'—the production of a pink colour on the addition of a mineral acid to a peptone water culture of the cholera vibrio—is due to the presence of both indole and nitrites in the culture. It is a non-lactose fermenter. Gelatin and serum are rapidly liquefied.

Antigenic Structure

On the basis of their O antigens, the cholera and cholera-like vibrios can be divided into six serological groups. The cholera vibrio belongs to subgroup 1 of this classification. The only other member of this subgroup—the El Tor vibrio—very closely resembles the cholera vibrio in biochemical properties. Three distinct antigenic subtypes of *V. cholerae*—the *Inaba*, *Ogawa* and *Hikojima* varieties—have been distinguished. These differ from one another in their content of minor antigens, on the basis of which they have been assigned the antigenic formulae AC, AB and ABC respectively. The cholera vibrio also possesses an H antigen which is shared by a number of non-cholera vibrios. This antigen is therefore of no value in identification.

Pathogenicity

The cholera vibrio is endotoxic, its toxicity resembling that of other Gram negative bacilli in being associated with the somatic antigen. From the work of Jenkin and Rowley, however, it would appear that the toxicity of the antigen is due mainly to its protein component. The vibrio autolyses very readily and, consequently, considerable amounts of the endotoxin are liberated during growth. Whether this substance is responsible for the toxic lesions produced in the intestinal mucosa in man has not at the moment been firmly established. The investigation of this problem has, unfortunately, been considerably hampered by the lack of a suitable experimental animal in which intestinal changes resembling those occurring in the human disease could be reliably produced. The cholera vibrio produces a neuraminidase (receptor-destroying enzyme) resembling the neuraminidase of the influenza virus (p. 497). No role in pathogenicity has so far been attributed to this enzyme, nor to a mucinase demonstrable also in culture filtrates and which can break down intestinal glandular mucin.

On intraperitoneal injection the cholera vibrio is rapidly lethal to guinea-pigs, mice and rabbits. A similar pathogenicity is, however, also shown by certain non-cholera vibrios. Virulence tests therefore do not by any means establish that an organism is *V. cholerae*, though if it is non-pathogenic to the guinea-pig it can be safely assumed not to be a cholera vibrio.

No animal under natural conditions suffers from cholera. By neutralization of the gastric juice with bicarbonate, combined with the injection of opium to inhibit peristalsis, Koch was able to induce a cholera-like disease in guinea-pigs. Young rabbits, too, can apparently be infected by intubation, and exudation of fluid is reported to occur following introduction of the vibrios into a ligated loop of rabbit intestine. However, these procedures have not so far been shown to be of significant value in elucidating the pathogenesis of cholera in man.

Cholera

Cholera is an acute disease marked by intense diarrhoea and vomiting. As a result there is a great loss of fluid which may, in severe cases, amount to as much as two-thirds of the plasma volume. The dehydration in turn leads to haemoconcentration, anuria and severe muscular cramps. In the absence of treatment, case mortality rates of the order of 60 to 70 per cent have been frequent. Death is usually due to renal failure. The choleraic stool has a characteristic appearance. It is almost completely fluid with flakes of mucus floating in it, the common term 'rice water stool' being a fairly good description of this appearance. The stool contains large numbers of cholera vibrios—in some cases up to 10^9 organisms per ml having been observed.

In recent years our ideas on the pathogenesis of cholera have been considerably revised. It was at one time thought that the toxins of the vibrio caused desquamation of the epithelial cells of the gut, and that this desquamation was the basic lesion. It has now been established that, on the contrary, this is entirely a post-mortem phenomenon. Biopsy examination during life has shown that the epithelium is, to all intents and purposes, normal in appearance.

The intestinal mucosa is not invaded and there is never a general bacteraemic spread of the organisms through the body. They appear in fact to mutiply largely on the luminal surface of the intestinal mucous membrane. The nature of the biochemical lesion in cholera has not been determined, but it is thought that some toxic product of the vibrio damages the sodium pump mechanism of the alimentary epithelium, to such an extent that there is gross loss of electrolyte and of fluid into the lumen. There is a possibility that some product of the organism may in addition have a toxic effect on the kidney.

The vibrios are rapidly eliminated, the great majority of cases ceasing to excrete them in about 3 weeks from the onset of the disease. It is doubtful whether a persistent carrier state ever develops; if it does it is extremely rare. Healthy persons who have been in contact with a case may, however, become infected and may excrete the organism for a short time without the development of clinical symptoms. Such subjects, known as contact carriers, are of considerable importance in maintaining cholera as an endemic infection. Occasionally contact carriers after carrying the organism for some time develop the clinical disease possibly as a result of a dietary indiscretion; in these circumstances they are sometimes referred to as precocious carriers.

Cholera is characteristically an epidemic disease. It was virtually unknown outside India before the nineteenth century, but since then many epidemics have occurred throughout the world—the most recent being in Egypt in 1947 and Thailand in 1958. In the Ganges delta in India it appears to have been endemic for centuries and this appears to have been the main source from which most pandemics have originated and from which infection of the rest of the Indian subcontinent has occurred. The magnitude of this endemic infection is shown by the fact that in East Pakistan alone there were approximately a quarter of a million deaths from cholera in the period 1948 to 1959. In India and Pakistan the disease achieves a maximum epidemic prevalence in the months April to June and October to December. A second great focus of endemic infection is in the Yangtse valley in China. Notable water-borne epidemics outside India were the London Broad Street pump epidemic of 1854, in which, for the first time, the role of water in the spread of cholera was brilliantly established by John Snow, and the Hamburg epidemic of 1892 which dramatically demonstrated the effectiveness of sand filtration as a method of controlling water-borne disease.

In endemic areas at non-epidemic periods the disease is probably maintained, like endemic dysentery, by casual and environmental contamination from both cases and carriers. In the transmission of the disease from one place to another the precocious or incubating carrier is of special importance.

There is some evidence to relate high cholera incidence to high atmospheric humidity, but this is not the only factor involved, and the reasons for the marked seasonal variations of the disease in endemic areas is not understood. Major epidemics of cholera appear to be due, almost invariably, to contaminated water supplies in which, particularly if alkaline, the vibrios may survive for a considerable time; this is, apparently, a frequent cause when water is stored in large tanks, as in certain tropical communities.

The El Tor vibrio can cause a diarrhoeal condition, sometimes known as paracholera, which is similar to, but much less severe than true cholera. The original home of the organism appears to have been in Celebes in Indonesia, to which it was for many years confined. In recent years, however, the vibrio has shown a remarkable increase in its potential for epidemic spread. Thus it achieved an extensive dissemination through the Far East in the period 1958 to 1961, invading East Pakistan in 1963 and Calcutta in 1964.

Diagnosis

A provisional diagnosis of cholera can frequently be made by direct microscopic examination of the stools; the occurrence of large numbers of vibrios in a 'rice water stool' is virtually conclusive evidence of infection. The vibrios may be sufficiently numerous in the faeces to permit the direct performance of agglutination tests with faecal material.

In isolating the organism it is essential that cultures, for which either faeces or a rectal swab may be used, should be carried out as soon as possible. If delay cannot be avoided, the specimen should be kept in a buffered saline mixture; for this purpose a borate saline mixture has been described as being satisfactory. The specimen should be inoculated into a tube of alkaline peptone water and on to an appropriate solid selective medium. After about 6 hours the peptone water will usually show an extensive surface growth which can then be subcultured onto the selective medium employed. A variety of selective media has been recommended for the isolation of the cholera vibrio. These include Dieudonné's alkaline blood agar, MacConkey's medium and Monsur's medium which contains tellurite, taurocholate and gelatin. On this the vibrio produces a colony with a black centre and surrounded by a definite halo as a result of gelatin breakdown.

Strict criteria are required for the identification as *V. cholerae* of a vibrio isolated from the faeces of a suspected carrier or from a sample of water. The main differential characteristics of *V. cholerae* are fermentation of saccharose and mannose but not of arabinose—a positive cholera red and a negative Voges-Proskauer reaction. In most cases an organism giving these reactions is found to be the cholera vibrio. The organisms should be agglutinated by an O sub-group I serum. Occasionally strains are rough on primary isolation and are therefore inagglutinable by O serum; this is particularly so in the case of strains isolated from water or from sporadic cases. The El Tor vibrio which may be found in the faeces of non-cholera patients is also agglutinated by subgroup I serum and may give all the biochemical reactions of the cholera vibrio. It may be differentiated from the cholera vibrio by the fact that it produces a soluble haemolysin for sheep and goat cells.

Serological tests on the patient's serum are of little value in diagnosis during the acute stage of the disease. They may, however, be of some value in establishing a retrospective diagnosis and in the detection of carriers. The tests are carried out with a *V. cholerae* O suspension.

Treatment

Though the cholera vibrio is sensitive to sulphonamides and to various antibiotics, chemotherapy appears to have little, if any, effect on the clinical course of the disease. It may, however, diminish the period of convalescent carriage and therefore reduce the risk of the patient being a source of further infection. The most important measures in treatment are those designed to make good the fluid loss. The adoption of such measures has, in recent years, effected a reduction in case mortality from about 70 per cent to about 20 per cent.

Prophylaxis

As in the case of enteric fever, a dramatic reduction in the incidence of cholera followed the introduction of the large-scale purification of water supplies and of sanitary methods for the disposal of excreta. These methods, combined with hygienic handling of food, should control epidemic spread of the disease; it may, however, be difficult to eradicate the disease from the remaining endemic foci.

A killed vaccine prepared from the Inaba and Ogawa strains is widely used for active immunization. Vaccination is employed for people going to countries where cholera is endemic, and also in mass immunization programmes in endemic zones. If possible, two injections should be given with an interval of 4 weeks between each. In mass immunization programmes only one injection may be feasible. The vaccine is much less toxic than TAB vaccine, with which it may safely be combined. Although the efficacy of vaccination has not been fully documented, there is reason to believe that it confers some degree of protection against infection. Unfortunately, the mortality of the disease in those who have contracted it in spite of vaccination is unaffected.

Other Vibrios

A number of *Vibrio* species can cause disease in animals, e.g. *V. foetus*, a microaerophilic species which can cause abortion in sheep and cattle. A few infections with this organism have been reported in pregnant women. *V. jejuni* and *V. coli* can give rise to diarrhoeal syndromes in cows and young pigs respectively. *V. metschnikovii* resembles the cholera and El Tor vibrios in being highly pathogenic for guinea-pigs on intraperitoneal inoculation, but is serologically distinct. It is responsible for a septicaemia disease in poultry.

Spirillum

This is a genus of small, actively motile spiral organisms morphologically resembling the spirochaetes. Spirilla differ from the latter, however, in being rigid and in owing their motility to polar flagella. Because of this they are classified with the Pseudomonadales. A number of species are found as free-living organisms in soil and water.

Spirillum minus

This is the only pathogenic member of the genus. It is a common parasite of the respiratory tract of rats in various parts of the world. It is a small, actively motile organism—measuring from 2 to 5μ in length usually with two or three complete spirals. It has not so far been maintained in culture on inanimate media and is consequently regarded by some workers as being more properly classed with the spirochaetes than with the bacteria.

Spirillum minus is the cause of a variety of rat-bite fever. In this condition after some weeks, the site of the wound, which may have healed, becomes inflamed and breaks down, the drainage glands become swollen, there is pyrexia, sudden in onset and remittent in type, and a purpuric skin rash. The spirilla are present in the blood but are few in numbers and are difficult to demonstrate. The easiest method of diagnosis is to inject blood intraperitoneally into a mouse or guinea-pig, in the blood of which the spirilla can be demonstrated after about 10 days by dark ground illumination.

This variety of rat-bite fever must be distinguished from that due to *Streptobacillus moniliformis* (Chapter 28). Both varieties respond to treatment with penicillin.

Pseudomonas aeruginosa (*Pseudomonas pyocyanea*)

Organisms of the genus *Pseudomonas* are widely distributed in nature occurring as free-living organisms in the soil, in water and in decomposing organic material. Bergey lists 149 named species, the majority of which are plant pathogens. A striking feature of the genus is the great diversity of compounds which can be utilized by different members for energy production. The only species pathogenic for man is *Pseudomonas aeruginosa*.

Cultural Properties

Pseudomonas aeruginosa is an actively motile, non-sporing, non-capsulated, Gram negative rod. It is a strict aerobe and grows readily on ordinary media at 37° C. It produces two pigments, pyocyanine, which is blue, and fluorescein which is greenish yellow and fluorescent. The pigments diffuse throughout the medium, giving the latter a bright green colour by which the organism is readily identified. On blood agar the colonies have a slightly honeycombed appearance with an irregular, undulating edge. The growth has a highly characteristic odour resembling that of trimethylamine; this odour is of value in indicating the presence of even a few colonies of *Ps. aeruginosa* on plates. Most strains break down glucose which is the only common sugar attacked with the production of acid but no gas. This is not strictly a fermentation but an oxidation and results in the production of gluconic acid. Gelatin is rapidly liquefied. Indole is not produced.

A filtrate of an old broth culture is capable, even in high dilution, of killing bacteria of various species. This property was formerly attributed to the action of an enzyme, pyocyanase, but appears to be mainly due to a yellow pigment, α-oxyphenazine. An unusual property of *Ps. aeruginosa* is its capacity to form hydrocyanic acid.

Pathogenicity

Pseudomonas aeruginosa appears to possess little power of initiating infection by itself. Not infrequently, however, it occurs as a secondary invader of infected tissues or of tissues which have been traumatized by operation or other manipulation. Children, and persons with diminished resistance, e.g. from administration of corticosteroids, are particularly susceptible to infection. As the species *Ps. aeruginosa* is highly resistant to the commonly used antibiotics, and because of its capacity to persist and even to multiply in unpromising environments, it has in recent years assumed considerable prominence as a cause of hospital infections, especially of infections of wounds and of the urinary tract. Most *Pseudomonas* infections of the urinary tract occur either as a sequel to operations, following catheterization or complicating chronic genito-urinary infections. Bacteriophage typing and pyocine sensitivity have been of considerable value in elucidating the epidemiology of these infections. Most appear to be due, as in the case of *Staph. aureus*, to hospital strains of enhanced infectivity and virulence.

Pseudomonas aeruginosa has a special preference for moist environments; it has been frequently isolated from disinfectant solutions—notably chloroxylenol and cationic detergents—to which it is often highly resistant. Its occurrence in eye drops and lotions is a particular hazard in ophthalmology since it may produce a postoperative ophthalmia which may lead ultimately to blindness. Other important sources of infection are bed-pans, urine bottles and water taps.

For the treatment of *Pseudomonas* infections, polymyxin B and polymyxin E (Colistin or Colimycin) are the agents of choice.

Pseudomonas pseudomallei (*Pfeifferella whitmori*)

Pseudomonas pseudomallei is a short, Gram negative, motile bacillus frequently showing bipolar staining. The optimum growth temperature is 37° C but the organism will grow well at 32° C. On agar it produces a cream coloured, opaque colony with an irregular edge. It ferments glucose, maltose, mannitol, lactose and saccharose with the production of acid but not gas and liquefies gelatin. *Ps. pseudomallei* shows some antigenic relationship with *Actinobacillus mallei* (p. 375) and is classified by some workers with this organism—the generic names *Pfeifferella*, *Malleomyces* and *Loefflerella* being variously used. It is pathogenic for guinea-pigs and rats and like *Act. mallei* produces a Straus reaction in the male guinea-pig.

Pseudomonas pseudomallei is a normal parasite of the respiratory tracts of many rodents. In man it produces melioidosis—a disease, usually of acute character, in which lesions resembling those of glanders occur in the lungs and other organs. Melioidosis is a rare disease and is confined to tropical countries. There is no effective treatment.

CHAPTER 23

THE PASTEURELLAE

Like the other genera of the Brucellaceae the pasteurellae are small, Gram negative, highly parasitic, aerobic, non-sporing bacilli. A chacteristic feature is their marked tendency to show bipolar staining.

Pasteurella pestis

Morphology

Pasteurella pestis is found in its most characteristic form in material taken from early plague lesions in man or animals. It is short and thick, 1 to 2μ by 0·5 to 1μ in size. It has rounded ends presenting a boat-shaped appearance, and may frequently appear almost coccal in outline. It occurs in the body either singly or in pairs, short chains being exceptional. In fluid media it tends to grow in long chains. Old lesions, old cultures, or young cultures on 'salt agar' (agar containing about 3 per cent sodium chloride) show ovoid, globular, club-shaped and snake-like involution forms. In the body and on serum agar at 37° C it possesses a capsule which is often, however, rather poorly defined. *Past. pestis* is non-motile.

Cultural Properties

The plague bacillus grows on ordinary media but growth is rather slow. The optimum growth temperature is 28 to 30° C but satisfactory growth occurs at 37° C. Growth from small inocula requires a low oxidation-reduction potential. On blood agar after 24 hours' growth the colonies are very small—0·1 to 0·2 mm in diameter—translucent and slightly viscid. It is non-haemolytic. If grown in broth on the surface of which a little oil or butter is floated the organism grows in a stalactite formation suspended from the under-surface of the oil.

For the differentiation of *Past. pestis* from other pasteurellae, the biochemical reactions of importance are failure to produce indole, positive methyl-red reaction, failure to break down urea and growth on MacConkey's medium. In addition it is lysed by a specific bacteriophage inactive against other pasturellae. On the basis of glycerol fermentation and nitrite production three epidemiological types, each of which shows a specific geographical distribution are distinguishable.

Antigenic Structure

Pasteurella pestis has a complex antigenic structure. Three different types of antigen have been described: (1) A heat-labile capsular protein antigen. This antigen is only produced in significant amounts when the organisms are grown at 37° C. It is the antigen responsible for the stimulation of protective antibody. (2) The plague toxin (see below). (3) A somatic antigen complex. One or more of the components of this complex are identical with somatic antigen components of *Pasteurella pseudotuberculosis*.

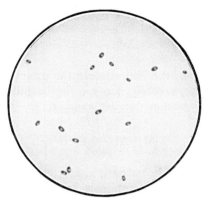

FIG. 25. *Past. pestis* FROM A YOUNG AGAR CULTURE (× 950)

Pathogenicity

The plague bacillus produces a protein endotoxin which can be converted by treatment with formalin into toxoid. The toxin will adsorb to tannic acid treated red cells, and antitoxin can consequently be titrated by the passive haemagglutination technique. The toxin has a damaging effect on the peripheral blood vessels. On intradermal injection in laboratory animals it causes a local oedema which may be followed by tissue necrosis. The toxin presumably plays a part in the production of the tissue lesions found in plague.

Laboratory animals, particularly guinea-pigs, rats and mice, are susceptible to infection. As a result of subcutaneous injection in the guinea-pig, there is a local lesion with marked oedema; the glands draining the area involved are enlarged and often show small pale areas of necrosis resembling, in naked eye appearance, miliary tubercles. The animal generally dies within a week of receiving the injection. The guinea-pig may also be infected by smearing the conjunctiva, or the nasal mucous membrane, or by rubbing the freshly shaved skin of the abdomen with material containing the bacilli.

Plague

Plague is primarily an infection of rodents, particularly of the rat, in which it generally takes the form of an acute and rapidly fatal septicaemia. A rat usually becomes infected by the bite of a flea which has previously bitten a rat suffering from plague septicaemia. Man is only incidentally infected and except in pneumonic plague the disease is not transmissible from man to man.

Human plague is a most serious disease. It occurs either in large-scale epidemics in towns or cities, this type being known as *urban plague*, or as sporadic cases in rural areas—the so-called *rural* or *sylvatic plague*.

Urban plague is now mainly a disease of tropical and sub-tropical countries and is spread to man from infected rats by rat fleas—the most important of these being *Xenopsylla cheopis*. The flea becomes infected when it bites an infected rat; the organisms then multiply in the proventriculus of the flea and are regurgitated into the wound when the flea bites a fresh victim. Infection may also apparently occur on occasion, through minute abrasions of the skin, from bacilli present in dust.

Epidemics of urban plague are always preceded by an outbreak (epizootic) in rats. Grey rats are usually the variety first infected, the disease then spreading to the black rat. Finally when the rat population is seriously reduced in numbers by the disease the fleas turn to man as an alternative host. Epidemics of plague occur only when the ambient temperature is in the range 10 to 30° C. At temperatures above 30° C fleas rapidly become non-infective. The human flea *Pulex irritans* appears to be incapable of transmitting the disease.

From time to time pandemics of plague have swept throughout the world and all communities appear at one time or another to have been infected. It is probable that the Black Death of the fourteenth century was a pandemic of plague, at first bubonic and later pneumonic, originating from a wild rodent reservoir in Southern Russia. India, however, appears to have been the focus of infection from which most pandemics have originated. The disease is now endemic in India, South-East Asia, parts of Africa and South America. From being one of the great scourges of mankind, plague is now, presumably as a result of control of the rodent and vector populations, of relatively infrequent occurrence. Thus, throughout the world, only approximately 1300 cases were recorded in 1962, whereas in India alone plague is believed to have been responsible for some 10 million deaths in the first 20 years of the century. This fall in the incidence of the human disease has unfortunately, however, been associated in certain parts of the world with progressive extension of the prevalence of *Past. pestis* in wild rodent populations.

Sylvatic plague appears as a sporadic disease occurring in rural areas—the sources of infection being various wild rodents, some 200 varieties of which have now been shown to be infected. In different parts of the world the infection predominates in different species. Thus, ground squirrels and voles are of particular importance in the U.S.A. and bandicoots in India. Amongst the rodent population the disease is spread by fleas and other biting insects. Human infection, however, more often occurs as a result of handling, or being bitten by, an infected animal, and has been found chiefly in workers in woods, in hunters and in children. In addition to giving rise to occasional human cases the wild rodent reservoir is of considerable importance as the continuing source of infection for the rat population, and its existence therefore constitutes a serious menace to man.

In man plague occurs in two clinical forms: *bubonic*, which is much the commonest variety, and *pneumonic*. Bubonic plague is characterized by the appearance of swelling and inflammation in the lymphatic glands draining the site of the bite. Since bites usually occur on the leg the inguinal glands are those most frequently involved. The pathological condition of the swollen glands, which are known as buboes, is one of intense inflammation with haemorrhages, leading eventually to necrosis. In the early stages the glands are packed with enormous numbers of coccoid, polar-staining bacilli, and a film prepared from the gland pulp may resemble a pure culture of the organism.

Pneumonic plague is characterized by a rapidly spreading bronchopneumonia of haemorrhagic type. Since the bacilli are present in large numbers in the sputum the disease is extremely infectious. As might be expected of a respiratory disease, epidemics are commonest in the colder months of the year. The disease probably originates in the first place from a patient suffering from bubonic plague in which the infection has localized, as a result of metastatic spread, in the lung. Pneumonic plague does not occur in epidemic form in India; epidemics appear to occur almost exclusively in Manchuria, Northern China and Mongolia.

Diagnosis

The demonstration of typical polar-staining bacilli in fluid aspirated from a bubo, or in the sputum of a case of suspected pneumonic plague, is strongly suggestive of infection. Isolation of the bacillus is readily achieved by inoculation onto blood agar, the plates being incubated at 30° C. Since the organism is highly infective, laboratory diagnosis should be attempted only by skilled and immunized personnel. Identification is by demonstration of the morphological and biochemical characteristics of the organism and of its agglutinability by specific antiserum. The susceptibility of *Past. pestis* to a specific bacteriophage is of value in differentiating this species from *Past. pseudotuberculosis*. A particularly detailed and careful examination, which should include a virulence test in guinea-pigs or white rats, is essential for the identification of organisms isolated from rats or from suspected human cases in non-plague areas.

The organism may also be isolated by direct inoculation of a guinea-pig. This should be attempted if few or no organisms are demonstrable in smears prepared from the bubo. If the material for examination has undergone extensive secondary bacterial invasion, some of it should be rubbed on to the shaved skin of the guinea-pig; if *Past. pestis* is present it will penetrate the skin and set up an infection. Infected guinea-pigs usually die within a week after inoculation when the characteristic local and general lesions may be demonstrated at post-mortem examination.

Pasteurella pestis can frequently be isolated from the blood in the early stages of the disease. For this purpose a broth containing cystine appears to give best results.

Treatment

Excellent results have been obtained with streptomycin in the treatment of plague. Chloramphenicol, the tetracyclines and sulphadiazine are also of value.

Prophylaxis

In countries where plague occurs the most important methods in its prevention are: the reduction of the rat population by the use of chemical rodenticides —dicoumarin, sodium fluoroacetate and α naphthyl-thiourea, the control of fleas for which DDT is of great value, and the early diagnosis of plague epizootics in rats.

Killed vaccines have been widely used for active immunization. They appear to give appreciable, if not complete, protection against infection and somewhat reduce the severity of the disease in those who, in spite of inoculation, contract it. The immunity is of short duration and revaccination at six-monthly intervals is necessary for those who continue to be exposed. A living vaccine prepared from a mutant of diminished virulence has also been employed. It has been found to confer much greater protection in animals than heat-killed vaccine. The vaccine, which is given in a single dose, appears to be particularly suited for mass immunization campaigns in native populations.

Pasteurella tularensis (*Francisella tularensis*)

Pasteurella tularensis is a very small Gram negative bacillus which exhibits very marked pleomorphism in culture. In the tissues it is found in large numbers inside the tissue cells, where it appears to be capsulated; capsulation has not however been demonstrated in culture. It is non-motile and non-sporing.

It will not grow on ordinary media but may be isolated, though with difficulty, by the use of special media, e.g. coagulated egg yolk or a medium containing glucose, rabbit blood and cysteine. It also grows well in the cells of the chorio-allantoic membrane of the developing chick embryo. It is antigenically homogeneous but shows some serological relationship with the brucellae and with *Pasteurella pestis*.

Tularaemia

Tularaemia is a plague-like infection of wild rodents. It appears to be widely distributed in the U.S.A. from which it was first reported, and is present also in Japan and in northern Europe. In most animals the disease appears to be spread mainly by ticks which can transmit the parasite transovarially. Human infection is uncommon and is usually due to the handling of infected animals, particularly rabbits and hares, the infection probably occurring mainly through abrasions of the skin. In the commonest type of infection a small papule which eventually breaks down to form an ulcer appears at the site of introduction of the organism, usually on the finger; the local lymph glands become enlarged and may undergo ulceration. Infection may also occur through the conjunctiva with associated involvement of the pre-auricular and cervical lymphatic glands. A generalized form of the disease also occurs probably as a result of respiratory or intestinal infection. At post-mortem examination there are widespread necrotic lesions in various organs.

Very successful results have been obtained in cases of tularaemia by treatment with streptomycin.

Killed vaccines are available and can be used for the immunization of persons whose occupation exposes them to the risk of infection. Vaccination appears to confer substantial immunity.

Diagnosis

The best method of isolating the organisms is to inject a guinea-pig intraperitoneally with material from the human lesions and obtain a culture from the necrotic foci which develop in the liver, spleen and lungs of the animal.

The agglutination test is of considerable value—diagnostic titres being usually found in the second week of the disease. The serum of tularaemia patients may also agglutinate *Br. abortus* to a fairly high level.

A delayed type of hypersensitivity may be demonstrated by the intradermal injection of a killed suspension of the organism. The skin test is usually positive during the first week of the disease. Hypersensitivity persists for a considerable period after recovery.

Other Pasteurellae

Pasteurella species are of considerable importance as animal pathogens. The most important of these are *Past. pseudotuberculosis* and *Past. septica*.

Pasteurella pseudotuberculosis is the cause of pseudotuberculosis—a disease which occurs in epizootic and enzootic form in a variety of animals. In the chronic type of the disease nodular lesions resembling those of tuberculosis occur in lymphatic glands, liver, spleen and lungs. In rodents the disease may occur in an acute form which resembles plague.

Pasteurella pseudotuberculosis differs from *Past. pestis* in the following respects: It is non-capsulated, motile in 18-hour cultures at 22° C, grows more luxuriantly, particularly on desoxycholate citrate medium, is non-pathogenic to white rats, and is insusceptible to *Past. pestis* bacteriophage. Serological differentiation of the two species, which are antigenically related, is not always satisfactory.

At one time human infection with *Past. pseudotuberculosis* was thought to be extremely rare; in the last decade, however, an increasing number of infections due to this organism have been reported. These infections may take the form of a severe typhoid-like disease with a high fatality rate or of a relatively mild condition involving the caecum and terminal ileum and their draining lymphatic glands and often simulating acute appendicitis. This latter condition has been observed mainly in children and young adults and is the more frequent type of human infection. The demonstration of agglutinins, using live suspensions of *Past. pseudotuberculosis*, appears to be of value in establishing the diagnosis.

Pasteurella septica is the cause of chicken cholera and of haemorrhagic septicaemia in various mammals. *Past. septica* is capsulated, non-motile at 22° C, produces indole, is unable to grow on desoxycholate citrate medium, and is pathogenic for white rats.

Pasteurella septica rarely infects man but the number of diagnosed human infections appears to be increasing. Many of these have been cases of localized wound infection following an animal bite but generalized infections, in some cases showing localization in the brain or lungs, have been reported.

CHAPTER 24

HAEMOPHILUS, BORDETELLA, MORAXELLA

Haemophilus

This is a genus of very small non-motile, non-sporing aerobic Gram negative bacilli of highly parasitic character. All are difficult to grow and to maintain in laboratory culture. The genus is differentiated from other brucellaceae primarily by its nutritional requirements. All species require one or other or both of two accessory growth substances—X factor or haematin and V factor or phosopho-pyridine nucleotide. Both of these factors are conveniently supplied in blood.

Haemophilus influenzae

Morphology

The morphology of this organism varies considerably. The type most frequently observed is a short coccobacillus measuring $1 \cdot 5 \times 0 \cdot 3\mu$. This is the type usually found in tissues and in body fluids. Sometimes the organisms are arranged in short chains suggesting streptococci. Some strains are more definitely bacillary and some are filamentous in type. The filaments in the latter often show irregularly placed swellings which may be as great as 2 to 3μ in diameter. There is a tendency for coccobacillary organisms to become filamentous on subculture. This is frequently, although not always, associated with an antigenic and colonial change analogous to S → R variation in the salmonellae and other Gram negative bacilli. The organisms tend to develop autolytic changes in culture. Degenerating forms stain poorly, sometimes showing bipolar staining. Fully virulent strains are capsulated.

Cultural Properties

Haemophilus influenzae is strictly aerobic, little if any growth occurring under anaerobic conditions. It requires both X and V factors for growth. On blood agar, colonies are just visible as very minute, clear, drop-like non-haemolytic dots at the end of 24 hours. Better growth is obtained on media in which the contents of the red cells have been liberated either by heat, as in the so-called 'chocolate' agar and in Levinthal's medium, or by tryptic digestion as in Fildes's medium. The latter two media have the advantage of being quite transparent; when grown on them capsulated strains yield iridescent colonies and non-capsulated strains non-iridescent colonies.

338

Morphologically typical coccobacillary strains and morphologically atypical filamentous strains can as a rule be distinguished by their colony appearance, the former giving smooth colonies and the latter slightly rough, granular colonies. Whether grown deliberately or accidentally in mixed culture with staphylococci, *H. influenzae* show the phenomenon of satellitism; this is a great increase in the size of the colonies in the immediate vicinity of a staphylococcal colony, and is due to the liberation of V factor from the staphylococcus. Biochemical reactions are of no importance in identification.

Haemophilus influenzae is a very delicate organism and dies out rapidly outside the body. It is particularly susceptible to drying. It is important therefore that culture should be carried out as soon as possible after the clinical material has been taken.

Haemophilus influenzae is of low pathogenicity for ordinary laboratory animals. In large doses by the intraperitoneal route it will cause death. This is, however, due to liberation of endotoxin rather than to invasion of the tissues. The endotoxin is probably chemically similar to the endotoxins of the enterobacteriaceae. Virulence is greatly enhanced if the organism is suspended in mucin, which appears to give considerable protection against the host's defences. Under these conditions small inocula will frequently produce a fatal infection.

Antigenic Structure

Capsulated strains can be divided into six serologic types—a to f—the type specificity of which depends on haptenic polysaccharides present in the capsule. Typing can be carried out either by the agglutination or capsule-swelling reactions. The capsules are readily lost in laboratory culture. Many of the strains isolated from normal throats and some of those obtained from lesions are non-capsulated on primary isolation. Type transformation of rough variants can be effected in the same way as with the pneumococcus.

Infections due to *Haemophilus influenzae*

Haemophilus influenzae owes its name to the belief, at one time widely held, that it was the cause of influenza. This belief arose from the frequency with which it was encountered in cases of influenza in the great pandemics of 1890 and 1918 to 1919. Many of the strains isolated were undoubtedly responsible for a secondary pneumonia complicating the disease, but others were almost certainly non-pathogenic commensals.

Haemophilus influenzae can frequently be isolated from the normal respiratory tract; these strains are usually non-capsulated and avirulent. The organism is frequently a secondary invader of the respiratory tract in influenza and is occasionally responsible for pneumonia complicating the disease. *H. influenzae* plays a role of great importance in the acute exacerbations occurring in the course of chronic bronchitis, and is apparently more frequently responsible for these exacerbations than any other organism.

Haemophilus influenzae is an important cause of acute pyogenic meningitis in children, ranking next in importance as a cause of this condition to meningococci and pneumococci. *H. influenzae* meningitis is sporadic in occurrence. The majority of infections occur in children under 2 years of age. In its pathogenesis the condition closely resembles meningococcal meningitis. The organism first sets up a focus of infection in the pharynx from which it invades the blood stream—meningeal involvement occurring as a result of this haematogenous spread. Occasionally the organism localizes in the joints, where it produces an acute pyogenic arthritis, or in the valves of the heart with the production of subacute bacterial endocarditis.

By direct spread from the nasopharynx, it may give rise to sinusitis, otitis media, and, in children, epiglottitis. In the last condition, the degree of oedema and inflammation produced may be so severe as to cause marked respiratory obstruction. *H. influenzae* is an occasional cause of acute conjunctivitis.

Diagnosis

In cases of *H. influenzae* meningitis the organisms can usually be demonstrated in Gram films of the centrifuged deposit from the cerebrospinal fluid, and as a rule show the typical coccobacillary morphology. They are characteristically found within the polymorphonuclear leucocytes.

Blood agar may be used for routine cultures from sputum, but when, as in meningitis, *H. influenzae* is sought specifically, its detection is rendered easier if one of the special media such as Levinthal's or Fildes's medium is used; these media, being transparent, permit the ready recognition of the characteristic iridescent colonies of capsulated strains. Their identity may be confirmed by the Neufeld reaction with specific antiserum, if this is available. The majority of infections are due to type b strains. If a specific antiserum is not available, the identification of *H. influenzae* may be achieved by demonstration of its specific growth requirements. In some cases, and particularly in cultures made from sputum, the phenomenon of satellitism may be observed and is of considerable value in identification.

In cases of *H. influenzae* meningitis it may be possible to detect the presence of type specific antigen in the cerebrospinal fluid by the ring precipitin technique.

Treatment

Chloramphenicol has so far been the antibiotic of choice in the treatment of meningitis on account of its ready diffusion into the cerebrospinal fluid. Clinical experience has shown that it is best combined with a sulphonamide. *H. influenzae* is also highly sensitive to ampicillin but this does not readily gain access to the cerebrospinal fluid. Its role in the therapy of *H. influenzae* meningitis has still to be determined. Both ampicillin and the tetracyclines have been used in the treatment and chemoprophylaxis of chronic bronchitis.

Haemophilus parainfluenzae and *Haemophilus haemolyticus*

These species, which are frequently found as respiratory commensals, produce colonies similar to those of *H. influenzae*. *H. parainfluenzae* resembles the non-capsulated strains of *H. influenzae* but differs in requiring V factor but not X factor for growth. It occurs as a respiratory commensal but can cause conjunctivitis and subacute bacterial endocarditis. *H. haemolyticus* requires both X and V factors and is haemolytic on blood agar.

Haemophilus ducreyi

This bacterium measures from 1·5 to 2·0μ by 0·5μ. In a soft chancre, and in the pus of a bubo, it commonly occurs in chains of from three to twenty bacilli, but solitary bacilli are seen either free or within pus cells. It is Gram negative, and frequently exhibits polar staining.

The organism is difficult to cultivate at first; a satisfactory medium consists of 3 per cent agar containing 25 to 30 per cent of defibrinated rabbit blood or rabbit, sheep or human blood which has been allowed to clot and to express its serum and has then been heated to 55° C for 15 minutes. In later cultures, X but not V factor is necessary for its growth.

The species is serologically homogeneous and may be specifically identified by the agglutination test.

Haemophilus ducreyi produces soft chancre or chancroid, a fairly common venereal disease, which may be confused with syphilis.

Patients with soft chancre develop a delayed-type skin reaction following intradermal injection of a killed suspension of the organism. Positive skin reactions may also be given by patients suffering from lymphogranuloma venereum. Hypersensitivity is demonstrable for many years after infection.

Haemophilus ducreyi shows the same susceptibility as *H. influenzae* to chemotherapeutic agents, but treatment with sulphonamides or streptomycin is preferred by most workers, since these drugs will not mask primary syphilitic lesions as may occur if the condition is treated with a drug active against *Treponema pallidum*.

Bordetella

The genus *Bordetella* differs from *Haemophilus* in not requiring X or V factors for growth.

Bordetella pertussis

Morphology

Bordetella pertussis is very similar to *H. influenzae* in morphology but is inclined to be more definitely bacillary and less pleomorphic. Capsules are demonstrable in young cultures.

Cultural Properties

Bordetella pertussis is difficult to isolate, requiring specially enriched media such as that of Bordet and Gengou, which is a glycerol potato extract agar containing a high concentration of defibrinated horse blood. The medium may be rendered considerably more selective by the addition, as recommended by

Lacey, of a diphenylamine (M & B 938) and of penicillin in a concentration of 0·25 units per ml. The colonies after 72 hours incubation are very small, glistening and with a pearly appearance. They are surrounded by a zone of haemolysis which has an ill-defined periphery. Although blood is required for its isolation *Bord. pertussis* can be grown in subculture on agar containing serum, albumen or charcoal. These substances do not supply a nutrient requirement but permit growth by neutralizing traces of oleic acid which are usually present in ordinary media and on glass ware, and to which *Bord. pertussis* is very sensitive. On prolonged subculture the organism will usually grow on ordinary agar.

Antigenic Structure

Bordetella pertussis is antigenically extremely complex, up to 14 different antigens having been recognized in various strains in agar gel diffusion tests. The most important of these antigens are the capsular and somatic antigens which function as agglutinogens, the heat-labile endotoxin, the histamine-sensitizing factor and the protective antigen. A number of heat-labile capsular antigens have been identified in individual strains; these occur in combinations of two or more and permit the recognition of a number of different serotypes. All the serotypes, however, share a common antigenic component—the type antigen 1. Because of this, antiserum compared against one strain of *Bord. pertussis* will agglutinate all other strains.

Capsular antigenic loss may occur by a reversible process, designated by Lacey as modulation, and by an irreversible process of mutation analogous to S → R variation amongst the salmonellae. As described by Lacey, modulation can be induced by altering the ionic composition of the growth medium. The normal capsulated form is designated X mode. Lacey distinguishes two non-capsulated forms or modes—I and C which differ from one another and from the X mode in somatic antigen composition. A common somatic antigen appears to be present in all three modes.

Freshly isolated strains of *Bord. pertussis* usually possess a haemagglutinin, active on the red cells of a variety of animal species. The haemagglutinin possesses significant activity only at high temperatures: 42 to 50° C. Haemagglutinin is demonstrable in culture supernatants, and can be extracted from the cell by simple washing; this suggests that it is present in the capsular layer. It is antigenic, and antibody to it can be measured by a haemagglutination inhibition test.

Like other Gram negative bacteria, *Bord. pertussis* possesses somatic antigens which consist of lipopolysaccharide protein complexes, the specificity of which is due to the polysaccharide component. Although endotoxic, the purified somatic antigens appear to have appreciably lower toxicity for experimental animals than the endotoxins of enterobacteriaceae. A heat-labile protein endotoxin has also been identified which appears to occur as an intracellular component. It is produced only by capsulated strains, and can be liberated by autolysis and by physical disruption of the cell. Although the toxin is strongly antigenic, antitoxin does not appear to be produced during the course of infection or as a result of artificial immunization. Because of this the role of the toxin in pathogenicity is equivocal.

A substance with the property of increasing sensitivity of mice to histamine occurs as a component of the cell wall. It is markedly heat labile, being destroyed in half an hour at 75° C. Like the toxin, it is found only in fully virulent capsulated organisms.

Immunization with a suitably prepared vaccine will produce a substantial degree of protection against pertussis. The nature of the antigen responsible for the stimulation of protective antibody is, however, still in doubt. It is clearly not identical with the somatic antigens, haemagglutinin, or the heat-labile endotoxin. Although it has physical properties similar to those of the histamine-sensitizing factor, the relative capacities of different preparations to stimulate protective antibody and to sensitize mice to histamine appear to vary independently. It has recently been suggested by Preston and Evans on the basis of intracerebral mouse protection tests, which appear to provide a valid index of the protective efficacy of pertussis vaccines for man, that the capacity to stimulate the production of protective antibody is a function of the capsular antigens. As against this identification, however, is the fact that organisms which possess no type-specific capsular antigens identified by agglutination tests, and belonging to Lacey's I and C modes, can nevertheless stimulate the development of protective antibody.

Whooping Cough

Bord. pertussis is an exclusively human pathogen. It is the cause of pertussis or whooping cough. Though present in large numbers in the respiratory secretions of infected patients it shows no tendency to spread elsewhere in the body. It is rarely recoverable from normal subjects.

Whooping cough is a disease of childhood. Its mortality has decreased considerably during recent years, but it is still one of the most serious of the epidemic childhood diseases. It is particularly dangerous in the very young child, over half the deaths occurring in the first year of life. It is probably more highly infectious than any other bacterial disease of the respiratory tract. Consequently children who have not been immunized and who come into contact with the disease are almost certain to contract it. Whooping cough is a disease of world-wide distribution and occurs mainly in epidemic form.

The clinical course of whooping cough can be divided into three stages. The first is a catarrhal stage, lasting about 14 days, during which the child has a mild but progressively increasing cough. The catarrhal stage is followed by the paroxysmal stage which lasts for a further fortnight; the typical paroxysmal cough is the most marked feature of this stage. The final or convalescent stage also lasts about 2 weeks.

In the early stages of infection, the organisms are mainly found in the trachea and the bronchi. In the later stages they invade the lung itself and may be observed in the alveoli. They may produce localized pneumonic changes in the lung tissue, but of more serious import is their capacity to predispose the lung to secondary invasion with pyogenic organisms. Atelectasis may result from blocking of the bronchioles with mucus and may lead to bronchiectasis, which causes serious and permanent damage to the lung tissue. Anoxaemia resulting from atelectasis and pulmonary infiltration is responsible for the convulsions which occur in a small proportion of cases. Whooping cough is sometimes followed by an encephalitis, the precise pathogenesis of which is unknown.

Diagnosis

Plates of Bordet and Gengou's medium, or some modification of it (p. 341), may be inoculated by spreading a specimen of sputum, by allowing the patient to cough on the plate and so distribute droplets containing the organism over its surface (cough plate method) or, best of all, by spreading material collected with a swab from the posterior nasopharyngeal wall. The latter can be obtained by West's postnasal swab—this is a curved swab which is inserted through the mouth to the nasopharynx—or better still by a perinasal swab inserted along the floor of the nose. The organisms are identified on the basis of morphology, colony form and agglutination by specific antiserum. The fluorescent antibody technique has been favourably reported on for the direct demonstration of the organism in nasopharyngeal swabs.

A slide agglutination test with a suspension of living organisms is sometimes used to detect antibody in the patient's serum. It has the limitation of giving a positive result only when the disease is well established—usually not before the third week. A complement fixation test is also used.

Treatment

The wide-spectrum antibiotics—chloramphenicol and the tetracyclines—are reported to be of value in the treatment of pertussis. They appear, however, to be effective only if given at an early stage of the disease, being of little value in cases of more than one week's duration. Good results have been claimed for treatment with gamma globulin from individuals who have been immunized with pertussis vaccine, but its value is not generally agreed.

Prophylaxis

A high degree of protection can be given against pertussis by immunization with a killed vaccine. The strains used must be carefully selected and must be fully toxic organisms which have not undergone $S \to R$ variation. Pertussis immunization is usually combined with immunization against tetanus and diphtheria (p. 289). In infants and young children reactions following vaccination are negligible. Severe reactions may, however, occur in children of school-going age. The development of an encephalopathy some hours after injection has been described, but fortunately is extremely rare.

It is claimed that gamma globulin obtained from adults injected repeatedly with pertussis vaccine is capable of conferring passive protection. The value of this procedure is *sub judice*.

Bordetella parapertussis

This organism which has been isolated from cases of mild whooping cough is very similar to *Bord. pertussis* in its cultural properties. Like the latter it produces a dermonecrotic toxin and is haemolytic on blood agar. It can be distinguished by the following criteria: it grows more luxuriantly on Bordet-Gengou medium on which it produces a brownish black discoloration; it produces catalase; though it possesses some antigenic components in common with *Bord. pertussis* the two species can be distinguished serologically.

Moraxella lacunata
(Morax-Axenfeld bacillus)

Moraxella lacunata is a very small, aerobic, non-motile, non-sporing, Gram negative bacillus which is the causative agent of a type of catarrhal conjunctivitis. In conjunctival exudates the organisms are characteristically found in pairs. *Moraxella lacunata* will not grow on ordinary agar and grows poorly on blood agar; it is most readily isolated on Löffler's serum on which, after 24 hours' incubation, it produces small colonies which are very difficult to see. The colonies are surrounded by a depression in the medium due to liquefaction of the serum. It does not require either X or V factors for growth. Like the neisseriae, *Moraxella lacunata* gives a positive oxidase reaction and is highly susceptible to penicillin.

CHAPTER 25

THE BRUCELLAE

The brucellae are very minute, Gram negative, non-motile, non-sporing rods which may be so short as to appear coccal in morphology. Capsules have been described as being present in freshly isolated strains, but if this is correct they are soon lost. Three species are recognized: *Brucella abortus, Brucella melitensis* and *Brucella suis*. Two other species—*Brucella ovis* and *Brucella neotoma*—have been proposed for strains isolated from rams and wood rats respectively but their inclusion in the genus has not yet been generally agreed.

Cultural Properties

The brucellae are aerobic, but primary growth from small inocula is improved by mild reducing conditions. They will grow on ordinary media but growth is slow. For isolation, enriched media—liver extract broth and liver extract agar—have been widely used, but more modern media—serum dextrose agar and Albimi agar—appear to give better results. Growth on artificial media is slow and colonies may not become visible for 48 hours. When freshly isolated the colonies are smooth, circular, convex and translucent, but these organisms readily undergo $S \rightarrow R$ variation to yield a slightly rough, yellowish brown colony.

Conventional fermentation tests are of little value in differentiating the different *Brucella* species. For this purpose the following criteria have been widely used: (1) Requirement for CO_2 on primary isolation. *Br. abortus* will grow on primary culture only in the presence of a high concentration—*circa* 10 per cent—of CO_2. (2) Production of H_2S. When grown on liver extract agar *Br. abortus* and American strains of *Br. suis* produce H_2S for at least 4 days. *Br. melitensis* and Danish strains of *Br. suis* either do not produce H_2S or produce a small amount detectable for one day only. (3) Sensitivity to certain dyes, of which thionine and basic fuchsin are the most generally useful. The dyes are usually incorporated in the growth medium; the optimum concentration of dye depends to some extent on the medium used but usually lies between $1/30,000$ and $1/60,000$ for thionine and between $1/25,000$ and $1/50,000$ for basic fuchsin. In recent years, however, an increasing number of isolates have been found which have shown atypical cultural and antigenic reactions. For the classification of these two further types of tests have been used.

1. Metabolic tests to determine the capacity of the organisms to oxidize a variety of amino acids and sugars. The substrates of most differential value in these tests are glutamic acid, ornithine, lysine and ribose. Glutamic acid is

oxidized by *Br. melitensis*, *Br. abortus* and most strains of *Br. suis*; ornithine and lysine only by *Br. suis* and ribose by *Br. suis* and *Br. abortus*.

2. Determination of the susceptibility of the organisms to a bacteriophage which is only significantly active against *Br. abortus*. On the evidence available these latter tests would appear to be more satisfactory than the classical biochemical, cultural and antigenic tests for species classification.

DIFFERENTIATION OF *Brucella* SPECIES

	Br. melitensis	Br. abortus	Br. suis
Usual reservoir	Sheep, goats	Cattle	Pigs
Require 5–10% CO_2	−	(+)	−
H_2S production	−	(+)	(++)
Growth in presence of			
Thionine	(+)	(−)	+
Basic fuchsin	+	(+)	(−)
Predominant antigen	(M)	(A)	A
Sensitivity to specific brucella phage	−	(+)	−
Oxidation of:*			
Glutamic acid	+	+	(+)
Ornithine	−	−	+
Ribose	−	+	+

Adapted from S. S. Elberg (1965).

Signs without brackets indicate invariable reactions. Signs within brackets indicate commonest reactions.

Variations within each species in respect of CO_2 requirement, H_2S production, dye susceptibility and predominant antigen permit differentiation of biotypes. The less common biotypes usually have a restricted geographic distribution.

* Other substrates used: L-lysine, D- and L-alanine, L-arginine, L-asparagine, L-arabinose, D-galactose, D-xylose.

Antigenic Structure

The behaviour of the brucellae in agglutination tests has been explained by Miles on the assumption that they possess two antigens, A and M, which are present in each of the species in different proportions, A being the dominant antigen in *Br. abortus* and *Br. suis*, and M the dominant antigen in *Br. melitensis*. Sera prepared against any of the species will contain antibody against both antigens but can be rendered monospecific for either antigen by controlled absorption with a strain in which the other antigen is the major component. Monospecific sera agglutinate only organisms in which the corresponding antigen is present as the major component, but a minority of strains are agglutinable by both antisera. Work in recent years has indicated that the antigenic composition of the brucellae is more diverse than was originally thought, some strains which are biochemically and culturally *Br. abortus*, reacting with anti-M but not with anti-A sera, and strains which are biochemically and culturally *Br. melitensis*, reacting with anti-A and not with anti-M sera. In addition, examination by the Ouchterlony plate method (p. 132) has shown the occurrence in the brucellae of a large number of antigens capable of precipitating with antibody. These tests have not so far revealed any species-specific antigens, and the relationship between the agglutinogens and the antigens demonstrable by the Ouchterlony method has not yet been defined. Some antigenic overlap has been demonstrated between the brucellae and *Vibrio, Pasteurella* and *Salmonella* species. This overlap must be remembered in the interpretation of diagnostic agglutination tests and antibody responses.

The brucellae undergo S → R transformation more quickly than do most other bacteria. Even when the change has not been completed, the three species are antigenically indistinguishable. The S → R change may occur without the development of spontaneous agglutinability in saline. In such a case it may be detected by incubation of a suspension of the organism with 1/1000 acriflavine at 37° C; if the strain is rough, it is agglutinated by acriflavine.

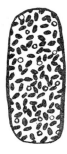 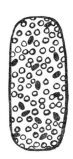

O = BR. ABORTUS ANTIGEN (A)
● = BR. MELITENSIS ANTIGEN (M)

FIG. 26. ANTIGENIC COMPOSITION OF BRUCELLAE
Left *Br. melitensis*   Right *Br. abortus*
Br. suis resembles *Br. abortus*, but with a lower A to M ratio.

Undulant Fever

The brucellae are primarily animal pathogens; cattle, goats and pigs are particularly affected and are the main source of human infections. Under natural conditions infection of goats and sheep is mainly due to *Br. melitensis*, infection of cattle to *Br. abortus* and infection of pigs to *Br. suis*. *Br. abortus* infection of cattle is widespread throughout the world. Infection of goats and sheep with *Br. melitensis* mainly occurs in Mediterranean countries. *Br. suis* infection of pigs though occurring in various parts of the world, mostly in a sporadic form, is found as an epizootic infection mainly in the pig rearing areas of the U.S.

In cattle, goats and sheep the brucellae are responsible, on primary infection, for a form of contagious abortion. When established in a herd, however, they give rise to chronic and latent infection with abortion as an infrequent manifestation. Infected animals excrete the organism freely in the uterine discharges, in the faeces and in the urine. In most cases the organisms localize in the mammary glands and are excreted in the milk; this is of particular importance in the transmission of infection to man. In pigs, however, abortion is infrequent and the mammary glands are rarely involved.

In man the brucellae give rise to three types of infection: (1) Latent infections, which can be detected only by serological methods. These appear to be common in persons whose occupation brings them into contact with infected animals. (2) Acute infections, the most prominent feature of which is a daily or diurnal remitting fever which is responsible for the name—undulant fever—by which they are commonly known. This type of fever occurs most typically in *Br. melitensis* infections. It has in the past been generally assumed that the fever is due to the liberation of brucellae into the blood stream from their sites of multiplication in the reticulo-endothelial system. This view is almost certainly incorrect. It is considerably more likely that it is due to the liberation of endogenous pyrogens from polymorphonuclear leucocytes. In addition to fever and toxaemia there may be a wide variety of symptoms referable to involvement of particular organs. Lymph nodes, liver and spleen—the chief sites of the reticulo-endothelial system are frequently enlarged. There may also be evidence of hepatitis, cholecystitis, subacute bacterial endocarditis or osteomyelitis. As a general rule *Br. melitensis* and *Br. suis* cause more serious clinical disease than *Br. abortus*. Pyogenic lesions are relatively frequent in infections caused by *Br. suis*. (3) Chronic low-grade infections usually showing periodic exacerbations. Pyrexia may be slight or absent—the common clinical manifestations being sweating, lassitude and joint pains. In this type of infection which usually occurs as a sequel to an acute infection the organisms can only rarely be isolated from the blood. In contrast to its occurrence in animals, abortion appears to be a rare event in man.

Brucellosis is primarily a disease of the reticulo-endothelial system, in which the organisms multiply with the production of a granulomatous tissue reaction. The brucellae have an unusual predilection for intracellular growth, and may be demonstrated inside phagocytic cells, endothelial cells and fibrocytes. Their intracellular location explains the difficulties found clinically in the satisfactory treatment of brucellosis by chemotherapeutic agents and also why the condition can persist for a long time in the presence of a high titre of circulating antibody. Evidence has been presented by Sulkin that in the cells of experimentally infected animals the brucellae persist as L forms; this might conceivably explain their persistence in the body in the presence of a high concentration of antibody. There is some evidence that spontaneous recovery from *Brucella* infection may be largely due to a cellular immunity analogous to that found in tuberculosis. This cellular immunity appears to require the co-operation of an unidentified serum factor. In the guinea-pig the immunity appears to be non-specific, being active also against other intracellular parasites, e.g. the tubercle bacillus and *Listeria monocytogenes*.

The brucellae appear to spread from the initial site of introduction, via lymphatic channels, to the local lymph glands in the cells of which they multiply. From the lymph glands they are discharged into the blood stream by which they are disseminated to other reticulo-endothelial sites throughout the body. They have a particular predilection for the placenta which they appear to reach via the lumen of the uterus. Their predilection for the placenta may possibly be due to the presence of erythritol which has been found to stimulate the growth of brucellae in culture. They multiply within the placental cells, and it is generally believed that abortion is due to a necrotizing action of the locally produced endotoxin.

Brucellosis is commonest in individuals, e.g. veterinarians and farmers, who work with infected animals. The organisms may gain entry to the body through abrasions in the skin, through the conjunctiva, through the alimentary tract and possibly also through the respiratory tract. Individuals of the general population may also become infected—almost invariably as a result of the ingestion of infected cow's or goat's milk, consumed in the raw state. In milk products, e.g. butter and cheese, the organisms die out rapidly and these are rarely if ever sources of infection. The incidence of overt brucellosis in persons known to have consumed infected milk is very low. This would seem to indicate a high degree of resistance in man to infection by the alimentary route.

Diagnosis

The most consistently successful method of diagnosis is by the demonstration of antibodies in the patient's serum. In a well-established case titres, in the Felix method, of up to 1 in 5000 are frequently found. In some cases of brucellosis the patient's serum shows the presence of a marked prozone, i.e. inhibition of agglutination in the higher serum concentrations in agglutination tests. In chronic infections agglutination titres may be low or absent. That in such cases the serum may nevertheless contain a high titre of a non-agglutinating antibody may be shown by the use of the antiglobulin test (p. 130). This antibody is mercapto-ethanol resistant, has a marked capacity to fix complement and can be shown in antiglobulin tests with antisera specific for the main immunoglobulin classes (p. 99) to be IgG, though some IgA which does not fix complement is also usually present. By contrast the agglutinating antibodies present in the sera of acute cases are of the IgM class though as can be shown by their mercapto-ethanol resistance considerable amounts of IgG are also normally present. In acute infections IgM antibodies appear before IgG antibodies and persist for longer periods after clinical cure. This chronological sequence and the predominance of IgG in chronic infections are probably due to the fact that IgG antibodies are produced only in response to a substantial antigenic stimulus such as would be represented by the continued multiplication of brucellae in the body.

The persistence of antibody after infection is variable. In some cases it falls rapidly to a low level but in others it persists at a high level for some years. It is possible that some of the latter cases are examples of persistent latent infection.

An attempt should also be made to isolate the organism from the blood. It is frequently stated that the chance of obtaining a positive blood culture is greatest if the blood is taken at the height of a pyrexial period. This is largely based on the assumption that the fever is due to the liberation of organisms into the blood from the reticulo-endothelial system. There is considerable doubt, however, as to whether this view is correct. It is probably more important to make persistent attempts to isolate the organism than to choose a particular time for doing so. Even then blood culture is often unsuccessful. Blood culture may be carried out using liver extract broth, glucose serum broth or by Castaneda's method, in which a mixture of blood and broth is poured over the surface of agar in a specially prepared bottle. Cultures should be incubated in an atmosphere of 5 to 10 per cent CO_2.

It may on occasion be possible to isolate the organisms from the bone marrow or from lymph glands. They have also been isolated from the cerebrospinal fluid, bile and urine.

The most satisfactory way of demonstrating the presence of *Br. abortus* in milk is by intraperitoneal or subcutaneous injection of a guinea-pig. The demonstration of agglutinins in the serum of the guinea-pig a few weeks after inoculation strongly suggests that the milk injected contained *Br. abortus*. Complete proof is afforded by killing the animal 2 months after inoculation and cultivating the organism from spleen and lymphatic glands. The milk of infected cows contains agglutinins, the demonstration of which is of considerable diagnostic value in animals which have not been inoculated with S19 vaccine (see below).

During the course of infection, a delayed type of hypersensitivity develops and may be demonstrated by intradermal injection of killed organisms or of various types of extract (*brucellin, brucellergin*). Skin tests have the same limitation as the tuberculin reaction (p. 364) as diagnostic procedures in that they give positive results not only if the patient is suffering from an active infection but also if he has had a prior infection. They are, however, of value in population surveys to determine the overall incidence of brucella infection. Many of the reagents which have been advocated for skin testing have the disadvantage, from the point of view of serological diagnosis, that they stimulate antibody production.

Treatment

The brucellae are susceptible to the wide-spectrum antibiotics. It is claimed that the best results in the treatment of brucellosis are given by combined antibiotic therapy. Although marked symptomatic improvement is readily achieved it has, however, been found difficult to ensure complete sterilization of the patient's tissues by antibiotic therapy. Relapses are frequent even after prolonged treatment and are probably due to the release of organisms from intracellular sites of multiplication in which they are inaccessible to chemotherapeutic agents.

Prophylaxis

Brucellosis in animals is difficult to control. Attempts may be made to build up brucella-free herds of cattle by eliminating all animals whose sera show a significant level of *Brucella* agglutinins but it is difficult to maintain them free from infection. Immunization with a live vaccine prepared from the attenuated S19 strain of *Br. abortus* confers a substantial degree of immunity and has been widely used for the prophylaxis of the disease in cattle. This strain has, however, appreciable virulence for pregnant animals and for man. As a result veterinary surgeons not infrequently become accidentally infected. In those with prior brucella infection accidental inoculation can produce severe allergic reactions. A considerable drawback to the S19 strain for animal immunization is its marked capacity to stimulate the production of agglutinating antibodies. When used widely in animals therefore it greatly diminishes the value of agglutination tests as diagnostic procedures. Recently, an attenuated strain, 45/20, has been introduced, which has the advantage of being non-agglutinogenic. Unfortunately, it is much less stably attenuated than S19. Consequently, recent work has been concerned with the preparation of suitable killed vaccines from this strain. The value of such vaccines in immunization programmes requires further assessment.

Brucellosis occurring in members of the general population who are infected by ingestion of infected milk may be eliminated by the pasteurization of all milk destined for human consumption. Vaccination of individuals whose occupation exposes them to infection has so far only been attempted in the U.S.S.R.

CHAPTER 26

THE MYCOBACTERIA

The mycobacteria are slender, non-capsulated, non-motile, non-sporing rods. They are very difficult to stain but when stained the stain cannot be removed by treatment with strong mineral acid. Because of this they are known as *acid-fast bacilli*.

The genus includes both pathogenic and saprophytic species. The former are more difficult to grow and are in general more acid-fast than the latter. The most important of the pathogens are the tubercle bacilli and the leprosy bacillus—*Mycobacterium leprae*.

Mycobacteria have a much higher lipid content than other organisms, the lipids, mainly phospholipids (or phosphatides) and various waxes, appear to occur primarily as components of the cell wall. On hydrolysis a variety of fatty acids have been obtained, some of which, branched-chain fatty acids—tuberculostearic, phthienoic, mycocerosic and mycolic acids—are apparently unique to the mycobacteria. It is probable that the high lipid content of the mycobacteria is responsible for many of their biological properties.

1. Acid-fastness is believed to be due to the presence of mycolic acid, a component of various wax fractions.

2. The lipids probably confer a low permeability to water-soluble compounds, which might explain the resistance of tubercle bacilli to chemical disinfection.

3. There is considerable evidence that the high lipid content of the tubercle bacillus plays a major part in determining the type of tissue reaction it evokes in the animal body. This renders it difficult to dispose of, as a result of which it stimulates a granulomatous foreign-body type of reaction. In addition the wax D component (p. 182), for some reason as yet unexplained, plays a decisive role in inducing delayed-type hypersensitivity.

Tubercle Bacilli

There are five distinct varieties of tubercle bacilli: human, bovine, avian, murine and piscine. Only the human and bovine varieties cause tuberculosis in man. These, though formerly assigned to the same species, are now usually designated as separate species—the human variety as *Mycobacterium tuberculosis*, and the bovine variety as *Mycobacterium bovis*. The avian, murine and piscine varieties produce lesions resembling those of human tuberculosis in birds, voles and fish respectively, and are now classified as separate species, *Mycobacterium avium*, *Mycobacterium microti* and *Mycobacterium marinum*, respectively.

In the description which follows we will be concerned only with the properties of *Myco. tuberculosis* and *Myco. bovis*.

Morphology

Mycobacterium tuberculosis is a thin, straight or slightly curved rod measuring from 2 to 5μ by 0·3μ. By contrast *Myco. bovis* tends to be somewhat shorter and thicker. The organisms may stain uniformly or present a beaded, irregularly stained appearance. In the tissues the bacilli occur singly, in pairs arranged at an angle, or in clusters of organisms usually lying parallel to one another. In cultures of virulent organisms clusters or 'cords' of parallel bacilli are a characteristic feature.

Tubercle bacilli are both acid- and alcohol-fast and are normally demonstrated microscopically by the Ziehl-Neelsen technique. They may also be demonstrated by fluorescence microscopy (p. 39). There is some evidence that when growing in the tissues non-acid-fast forms of the organism occur.

Cultural Properties

Tubercle bacilli grow slowly, their average generation time being about 24 hours, and prolonged incubation of cultures is therefore necessary. On primary culture colonies are not usually visible in less than 10 to 14 days. They are strict aerobes and grow best at 37° C.

For isolation, coagulated egg media, e.g. Löwenstein's medium, are those most frequently employed. Although special media are required for their isolation, tubercle bacilli are not nutritionally exacting. On subculture they grow well on simple synthetic media incorporating an ammonium salt or amino acid, e.g. asparagine, as nitrogen source, and glucose, provided a large inoculum is employed. They will not grow in such media, however, from small inocula; this is apparently because they are highly susceptible to the toxic action of very small amounts of various substances, particularly of fatty acids, which may occur as impurities in reagents and on glassware. The toxic action of these substances can be neutralized by the addition of serum or serum albumen. A simple fluid medium containing albumen and a synthetic fatty acid ester, known commercially as Tween 80 (sorbitan mono-oleate), is widely used in experimental work and in sensitivity testing. Tween 80 stimulates the growth of the organism and also causes it to grow in a dispersed fashion rather than in the clumps found in the ordinary fluid media.

On primary culture *Myco. tuberculosis* and *Myco. bovis* show characteristic differences in cultural characteristics. On egg media the human type produces a dry wrinkled warty growth. The individual colonies have a thin uneven edge and tend to spread out over the surface of the medium. *Myco. bovis* grows much less luxuriantly and yields a growth which is more powdery and less cohesive than that of *Myco. tuberculosis*. The individual colonies have entire even edges and show little tendency to spread over the surface of the medium. This type of growth is referred to as *dysgonic* in contrast to the more profuse growth of *Myco. tuberculosis* which is described as *eugonic*. The types differ also in the way in which they respond to the presence of glycerol. Glycerol in a concentration of 0·75 per cent has a stimulating effect of the growth of the human type but has no such effect on the growth of the bovine type. In fact the growth of some strains of *Myco. bovis* may be slightly inhibited. These differences are reliably demonstrable only on primary culture—on subculture the growth of *Myco. bovis* tending to resemble that of *Myco. tuberculosis*. Growth characteristics cannot

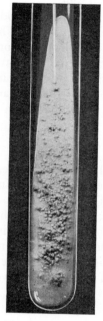

FIG. 27. CULTURE OF TUBERCLE BACILLUS (HUMAN VARIETY) ($\times \frac{1}{2}$)

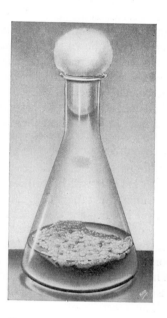

FIG. 28. CULTURE OF TUBERCLE BACILLUS (HUMAN VARIETY) ON SURFACE OF GLYCEROL BROTH

be relied on exclusively for the differentiation of the two species since some strains are culturally atypical. The species may be differentiated by pathogenicity tests. Both are pathogenic for guinea-pigs, which develop a local caseous lesion and signs of disseminated tuberculosis, but *Myco. bovis* alone is highly pathogenic for rabbits. The niacin test is also of considerable value in species differentiation. This compound is readily demonstrable in cultures of *Myco. tuberculosis* but not, or only to slight extent, in cultures of *Myco. bovis*.

Antigenic Structure

A variety of antigenic components, both proteins and polysaccharides have been identified in tubercle bacilli. Of these the most important are the protein antigens, known collectively as *tuberculoprotein* or *tuberculin* and which are capable of eliciting the allergic reactions demonstrable in the tuberculin test. Slight antigenic differences can be shown between the tuberculins of *Myco. tuberculosis* and *Myco. bovis* but they are nevertheless so similar that they behave virtually identically in skin tests. Protein antigens which cross-react serologically with the tuberculoproteins of these species are also present in *Myco. avium*, leprosy bacilli and saprophytic mycobacteria. Most of the tuberculoproteins capable of eliciting the tuberculin reaction appear to occur as cell wall components. At least one cytoplasmic protein, however, will elicit skin reactions in animals hypersensitive to tuberculin, and there is some evidence that this gives a more species-specific reaction than the proteins of the cell wall.

Tubercle bacilli have been examined serologically by a variety of methods—agglutination, complement fixation and the Ouchterlony technique. These studies have shown that the mammalian type bacilli form a serologically homogeneous group readily distinguishable from saprophytic and atypical mycobacteria, but nevertheless sharing antigens with them. Serological tests have not been of practical value, however, in the identification and differentiation of mycobacteria, since they do not permit the degree of resolution which can be achieved by cultural methods.

Pathogenicity

The pathological changes occurring in tuberculosis will not be considered in detail here. It will be sufficient to recall that in the tissues of infected animals and man the tubercle bacillus causes the production of a characteristic and unique lesion—the tubercle. In its typical form the tubercle shows a peripheral zone of fibroblasts and lymphocytes, an inner zone of epithelioid cells, and in its centre one or more giant cells. As it increases in size necrosis of the central portion occurs. The necrotic material is not normally digested; consequently it has a cheesy appearance and consistency on account of which it is known as caseous, i.e. cheesy material.

The reaction of the tissues to tubercle bacilli is basically similar to their reaction to foreign bodies which cannot be broken down by normal disposal procedures. In the case of the tubercle bacillus this type of response is primarily determined by its high lipid content. This view is supported by the finding that tubercle-like lesions can be produced in experimental animals by the injection of lipid fractions obtained from the bacillus. The necrotic changes found in the tubercle are clearly the result of tuberculoprotein hypersensitivity which develops during the course of the infection. Since there is no evidence that the tissue cells are themselves sensitized, the mechanism by which they are damaged is obscure. It is possible that, during the course of infection, tuberculin may be adsorbed to the surface of the cell, and that the cell is damaged by interaction of the tuberculin on its surface with sensitized lymphocytes and/or macrophages. Alternatively, the tissue damage may be the result of a direct reaction between tuberculin and the sensitized lymphocytes and macrophages; as a result some toxic substance may be produced which has a direct action on the tissue cells or may affect these indirectly by damaging the blood vessels.

Normally, when necrosis of tissue occurs the necrosed tissue is digested by tissue proteolytic enzymes. In caseous lesions, however, this normal proteolysis is inhibited, presumably due to the inhibition of tissue proteases. It has been suggested that the inhibitor is a lipid component of the bacillus.

Although the phosphatide and tuberculoprotein of the tubercle bacillus may account for the microscopic anatomy of tuberculous lesions they are present in attenuated bacilli which are unable to establish a progressive infection. Some other factor or factors must therefore be required for virulence. The nature of this virulence factor is, however, still in dispute. In this connexion the isolation by Bloch from virulent bacilli, by extraction with petrol ether, of a lipid claimed to have a toxic action on tissue cells and leucocytes and capable of inhibiting leucocyte migration has aroused considerable interest. Since extraction with petrol ether disrupts the cords invariably found in virulent cultures the lipid has been designated 'cord factor'. 'Cord factor' is a component of the wax fraction of the tubercle bacillus, and has been identified as a complex of mycolic acid and trehalose. Since, however, the factor is present in attenuated tubercle bacilli and saprophytic mycobacteria its role in virulence is not clear.

Killed tubercle bacilli have considerable toxicity for experimental animals on injection but a similar toxicity is shown by the saprophytic mycobacteria. This toxicity presumably contributes to the overall effect of tuberculosis infection.

Tuberculosis

Tuberculosis is a disease of world-wide prevalence and is responsible for more serious illness than any other of the infectious diseases. Over the last century, however, its incidence in most countries has diminished enormously. Thus the mortality in England and Wales in 1855 was 3626 per million; by 1960 it had fallen to 75 per million. Some of this fall has undoubtedly been due to an improvement in social conditions, but in recent years the improvement has been mainly due to the introduction of chemotherapy, effective case finding and prophylaxis by BCG vaccination. Ultimately, it should be possible by the application of these measures to achieve complete eradication of the disease.

In communities where there is a high prevalence of the disease the majority of people make their first contact with the tubercle bacillus in childhood and as a result develop a primary childhood infection—generally of pulmonary type. This type of infection has a high tendency to spontaneous cure. In those who have recovered from it, it leaves an appreciable but by no means complete resistance to reinfection. At the same time it renders the tissues hypersensitive or allergic so that they react quite differently to future contact with the tubercle bacillus. This change in reactivity is demonstrable by the various types of tuberculin test. Until recently a high rate of childhood infection has been the rule in the British Isles and in most European countries. Thus it has been a frequent finding that 90 to 100 per cent of young adults in urban areas have given a positive tuberculin reaction. In these circumstances most cases of adult tuberculosis have been due to reinfection of individuals who had recovered from, but were sensitized by, a primary childhood infection. With the marked fall in the prevalence of the disease in recent years, however, this position is rapidly changing. Childhood infection is now much less frequent and many people are in consequence becoming infected for the first time in adult life.

Pulmonary tuberculosis is the commonest form of the disease; it is almost invariably due to the human-type bacillus. Infection appears to occur mainly by inhalation of droplets or droplet nuclei from an infected case. Tubercle bacilli remain viable in contaminated dust for a considerable time, and it was at one time thought that this was an important, possibly the major source of infection. Dust particles, however, appear to be almost invariably greater than 5μ in diameter—the upper limit of size above which particles are normally incapable of gaining access to the alveoli to initiate a pulmonary infection.

It is believed that some of the pulmonary infections occurring in adult life are endogenous in origin, i.e. that they arise from organisms persisting in the apparently healed lesions of a primary childhood infection. These organisms might be activated by a variety of debilitating factors. It is also possible that a slight contact with the tubercle bacillus insufficient in itself to give rise to progressive infection might activate a latent lesion by producing a focal allergic reaction.

The pulmonary lesions in childhood infection show some striking differences from those in the adult. They are usually relatively slight and in most cases undergo fairly rapid resolution. In a small proportion of cases, however, the disease is not arrested and assumes a rapidly progressive form. In the adult on the other hand the lesions are much more chronic and with little tendency to spontaneous cure. There is also considerable destruction of tissue with caseation and cavity formation. In childhood there is invariably an involvement of the mediastinal glands; in the adult this mediastinal involvement does not occur. These differences are usually attributed to the operation in the adult of allergy and immunity resulting from childhood infection. Nowadays, however, first infection occurs more frequently in adult life than formerly and in most of these cases the lesions are still those of classical adult type. This may be due to the fact that immunity and allergy develop more rapidly in the adult than in the child.

Infection with bovine bacilli is almost invariably due to the consumption of milk from an infected cow. In European countries and in America it is now, as a result of the effective control of the disease in bovines, very uncommon. These infections occur mostly in children, and usually present as abdominal tuberculosis with involvement of mesenteric glands.

Once a focus of infection has become established in the tissues the disease can spread by direct extension, through natural channels, by the lymphatics and by the blood. As a result of direct extension, microscopic tubercles coalesce to form tubercles visible to the naked eye. These in turn coalesce to form large areas of caseation. Direct extension of the infection is facilitated by transport of bacilli from diseased tissue to normal tissue by phagocytic cells. The transported bacilli then set up secondary foci of infection. Direct extension of the lesion, if unchecked, ultimately results in gross destruction of the organ involved. Lymphatic spread is best exemplified in the spread to the hilar glands, which is an invariable occurrence in the primary pulmonary infections of childhood. Haematogenous spread may be of a massive character with the development of multiple metastic lesions which occur primarily in the lungs, and often in other organs as well. This type is known as miliary tuberculosis, since the multiple lesions in the lungs appear like millet seeds. Massive haematogenous dissemination usually occurs as a result of ulceration of a lesion into a vein.

Frequently the haematogenous spread is of a less dramatic type and single metastatic foci are set up in a variety of organs. These are found most frequently in bones, joints, brain, meninges and the kidneys. The initial focus of infection may, in these cases, be quite overshadowed by the clinical features of the metastatic lesion, and may in fact have resolved before the appearance of the latter. Both lymphatic and haematogenous spread occur mainly as complications of primary tuberculosis.

Age is an important factor in determining the severity of the disease. In children of less than 5 years, and particularly in infants, the mortality is high. In children of from 5 to 15 years the mortality is low and asymptomatic latent infection is usual: this is the age group of typical childhood primary tuberculosis. These differences appear to be due entirely to differences in physiological susceptibility; the milder disease in the older child is not due to acquired immunity. After 15 years of age the mortality from the disease again increases.

In experimental animals genetic factors are of considerable importance in determining susceptibility to tuberculosis. Evidence that a genetic factor is also of importance in man is provided by the finding that in twins of which one is infected infection of the second twin is commoner when they are identical than when they are non-identical. There is also epidemiological evidence that resistance to infection is greatly diminished by malnutrition. In Great Britain and Germany there was a considerable increase in the incidence of the disease in both world wars, an incidence which is usually attributed to a lowering of nutritional status. That nutrition affects susceptibility receives considerable support from experiments of Dubos, who found that the susceptibility of mice to experimental infection could be greatly increased by feeding them on a protein poor diet. Mice in a state of nutritional deficiency may even develop progressive lesions following inoculation of the attenuated BCG strain. A very marked predisposition to tuberculosis is found in patients suffering from silicosis, a disease in which a progressive fibrosis of the lungs occurs as a result of the inhalation of particles of silica.

Allergy in Tuberculosis

The development of allergy in the course of tuberculosis infection was first demonstrated by Koch, and the reaction of the tuberculous animal to reinfection is in consequence known as Koch's phenomenon. When a normal guinea-pig is injected subcutaneously with a suspension of tubercle bacilli a slight local nodule forms within some hours and disappears in a few days. After about 10 to 14 days a hard nodule appears, which breaks down to form an ulcer. The infection spreads to the local lymphatic glands, which become large and caseous, and ultimately becomes disseminated through the body. If, on the other hand, a tuberculous guinea-pig, which has been infected some 4 to 6 weeks previously, is injected, a small area of swelling develops within about 48 hours and rapidly progresses to form a shallow ulcer. The ulcer heals within a short time and there is no involvement of the local lymphatic glands. Koch found also that similar local inflammatory reactions could be produced in tuberculous guinea-pigs by the injection of killed bacilli or of small amounts of tuberculin. Following the injection of tuberculin the tuberculous animal develops a severe and often fatal systemic reaction. In addition to this general reaction there occurs also a local reaction at the site of the injection and a marked focal reaction around the tuberculous lesions in the tissues, the main feature of which is a gross enlargement of the capillaries.

These reactions of the tuberculous animal are due to allergy to tuberculoprotein which is acquired during the course of the initial infection. Allergy may also be induced by the injection of killed tubercle bacilli but not by the injection of tuberculoprotein per se. It can, however, be produced by injection of tuberculoprotein together with a wax extracted from the bacillus (p. 182).

In man, as in the guinea-pig, allergy to tuberculoprotein develops as a result of tuberculous infection. After recovery from infection the allergic state persists for many years even in the absence of further contact with the tubercle bacillus. It may be demonstrated in a variety of ways in all of which tuberculoprotein is applied to or injected into the skin. These procedures are known as tuberculin tests and are widely used both to indicate that an individual has at some time suffered from a tuberculous infection and to a lesser extent for the diagnosis of a current infection (p. 365).

For tuberculin testing tuberculoprotein is used either in the form of Old Tuberculin or PPD. The name Old Tuberculin is the name applied to a preparation obtained by the original method of Koch. It consists of a filtered glycerol broth culture of the tubercle bacillus concentrated to one tenth of its original volume by evaporation. PPD is a highly purified preparation of tuberculoprotein prepared from the growth of the bacillus in a special synthetic medium. Since it is purer than Old Tuberculin and therefore less likely to give rise to non-specific reactions PPD is now the reagent of choice for skin testing.

Of the various methods of tuberculin testing available, the Mantoux test, in which graded amounts of tuberculin or of PPD are injected intradermally and the Heaf test in which the reagent is introduced into the skin by a multiple puncture spring release gun are the most precise and the most reliable. The Heaf test is technically simpler than the Mantoux test and being equally precise is being increasingly employed as a routine procedure. In both, a positive reaction is indicated by the development of areas of redness and swelling in the skin around the sites of introduction of the tuberculoprotein, reaching a maximum usually about 72 hours after the performance of the test.

A false negative reaction is sometimes given in the tuberculin test. The test is frequently negative in cases of advanced tuberculosis, in miliary tuberculosis, and in children following excessive exposure to sunlight or during the course of one of the exanthemata. A negative reaction may also be obtained in the early stages of infection, before the allergic state has developed sufficiently to give a positive reaction.

Immunity

There is no doubt that, as a result of tuberculous infection, a specific immunity develops. Thus in communities in which tuberculosis is widely prevalent, people who have sustained a primary infection in childhood and who, as a result, give a positive tuberculin reaction, are much less likely to contract the disease on subsequent exposure than those who give a negative reaction. It should be noted, however, that in environments in which tuberculosis is not widely prevalent, tuberculin-positive persons have a higher chance of developing the disease than have those who are tuberculin negative. This can be attributed to the fact that, under these conditions, the development of the disease in adult life is most frequently due to the reactivation of a primary lesion. In addition it is clear that immunity can be produced not only by infection but also as a result of immunization with a live attenuated vaccine (p. 367).

Although the existence of immunity is undisputed, there is considerable doubt as to the mechanism responsible. This will be considered under two headings.

1. The Role of Humoral Antibody

So far there is no positive evidence that immunity against tuberculosis is in any way dependent on humoral antibodies. (a) Normal animals cannot be protected by passive transfer of serum from immune or infected animals. (b) Antibodies identical with those produced by BCG vaccination can be produced in animals by inactivated vaccines which are unable to confer immunity. (c) In man immunity develops normally in cases of hypogammaglobulinaemia. (d) The tubercle bacillus appears to be completely resistant to the bactericidal effects of antibody and complement and to phagocytosis by polymorphonuclear leucocytes.

2. Cellular Immunity

The view that there may be a specific cellular immunity in tuberculosis was first proposed by Lurie who found that, when introduced into the anterior chambers of the eyes of normal rabbits, mononuclear cells from infected rabbits showed a resistance to infection not possessed by mononuclear cells from normal animals. Although there have been some reports to the contrary, the concept of a cellular immunity dependent on increased macrophage resistance is now generally accepted. There has been some difference of opinion, however, as to whether this resistance depends solely on the macrophages. Thus Fong and Elberg have obtained evidence that in the guinea-pig, macrophage immunity requires for its expression the co-operation of an unidentified serum factor, which they found in higher concentration in the sera of immune than of non-immune animals. The immunity of macrophages developed as a result of tuberculous infection is to an appreciable extent non-specific, extending in experimental animals to other intracellular parasites, e.g. to the brucellae and Listeria monocytogenes.

In view of the accumulating evidence that, in delayed-type hypersensitivity, macrophages as well as lymphocytes participate in the hypersensitive state—as manifested in the inhibition of their migration from explants in the presence of antigen (p. 184)—it is tempting to relate macrophage immunity to macrophage sensitization. This view is further strengthened by the finding that macrophages from animals with delayed hypersensitivity show, on contact with the sensitizing antigen in vitro, an increase in lysosomal activity, as manifested by an increase in the activity of hydrolytic enzymes. Such an increase has been demonstrated in macrophages from tuberculous animals. An increase in lysosomal activity might well be responsible for an increase in bactericidal activity against intra-cellular bacteria. The increase in lysosomal activity might occur as a result of combination of antigen with antibody-like groupings on the surface of the macrophage, or it might, in some way, be the result of contact of antigen with sensitized lymphocytes. On either basis the induction process would possess immunological specificity. Once the increased bactericidal activity had been established, however, it might be expected to extend to all intracellular parasites.

In addition to a possible cellular component, it seems likely that the inflam-matory reaction which develops in the hypersensitive individual on contact with the tubercle bacillus would tend to localize the infection, and that, parti-cularly if it progresses to caseation, a local environment, unfavourable to multi-plication of the bacillus, would be created.

There are, however, certain difficulties in associating immunity with hyper-sensitivity.

1. It has been shown by Rich that it is possible to desensitize an allergic animal, as demonstrated by loss of cutaneous reactivity, without affecting its immunity. As against this, however, loss of cutaneous reactivity may not indicate total loss of hypersensitivity. Thus animals which have lost their cutaneous reactivity may still be killed by intravenous injection of tuberculin.

2. It has been found by Raffel that it is possible to sensitize an animal by injection of tuberculoprotein together with a wax fraction of the organism, presumably wax D (p. 353), without stimulating immunity. This may have been however because the antigenic stimulus was not sufficiently intense.

3. There is no correlation, either in animals or in man, between the extent of the hypersensitive state, as manifested by the strength of cutaneous tuber-culin reactions, and the immune state. In fact in the British Medical Research Council trial (MRC Report, 1956), it was found that children who gave strongly positive tuberculin reactions were much more likely to develop tuberculosis subsequently than those who gave weakly positive reactions, while children inoculated with vole bacillus vaccine, so that they exhibited a low grade cutaneous reactivity, were as well protected as children who developed a more intense cutaneous reactivity as a result of BCG vaccination. These findings do not, however, invalidate the association of hypersensitivity with immunity; they could be explained on the grounds that an excessive inflammatory reaction might facilitate wider dissemination of the bacilli by opening up the blood and lymphatic channels.

Diagnosis

Only a brief outline of the various techniques used in the laboratory diagnosis of tuberculosis will be undertaken.

The material to be examined depends on the site of the infection: in suspected tuberculous meningitis the cerebrospinal fluid, in suspected genito-urinary infection the urine and in suspected pulmonary tuberculosis the sputum. In certain cases of suspected pulmonary infection, however, it may not be possible to obtain a specimen of sputum. This particularly happens with young children who frequently swallow any sputum produced. In such cases tubercle bacilli may be demonstrable in the faeces or in material obtained by gastric lavage or by the use of a laryngeal swab.

Three methods are used for the demonstration of tubercle bacilli: (*a*) microscopy, (*b*) culture, (*c*) animal inoculation. Ideally all three methods should be used. Although, in general, culture and animal inoculation are more sensitive than microscopy, they may give negative results in patients harbouring bacilli resistant to INAH. Positive microscopic results associated with negative culture may also be found during the course of chemotherapy, just prior to the stage of total elimination of the bacilli. At this stage the bacilli demonstrable are presumably of diminished viability.

Microscopy

Films should be prepared from all materials suspected of containing tubercle bacilli and an attempt made to demonstrate the organisms microscopically. Great care must be taken in microscopic diagnosis because of the danger of confusing saprophytic acid-fast bacilli which may be present in reagents or on glassware with tubercle bacilli. It is essential therefore that all containers used in the collection of specimens should be thoroughly cleaned, new cleaned slides should be used for the preparation of films and all stains should be made up in distilled water. For the collection of specimens of sputum waxed cardboard cartons which can be discarded are strongly recommended.

Two microscopic procedures are available: the Ziehl-Neelsen method and fluorescence microscopy (Chapter 2). In most laboratories the Ziehl-Neelsen method is the one routinely used but in laboratories carrying out a large number of daily examinations fluorescence microscopy is frequently preferred since it permits a more rapid examination of films. Positive results obtained by fluorescence microscopy can be confirmed by restaining the film by the Ziehl-Neelsen method but experienced workers do not as a rule find this necessary.

Sputum may be examined directly or after concentration for which Petroff's method (see below) may be used. Fluids, e.g. cerebrospinal fluid, pleural fluid and urine, should be centrifuged and films made from the deposit. In the case of cerebrospinal fluid films should also be prepared from the fine web-like clot which is often present.

As a general rule the finding of acid alcohol-fast bacilli of typical morphology in sputum or in material coming from the interior of the body, viz.: cerebrospinal fluid, pleural fluid or pus from an unopened abscess can be taken as conclusive evidence of tuberculosis.

Great care must, however, be taken in the microscopic identification of acid alcohol-fast bacilli found in urine, as tubercle bacilli. If the urine has not been taken by catheter, smegma bacilli may be present and may be morphologically indistinguishable from tubercle bacilli. They should, however, be found only rarely in mid-stream specimens if these have been properly taken; nevertheless if acid-fast bacilli are present, the examination should be repeated on a catheter specimen.

Culture

The medium most widely used for the isolation of tubercle bacilli is the Löwenstein-Jensen medium incorporating 0·75 per cent. glycerol. At least two tubes of this medium should be inoculated from each specimen. Many bacteriologists consider it advisable to inoculate one or more tubes of Dorset's egg medium as well on the grounds that the bovine type of tubercle bacillus may be inhibited by the concentration of glycerol in the Löwenstein-Jensen medium. Cultures are examined at intervals and any suspicious colonies stained by the Ziehl-Neelsen method. They should not be discarded as negative in less than 8 weeks.

Saprophytic acid-fast bacilli and atypical mycobacteria also grow on egg media, and may show considerable colonial and microscopic resemblance to tubercle bacilli. Because of this an organism should not be accepted as a tubercle bacillus until it has been subjected to further tests, the most important of which is guinea-pig inoculation. INAH-resistant strains of tubercle bacilli are, however, usually of low virulence for guinea-pigs, producing at most a local lesion. They require particularly careful examination to differentiate them from atypical mycobacteria (p. 369).

For the isolation of tubercle bacilli from sputum, the sputum is first treated to break down the mucus present, either by incubation with proteolytic enzymes or trisodium phosphate, or with agents such as sodium hydroxide or sulphuric acid which, as well as breaking down mucus, also kill commensal bacteria. Of these methods, alkali treatment, as in Petroff's method, is probably the most widely used. The method may also be used for the treatment of pus and deposits from fluids contaminated or infected with other organisms. Deposits from uncontaminated fluids may be inoculated without treatment.

Guinea-Pig Inoculation

For normal drug-sensitive strains guinea-pig inoculation has much the same sensitivity as culture. The material to be inoculated is treated as for culture and is injected either subcutaneously or intramuscularly into the animal's thigh. For routine diagnostic work the animal is killed after 8 weeks and a post-morten examination is then carried out. In positive cases films should be made from the local caseous lymphatic glands and stained by the Ziehl-Neelsen method. Guinea-pig inoculation should not be regarded as an alternative to culture, since many INAH-resistant strains are avirulent for guinea-pigs.

Other Methods

There are no satisfactory serological methods for the diagnosis of tuberculosis. A red cell agglutination test, in which the patient's serum is tested for its capacity to agglutinate cells which have been coated with a polysaccharide antigen present in Old Tuberculin, has been used; it is not reliable, however, since it gives negative results in cases of active tuberculosis and, like the tuberculin test, indicates at most, when positive, that the subject has at one time been infected.

The tuberculin test is primarily used to indicate past infection with the tubercle bacillus—its main practical applications being (*a*) as a preliminary to

BCG vaccination (see below) and (*b*) in epidemiological surveys to determine the incidence of latent tuberculosis. In certain circumstances, however, the test has considerable diagnostic value. As a general rule, except under the conditions previously noted, a negative reaction can be taken as indicating the absence of tuberculous infection. The value of a positive reaction in indicating current infection depends on two factors: (1) the age of the person and (2) the degree of prevalence of tuberculosis in the community. In infants and in young children the test is of considerable diagnostic value—the younger the child the greater the value, since the younger the child the less likely is it to have had a prior infection. A positive reaction in a child of less than two can, in any community, be taken as conclusive evidence of the presence of active tuberculosis. In the adult, however, the position is different. In communities where there is a high prevalence of tuberculosis a positive reaction usually means only that the person was at one time infected. The lower the prevalence of the disease, however, the greater is the probability that a positive reaction indicates current infection.

Treatment

A number of chemotherapeutic agents are active against the tubercle bacillus and have given dramatic results in treatment. The most important of the agents used are streptomycin, PAS and INAH. The most effective of these are streptomycin and INAH which are bactericidal; PAS is purely bacteriostatic. Tubercle bacilli, however, readily become resistant to streptomycin and INAH but, as discussed in Chapter 10, the development of resistance is greatly diminished when a combination of two or more of the drugs is employed. In practice, the best results have been obtained with regimens in which treatment has started with all three drugs. The regimen can be modified subsequently, according to the results of sensitivity tests.

With effective chemotherapy it is now clear that, when the organisms are originally sensitive, it should be possible to obtain a bacteriological cure in virtually every case. This has been shown clearly in a trial, organized by the International Union against Tuberculosis, in which all patients who were maintained on a regimen of streptomycin, INAH and PAS for 6 months, followed by PAS and INAH for a further 6 months, became bacteriologically negative. In the past, however, the therapy of tuberculosis has not been as successful as this, and the development of resistance, even with combined therapy, has been not infrequent. Thus in a random sample carried out by the British Tuberculosis Association in 1960, it was estimated that, in Britain, there were then 3500 patients infected with tubercle bacilli resistant to one or more of the major drugs, and 1800 with bacilli resistant to all three. These results can undoubtedly be attributed to inadequate treatment. It has been suggested that host factors may also be of importance in the genesis of therapeutic failures and in permitting the emergence of resistant strains. Such factors would include the presence of open thick-walled cavities in which bacilli multiply rapidly because of free access of oxygen, and into which there may be a slow penetration of drug and, in the case of INAH, rapid metabolism of the drug by rapid inactivators (p. 220). It would appear, however, from data presented by Mitchison, that the presence or absence of cavitation is only of importance with inadequate therapeutic regimens, and provided that sufficient INAH is given, there is no difference in success rate between rapid inactivators of INAH and slow inactivators.

It is a general finding that in the later stages of treatment, on what is obviously an effective chemotherapeutic regimen, patients continue to excrete tubercle bacilli which, on subsequent sensitivity testing, are found to be sensitive. These bacilli could either be located in some focus of infection into which the drugs had failed to penetrate or they could be sensitive organisms which have remained in a dormant or non-metabolizing state—'persisters'—because of which they are insusceptible to the action of the drug. The latter appears to be the more usual alternative. There is some evidence that this problem is minimized when high doses are used in the early stages of treatment.

With the emergence of drug-resistant strains it has been a matter of some importance to determine whether these have the same virulence or pathogenicity for man as drug-sensitive strains. With the exception of the INAH-resistant strains this appears to be the case. The latter are not only of diminished viability in culture but also, depending on the level of resistance, of lowered virulence for the guinea-pig. In general there is a correlation between the level of INAH resistance, loss of guinea-pig virulence and loss of capacity to produce catalase and peroxidase—a loss which, by increasing the bacilli's sensitivity to hydrogen peroxide, might explain their lowered viability on culture. As regards their effect on man, the evidence suggests: (1) That they have a somewhat lower infectivity, since the frequency of INAH-resistant primary infections are much lower than the number of cases disseminating INAH-resistant bacilli, and (2) That they have a lower virulence, since the survival of patients harbouring resistant strains has been longer than would have been expected in the absence of chemotherapy. There is, however, no evidence that the development of INAH resistance is more likely to lead to spontaneous cure.

When resistance develops to the major antituberculous drugs indicated above, the following, which are used in various combinations have been found to be of most value: ethionamide, pyrazinamide, cycloserine and viomycin. It is recommended that treatment should be continued for not less than 2 years.

If at all possible sensitivity tests should be carried out on organisms isolated before the beginning of treatment. At present the majority of organisms isolated from fresh cases of tuberculosis, i.e. cases which have received no previous chemotherapy, are fully sensitive to the three major antituberculous drugs. Nevertheless a proportion of fresh isolates—about 5 per cent in the British Isles—are resistant to one or other of these drugs. The proportion does not seem to be increasing, almost certainly because of the much more rigid and effective therapeutic regimens now adopted. In Africa, however, the incidence of primary resistance is much higher and presumably reflects the less satisfactory conditions under which treatment must often be carried out.

When the organisms are initially sensitive there is little point in carrying out sensitivity tests in the course of treatment. In fact these may give misleading results when the patients develop what is known as *transitional resistance*. This is found when there is a large initial population of tubercle bacilli which, because of its size, may contain organisms resistant to one or other of the drugs employed. These resistant organisms will be disposed of less rapidly by the other drugs used than will the bulk of fully sensitive bacilli. In such cases culture would appear to yield a preponderantly resistant population. These organisms do not, however, constitute a therapeutic problem since they will eventually be disposed of by the drug or drugs to which they are sensitive. For the control of treatment, simple smear examination, using a standardized technique which will permit a valid quantitative assessment of the number of organisms present, and cultural examination provide in most cases all the information required.

Prophylaxis

Neither dead vaccines of tubercle bacilli nor tuberculin will stimulate immunity against tuberculosis. Immunity can, however, be produced by the use of a living vaccine, consisting of a strain of bovine bacilli, *Bacille Calmette-Guérin* (more commonly known as BCG) attenuated by prolonged culture on a bile-containing medium. The BCG strain in not completely avirulent. It will grow to a limited extent in the tissues; in fact its immunizing effectiveness appears to depend on its being able to do so. It is, however, attenuated to the extent that it does not normally initiate a progressive infection. The BCG vaccine strains currently employed differ considerably in their degree of attenuation. Consequently their immunizing potency must be kept continually under review, particularly to ensure that they do not become over-attenuated.

The vaccine is introduced, usually in the deltoid region, by intradermal inoculation or by the multiple puncture method. Following intradermal inoculation a small nodule develops and is usually well established in about three weeks. This local lesion may progress to ulcer formation, but the process is quite benign and the ulcer heals by scar formation. In a few cases there is an associated enlargement of the cervical and axillary lymph nodes which may, although very rarely, progress to abscess formation. To date 5 cases have been recorded in which the BCG strain has given rise to a progressive infection—but the risk of this occurring must be regarded as infinitesimal. BCG vaccination can, in fact, be regarded as being as safe as any other prophylactic measure. The risk against which it protects is currently in most communities immeasurably greater than any risk attendant on the vaccination process.

Contra-indications to BCG vaccination are measles, pertussis, eczema or tuberculosis. Moreover, BCG vaccine should not be given to patients under prolonged cortisone treatment, nor at the same time as any other inoculation.

A tuberculin test must be carried out as a preliminary to vaccination—only those who are tuberculin negative being inoculated. In the case of young children, particularly those who have been in contact with a case of tuberculosis, it is desirable also to carry out a second tuberculin test 6 weeks after the first, the child having been removed from all contact with the disease during the intervening period. The double test minimizes the possibility that the child is infected at the time of inoculation. If the child were infected a short time prior to the first test, he might give a negative reaction because the allergic state had not had sufficient time to develop. After a further 6 weeks, however, the allergic state should have developed sufficiently to give a positive reaction. After a satisfactory intradermal inoculation the reaction should be positive at the end of 6 to 8 weeks. A tuberculin test is not, however, necessary, inspection of the lesion being sufficient to show that the vaccine has taken.

We are not yet in a position to assess fully the effects of BCG vaccination, but from the data so far available it is clear that it gives a considerable amount of protection against the disease. Thus in extensive trials which have been carried out by the Medical Research Council in children in industrial areas in England vaccination was found to confer approximately 85 per cent protection over a follow up period of 6 to 7 years. These data, of course, only show that vaccination protects against a primary infection. It is not to be expected that it will protect against exogenous post-primary infection. However, even if the main effect of vaccination is only to reduce the incidence of primary infection, it would be of enormous value, since by so doing it not only reduces the total amount of tuberculosis in the community but also produces a primary infection that is without the risk of progressive disease. The value of BCG vaccine is greatest in communities which have a high normal incidence of tuberculosis. In communities where, possibly as a result of vaccination, the incidence of the disease is low, there is a considerable case for not attempting general vaccination. In such communities the disease can be controlled by effective case finding and chemotherapy. Under these conditions the tuberculin reaction can be used as a diagnostic test, whereas if there were general vaccination it would have no such value. Whatever the policy towards general immunization persons in special risk categories, viz. nurses, medical students, laboratory workers and children from a tuberculous environment, should certainly be vaccinated.

The duration of the immunity produced following BCG vaccination is not known with certainty. It probably varies in different communities depending on the chance of the immunized individual being exposed to the tubercle bacillus. Individuals who live in communities where tuberculosis is prevalent might from time to time be exposed to contact with the bacillus, which would provide an antigenic stimulus sufficient to maintain their immunity at high level, but because of vaccination would be protected from infection. Because of this 'topping up' of immunity a single vaccination might therefore result, in such an environment, in a more or less permanent immunity.

A living vaccine derived from the vole type of tubercle bacillus, discovered by Wells, has also been used for active immunization. The immunity produced by the vole vaccine appears to be at least as great as that produced by BCG, but the vaccine has so far been used only on an experimental scale. As compared with BCG vaccine the vole bacillus vaccine has the disadvantage, however, that it produces a more marked local reaction and has in some cases given rise to lupus-like lesions at the site of inoculation.

Many communities have succeeded in greatly diminishing the incidence of bovine tuberculosis and some in eliminating the disease altogether by improvement in milk hygiene. For this purpose the most important measure is pasteurization which, if properly carried out, can be completely relied upon to kill any tubercle bacilli present in the milk. The safety of milk can be further ensured by the building up and maintenance of tuberculin tested herds.

Atypical Mycobacteria

This term is applied to a heterogeneous collection of mycobacteria which, in recent years, have been isolated from various clinical sources. They differ from tubercle bacilli in being non-pathogenic for guinea-pigs, producing at most a local lesion at the site of inoculation. Most are highly resistant to INAH. Most differ, however, from INAH-resistant guinea-pig avirulent tubercle bacilli in being active producers of catalase, the catalase produced being unlike that of the tubercle bacillus in being resistant to heating at 60° C. A variety of other tests have been used for distinguishing atypical mycobacteria from tubercle bacilli, and may need to be used in doubtful cases.

Only one species, *Mycobacterium kansasii*, is clearly defined. This is a photo-chromogen which develops an intense orange pigmentation after exposure to light; this pigmentation is only produced by actively growing cultures. *Myco. kansasii* is virulent for mice. In man it produces pulmonary lesions indistinguishable from those of chronic pulmonary tuberculosis. It is usually resistant to streptomycin and PAS, as well as to INAH.

Two other groups of atypical mycobacteria have been implicated in human disease: (1) The scotochromogens. These develop pigmentation when growing in the dark. They are non-pathogenic for mice and are usually streptomycin resistant. They have been isolated from cases of cervical adenitis in children. (2) Non-pigmented slow-growing mycobacteria—the so-called Battey bacilli. These are also streptomycin resistant, and may or may not be virulent for mice. In man they can produce tuberculosis-like pulmonary lesions.

A further group of atypical mycobacteria which grow rapidly and are non-pigmented, and which may or may not produce lesions in mice, have not so far been implicated in human disease.

Mycobacterium leprae

In infected tissues, leprosy bacilli appear as acid-fast bacilli, morphologically resembling tubercle bacilli. Because of this they have been assigned to the *Mycobacterium* genus as *Myco. leprae*. The protection against leprosy recently shown to be given by BCG vaccination supports the validity of this classification.

So far no organism with any real claims to be regarded as the leprosy bacillus has been isolated by laboratory culture. Its propagation in the footpads of mice has, however, been reported recently. Under these conditions the organism has a long generation time of 12 to 13 days, a finding consistent with the chronicity of the lesions characteristic of leprosy in man. No other laboratory animal has been reported as susceptible.

Leprosy

Leprosy is divided into two varieties—the lepromatous and the tuberculoid, which differ in the type of tissue lesion produced. This in turn depends on differences in the resistance of the patient. In the lepromatous type, in which resistance is low, there is a diffuse inflammatory reaction, the granulation tissue showing extensive infiltration with mononuclear type cells, and the presence of giant cells. Leprosy bacilli are usually present in large numbers, occurring either in groups of parallel bacilli or in large globular clumps known as globi. In the tuberculoid type, in which the resistance of the patient is high, the lesions are characteristically fibrotic with relatively few inflammatory cells and very scarce bacilli. The main lesions in leprosy are in the skin and nerves. In individual patients the disease is often predominantly cutaneous or predominantly neural. The cutaneous lesions occur mainly in exposed parts of the body—the face, hands, arms and legs. In the lepromatous type the lesions are nodular and frequently ulcerate and become secondarily infected. In the tuberculoid type they are raised erythematous macules. The neural lesions affect particularly the sensory nerves, leading to anaesthesia, deformities and trophic changes; they are usually of tuberculoid type. The mucous membrane of the nose is frequently involved, particularly in the lepromatous type, and bacilli may be demonstrable in the nasal secretions. Though mainly a superficial disease, invasion of the blood stream may occur, and the organisms may spread to the viscera.

Characteristically, leprosy is a disease of communities in which standards of hygiene are low. Its infectivity is low, and both close and prolonged contact are necessary for infection. Susceptibility is maximal in childhood and most infections occur before adult life. The extreme chronicity of the disease is matched by the long incubation period, usually from 2 to 4 years. Not infrequently infection contracted in childhood is not manifested clinically until adult life. Subclinical infection is not uncommon, and the disease can regress spontaneously.

Diagnosis is usually made by the demonstration of bacilli in material obtained by skin biopsy, or in scrapings from the nasal mucosa.

Diaminodiphenyl sulphone (DDS) is the drug of choice in the treatment of leprosy. Treatment must be continued for several years sometimes throughout the life of the patient. DDS must be administered with care since it is highly toxic. Experiments in mice infected by the footpad route suggest that INAH and a combination of INAH and PAS may be of value in treatment but this has not, however, been demonstrated in the human disease.

Lepromin Reactions

A delayed-type hypersensitivity may be demonstrated by a skin test somewhat similar to the tuberculin test, and known as the *lepromin* test. Lepromin is an autoclaved extract of infected leprous tissue from which the larger particles have been removed by centrifugation. Two types of reaction are demonstrable. The Fernandes reaction, which is strictly analogous to a positive tuberculin reaction, reaches a maximum in 2 to 4 days. As the reaction fades it is succeeded by a nodular infiltration of the skin which is maximal in from 3 to 4 weeks; this is known as the Mitsuda reaction. The Fernandes reaction, but not the Mitsuda reaction, is also produced by purified protein preparations derived from the bacilli. These skin reactions have little diagnostic value since they may develop as a result of tuberculous infection, and following administration of BCG vaccine. Leprosy patients do not, however, develop tuberculin hypersensitivity. Although of little use in diagnosis, the lepromin test has considerable prognostic value. The Mitsuda component, which in this context is the important reaction, is usually negative in lepromatous infections, indicating a poor prognosis, and positive in tuberculoid infections, indicating a good prognosis.

The precise immunological basis of the Mitsuda reaction is unknown. It does not appear to be a classical delayed-type hypersensitivity, on the model of the tuberculin reaction, but seems to have much in common with the hypersensitivity demonstrable by the Kveim test in sarcoidosis and the cutaneous hypersensitivity which develops as a result of exposure to beryllium and zirconium. Since the reaction is only produced by antigens containing particulate material derived from the tissues, it is possible that it may to some extent be due to altered tissue antigens. In relation to this possibility it is of interest that patients with lepromatous leprosy who exhibit a negative Mitsuda reaction appear to have a considerably diminished capacity for homograft rejection.

EFFECT OF BCG VACCINATION IN PROPHYLAXIS OF LEPROSY

Uganda trial 1960 to 1964

Cases of leprosy discovered at follow-up 2 to 3 years after beginning of trial

Tuberculin status at intake	Unvaccinated			BCG Vaccinated			
		Cases of leprosy			Cases of leprosy		Per cent reduction by vaccination
	Total	No.	per 1000	Total	No.	per 1000	
Negative	2930	20	6·8	2844	4	1·4	79
Weak positive	5141	69	13·4	5247	14	2·7	80
Strong positive	1081	9	8·3	—	—	—	—

(Brown, J. A. K. and Stone, M. M., *Brit. med. J.* 1.1.1966)

Protection against leprosy by BCG vaccination is approximately the same as against tuberculosis. Disease occurring was of *tuberculoid* variety. Vaccination might not give same protection against *lepromatous* leprosy.

BCG Prophylaxis

The finding that persons giving a positive Mitsuda reaction are less likely to develop leprosy than those giving a negative reaction, together with the observation that BCG vaccination can induce lepromin hypersensitivity, has led to the hope that BCG vaccination might have a protective effect against leprosy. A recent trial in Uganda has confirmed this expectation. A group of children giving negative or weakly positive tuberculin Heaf tests were assigned to vaccinated and non-vaccinated groups. After a two-year follow-up period, the incidence of leprosy in the non-vaccinated children was 11 per 1000, and in the vaccinated children, 2·2 per 1000. This degress of protection was maintained in a second follow up for a further period of 14 months. In the unvaccinated children protection was clearly related to tuberculin positivity when adjustment was made for the age composition of the population. In addition it was found that the degree of protection afforded by vaccination was not related to age, a finding which suggests that the incubation period of the disease may not be as long as has been previously thought.

Mycobacterium ulcerans

This organism is responsible for a disease characterized by the occurrence of granulomatous ulcers in the skin and subcutaneous tissues, particularly of the arms and legs. Visceral involvement is unknown. The condition, which is uncommon, has been reported from Australia, West Africa and Mexico.

Mycobacterium ulcerans differs from the tubercle bacillus, which in many respects it resembles, in having an optimum growth temperature in the range 25 to 35° C. Like the tubercle bacillus growth is slow. Rats and mice may be infected with the development of ulcerative lesions of the extremities but the organism is non-pathogenic for guinea-pigs. The superficial and peripheral distribution of the lesions can be related to the temperature requirements of the organism, the lesions occurring in those areas of the body whose temperature is normally less than 37° C.

Mycobacteria closely resembling *Myco. ulcerans* and with the same pathogenic propensities have been reported from Sweden. Infection has been traced to swimming baths and the organism has in consequence been designated *Myco. balnei*.

Non-pathogenic Mycobacteria

Saprophytic non-pathogenic mycobacteria are widely distributed in nature, occurring in the soil, on grass and in water. The occasional presence of organisms of this type on rubber corks and in tap water could cause confusion in the microscopic diagnosis of tuberculosis. The saprophytic mycobacteria resemble the tubercle bacillus morphologically but differ in that they grow well at room temperature and on nutrient agar.

Mycobacterium smegmatis

This non-pathogenic mycobacterium is of greater practical importance than those described above. It occurs in smegma and is occasionally found in urine in which it may be confused with the tubercle bacillus. As a rule *Myco. smegmatis* is less acid-fast than the tubercle bacillus and many strains are decolorized by alcohol, but strongly acid alcohol-fast strains occur. The organism grows readily on nutrient agar and has an optimum growth temperature of 37° C.

CHAPTER 27

ACTINOMYCETES, ACTINOBACILLUS

The actinomycetes are a group of organisms intermediate in properties between bacteria and fungi. They are Gram positive, branching filaments, non-sporing, non-motile and non-capsulated. As with the fungi the filaments interlace to produce a tangled mycelial growth. Two genera are distinguished: *Actinomyces* and *Nocardia*.

Actinomyces

The genus *Actinomyces* consists of anaerobic or micro-aerophilic non-acid-fast species of highly parasitic nature. Three species are distinguished: *A. bovis*, the cause of actinomycosis or lumpy jaw in cattle, *A. baudettii*, the cause of actinomycosis in cats and dogs and *A. israelii*, the cause of actinomycosis in man.

Actinomyces israelii

In the tissues *A. israelii* occurs in the form of yellowish granules which are usually readily visible to the naked eye. These granules, known as sulphur granules, are in fact colonies of the actinomycete. The centre of the granule consists of a dense felted mass of branching Gram positive filaments each about $0 \cdot 5 \mu$ in diameter. In older colonies the filaments fragment to yield bacillary and coccal forms. At the edge of the granule they terminate in radially disposed, pear-shaped bodies, or clubs—almost certainly formed by the deposition of lipid from the tissues around the end of the filaments. In contrast to the filaments the clubs are Gram negative. In young colonies the clubs are very delicate and are very readily broken up or dissolved in water.

Actinomyces israelii is difficult to isolate and even more difficult to maintain in laboratory culture. Isolation may be attempted by inoculation of the granules, preferably after washing in sterile water to remove contaminants, onto blood agar or brain-heart infusion agar. Plates are incubated anaerobically, preferably in the presence of 5 per cent CO_2. In addition, the washed granules should be incorporated in a glucose or serum agar stab in which, after a few days' incubation, micro-aerophilic colonies appear in a zone from $0 \cdot 5$ to 2 cm below the surface of the medium. On the surface of solid media *A. israelii* produces irregular, warty colonies adherent to the medium. The organisms present in these colonies have a mainly bacillary morphology—although branching filamentous forms are occasionally seen—which by its club shape, irregular staining and angular arrangement shows considerable resemblance to the corynebacteria. Clubs are not found in cultures.

Actinomycosis

Actinomyces israelii is a strict parasite. It is frequently present in the mouths of normal individuals, where it is found mainly around the teeth and in the tonsillar crypts. It normally lives a harmless parasitic life in the mouth and, with other mouth actinomycetes, may play a part in the formation of dental tartar. It is believed that the development of an allergy to the organism may be a necessary preliminary to successful invasion of the tissues. Trauma is an important predisposing factor in the development of lesions around the mouth.

Actinomycosis, though of world-wide distribution, is an uncommon disease. It occurs in three main clinical forms: (1) Cervico-facial actinomycosis. In this,

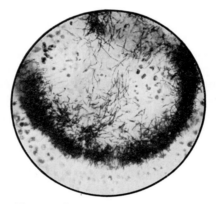

FIG. 29. COLONY OF *Actinomyces israelii*
IN LIVER (× 500)

which appears to be the commonest variety, the lesions occur mainly in the cheek and submaxillary regions. (2) Thoracic actinomycosis, in which the lesions occur in the lungs. (3) Abdominal actinomycosis. In this type the lesions are usually in the neighbourhood of the caecum. From these the organisms may pass by the portal vein to the liver which may as a result become riddled by actinomycotic abscesses. Histologically the lesions of actinomycosis are granulomatous in character, usually with considerable suppuration and the formation of discharging sinuses. A striking feature of the disease is the absence of involvement of the local lymphatic glands.

In actinomycotic lesions, along with *A. israelii*, a small Gram negative bacillus *Actinobacillus actinomycetemcomitans* is also frequently found, often in considerable numbers. This organism, which is one of the brucellaceae and can be cultivated under aerobic conditions, appears to be very similar in properties to *Actinobacillus lignieresii*, the cause of woody tongue in cattle.

Although *A. israelii* is sensitive to penicillin and a number of commonly used antibiotics, antibiotic therapy is not always successful. On the whole the tetracyclines appear to give the best results. This is possibly because they are active also on *A. actinomycetemcomitans* which is resistant to penicillin.

Nocardia

The genus *Nocardia* comprises a group of aerobic actinomycetes which are widely distributed in the soil where they live a purely saprophytic life. Many are acid fast.

They grow readily on agar media. Occasionally they are pathogenic to man, in whom they give rise to chronic granulomatous lesions in which, as in actinomycosis, granules consisting of colonies of the organism are frequently demonstrable.

Nocardiosis occurs in two clinical forms—systemic nocardiosis and mycetoma. In systemic nocardiosis, lesions occur mainly in the lungs but there may be haematogenous spread to other organs, particularly the brain. The condition is uncommon and is most frequently due to *N. asteroides*, an acid-fast species which, on agar media, produces an orange star-shaped colony from which the species derives its name. Mycetoma is a chronic granulomatous condition, mainly localized to the region of the foot (Madura foot), which occurs in certain tropical countries. It is most frequently due to *N. madurae*, a non-acid-fast species, but may also be caused by several species of filamentous fungi. Infections due to the latter are usually referred to as maduromycosis.

Sulphonamides have given excellent results in the treatment of *Nocardia* infections, if given early in the disease. In mycetoma, chemotherapy is combined with surgical treatment. Infections due to filamentous fungi are not susceptible to chemotherapy.

Actinobacillus mallei (*Pfeifferella mallei*)

Actinobacillus mallei, the causative organism of glanders, is a non-motile, non-capsulated, non-sporing Gram negative bacillus, which sometimes occurs in the form of long, slightly branched filaments. It is aerobic and grows moderately well, but rather slowly, on ordinary media. For purposes of isolation, blood agar is quite satisfactory.

Guinea-pigs are highly susceptible. In male animals, following intraperitoneal inoculation, marked inflammatory changes are found in the tunica vaginalis of the testis. This is known as the Straus reaction. Guinea-pig inoculation, preferably by the subcutaneous route, may be used as a method of isolation, the organism being recoverable from the regional lymphatic glands.

Glanders

Glanders is a disease essentially of the horse family, man being only occasionally and incidentally infected. The disease in both animals and man is characterized by the occurrence in infected tissues of granulomatous nodules composed of leucocytes, epithelioid cells and connective tissue. Pus is not usually produced, but the central cells generally degenerate and disintegrate and the nodules become soft and break down, forming ulcers. In the more chronic nodules the connective tissue development is exaggerated and the leucocytic invasion is less marked. Bacilli are fairly plentiful in the acute lesions, mostly extracellular, but a few lie within the leucocytes. It may be impossible to find any in old chronic cases. Glanders is now virtually unknown in horses in the British Isles but still occurs in Eastern Europe and in parts of Asia.

Infection with *Act. mallei* is rare in man and is found mainly in those whose work involves close contact with horses—the organism usually gaining access through wounds and abrasions. Cultures of the organism are, however, very highly infective and have given rise to a number of laboratory infections.

In man, glanders may be either acute or chronic. The primary lesion is generally in the skin, more rarely in the mucous membrane of the nose, mouth or eye and is associated with inflammation of the draining lymphatic vessels. In acute cases there is pyrexia, very severe prostration and usually a generalized pustular rash. In chronic cases secondary foci occur throughout the body.

Satisfactory results have been claimed in the treatment of glanders with sulphadiazine. In the absence of treatment, glanders is almost invariably fatal.

Serological tests may be used for diagnosis of the disease in infected animals—the complement fixation test being the most reliable. During the course of glanders a delayed type hypersensitivity which may be detected by the *mallein* test develops. Mallein is a concentrated and filtered glycerol broth culture of the organism, and for the test may be introduced by the subcutaneous, intradermal or conjunctival routes. The test should not be employed for the diagnosis of glanders in man as it may cause very severe reactions.

CHAPTER 28

L FORMS, MYCOPLASMA, STREPTOBACILLUS LISTERIA, ERYSIPELOTHRIX, BARTONELLA

Bacterial L Forms

Many bacteria, when grown in the presence of inimical environmental agencies, give rise to variants which have lost their capacity to synthesize a cell wall but are still capable of multiplication. These variants, because of their resemblance to the L1 forms which arise spontaneously in cultures of *Streptobacillus moniliformis* (p. 381), are known as L forms. A variety of agents have been found to be effective in the production of L forms—penicillin and other antibiotics which inhibit cell wall synthesis, the amino acid glycine, antisera and a high salt concentration. Of these penicillin has been most used. As a rule L forms, when first isolated, are unstable and tend to revert under normal conditions to the normal form. On serial subculture, however, stable L forms, which do not tend to revert to the normal form, are produced.

Since, like protoplasts L forms are osmotically unstable they will grow only on media of high osmotic tension. This is most readily achieved by the incorporation of serum in a concentration of *circa* 20 per cent. Serum probably also acts as an adsorbent for substances which might be toxic to the L form. On solid media most L forms produce a characteristic fried-egg type of colony, the dense central portion of which is due to growth into the medium, and the less dense periphery to growth on its surface.

The morphological elements in these colonies vary in size from minute coccal bodies, about 300 mμ in diameter, to large irregular structures about the size of a leucocyte. The large bodies are more numerous towards the periphery of the colonies where they tend to accumulate large intracellular globules filled with cholesterol. Filtration data have established the small bodies as the minimal reproductive units. Their relationship to the larger bodies, however, is not completely clear. Most microbiologists favour Tulasne's view that the small bodies increase in size to form the large bodies, and that these fragment ultimately to give rise to a new generation of small bodies. As might be expected from their lack of cell wall, L forms are soft and extremely fragile and are broken up when films are prepared by ordinary methods. They can, however, be stained satisfactorily in situ or by the use of impression preparations.

The precise mechanisms involved in the production of L forms are not clear. The simplest view is that they are mutants which lack the capacity to synthesize a cell wall but which are still capable of division and are therefore selected in the presence of agents, e.g. penicillin, which inhibit cell wall synthesis. In this case the gradual development of stable L forms would appear to indicate that these must arise as a result of a series of consecutive mutations. Precisely how L forms differ from protoplasts (p. 5) is unknown—these resemble the L form in lacking a cell wall but are incapable of multiplication, although they can increase in size. It is possible that the treatment involved in the preparation of protoplasts, as well as removing the cell wall, eliminates some structure required for cell division, while in L forms this structure is retained.

In general, bacterial L forms are avirulent for experimental animals susceptible to the parent form. An important exception to this, however, is the L form of the cholera vibrio which is fully pathogenic for mice. This finding would suggest that the endotoxin of the cholera vibrio plays only a subsidiary role in the pathogenicity of the vibrio for the mouse.

At the moment it is not possible to state the extent to which L forms develop in the animal body during the course of infection. It is conceivable that transformation to the L form might allow the organism to resist the natural defences of the body. Some evidence has been presented that this may occur to brucellae in the bodies of experimental animals.

Mycoplasma

The generic name *Mycoplasma* is now applied to organisms previously described as pleuropneumonia (PPO) and pleuropneumonia-like organisms (PPLO). In microscopic and colonial morphology, mycoplasmas are virtually indistinguishable from bacterial L forms. The main differences are the smaller size—125 to 150 mμ—of their minimal reproductive unit and, in the case of the parasitic species, the existence of a nutritional requirement for sterol. Because of their resemblance to induced bacterial L forms, it has been suggested that mycoplasmas may be stable L forms which have arisen spontaneously from various bacterial species.

Mycoplasmas occur both as saprophytes and as parasites. Saprophytic mycoplasmas have been isolated mainly from soil and sewage, and parasitic mycoplasmas from human and other animal sources. In animals they appear to have a predilection for the respiratory and genito-urinary tracts and for the joints. Mycoplasmas from human sources fall into six major antigenic groups. Techniques used in their differentiation are: complement fixation, immunofluorescence, precipitation in agar gel, haemagglutination inhibition—using tannic acid treated red cells sensitized by extracts of the organisms obtained by sonic disruption—and growth inhibition by specific serum. Mycoplasmas differ from bacteria in that homologous antibody will inhibit growth in the absence of complement—a property which they share with the leptospirae.

As they lack a cell wall, mycoplasmas are insusceptible to the action of penicillin; they are, however, highly susceptible to the tetracyclines.

The only mycoplasma of proved pathogenicity for man is *Mycoplasma pneumoniae*, which has been isolated from cases of primary atypical pneumonia

(PAP). Mycoplasmas have been found frequently as contaminants of tissue cultures. The majority of these strains have been strains of human origin and produced no change in the cells of the culture. Some, however, produce a cyto-pathogenic effect (p. 434), because of which a mistaken diagnosis of virus infection may be made. It is therefore essential that in identifying a transmissible agent which produces cytopathogenic effects on tissue culture as a virus, the possibility of *Mycoplasma* contamination should be excluded. In cases of tissue culture contamination that have been studied in detail, the cytopathogenic effect observed has been attributed to a depletion of the arginine in the nutrient medium by the mycoplasma. Apart from *M. pneumoniae*, mycoplasmas have been suspected as being the causes of a number of conditions: upper respiratory tract infection, genito-urinary tract infection—particularly non-specific urethritis—arthritis, and leukaemia. The possible aetiological role of myco-plasmas in upper respiratory tract infection is supported by the development of laryngitis and tonsillitis in artificially infected human volunteers, the incidence of successful experimental infections being highest in those who prior to infec-tion showed no serum antibody to the *Mycoplasma* employed. A presumptive association of mycoplasmas with non-specific urethritis has been suggested by the frequency with which they have been isolated from patients with this disease, together with the demonstration that complement fixing antibodies are found more often, and in higher titre, in such patients than in uninfected controls. The role of mycoplasmas in human conditions other than pneumonia has, however, still to be determined.

The isolation of mycoplasmas from the bone marrow of cases of leukaemia has been described by two groups of workers. In one report, mycoplasmas were isolated in human embryo kidney cell tissue cultures, in which they produced cytopathogenic effects—as a result they were at first thought to be viruses. Although the strains isolated appeared to be identical, and differed antigenically from previously reported human strains they appeared to share antigens with a rodent strain of *Mycoplasma*. In the second report a *Mycoplasma* was isolated by direct inoculation onto an agar medium, and was found to be a slightly atypical strain of *Mycoplasma orale*, a recognized mouth commensal. The significance of these observations is in doubt, and for the moment it must be presumed that the mycoplasmas were present only as secondary in-vaders which found that leukaemic marrow satisfactorily met their nutritional requirements.

Primary Atypical Pneumonia

The use of penicillin in the treatment of pneumonia, particularly during World War II, was primarily responsible for the realization that many pneu-monias were not of bacterial origin. Many of these non-bacterial pneumonias present a characteristic clinical and radiological appearance to which the name *primary atypical pneumonia* has been applied. In this condition cough is a prominent feature, but there is no leucocytosis as occurs in bacterial pneumonia and X-ray examination shows the presence of characteristic lung opacities which are usually much more extensive than would be expected from the physical examination and clinical condition of the patient.

Many cases exhibiting this syndrome were found, during the course of their illness, to develop agglutinins active against human red cells in the cold, i.e. at 0 to 4° C. A somewhat smaller proportion show the presence of agglutinins active against a non-haemolytic streptococcus, *Streptococcus MG*. The unduly long incubation period (for an acute respiratory disease) of two weeks suggested that cases developing cold agglutinins might belong to a single aetiological group. That this was in fact the case was shown by Eaton and his associates who isolated an agent—in the chick embryo—which they found to be capable of producing pulmonary consolidation in cotton rats and hamsters. The aetiological role of this agent was finally established, using the fluorescent antibody technique, by the demonstration of antibody to it in the sera of a high proportion of persons exhibiting the PAP syndrome, and, also, by the demonstration of its capacity to produce febrile respiratory disease and pneumonia in human volunteers lacking demonstrable antibody.

At first the agent was thought to be a virus, though its susceptibility to tetracycline and streptomycin seemed to be incompatible with this identification. Its final characterization as a *Mycoplasma* was accomplished by its propagation, by Chanock et al., on a cell-free agar medium containing 20 per cent horse serum and 2·5 per cent fresh yeast extract. Sera from pig, cow or rabbit could be substituted for horse serum. As well as creating osmotic conditions suitable for growth, serum supplies cholesterol and other unidentified growth factors. The essential components in the yeast extract are dialysable but have not been specifically identified.

Mycoplasma pneumoniae grows more slowly than other mycoplasmas isolated from human sources, colonies on primary isolation appearing in from 6 to 20 days. They have a characteristic mulberry surface, and lack the fried-egg appearance of most other mycoplasma colonies. Other criteria of importance in identification are: (*a*) Fermentation of glucose and other sugars, and (*b*) Rapid haemolysis of guinea-pig erythrocytes. To demonstrate this the erythrocytes are incorporated in an agar overlay after colonies have developed. A haemolytic zone develops around the colony after 24 to 48 hours' incubation. The haemolysin appears to be highly labile and to require oxygen for its activity. Final identification is by serological methods (p. 378). *M. pneumoniae* shows a slight antigenic relationship to other mycoplasmas, apparent, however, only with the very sensitive passive haemagglutination technique.

In addition to producing PAP, *M. pneumoniae* can also cause upper respiratory tract infection and inapparent or latent infection. It has been estimated that at least 90 per cent of cases of mycoplasma infection do not progress to the pneumonic stage. *Mycoplasma* pneumonia is not highly infectious and, unlike influenza, occurs uniformly throughout the year. The disease is most frequent in adults of from 20 to 30 years of age. Diagnosis is best achieved by serological methods. The demonstration of cold agglutinins for human group O red cells, and of agglutinins for the MG streptococcus are probably the most widely used serological tests. A considerable number of patients, however, fail to develop these antibodies. The frequency with which they are demonstrable varies considerably in different epidemics, and in general both their frequency and their titre appears to be related to the severity and duration of the disease. Of the tests employing *M. pneumoniae* antigen the immunofluorescent technique using chick-embryo lung antigen appears to be the most satisfactory. The indirect haemagglutination test shows the highest antibody titres but the antibody level may have reached a maximum at the time of onset of symptoms.

The development during the course of PAP of cold agglutinins and agglutinins for the MG streptococcus is of considerable immunological interest. The development of cold agglutinins may be related to the fact that *M. pneumoniae* has been shown capable of inactivating the *i* antigen which is present on most human red cells. It is possible that red cells modified in this way may be able to stimulate auto-immune antibodies. The development of MG agglutinins at first suggested that the mycoplasma might be an L form of the MG streptococcus. Since the MG streptococcus and *M. pneumoniae* do not appear to have antigens in common it is doubtful whether this could be the case.

In addition to the above reactions the sera of atypical pneumonia patients frequently fix complement in the presence of various tissue antigens and give false positive reactions in reagin tests for syphilis. It would seem therefore that the *Mycoplasma* infection might, in some non-specific way, initiate abnormal responses from the antibody-producing machinery. This raises the interesting possibility that in various syndromes in which auto-immune responses have been found (p. 124) there might be a concomitant *Mycoplasma* infection.

The tetracyclines have proved to be of considerable value in serologically positive *M. pneumoniae* infections.

An inactivated vaccine capable of stimulating antibody production in human volunteers has been prepared, but its efficacy in the prophylaxis of natural *M. pneumoniae* infection has still to be determined.

Streptobacillus moniliformis

Streptobacillus moniliformis is a Gram negative, non-capsulated, non-sporing, non-motile organism which, under normal conditions of growth, gives rise to L forms. It will grow only on media containing a high concentration, 20 to 30 per cent, of serum or other body fluid. Growth is best at 37° C and under aerobic conditions. On solid media it produces two types of colony each with a characteristic microscopic morphology: (1) A granular colony growing on the surface of the agar and usually measuring, after 2 or 3 days' incubation, from 3 to 5 mm in diameter. (2) At the periphery of and underneath the surface colonies are the L-form colonies. These are very small microscopic colonies which grow into the substance of the agar. The colonies, which grow more slowly than the surface colonies and develop better at room temperature than at 37° C, have a dense centre and a clear edge. The organisms present in these colonies resemble those found in bacterial L form colonies (p. 377).

In the surface colonies the organisms occur as short bacilli—these predominate in young cultures—or as long filaments which may measure up to 150μ in length. As the filaments age they undergo fragmentation into bacillary and coccal elements which frequently present a Morse code like appearance. In addition, the filaments usually show the presence of large, oval or spindle-shaped swellings which may measure up to 20μ in diameter. These swellings, which are responsible for the species designation *moniliformis*, are presumably preliminary stages in the formation of the L forms.

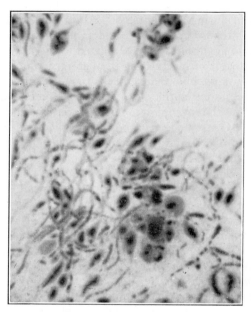

FIG. 30. STREPTOBACILLUS MONILIFORMIS
(*Dr. E. Kleineberger-Nobel*)

Rat-bite Fever

Streptobacillus moniliformis is a normal parasite of the nasopharynx of the rat and is responsible for a variety of rat-bite fever in man. The bite heals normally, but following an incubation period of about 10 days the site of the bite becomes inflamed with the development of a local lymphangitis and lymphadenitis and the appearance of septicaemic symptoms. Endocarditis and arthritis may occur as complications. The organism can also gain entry through the gastrointestinal tract, but this mode of infection appears to be very rare.

Some cases of rat-bite fever respond well to penicillin but the tetracyclines, which are active against the L forms as well as the bacillary form, appear to give better results.

Isolation is most readily achieved by inoculation of the blood into a good infusion broth to give a final blood concentration of 20 per cent.

Listeria and Erysipelothrix

These genera resemble each other closely and are both assigned to the family

Corynebacteriaceae. Only one species is recognized in each genus. Both are widely distributed in nature as pathogens of a variety of animal species.

Listeria monocytogenes. This is a Gram positive, non-sporing aerobic bacillus. It is sluggishly motile exhibiting a characteristic end over end or 'tumbling' motility. It will grow on nutrient agar, but growth is considerably improved by the addition of glucose, blood or serum. The colonies, which are small, are demonstrable after 24 hours' incubation at 37° C. The organism occurs in both smooth and rough colony types. Smooth colonies consist of normal bacillary elements, but in the rough colonies long filamentous forms are predominant. Most strains are haemolytic on blood agar.

Listeria monocytogenes is responsible for a natural infection occurring in sheep, cattle, rabbits, guinea-pigs and other animals. In smaller animals the infection takes the form of a septicaemia which is associated with areas of focal necrosis in the liver. The presence of a monocytosis—which gives the organism its name—is a characteristic feature. In cattle, sheep and goats the infection takes the form of a meningoencephalitis; in these animals a monocytosis is unusual.

In man, as in cattle, *Listeria monocytogenes* may cause meningoencephalitis, but the condition is very rare and only a limited number of cases have been reported. In these cases a monocytosis was observed in the peripheral blood. The mode of infection has not been discovered. A generalized infection in infants associated with focal necrosis of the liver and spleen has also been described. The disease which is known as granulomatosis infantiseptica has a high mortality rate. The infection is believed to be transmitted from the mother to the foetus in utero. In contrast to the disease in the infant the infection in the mother is usually mild and may be asymptomatic. *Listeria monocytogenes* has been isolated from the blood in several cases of infectious mononucleosis but is not accepted as a cause of this condition.

Erysipelothrix rhusiopathiae is very similar to *Listeria monocytogenes* in its properties. It differs from *Listeria* antigenically, in certain biochemical reactions and in being non-motile. On primary isolation it tends to be microaerophilic.

Erysipelothrix rhusiopathiae is responsible for a natural infection in a variety of animals which is characterized by septicaemia and the presence of focal lesions in the liver. In swine it causes the condition known as swine erysipelas. The organism also occurs as a commensal on the skin and scales of various types of fish.

Human infection is not uncommon. It occurs mainly in those whose work involves the handling of fish, meat or poultry—the organism gaining access through abrasions of the skin. At the site of inoculation a purplish red oedematous area develops. The lesion spreads by peripheral extension while at the same time clearing in the centre. The condition has some resemblance to erysipelas and is on this account known as erysipeloid. The disease is a mild one with a low fatality rate, but relapses are frequent. Isolation of the organism from the skin lesions is difficult and is only likely to be successful with material taken by skin biopsy. Penicillin appears to be the most effective chemotherapeutic agent.

Bartonella bacilliformis

The genus *Bartonella* belongs to the family Bartonellaceae, a group of organisms which are parasites of the red blood cells of a variety of animal species. The Bartonellaceae are classified by Bergey in the order Rickettsiales but differ from the other members of this order in being able to grow on inanimate laboratory media.

Bartonella bacilliformis is a small Gram negative, motile, non-sporing organism. It exhibits marked pleomorphism, particularly in the blood of infected individuals in which bacillary, coccal and even ring forms may appear.

The organism is aerobic and grows optimally at about 28° C. 'Sloppy' agar containing 10 per cent rabbit serum and a low concentration of rabbit haemoglobin is the medium most frequently used for its isolation. In this medium, growth becomes apparent in about 10 days as a narrow band about 1 cm wide just beneath the surface of the agar.

Bartonella baciliformis appears to be restricted in distribution to the mountainous parts of Peru, Ecuador and Columbia, where it gives rise to latent infection in a considerable proportion of the population. In these people the organism is present in the blood, from which it may be isolated. In a small proportions of infected individuals it gives rise to overt disease, producing two symptomatically distinct clinical syndromes—Oroya fever and Verruga peruana.

Oroya fever is a febrile haemolytic anaemia; it is a serious disease and in the absence of treatment has a high fatality rate. The parasite may be demonstrated in the peripheral blood both in red cells and in the cytoplasm of mononuclear leucocytes. The organisms are also widely distributed throughout the body and are demonstrable in the endothelial cells lining lymph and blood capillaries. The infected endothelial cells are grossly distended and bulge out markedly into the lumen of the vessel. *Bartonella bacilliformis* has not been shown to possess a haemolysin, and the mechanism by which it causes haemolysis is not known.

Verruga peruana is a much less serious condition than Oroya fever. It is characterized by warty granulomatous lesions in the skin. The organisms are demonstrable in the skin lesions, particularly in the proliferating endothelial cells which are invariably present. The condition usually develops as a sequel to an attack of Oroya fever, but may appear as the only manifestation of infection. No differences have been demonstrated between the strains of *Bartonella* responsible for these two conditions. Consequently it is believed that the relatively mild character and the symptomatology of Verruga peruana are determined by immunity to the parasite. The identity of the aetiological agents of Verruga peruana and Oroya was first demonstrated in 1885 by Carrion, who submitted himself to inoculation with material from a Verruga patient and died 6 weeks later from Oroya fever.

The organism is transmitted by sandflies—*Phlebotomus*—which bite only at night. Consequently prophylaxis—by the use of DDT and the application of measures to prevent the attack of night-biting insects—is relatively simple and effective. Diagnosis is by microscopic demonstration and isolation of the parasite. In both conditions isolation is most readily achieved by blood culture. Penicillin has been found to be of considerable value in the treatment of Oroya fever, but is of little value in the prevention or treatment of Verruga peruana.

Calymmatobacterium granulomatis (*Donovania granulomatis*)

This organism is the cause of granuloma inguinale, a chronic granulomatous venereal disease which occurs only in tropical countries. The organism is demonstrable within mononuclear cells obtained from the lesions in which it appears as a Gram negative capsulated bacillus. It has been grown in the yolk-sac of the chick embryo and, under in vitro conditions, in egg yolk. It appears to have some antigenic relationship to *Kl. rhinoscleromatis* (p. 293).

CHAPTER 29

THE CLOSTRIDIA

The genus *Clostridium* is a genus of Gram positive, anaerobic, sporing bacilli. The natural habitat of the clostridia is the soil. From the soil they may gain access to the intestinal tracts of animals and man, from which certain species can frequently be isolated. The genus is a very large one, 93 different species being described by Bergey. Only a few of the species described are pathogenic for man.

BIOCHEMICAL REACTIONS OF CERTAIN CLOSTRIDIA

	Species	Glucose	Lactose	Sucrose	Milk	Gelatin	Serum
Mainly Saccharolytic	Cl. perfringens	AG	AG	AG	AG	+	−
	Cl. septicum	AG	AG	AG	Ag	+	−
	Cl. novyi	AG	−	−	Ag	+	−
	Cl. fallax	AG	AG	AG	Ag	−	−
	Cl. tertium[1]	AG	AG	AG	Ag	−	−
Mainly Proteolytic	Cl. bifermentans	AG	−	−	D	+	+
	Cl. botulinum[2]	AG	(AG)	−	D	+	+
	Cl. histolyticum	(A)	−	−	D	+	+
	Cl. sporogenes	AG	−	−	D	+	+
	Cl. tetani	−	−	−	−	+	−

[1] *Cl. tertium* grows appreciably under aerobic conditions.
[2] Changes produced by type A and most type B strains.
A = Acid. G = large amount of gas. g = small amount of gas. D = digestion. + under serum and gelatin = liquefaction. ( ) = not produced by all strains.

The clostridia differ morphologically from the aerobic sporing bacilli in that in most cases the spore is normally wider than the body of the bacillus. Some, notably *Clostridium sporogenes*, spore readily; with others, particularly *Cl. perfringens*, sporing is infrequent. In general, spore formation is diminished in the presence of fermentable carbohydrate. In the pathogenic species, except for *Cl. tetani*, the spore is central or subterminal in position; *Cl. tetani* possesses a terminal spore. All the pathogenic species are motile with the exception of *Cl. perfringens*, which is also the only species to produce a capsule.

On the basis of their biochemical behaviour most of the pathogenic clostridia can be divided into two contrasting groups.

1. Predominantly saccharolytic organisms. These are active fermenters of

sugars, do not digest serum, produce a pinkish colour in Robertson's meat medium, which is not decomposed and yield cultures which frequently have a smell reminiscent of rancid butter—due to the presence of higher fatty acids such as butyric acid.

2. Predominantly proteolytic organisms. These are not as active sugar fermenters as the first group. They digest serum, produce a black colour in meat which is extensively decomposed and their cultures have a putrefying smell due mainly to the liberation of hydrogen sulphide from proteins.

Clostridium tetani does not fall into either of these groups being only mildly proteolytic and not at all saccharolytic.

The biochemical activities of most importance in species differentiation are the fermentation of glucose, saccharose and lactose, appearance of the growth in Robertson's meat medium, and effect on gelatin, serum and litmus milk. Clostridia may reduce the indicators present in sugar media and consequently false negative fermentation reactions may be obtained. The correct reaction is apparent if further indicator is added to the medium prior to reading the results of the test.

The pathogenic clostridia are very active exotoxin producers, and it is to this property that their pathogenicity is mainly or entirely due. The demonstration of the appropriate toxin and its neutralization by specific antitoxin are essential for the identification of the pathogenic species. For this purpose guinea-pigs and mice, which are highly susceptible to the toxins of the clostridia, are commonly employed.

The identification of the pathogenic clostridia usually affords little difficulty. Since, however, clinical material frequently contains more than one species of *Clostridium* and since some species tend to swarm on solid media it is often difficult to isolate single species in pure culture. The material should be plated directly on to a well dried blood agar plate; thorough drying of the surface should prevent swarming. This may also be achieved by the use of a high concentration of agar—from 4 to 6 per cent. Willis and Hobb's medium (p. 45) is of considerable value for the isolation of clostridia because of its selective and differential properties. Tubes of Robertson's meat medium should also be inoculated for enrichment purposes. After inoculation one tube is incubated unheated and a second after heating to 80° C for 10 minutes. Subculture from meat medium is often successful in isolating a *Clostridium* when direct plating is negative. Identification of the non-pathogenic clostridia, particularly of the proteolytic varieties, may be extremely difficult. The demonstration of antibody in the patient's serum is of no value in the diagnosis of clostridial infections.

Clostridium tetani

Morphology

Clostridium tetani is a slender bacillus with a round terminal spore which gives the organism a 'drumstick' appearance. Spores are produced in the body as well as in culture. The drumstick appearance is not a completely reliable diagnostic criterion since it is also shown by certain non-pathogenic clostridia, notably *Cl. tetanomorphum*.

Cultural Properties

Clostridium tetani produces a delicate irregular colony with fine offshoots. If the medium is moist, the growth is in the form of a thin film which spreads over the surface except in the case of occasional non-motile strains which produce isolated colonies. This swarming capacity is made use of in Fildes's method for the isolation of *Cl. tetani* in which primary cultures in peptic blood broth after heating to kill non-sporing organisms are inoculated into the condensation water of a blood agar slope. It may then be possible to obtain a pure culture from the edge of the swarming film of growth which may have spread a considerable distance up the surface of the slope.

On the basis of its flagellar antigen composition the species can be sub-divided into ten antigenic types. One of the types—type VI—is non-flagellated. All the antigenic types have a common O antigen.

Pathogenicity

Clostridium tetani produces a very powerful exotoxin which has a selective action on the central nervous system. There is a considerable body of evidence that the toxin acts centrally, i.e. on the nerve cells in the brain and spinal cord, rather than on the peripheral nerves. Its central action results in an exaggerated reflex motor response to sensory stimuli. The precise mechanism by which it produces this effect is unknown, but there is evidence suggesting that it may act

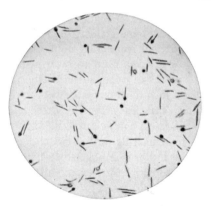

FIG. 31. *Cl. tetani* FROM AN AGAR
CULTURE (× 800)

by inhibiting the synthesis and liberation of acetylcholine. This would have the effect of freeing the reflex pathways in the cord from central control.

The toxin is protein in nature and has been obtained in crystalline form. It is destroyed by heating to 65° C for 5 minutes, by the action of acid and by proteolytic enzymes. It is therefore inactivated in the stomach and the intestinal tract and is consequently without effect if ingested. It is extremely potent—1 mg of a purified preparation containing around 6×10^6 mouse lethal doses. Culture filtrates differ considerably in potency but an active filtrate may contain as much as 10^5 mouse lethal doses per ml.

Filtrates of *Cl. tetani* also contain an oxygen-labile haemolysin which resembles and is immunologically related to streptolysin O. The haemolysin is produced by strains of the organism which fail to produce the neurotoxin. No role has been assigned to it in pathogenicity.

Tetanus

The tetanus bacillus is widely distributed in the superficial layers of the soil in all parts of the world, but is more often found in richly cultivated land than in virgin soil. It is commonly present in the faeces of herbivora, particularly of horses, and, in some countries, e.g. in China, in the faeces of man.

Tetanus is due to infection of a wound—particularly of a deep penetrating wound or one in which there has been considerable destruction of tissue or which has been contaminated with soil—by tetanus spores. Wounds contracted in warfare are particularly liable to infection with tetanus bacilli. Infection of such wounds with pyogenic organisms increases the risk of tetanus still further. These factors predispose to the disease by creating an anaerobic environment in the wound suitable for the growth of the organism. Thus extensive laceration by interfering with the blood supply causes necrosis with resultant anaerobiosis, and soil lowers the oxidation-reduction potential of the tissues, mainly through the action of its calcium salts. Tetanus may, though infrequently, follow a trivial wound—particularly in children, who are more susceptible than adults—or may result from the infection of a burn or of a vaccination site (p. 486). In primitive communities tetanus neonatorum due to infection of the umbilical stump is not uncommon. In the past a number of infections have been traced to the use at operations of improperly sterilized catgut but as reliably sterile catgut is now available commercially this mode of infection should no longer occur. On occasion tetanus following operations has been ascribed to contamination of the operation wound by non-sterile instruments or other materials brought in contact with the wound or by the dust of the operating threatre from which tetanus bacilli have occasionally been isolated.

The bacilli inflict very little local injury, and there is normally no invasion of tissues, although they have, on a few occasions, been isolated from the spleen. The symptoms of tetanus are due entirely to the action of the neurotoxin, produced in the wound, on the central nervous system.

There has been considerable controversy as to the route by which the toxin gains access to the central nervous system. If toxin is injected into the limb of an experimental animal and the nerves supplying the limb are divided, tetanus does not occur. The toxin must therefore pass via the nerves. Both axonal spread and spread by the perineural lymphatics have in the past been strongly supported as the probable route. There is more convincing evidence, however, that the toxin travels in the fluid between the nerve fibres—its upward passage being accelerated by pressure on the nerves from muscular contractions.

The first symptom of tetanus is usually a tingling sensation in the vicinity of the wound. This is followed by the development of the characteristic muscular spasms occurring first in the proximity of the wound, then in the masseter muscles of the jaw, and ultimately involving all the voluntary musculature. Spasm of the masseter muscles is frequently the first obvious sign of the disease, and is responsible for its popular designation—'lock-jaw'. Death is due to cardiac and respiratory failure resulting from involvement of vital centres in the brainstem. In mild cases, particularly in individuals who have received prophylactic antitoxin, spasms localized to the muscles in the proximity of the wound may be the only manifestation of the disease.

Treatment

The results obtained with antitoxin alone in the treatment of tetanus have been disappointing. This is probably due to the fact that by the time symptoms appear the toxin is so firmly bound to the nervous tissue that it cannot be removed by antitoxin. With current therapeutic regimens in which antitoxin and heavy sedation are combined with thorough surgical cleaning of the wound and chemotherapy to control secondary bacterial invasion, the prognosis has, however, greatly improved. In general the chance of success varies with the incubation period. If this is less than 5 days the patient usually dies; if the incubation period is longer than 5 days most cases should recover.

Prophylaxis

Active immunization against tetanus is carried out by the subcutaneous or intramuscular injection of toxoid. Reactions are rare and usually mild. A full course of injection consists of 2 injections each of 1 ml of toxoid with an interval of not less than 6 weeks between each injection followed 6 to 18 months later by a third injection. Active immunization has been mainly used for individuals, especially service personnel, who are particularly at risk but as tetanus is now a more frequent cause of death than diphtheria there is a good case for routine immunization for all members of the population in infancy or childhood. For this purpose the toxoid is frequently given as a component of triple vaccine (p. 162).

It is of the utmost importance that all patients with wounds should receive adequate and immediate prophylactic treatment. There is, however, some doubt as to what is the best such treatment to employ. For many years the procedure followed by the British Army authorities—the value of which was first established in troops wounded on active service in the 1914–18 war—was widely adopted as a basis for the prophylaxis of civilian personnel. This consisted in the administration of tetanus antitoxin (ATS) to non-immune persons, with a booster dose of tetanus toxoid to those who were deemed to be immune. Immune persons were defined as those who had received two doses of tetanus toxoid within 6 months before the accident, or 3 doses—i.e. a full course—of toxoid within 5 years before the accident. In recent years, however, the acceptability of this regimen for civilians has been challenged by a number of workers. The grounds on which this challenge is based are: (1) The high incidence of reactions following the administration of ATS prepared in the horse. Under the conditions of active service the risk of death from an anaphylactic reaction might be much less than that of death following tetanus. This, however, does not necessarily apply to a civilian population. (2) In subjects who have received a previous injection of antitoxin the antitoxin is rapidly eliminated as a result of an immune response. Because of this the patient is protected only for a fairly short time. (3) Many cases of tetanus, particularly in children, occur as a result of minor wounds. These wounds admittedly carry a lower risk of tetanus than severe wounds but are much more numerous in incidence; in Cox and Knowelden's survey, which covered a 7-year period, minor wounds were responsible for the majority of cases of tetanus investigated. This disparity must, to some extent, be due to the fact that only the more serious wounds were reported and adequately treated, while trivial wounds were either not reported or were not regarded as requiring specific tetanus prophylaxis.

On these grounds Cox and Knowelden recommended the total abandonment of ATS. Instead they proposed, together with the thorough cleaning of the wound, the administration of penicillin and, regardless of the state of immunity of the patient, an injection of tetanus toxoid. This would be followed, for those who were not previously immunized, by a complete course of active immunization. Following the adoption of this regimen they found no significant increase in the incidence of tetanus. Many authorities are, however, reluctant to abandon the use of antitoxin completely, and consider it should be given if the wound is thought to carry a particularly high risk of tetanus—especially if there has been an appreciable delay in treatment. As an alternative to horse antitoxin, human gamma globulin obtained from persons who have been immunized with tetanus toxoid, could, if available, be employed. If the number of cases to which anti-toxin is given were small the general substitution of human antitoxin for horse antitoxin, which would eliminate the risk of an anaphylactic reaction, would be feasible. Human antitoxin has been found by Suri and Rubbo to persist much longer in the circulation than horse antitoxin, and since it can be used in low doses it does not interfere with the immunological responses to toxoid administered at the same time. It remains to be seen whether the increase in severe anaphylactic reactions to penicillin, following the adoption of such a programme, would more than outweigh the number of reactions to antitoxin. In this connexion it has been suggested that antibiotic should be given only to non-immune subjects. As an alternative to penicillin, erythromycin or tetracycline to both of which tetanus bacilli appear to be uniformly sensitive may be employed.

In the prophylaxis of tetanus, whatever specific prophylaxis is employed, a thorough surgical toilet of the wound removing all devitalized tissue and foreign material is of the greatest importance. In addition local antibiotic treatment of the wound, e.g. in dusting powder is recommended.

Clostridium botulinum

Clostridium botulinum, the cause of botulism in man and of similar intoxications in various animals, is a large thick bacillus with oval, central or subterminal spores. Six distinct types of *Cl. botulinum*—A, B, C, D, E and F are described. The types differ in producing antigenically distinct exotoxins and in certain biochemical properties. *Cl. botulinum* occurs more frequently in virgin than in cultivated soil.

Cultural Properties

Different strains of *Cl. botulinum* differ in their temperature optima. Some have an optimum at or about 37° C; this appears to be the case for those most frequently responsible for botulism in man. Others have an optimum in the range of 20 to 30° C. The colonies have a variable appearance but are uniformly haemolytic. On the basis of their biochemical characteristics strains of *Cl. botulinum* are divided into proteolytic (ovolytic) and non-proteolytic (non-ovolytic) groups. All type A and some type B strains belong to the proteolytic group. These strains are classified by Bergey as *Cl. parabotulinum*.

Pathogenicity

Though antigenically distinct the toxins of the various types have apparently an identical pharmacological action. Like the tetanus toxin they act specifically on the central nervous system and possibly by the same biochemical mechanism, i.e. by interfering with the release of acetylcholine. They differ from tetanus toxin, however, in that they act peripherally at the myoneural junction, and presumably interfere with the final stage in the transmission of the nerve impulse. Their effect is therefore very similar to that produced by curare.

The toxins are not inactivated by the gastric hydrochloric acid or by the proteolytic enzymes of the intestinal tract. From the intestinal tract they are absorbed into the blood, and from the blood gain access to the central nervous system. It is thought that the absorption of toxin through the alimentary mucosa requires a preliminary dissociation of the large toxin molecule into smaller fragments.

The different toxins differ in their lethality for different animal species. This probably explains why, under natural conditions, certain *Cl. botulinum* types are associated with disease of particular animals. The great majority of cases of botulism in man are due to type A strains, a minority to type B and a few to type E.

Type A and type B toxins have been isolated as crystalline proteins. The type A protein has a molecular weight in the undissociated state, of about 1,000,000. The toxins are fairly resistant to heat, withstanding exposure to 80° C for some time; they are, however, rapidly destroyed at 100° C. They are extremely potent. 1 mg of the purified toxin has been estimated to contain about 20×10^6 mouse minimum lethal doses and would constitute a lethal dose for 1000 tons of guinea-pigs.

Botulism

Botulism is an intoxication not an infection; it is due to the ingestion of toxin preformed in food by the growth of the organism. Since the organism is strictly anaerobic it is most likely to grow in food which has been canned or bottled. Nowadays, however, the risk from commercially canned food is virtually nonexistent, since in commercial processing the food is heated sufficiently to ensure the destruction of any spores which might be present. Consequently most cases occurring now are caused by food which has been preserved at home. In highly acid foods, e.g. fruits, with a pH of less than 4·5, germination of the spores is inhibited. The danger of botulism from such foods is therefore negligible. Vegetables are now the greatest hazard because of the readiness with which they may become contaminated by spores present in the soil.

Botulism differs from other forms of food poisoning in that gastro-intestinal symptoms are very slight. The action of the toxin on the parasympathetic nervous system is responsible for the most prominent symptoms, involvement of the eye muscles with protrusion of the eyeballs, ptosis, loss of accommodation, dilated pupils, as well as aphonia and dysphagia. Fever is generally absent and consciousness is retained. Symptoms usually appear within 24 hours of eating the food and death, due to respiratory or, more rarely, to cardiac failure, occurs 4 to 8 days later. The severity of the symptoms depends on the amount of food (and therefore toxin) consumed. This fact may explain the differences in the fatality rates in different outbreaks which average about 65 per cent. The toxin can be absorbed through the respiratory tract, and its presence in aerosols constitutes a serious hazard for laboratory workers.

Antitoxin has been used therapeutically in the disease in man in a few cases, but it is of little or no value.

Diagnosis

Diagnosis is usually made on clinical grounds and, from the character of the disease, presents little difficulty. Bacteriological confirmation is not possible by the isolation of the organism from the body but an attempt should be made to demonstrate the organism and its toxin in the suspected food.

Prophylaxis

Prophylaxis is chiefly a matter of the hygienic preparation of foodstuffs. Since the toxin which is the cause of the disease is thermolabile, the heating of any food, which may be suspected, to 100° C for a few minutes immediately before use, will make it quite safe. Anaerobic conditions are, of course, most perfect in canned and bottled foods, and these should be rejected if they are not in perfect condition, as judged both by the eye and by the nose. Since gas is produced by the growth of *Cl. botulinum* all canned foods should be discarded if the tin is blown. The ends of blown tins are convex and give a drum-like note on percussion. Blowing of tins is not necessarily, and is nowadays in fact rarely, due to the growth of *Cl. botulinum*. It can be caused by a variety of other organisms, particularly by thermophilic anaerobes, and may also result from chemical interaction between acids present in the food and the metal of the tin. It should be remembered, however, that food in which *Cl. botulinum* has grown may show no obvious signs of decomposition. Because of the very real danger of botulism from home preserved foods, home preservation should be restricted to the preservation of fruits.

Though of little or no value in treatment antitoxin appears to be of considerable value in prophylaxis and when a case of botulism has occurred should be given to all individuals partaking of the food responsible. Toxoids have been prepared from type A and type B toxins by treatment with formalin and can be used for the active immunization of laboratory personnel working with *Cl. botulinum*.

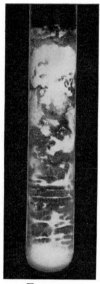

FIG. 32. STORMY FERMENTATION OF MILK BY
Cl. perfringens ($\times \frac{1}{2}$)

The Clostridia of Gas-gangrene

A great variety of clostridial species have been isolated from cases of gas-gangrene. Many of these, however, are purely saprophytic or are present as secondary invaders. The most important species and those primarily responsible for the condition are *Cl. perfringens*, *Cl. novyi* and *Cl. septicum*. Each of these is an active toxin producer and, although frequently present along with other species, can cause gas-gangrene by itself. *Cl. perfringens* is the species most frequently found, being present in about 60 per cent of all cases.

Clostridium perfringens (*Cl. welchii*)

Morphology

Clostridium perfringens is a large, Gram positive, non-motile, bacillus with square-cut or slightly rounded ends, usually measuring from 4 to 8μ by 0·8 to 1·2μ. Capsules are present in the tissues, but are found in cultures only when the medium contains serum. The organism produces oval subterminal spores which are of smaller diameter than the bacillus. Spores are not seen in the tissues and are not produced in media containing any carbohydrate fermented by the bacillus. Special media have been described, however, e.g. Ellner's medium, which will stimulate spore formation in culture.

Cultural Properties

Clostridium perfringens is a strict anaerobe. On blood agar it produces round, smooth, colonies with an entire edge and is haemolytic. _Cl. perfringens_ is actively saccharolytic but exhibits little proteolytic activity. A very characteristic change—the so-called 'stormy fermentation'—is produced in milk cultures. There is coagulation of the casein into a clot, which floats in an almost clear whey and the clot and layer of cream are torn and riddled as a result of the active evolution of gas.

The species is antigenically heterogeneous.

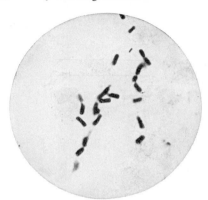

FIG. 33. _Cl. perfringens_ IN MUSCLE
(× 950)

Pathogenicity

Clostridium perfringens is a very prolific exotoxin producer. In the species as a whole a total of eight toxins, lethal for mice on intravenous inoculation, have been identified. On the basis of the major lethal toxins they produce, strains of _Cl. perfringens_ can be assigned to one or other of six subtypes A, B, C, D, E and F. In addition to the lethal toxins a number of extracellular enzymes —collagenase, proteinase, hyaluronidase, desoxyribonuclease and neuraminidase are also identifiable in culture filtrates. Some of these also tend to show a characteristic type distribution.

Only types A and F are pathogenic for man and only type A is involved in the production of gas-gangrene. Type A strains have also been implicated as causes of a variety of bacterial food poisoning. In distinction from normal type A strains, strains isolated from cases of food poisoning have been found to be non-haemolytic, only weakly toxigenic and produce spores with an unusually high degree of heat resistance. Meat which has been kept in a warm environment after cooking is the main source of these strains. In fact heating appears to activate spore germination. Type F strains have been found to be responsible for certain cases of human enterotoxaemia; this is a serious but uncommon condition in which there is a severe sloughing enteritis involving both the large and small intestines. Types B, C and D produce similar syndromes in various animals—particularly in sheep.

The most important of the toxic substances produced by type A strains is the α toxin. This is a lecithinase which breaks down lecithin to yield a glyceride and phosphoryl choline. To distinguish it from lecithinases from other sources, e.g. snake venom haemolysins, which have a different mode of attack, it is

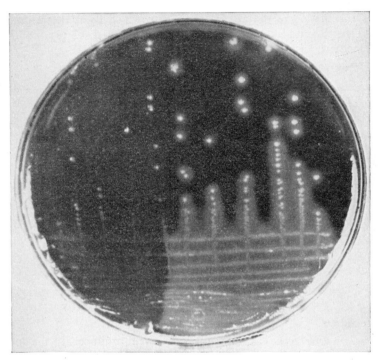

FIG. 34. *Cl. perfringens.* NAGLER REACTION ON SERUM AGAR

known as lecithinase C. It is the only bacterial toxin whose chemical action is precisely known. When injected into animals it causes necrosis of tissue cells and is lethal if given in sufficient amounts. It also haemolyses red cells by breaking down the lecithin of the red cell membrane. In its haemolytic action the α toxin shows the hot–cold effect which is also exhibited by the staphylococcal β lysin. Other types of *Cl. perfringens* also produce α toxin, but in much less amount than type A.

The α toxin may be demonstrated by the Nagler reaction. For this the organism is grown on plates containing 20 per cent human serum or egg yolk; as a result of lecithinase activity lipid is deposited around the colony, giving rise to a readily visible zone of opalescence. If antitoxin is spread over half the plate, it inhibits lecithinase activity and therefore prevents the development of opalescence on that half of the plate. Lecithinase activity and its specific inhibition by antitoxin may also be demonstrated by growing the organism in broth containing serum or egg yolk. Calcium and magnesium ions are necessary for lecithinase activity. *Cl. novyi* and *Cl. bifermentans* also produce lecithinase. The lecithinase produced by *Cl. bifermentans* is antigenically identical with that of *Cl. perfringens* and is neutralized by *Cl. perfringens* antitoxin.

The α toxin is the agent of primary importance in the pathogenicity of *Cl. perfringens*. Since lecithin is a normal component of cell membranes, the toxin is obviously in a position to cause grave damage to tissue cells. There is also evidence that it can interfere with cellular metabolism by its action on essential lipoproteins. Furthermore, by its local destructive action the α toxin creates conditions favourable to further growth of the organism. The α toxin may not, however, be solely responsible for the marked toxaemia found in gas-gangrene. Patients who fail to respond to treatment with very large amounts of antitoxin can frequently be saved by surgical removal of the affected tissue. This suggests that the organism produces some further but as yet unidentified toxic substance by its growth in the tissues.

Other substances produced by *Cl. perfringens* type A, and which may play some part in its pathogenicity are the θ toxin—an oxygen-labile haemolysin resembling streptolysin O, hyaluronidase, desoxyribonuclease and collagenase. Collagenase breaks down collagen fibres and therefore presumably contributes to the disintegration of muscle which is the most dramatic feature of *Cl. perfringens* infection.

Clostridium septicum

Clostridium septicum is a straight or slightly curved bacillus, measuring from 3 to 8μ by 0·4 to 0·8μ, but very much longer forms are frequently seen, both in the tissues and in culture. It is feebly motile. It produces oval, central or subterminal spores which are, however, rarely seen in infected tissues. *Cl. septicum* has a marked tendency to produce involution forms, the commonest of which is a large swollen form, sometimes known as a citron body.

Clostridium septicum is a saccharolytic anaerobe. On blood agar it usually produces a large colony with an irregular surface and with coarse projections at the edge. Some strains produce colonies very similar to those of *Cl. tetani*.

Pathogenicity

Clostridium septicum has considerable invasive powers and has frequently been isolated from the blood stream. It produces an exotoxin which is lethal on injection into animals and is specifically neutralized by antitoxin. The mouse minimum lethal dose of a toxic filtrate is about 0·005 ml. Filtrates of *Cl. septicum* have haemolytic properties which are believed to be due to the lethal toxin. *Cl. septicum* also produces hyaluronidase, collagenase and desoxyribonuclease.

Clostridium novyi (Cl. oedematiens)

This bacillus, which measures from 3 to 10μ by 0·8 to 1·0μ, resembles *Cl. perfringens* in appearance, but is usually rather longer. Spores, which are oval, thicker than the bacilli and subterminal, are freely produced in culture, even in the presence of fermentable carbohydrate.

Clostridium novyi is a saccharolytic anaerobe. It is one of the strictest of the anaerobes. On solid media it produces a colony similar to that of *Cl. septicum*. Type A strains produce a characteristic iridescence when grown on egg yolk agar.

Pathogenicity

Clostridium novyi is a more active toxin producer than either *Cl. perfringens* or *Cl. septicum*—the mouse minimum lethal dose of a toxic filtrate being about 0·0002 ml. The toxin which has been obtained in a highly purified form is lethal and necrotizing but is not haemolytic; it produces a gelatinous oedema by its action on muscle. Other toxic components identified in culture filtrates of *Cl. novyi* include two distinct lecithinases which differ antigenically from the α toxin of *Cl. perfringens*, an oxygen-labile haemolysin resembling streptolysin O and a lipase. On the basis of the toxins they produce, strains of *Cl. novyi* are divided into four types, A, B, C and D. The lethal toxin is produced by types A and B. Most human infections appear to be due to type A. Types B, C and D are responsible for various diseases in animals.

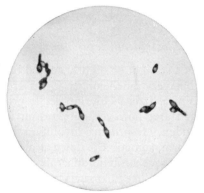

FIG. 35. *Cl. sporogenes* FROM A BROTH
CULTURE (× 950)

Gas-gangrene

Like tetanus, gas-gangrene is due to infection of severe and contaminated wounds. It occurs particularly as a result of wounds in which there has been considerable destruction of muscle, especially of the buttock and thigh. As in the case of tetanus the source of infection is usually the soil, particularly soil which has been contaminated with animal excreta. Clostridial wound infections may also occur after surgical operations in which an adequate aseptic technique has not been maintained. This type of infection, although rare nowadays, was the most serious sequel of operations, particularly of hindquarter amputations, in pre-Listerian surgery.

Most of the systematic work on the bacteriology of gas-gangrene has been concerned with the infection of war wounds. In the North African Campaign of World War II MacLennan found that clostridia could be isolated from 20 to 30 per cent of all such wounds. In the majority of cases the organisms were confined to the surface of the wound and were responsible for, at most, some slight delay in healing. The more serious clostridial infections he classified into two groups—anaerobic cellulitis in which there is considerable gas production in the tissues but the muscles remain normal, and anaerobic myositis or myonecrosis in which there is considerable destruction of muscle. In MacLennan's series these conditions were comparatively infrequent—anaerobic cellulitis occurring in about 5 per cent of wounds infected with clostridia and anaerobic myositis occurring in only 1·5 per cent.

In addition to the primary gas-gangrene organisms which have been considered above other clostridial species, notably *Cl. histolyticum*, *Cl. sporogenes*, *Cl. tertium*, *Cl. fallax* and *Cl. bifermentans* may be present in infected wounds. The presence of these organisms has a considerable adjuvant effect in the production of gas-gangrene by creating conditions in the wound suitable for the growth of the primary pathogens. This is probably particularly true of *Cl. histolyticum* which can actively digest living tissue and of *Cl. bifermentans* some strains of which are strongly toxigenic. (These strains are usually referred to as *Cl. sordelii*.)

Treatment and Prophylaxis

The essential measures in the treatment of gas-gangrene are: (1) The removal of all infected tissue. (2) Administration of antitoxin. A polyvalent antitoxin containing *Cl. perfringens*, *Cl. septicum* and *Cl. novyi* antitoxins is usually employed. In severe cases large doses are given every 4 to 6 hours by the intravenous route. Since it is not possible to identify the infecting organisms on clinical grounds a polyvalent antitoxin must be employed. (3) Chemotherapy. The best results have been obtained with a combination of penicillin and sulphadiazine. The tetracyclines or chloramphenicol, which are highly active against clostridia, may also be employed.

In the prophylaxis of gas-gangrene the most important single measure is the early surgical toilet of the wound. Antitoxin may also be used in prophylaxis but has been largely replaced by prophylactic penicillin. It should be noted that tetanus prophylaxis must be carried out in all persons with severe wounds of such a type as to favour the growth of clostridia.

Active immunity may be produced in animals against the toxins of the gas-gangrene clostridia by immunization with the appropriate alum precipitated toxoids. These, however, have not been used for active immunization in man. It is unlikely that they would be of much value in the prophylaxis of gas-gangrene since the antitoxin response is too slow in appearance to influence significantly the course of the infection.

CHAPTER 30

SPIROCHAETES

The order Spirochaetales comprises a group of spiral, actively motile, flexuous organisms. They are non-flagellated, their motility being due to gyratory and bending movements. Morphologically the spirochaetes are more complex than bacteria—the pathogenic varieties possessing a centrally situated contractile filament to which the body of the spirochaete is attached in a helical fashion. The pathogenic spirochaetes are also much thinner than bacteria. Consequently they are far more difficult to see and in wet preparations are visible only under dark ground illumination. Except for the borreliae they stain poorly with aniline dyes. They can, however, be stained with Giemsa's stain or by silver impregnation methods, e.g. Fontana's or Levaditi's.

Three genera of pathogenic spirochaetes are distinguished—*Borrelia*, *Treponema* and *Leptospira*. These are differentiated on morphological grounds. Of these genera only the leptospirae are cultivable in inanimate media.

THE BORRELIAE

Borreliae differ from other spirochaetes in possessing larger, more open coils and in being more readily stainable. Two groups are associated with disease in man—the borreliae of relapsing fever and *Borrelia vincentii*.

A variety of species of *Borrelia* have been described as being responsible for different geographical types of relapsing fever but it is doubtful whether each should be regarded as a separate species. Two main species are distinguishable— *Borrelia recurrentis*—the cause of European louse-borne relapsing fever and *Borrelia duttonii*—the cause of African tick-borne relapsing fever. Although differing in the insect vectors by which they are spread under natural conditions and in their antigenic properties these two species are very similar in their laboratory characteristics. Of the two *Borr. duttonii* is the more pathogenic for laboratory animals.

Borrelia recurrentis (*Borrelia obermeieri*)

Borrelia recurrentis measures from 8μ to 20μ in length and $0\cdot3\mu$ to $0\cdot4\mu$ in diameter. Its spirals may number from three up to as many as ten in the long forms. They are fairly regular and well marked but during life do not rigidly hold their shape, the whole organism bending and straightening itself. The amplitude of the spirals is from 1 to 2μ and the distance between the crests of each spiral about 3μ. *Borr. recurrentis* stains fairly well with aniline dyes but much better with Giemsa's or Leishman's stain. When stained by Gram's method it is Gram negative. The axial filament of *Borr. recurrentis* appears to consist of several closely packed fibrils.

Borrelia recurrentis has been cultivated in hydrocele or ascitic fluid containing a piece of fresh rabbit kidney but serial subculture has not been possible by this or any other in vitro method. It can, however, be propagated by inoculation onto the chorioallantoic membrane of the developing chick embryo. Following inoculation the spirochaetes invade the embryo and may be demonstrated in its blood.

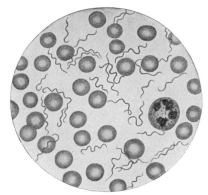

FIG. 36. *Borrelia recurrentis* IN A BLOOD
FILM

Relapsing Fever

Louse-borne relapsing fever may occur in sporadic or epidemic form—the latter occurring under conditions which favour louse infestation, e.g. cold and overcrowding. Consequently epidemics of louse-borne relapsing fever are frequently associated with epidemics of louse-borne typhus. Lice become infected on biting but for a few days after biting are non-infective. During this period the spirochaete multiplies in the body of the louse, eventually finding its way into the coelomic cavity. Infection may be caused by the feeding of the insect but more commonly by contamination of the wound with the coelomic fluid of lice which have been crushed in its vicinity. Transovarian passage of the spirochaete does not occur in lice which can therefore only become infected by biting. There is no known animal reservoir of infection.

In contrast to louse-borne relapsing fever the tick-borne variety occurs as a sporadic disease. The parasite is transmitted transovarially in the tick, and ticks are therefore probably the main natural reservoir of infection. It is possible, however, that there may also be a reservoir of infection in various wild animals, particularly in wild rodents. Some species of ticks are able to transmit infection by biting but with others infection is due to contamination of the bite with the secretions of the coxal glands.

Clinically the tick-borne and louse-borne varieties of relapsing fever are indistinguishable. The onset of the disease is acute with the appearance of fever about 3 to 10 days after infection. The fever usually lasts for about 4 days and then suddenly subsides; after about a week another bout of fever occurs and equally suddenly gives place to a normal temperature. In all, three to ten bouts of fever may occur each of less severity and of shorter duration than the preceding one. The mortality is low in sporadic cases but may be as high as 50 per cent in epidemics.

The spirochaete appears in the blood in cases of relapsing fever shortly before the temperature begins to rise, and the number increases until the fever is at its height. They remain numerous throughout the greater part of the period of pyrexia, but shortly before the crisis they disappear, and none can be found until the beginning of the relapse. There is some evidence that the spirochaetes which survive the crisis do so because they have undergone a change in antigenic type and that each relapse is associated with a further antigenic change.

The tetracyclines, especially chlorotetracycline, are the drugs of choice in treatment. Penicillin also appears to be effective.

Diagnosis

The diagnosis is most readily made by the demonstration of the borreliae in blood films stained by Giemsa's or Leishman's methods or by carbol fuchsin or by the examination of preparations under dark ground illumination. Sometimes the diagnosis of relapsing fever is first suggested during the performance of a blood count when the red cells are found to exhibit an unexpected motility as a result of being jostled by spirochaetes.

Mice and rats are susceptible to both tick- and louse-borne strains, while guinea-pigs are susceptible only to tick-borne strains. For diagnostic purposes the white rat is the most suitable animal; after inoculation of blood from a case, organisms usually appear in its circulation within 48 hours, and can be demonstrated in stained films.

The Wassermann reaction may be positive in both types of relapsing fever; in the louse-borne variety the Weil–Felix reaction may also be positive against Proteus OXK. There are, however, no specific serological diagnostic tests.

Borrelia vincentii

Borrelia vincentii measures from 5 to 25μ in length and has a variable number of loose irregular spirals. It stains readily with aniline dyes, and in wet preparations is actively motile. It occurs as a normal mouth commensal but is present in particularly large numbers in Vincent's angina—an ulcerative condition of the gums and throat—and in acute ulcerative gingivitis. It is generally found in association with fusiform bacilli (*Fusobacterium fusiforme*) (p. 299). A combination of the two organisms is also found in tropical ulcer and in gangrenous conditions of the lung. It has been suggested that they are merely secondary invaders, and that the primary condition may be a virus infection or the result of a dietary deficiency.

Borrelia vincentii has been grown under anaerobic conditions in media containing ascitic fluid. The organism is very difficult to grow in pure culture. Better growth is obtained in mixed cultures with fusobacteria.

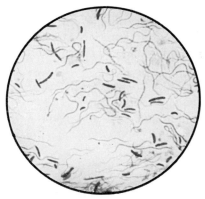

FIG. 37. SPIROCHAETES AND FUSIFORM BACILLI FROM THE THROAT OF A CASE OF VINCENT'S ANGINA (× 950)

THE TREPONEMATA

Treponema pallidum

This organism, which is usually about 8μ in length, may measure from 3 to 18μ, and is extremely slender, rarely exceeding 0·25μ in thickness. It is characterized by sharp, deep, regular spirals, the number of which depends on the length of the individual organism. The size of each spiral is fairly constant, a distance of about 1μ separating the crest of one from that of the next, while the depth of the curve is approximately 1μ. The axial filament of *Tr. pallidum* is composed of 3 very thin fibrils; these can be seen in electron micrographs of organisms which have been digested with trypsin or pepsin. This treatment dissolves the body of the spirochaete but leaves the fibrils unaffected. The filament protrudes at each extremity of the spirochaete as a fine terminal thread which is readily visible in dark ground preparations. The body of the organism is surrounded by a thin boundary membrane or periplast. There is some evidence that it also possesses a capsular layer consisting of hyaluronic acid. *Tr. pallidum* is fairly actively motile with what is sometimes described as a stately motility. It cannot be demonstrated by ordinary staining procedures but can be demonstrated by Giemsa's stain, Fontana's stain or by the India ink method. In the tissues it may be demonstrated by Levaditi's method. In exudates the organism is usually demonstrated by dark ground illumination.

So far *Tr. pallidum* has not been cultivated in inanimate laboratory media. It can, however, be grown in vivo in the testis and, less profusely, in the shaved skin of the rabbit. It can be propagated similarly but less readily in the hamster. Suspensions of *Tr. pallidum* from infected rabbit testis maintain their viability and activity for some time if kept in special media under highly anaerobic conditions. Suspensions prepared in this way are used in the *Treponema* immobilization test.

Treponema pallidum has a very low resistance to inimical agencies and dies out rapidly outside the body. It is very susceptible to the action of heat being destroyed in 1 hour at 42° C. Under optimal environmental conditions, however, it will survive in the cold for an appreciable time. It has been reported to be viable in refrigerated serum for about 24 hours and in tissues of the cadaver for a period of up to 5 days.

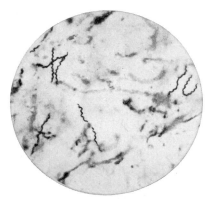

FIG. 38. *Treponema pallidum* IN A LYMPH
GLAND. WARTHIN'S STAIN (× 800)

Syphilis

Syphilis is most commonly acquired in sexual intercourse, but non-venereal infections also occur. It is unlikely that the organism can penetrate the unbroken skin or mucous membrane, but contact of the slightest break in the surface with material containing the organism may be sufficient to cause infection. A most important type of innocent or non-venereal infection is that seen in congenital syphilis, the disease being acquired in utero from an infected mother.

The clinical evolution of syphilis is divided into three stages—primary, secondary and tertiary. The typical primary lesion is an indurated ulcer or *chancre* which appears in from 9 to 90 days after infection. In venereal infections the primary lesion is usually on the genitalia. Extragenital non-venereal lesions may occur but are uncommon. Although the clinically obvious lesion of the primary stage is localized, the organisms at this stage are nevertheless distributed widely through the body, as a result of lymphatic and blood spread. Lymphatic spread to the local glands probably occurs within a few hours of infection.

The main characteristic of the secondary stage is the appearance of multiple lesions in the skin and mucous membranes. In some cases there are also clinical signs of involvement of the central nervous system. About 50 per cent of patients progress to the tertiary stage, which may only appear after the lapse of several years. This stage is characterized by a variety of chronic lesions which may occur in any organ. In the remaining 50 per cent of patients the disease either persists without clinical manifestation or undergoes apparent spontaneous cure.

Treponema pallidum occurs in greatest numbers in the primary lesion, the chancre, and its identification in that situation is the earliest and simplest method of diagnosing the disease. The treponemata may usually be found without difficulty in secondary lesions but are few in number in the lesions of the tertiary stage. Because of this, many workers consider that the intense tissue reaction found in tertiary lesions may be the result of an allergy to the treponema, possibly stimulated by reinfection.

Syphilitic infection confers some degree of immunity. This immunity is sufficiently developed to protect against further infection only if the disease has persisted at least as far as the secondary stage. Immunity to reinfection appears to be due to the antibody demonstrable in the treponema immobilization (TPI) test. Unlike reaginic antibody this antibody is capable of sensitizing the organism to the killing action of complement.

Diagnosis

In the primary stage a diagnosis of syphilis is made by demonstration of the spirochaete in the chancre by dark ground examination (p. 34). Other spirochaetes may also be present in the genitalia, but these are for the most part thicker with coarser and less regular curves than those of *Tr. pallidum*. In addition *Tr. pallidum* usually exhibits, when in motion, an angular bending of the body which is highly characteristic.

Serological tests are of paramount importance in the diagnosis of syphilis. The tests employed fall into two groups: *reagin* tests and *treponemal* tests.

1. Reagin Tests

These are tests which measure antibody to the *cardiolipin* antigen. This substance, which has been characterized as a diphosphatidyl glycerol, is a normal mammalian tissue component, heart muscle being a particularly potent source, but appears to occur also as a component of *Tr. pallidum*. In the standard serological tests for syphilis highly purified preparations of cardiolipin have, to a considerable extent, replaced the cruder preparations formerly employed. The reactivity of the antigen is considerably increased by the addition of lecithin and cholesterol, and these substances are therefore included in the formulations of cardiolipin currently employed. Cardiolipin antigen has been synthesized, and in preliminary studies synthetic antigen has given results similar to those of the natural product. Reagin tests are of two types—the Wassermann test which is a complement fixation test and various types of flocculation test, of which the best known and the most used is the Kahn test. Other flocculation tests in common use differ only in technical details from the Kahn test.

Reaginic antibody is not normally detectable until at least one week after the appearance of the chancre; thereafter positive serological results are obtained with increasing frequency until in the florid secondary stage positive reactions should be obtained in all cases. In late syphilis the antibody is usually, but not invariably, demonstrable. In cases showing involvement of the central nervous system reagin tests are usually positive in the cerebrospinal fluid as well as in the blood. A positive reaction in the cerebrospinal fluid, however, does not necessarily indicate neurosyphilis since antibody may be present as a result of 'leaking through' from the blood. It should be noted that if any bleeding occurs during the taking of cerebrospinal fluid the fluid may give a false positive reaction for antibody if the blood is serologically positive. In the diagnosis of neurosyphilis, cell counts and protein estimations should also be carried out on the cerebrospinal fluid—the number of cells present and the protein content being a guide to the activity of the syphilitic process. In the diagnosis of congenital syphilis it must be remembered that syphilitic antibody may be present in the foetal blood, giving rise to positive reagin tests, as a result of passive transfer from the mother rather than as the result of foetal syphilitic infection. Passively transferred antibody has usually disappeared within 2 months after birth though rarely it may persist for up to 5 months. Serial quantitative antibody estimations are of great importance in congenital cases since if the antibody present is passively transferred its titre will diminish with time while that due to congenital infection will persist or its titre may increase. Cord blood is quite unsuitable for serological testing since it is usually heavily contaminated and as a result frequently gives false positive results.

In tests carried out on treated patients the duration of sero-reactivity depends on the stage of the disease at which treatment was initiated. If treatment was started in the seropositive primary stage reagin tests usually become negative in about 6 months; if treatment was started in the secondary stage the tests usually become negative in about from 12 to 18 months. These figures, however, are subject to considerable individual variation. As a rough rule reaginic antibody persists after therapy for about twice as long as the condition has been present before therapy. In some cases of long duration before the initiation of treatment the tests may not become negative during the patient's life. These constitute the so-called 'Wassermann fast' cases.

The major difficulty in the serological diagnosis of syphilis by the use of reagin tests is the occurrence of false positive reactions. These reactions, which are usually known as biological false positives, fall into two types—acute and chronic. Acute false positive reactions are those in which the false positivity is of relatively short, i.e. a few weeks' or a few months', duration. Almost any acute infection can produce this type of reaction, malaria being particularly outstanding in this respect. Acute false positive reactions are also encountered as a result of smallpox vaccination, during pregnancy, or following prolonged ether anaesthesia. Chronic false positive reactions are much less frequently encountered. They usually persist for long periods, frequently for life, and are not associated with the precipitating causes responsible for acute false positive reactions. A high proportion of patients giving chronic false positive reactions have been found to be suffering from one of the so-called collagen diseases, e.g. disseminated lupus erythematosus, rheumatoid arthritis or rheumatic fever. It is possible that in these conditions the reaginic antibody is present as the result of a process of auto-immunization, the patient developing antibody against his own tissue lipids. Chronic false positive reactions, in the absence of demonstrable disease, appear to increase in frequency with increasing age. This might possibly indicate an increase in auto-immunization with advancing age—an increase which could conceivably have some significance in the ageing process.

2. Treponemal Tests

These are tests in which the antigen employed is of treponemal origin. A great variety of treponemal tests have been described, the most valuable of which are the treponema immobilization (TPI) test, the fluorescent treponemal antibody (FTA) test—in both of these the antigen employed is *Tr. pallidum*—and the Reiter protein complement fixation (RPCF) test.

The TPI test was first described by Nelson and Mayer in 1949. In this test serial dilutions of the patient's serum are mixed with a suspension of *Tr. pallidum* obtained from infected rabbit testis. The mixtures are then incubated at 37° C and examined by dark ground illumination; if the patient's serum contains antibody it will immobilize the spirochaete. The test is technically difficult and is available only in specialized reference laboratories.

It is now generally agreed that the specificity of the TPI test is extremely high and a survey of a very large number of micro-organisms has failed to reveal any which possess antigens capable of stimulating *Treponema* immobilizing antibody. As a diagnostic procedure, apart from its difficulty, the TPI test has two disadvantages: (1) It does not become positive as early as do reagin tests. (2) In treated cases positive reactions persist for a considerably longer time after cure. The test is therefore of limited value as a diagnostic test in the early stages of syphilis, and, in treated cases, as a test for cure.

The FTA test is a fluorescent antibody test carried out by the antiglobulin or sandwich procedure. A film prepared from a suspension of *Tr. pallidum* is first exposed to the serum under test, washed, and then exposed to a fluorescent antibody against human gamma globulin. The FTA test measures two distinct antibodies: (1) a genus-specific antibody probably identical with that detected in the RPCF test, and (2) an antibody specific for *Tr. pallidum*. The latter appears to be distinct from the immobilizing antibody detected in the TPI test. The FTA test has still to be fully evaluated, but it would appear to show a greater measure of agreement with the TPI test than reagin or RPCF tests. There is some evidence that, if the FTA test is carried out with serum which has first been absorbed with disintegrated Reiter treponemes, it has a specificity as high as that of the TPI test, and that it is at the same time more sensitive for the detection of early infections.

The antigen used in the RPCF test is a protein extracted from the Reiter strain of non-pathogenic *Treponema*. The antibody reacting in the test appears to develop somewhat earlier than *Treponema* immobilizing antibody but later than reaginic antibody. Its duration after cure appears to be intermediate between that of reagin and *Treponema* immobilizing antibody. Like the TPI test, therefore, it is of limited value as a test for cure. Because of its technical simplicity, however, it is much more suitable for routine use. Most workers familiar with the test feel that it should be included along with reagin tests as a routine procedure. It gives much fewer false positive reactions than the latter but its sensitivity is somewhat less than the TPI or FTA tests.

Treatment

For many years organic arsenical compounds and preparations of bismuth were the only drugs available for the treatment of syphilis. They were highly effective but their use has been rendered obsolete by the introduction of penicillin—a drug which is actively spirochaeticidal, virtually non-toxic and effective after a much shorter period of treatment. Unfortunately, a small proportion of patients treated with penicillin relapse after apparent clinical cure. It has been suggested that these failures may be due to the persistence of spirochaetes in a quiescent state in which they are insusceptible to the action of the drug. Cephaloridine is also effective and has been recommended for the treatment of patients allergic to penicillin.

Treponemata of the Endemic Treponematoses

The endemic treponematoses constitute a group of non-venereal treponemal infections which are endemic in various parts of the world. They are transmitted by close contact and only occur in communities with low standards of hygiene. In such communities infection normally occurs early in life and is usually contracted from an infected parent. Congenital infection does not appear to occur. Three distinct types of endemic treponemal infection are recognized: Yaws, due to *Treponema pertenue*, pinta due to *Treponema carateum* and endemic syphilis.

The treponemata responsible for these conditions are morphologically indistinguishable from *Tr. pallidum* and like the latter are non-cultivable on inanimate laboratory media. Their antigenic resemblance to *Tr. pallidum* is shown by the fact that the sera of infected patients contain both *Treponema* immobilizing and reaginic antibodies.

Yaws

Yaws is almost exclusively a disease of tropical countries, occurring in a belt extending roughly from the Tropic of Cancer to the Tropic of Capricorn.

The primary lesions of yaws occur on exposed areas, usually on the lower legs or the feet; these appear as painless papules which progress to ulceration. In the secondary stage, which usually supervenes after an interval of two or three months from the onset of the disease, widespread lesions similar in appearance to the primary lesions appear in the skin and mucous membranes. Corresponding to the tertiary stage of syphilis, ulcerative lesions in the skin and bone appear as late manifestations. The disease is contracted by direct contact with the ulcerating lesions in which the treponemata are present in large numbers.

Like *Tr. pallidum*, *Tr. pertenue* can be propagated in rabbits and hamsters. According to Turner and Hollander there are slight but significant differences in the pathogenicity of the two species, *Tr. pertenue* strains producing on the whole less indurated lesions in rabbits and more spreading lesions in hamsters than *Tr. pallidum*.

Pinta

Pinta appears to be almost exclusively a disease of Central and South America. The first sign of the disease is the appearance on an exposed area of the body of a primary papule or 'pintid'. Unlike the primary lesion of yaws this does not progress to ulceration. It is usually followed in from 5 to 18 months by the appearance of crops of flat erythematous skin lesions which ultimately become hyperkeratotic and depigmented.

Treponema carateum has not so far been serially propagated in laboratory animals but the disease has been transmitted to human volunteers by inoculation.

Endemic Syphilis

In the eighteenth and nineteenth centuries endemic syphilis was widespread in Europe. It was known by a variety of names, e.g. sibbens in Scotland, button scurvy in Ireland. It now occurs mainly in certain parts of Africa and in the Middle East, particularly in the more primitive communities. In its major clinical manifestations endemic syphilis is indistinguishable from venereal syphilis but differs from the latter in the rarity of a clinically obvious primary lesion.

Many workers consider that endemic syphilis is caused by *Tr. pallidum* and that it is epidemiologically the precursor of venereal syphilis—its non-venereal transmission being due to low hygienic standards. With improvement in hygienic conditions the venereal route would remain as the only method of transmission. Turner and Hollander have found, however, that in their pathogenicity for animals and in their immunological properties strains of treponemata isolated from cases of endemic syphilis are intermediate in characteristics between *Tr. pertenue* and *Tr. pallidum*. If this is correct it would seem that the transformation of syphilis from a non-venereal into an exclusively venereal infection is associated with some change in the properties of the treponema.

Non-Pathogenic Treponemata

Non-pathogenic treponemata are frequently present about the genitalia and in the mouth; they can be distinguished morphologically from *Tr. pallidum* but the differentiation requires considerable experience.

The Reiter strain of non-pathogenic treponeme is of importance as the source of antigen for the RPCF test (p. 407). Unlike the pathogenic treponemata this organism can be grown in media containing serum. Although originally isolated from a case of syphilis it differs sharply from *Tr. pallidum* in morphology and in being non-pathogenic for rabbits or hamsters.

THE LEPTOSPIRAE

A variety of leptospirae cause disease in man. All are naturally pathogenic for, or parasitic on, various animal species from which man is occasionally infected. Wild rodents are almost certainly the main animal reservoir. The various species may be differentiated in the laboratory by serologic methods; the differentiation is difficult, however, since they show a considerable degree of antigenic overlap.

The most important species are *Leptospira icterohaemorrhagiae* and *Leptospira canicola*. These are of world-wide distribution and are the only types prevalent in the British Isles. In their pathogenic properties, however, both for experimental animals—of which guinea-pigs are particularly susceptible—and for man, they are virtually indistinguishable.

Non-pathogenic leptospirae are frequently found in stagnant water. They are a heterogeneous group but are usually assigned to a single species *Leptospira biflexa*.

Leptospira icterohaemorrhagiae

Leptospira icterohaemorrhagiae measures 5 to 20µ in length and about 0·15µ in width. The spirals have an amplitude of about 0·5µ and measure 0·5µ from crest to crest. It is so fine and its spirals are so small, regular and close-set that, unless examined very carefully with high magnification, it may appear to consist of a chain of granules. Its greatest point of distinction from other spirochaetes is that one or both ends are sharply curved, forming terminal hooks. In wet preparations it is seen to whirl and spin at great speed.

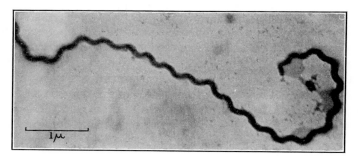

FIG. 39. *Leptospira icterohaemorrhagiae* (Electron micrograph)

Fletcher's medium, containing diluted rabbit serum, peptone and 1 per cent agar, is a highly satisfactory medium for routine cultivation. Unfortunately, some rabbit sera are not suitable for this medium since they inhibit the growth of the organism; a stock of rabbits known to produce satisfactory sera should therefore be maintained. Special media are used for the preparation of leptospiral suspensions for agglutination tests. The most widely used of these, Korthof's medium, contains various salts, peptone, rabbit serum and haemoglobin. *L. icterohaemorrhagiae* may also be grown on a semi-solid agar medium containing serum. This medium is useful for laboratory propagation of the organism since it requires subculture less frequently than do fluid media. The optimum temperature of growth is from 28° to 32° C.

Leptospirosis

The classical manifestation of leptospiral infection—Weil's disease, sometimes known as epidemic jaundice—is most frequently caused by *L. icterohaemorrhagiae*. It is characterized by the occurrence of pyrexia, gastro-intestinal symptoms, haemorrhages, either into the tissues or from mucous membranes and albuminuria. Conjunctivitis is an early and characteristic feature. A high proportion of leptospiral infections are anicteric; this is especially so of infections due to *L. canicola*. In some cases and especially in *L. canicola* infections the organisms localize in the central nervous system producing the symptoms of an aseptic meningitis which is clinically indistinguishable from aseptic meningitis caused by the enteroviruses. Leptospiral infection also occurs frequently in a mild form which can be recognized only by serological methods.

The parasites are present in the blood stream during the first week of the disease. From the second week onwards, they are demonstrable in the urine in which they may continue to be found for several weeks after convalescence.

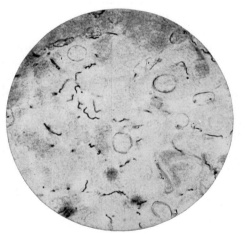

Fig. 40. *Leptospira icterohaemorrhagiae* IN SECTION OF KIDNEY OF AN INFECTED GUINEA-PIG (× 1200)

Human infection is most frequently due to contact with water contaminated by the urine of infected animals. Infection with *L. icterohaemorrhagiae* is usually derived from rats, and therefore occurs mainly in persons whose occupation brings them into contact with water which has been contaminated with rat urine. (Sewer workers, miners and those employed in cleaning fish and preparing tripe.) Infection can also occur as a result of bathing in infected water, usually that of a canal or river. Infection probably occurs mainly through cuts and abrasions of the skin but the organism can probably gain access to the tissues also through the conjunctiva or through the mucous membrane of the nose and mouth. Infections due to *L. canicola* are contracted mainly from dogs, for which the organism is a natural pathogen. In this case infection presumably occurs through contamination of the hands with the animal's urine. Other domestic animals may also harbour leptospirae but appear to be infrequent sources of infection.

Penicillin is highly active against the leptospirae in vitro, but has given disappointing results in treatment. Immune serum prepared by immunization of horses is reputed to be of value in infections due to *L. icterohaemorrhagiae* if given early in the disease.

Diagnosis

In the diagnosis of leptospiral infection serological tests are of primary importance. The following types of test are employed. (1) The agglutination lysis test. This test employs as antigens living suspensions of leptospirae and permits the titration of both agglutinating and lytic antibodies. (2) The agglutination test using formalin killed suspensions. This test only detects agglutinating antibodies. In both these tests the results are read by dark ground microscopy. Other tests which have been used are the red cell sensitization test and the complement fixation test. The latter is difficult to standardize but has recently been favourably reported on. In Britain suspensions of both *L. icterohaemorrhagiae* and *L. canicola*, which are the prevalent species, are used as antigens in the serological tests. Because of antigenic relationship between these two organisms some antibody against the heterologous antigen is usually found, particularly in the early stages of the disease. In the later stages of infection the titre is much higher against the homologous antigen. If possible a rising titre of antibody should be demonstrated.

Isolation of the organism may be attempted by the intraperitoneal inoculation of a guinea-pig with the patient's blood in the first week, or, later, with the centrifuged deposit of the patient's urine. Leptospirae may be demonstrable in the peritoneal cavity within a few days of inoculation. When this occurs some of the blood of the animal is taken by cardiac puncture and inoculated into a suitable medium. Since some human strains have little pathogenicity for animals direct culture from the same materials should be attempted. Microscopic examination of the deposit from the urine with the dark field condenser is often sufficient, but care must be exercised since other spirochaetes may be present. If the urine is acid in reaction the organisms disintegrate rapidly. Dark ground examination of the blood is not reliable since red blood cell fragments may present an appearance very similar to leptospirae.

CHAPTER 31

THE GENERAL PROPERTIES OF VIRUSES

As currently defined, viruses are a group of micro-organisms differing from bacteria in the following respects. (*a*) They are very much smaller. The human pathogenic viruses range in size from the small viruses of the arbo group, which measure about 20 mµ in diameter, to the large viruses of the pox group which measure from 250 to 300 mµ in their longest axis. Since the limit of resolution of the ordinary light microscope is about 250 mµ it is only the viruses at the upper end of this range which can be demonstrated by ordinary microscopic methods. (*b*) They cannot be cultivated on inanimate laboratory media. Viruses are obligatory intracellular parasites and will grow only within other living cells. Their obligatory parasitism is essentially a consequence of their small size. They are in fact so small that they cannot accommodate the enzymatic machinery which would allow them to maintain an independent free-living existence. They can reproduce only if they can make use of the metabolic machinery of the host cell for the production of the raw materials required for the synthesis of virus components. They are therefore not independent organisms in the sense in which bacteria are independent organisms.

The criteria considered above have for many years been regarded as sufficient for the definition of the viruses. The definition is too wide, however, since it admits the inclusion as viruses of micro-organisms—the rickettsiae and chlamydiae—which are now more usually regarded as very small bacteria. In current usage therefore the term virus includes the following additional criteria. (*a*) They possess only a single type of nucleic acid—which may be either RNA or DNA. (*b*) They do not multiply by binary fission. Instead, when a virus infects a cell the viral capsid is broken down with the liberation of the viral nucleic acid. The latter then proceeds to replicate, and its genetic information is translated into the synthesis of virus-specific protein. Because of this loss of virus integrity, there is—following infection and concomitant with the breakdown of the virus particle and before the synthesis of new virus—a phase during which infective virus cannot be recovered from the cell. This is known as the *eclipse* phase.

The obligatory parasitism of the viruses has aroused considerable speculation and controversy concerning their evolutionary status. One view which has been widely held is that they have arisen by a process of retrograde evolution from bacteria. As has been pointed out before (Chapter 1), it is possible to trade a gradual loss of synthetic ability in bacteria as we pass from the less to the more highly parasitic types. It is therefore possible that at least some viruses are forms of life in which this process has been carried to a stage where the organism is completely devoid of independent synthetic power.

A second possibility suggested by analogy with bacteriophage, and episomes is that viruses are derived ultimately from self-reproducing constitutents of the cells of higher organisms which have in some way acquired an independent status. Thus is seems not impossible that certain of the DNA viruses may at some time have originated from the host cell nucleus and that the RNA viruses may have originated from host cell cytoplasmic components, e.g. the microsomes. As yet, however, no one has demonstrated the transformation of any host cell component either of nuclear or microsomal origin into a virus.

A possible diarch origin for animal viruses is supported by studies on DNA base composition by the technique of doublet analysis. This has shown that for a number of small DNA viruses—all papovaviruses—the viral DNA shows a close similarity in design to that of the host cell DNA while the DNA of large DNA viruses—vaccinia, herpes, adeno—shows considerable differences from that of the host cell. It is possible that where the DNA of the virus resembles that of the host cell the virus has at some time in the distant past originated from the host cell DNA. On the other hand where the viral DNA differs from that of the host the virus may possibly have arisen from a completely different host species—possibly a bacterium.

Microscopy

Although the majority of viruses cannot be seen by ordinary microscopic methods, the light microscope nevertheless has some important applications in virology.

1. The large viruses of the pox group are just above the limit of resolution with ordinary light and can be demonstrated by the use of staining procedures which, as a result of deposition of stain on the surface of the particle, increase its apparent size.

2. The fluorescent antibody technique (p. 39) has been of considerable value for the demonstration of viral antigens in tissues. Antigenic components of the smallest viruses can be demonstrated by this technique.

3. For the demonstration of virus inclusion bodies (p. 438).

The great advances of recent years in our knowledge of the structure of virus particles have been achieved through the use of the electron microscope. In this instrument a beam of electrons is used instead of light rays, and because of the very short wavelength of the electron the limit of resolution is enormously increased. The electron microscope is capable of resolving particles with diameters as low as 1 mμ, and its use has consequently brought even the smallest viruses into the visible range.

Although positive-staining methods, particularly the shadow-casting procedure, have been valuable in revealing overall virus morphology they are incapable of providing information on virus substructure. For this purpose the greatest single advance has been the introduction of the negative-staining technique of Brenner and Horne. In this technique the virus-containing material is mixed with a neutral solution of phosphotungstate. The latter forms an electron dense glass around the particle, producing a reversal of contrast in the final image. The method not only allows visualization of the virus particle but also permits the demonstration of its structural sub-units; it is strictly analogous to the negative-staining techniques used in the demonstration of bacteria.

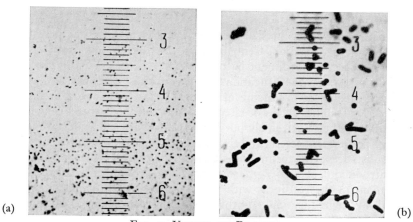

(a)   (b)

FIG. 41. VIRUSES AND BACTERIA

(a) Elementary bodies of vaccinia virus from conjunctiva of rabbit; (b) Staphylococci and *E. coli*. Both (a) and (b) stained by Paschen's stain. Both × 1200. Each division on micrometer scale = 1·1μ

Electron microscopy can also be used for counting the number of virus particles in a suspension. For this purpose the suspension is mixed with a suspension of polystyrene latex particles of known concentration. From the relative numbers of latex particles and of virus particles seen in the mixture the concentration of virus in the original suspension can be estimated.

Purification of Viruses

The starting point in virus purification is usually an infected tissue, the cells of which have been broken down by a process of homogenization. Where available, infected fluids, e.g. allantoic fluid or tissue culture fluid, may also be used. They constitute as a rule a purer source of virus than tissue homogenates. Purification of virus from an infected tissue presents considerable technical problems since the concentration of virus rarely amounts to more than 10^{-8} to 10^{-9} of the wet tissue. Because of this the preparation of highly purified virus normally requires the combined use of a number of different procedures. Even then it is difficult to be completely sure that the virus is completely free from tissue components, some of which may remain adsorbed to the virus surface throughout the purification procedure.

The more important techniques currently employed for purification are the following.

1. Filtration

This may be used to separate virus from larger particles, and has been of particular value in the preparation of viral suspensions free from tissue fragments, cells and contaminating bacteria. Before the introduction of electron microscopy, filtration through collodion membranes was very valuable for the estimation of virus size.

2. Centrifugation

The marked disparity in size between bacteria and viruses permits their separation by centrifugation. Centrifugation in relatively low centrifugal fields of 1000 to 2000 g will sediment bacteria but not viruses. Viruses can be sedimented by very rapid centrifugation. For this purpose elaborate and expensive centrifuges capable of producing centrifugal fields of 20,000 g or higher are employed. By suitable cycles of alternate slow- and high-speed centrifugation it is possible to obtain extremely pure preparations of virus which are free both from large particles—bacteria and tissue debris—and from smaller particles and soluble substances; this technique is known as *differential centrifugation*.

The introduction of *density gradient centrifugation* has resulted in an enormous improvement in the readiness with which particles of different sizes may be separated by centrifugation. In this procedure the material is centrifuged through an aqueous solution of a high density solute, the concentration of which increases progressively from the top to the bottom of the solution. The substances most used for gradient preparation are sucrose, glycerol, with which the concentration gradient is preformed by layering and caesium chloride and rubidium chloride with which the concentration gradient is formed during centrifugation. The rate of sedimentation of the particle through the gradient depends on its size, shape and density. If centrifugation is continued for long enough the particle eventually comes to rest in a zone determined only by its density. Density gradient centrifugation is carried out in plastic tubes from which the different zones can be withdrawn through holes pierced in the bottom of the tube.

3. Precipitation

Many substances capable of precipitating proteins may be used to precipitate viruses from tissue suspensions; ammonium sulphate and methanol have been of particular value. For the removal of contaminating proteins protamine sulphate has been widely used; this precipitates the protein but leaves the virus particles in suspension. Iso-electric precipitation in which the pH is adjusted to the iso-electric point of the virus is also valuable. The virus may however be precipitated at the iso-electric point of protein impurities, to which it is adsorbed on precipitation. A combined immunological and enzymic method may be used by which the virus is precipitated with specific antiserum, the precipitated virus then being freed from antibody by tryptic digestion to which most viruses, though possessing protein capsids (p. 417), are resistant.

4. Adsorption–Elution Procedures

A biological elution method is of considerable value for the preparation of pure suspensions of the myxoviruses. The virus is adsorbed onto red cells in the cold, and allowed to elute through the action of the virus enzyme at 37° C (p. 496). Adsorption–elution procedures employing ion exchange resins, such as DEAE cellulose, and inorganic adsorbents, such as calcium phosphate and diatomaceous silica, are also extensively used.

Other methods which may be used in viral purification are: (a) Treatment with organic solvents—ether or fluorocarbons. These are of value in removing tissue lipids from non-lipid-containing viruses. Lipid-containing viruses such as the myxoviruses and arboviruses are, however, broken down by treatment with lipid solvents. (b) Zone electrophoresis. This permits the separation of particles on the basis of charge. (c) Separation in two-phase systems using water-soluble polymers, in which the viruses are distributed in the two phases in concentrations differing from those of the impurities.

THE STRUCTURE OF VIRUSES

Not unexpectedly, the chemical complexity of viruses depends on their size, the smaller viruses consisting only of nucleic acid and protein. The protein constitutes a coat for the virus nucleic acid, protecting it from inactivation by otherwise inimical substances, e.g. tissue nucleases, which may be present in the environment. Once the virus has gained access to the cell the protein coat plays no further part in viral multiplication. In some cases, however, the protein coat clearly plays a part in initial attachment of the virus to susceptible cells. Such a function has, for example, been postulated for the poliomyelitis protein coat. In this case the coat also imposes a limitation on infectivity since the intact virus will not infect cells lacking receptors which bind with the coat protein, although such cells can be infected by protein-free viral nucleic acid. The protein coat of a virus is generally referred to as a *capsid*, and the combination of nucleic acid and capsid as the *nucleocapsid*. In some cases the nucleocapsid constitutes the entire virus. In others it is in turn surrounded by an outer layer or *envelope* which accumulates as the virus passes through or emerges from the host cell, and much of which seems to be derived directly from host cell membranes.

In the smaller viruses the capsid, as originally postulated by Watson and Crick, is built up, in the interests of genetic economy, from a number of identical subunits. Such a subunit structure restricts the amount of genetic information required for capsid synthesis, the information needed being simply that involved in the synthesis of the subunit. This economy is necessary, since the nucleic acid of the smaller viruses is in itself insufficiently large to code for more than a few medium-sized proteins, and this range must include, in addition to structural proteins, enzyme proteins involved in the replication of the viral genome. It is now known in fact that certain viruses, e.g. the small tobacco necrosis, the Rous sarcoma virus (p. 529) and the adeno-satellite virus do not carry all the information necessary for their own replication, and that they can multiply in the cell only with the co-operation of a larger 'helper' virus which codes for the missing functions.

Construction from prefabricated subunits makes possible a process of self-assembly of the viral capsid in which the subunits themselves come together to form a capsid, in a manner analogous to crystallization. The form of the capsid will in this case be a function of the geometry of the subunits. In the capsid structure the subunits will be held together by intermolecular forces, without the formation of covalent bonds, and the final position they take up will be that characterized, as in crystal formation, by a minimum of free energy. Because of this requirement the resultant structure will have considerable stability. Self-assembly is obviously a highly economical process since it eliminates the necessity for a multiplicity of enzymatic steps which might otherwise be required. It is in addition a highly efficient method for the construction of a complex structure since it is self-checking, subunits which may have structural defects being automatically rejected. There is evidence that a similar process of self-assembly is involved in the synthesis of bacterial flagella from flagellin subunits (p. 9). In the completed capsid, bonding between the nucleic acid and the overlying protein subunits contributes to the stability of the final structure. Nevertheless the relationship between the capsid and nucleic acid is not a highly specific one, the same capsid structure being capable of accommodating different molecular species of nucleic acid.

The subunit composition of the capsid is also important in relation to the release of the viral nucleic acid in infected cells. The removal of the protein coat is clearly a simpler process if it involves only the disassembly of non-covalently bonded subunits than if it involves the degradation of an integral protein sheath. In the case of the icosahedral viruses the removal of only a relatively few subunits might result in the release of the contained nucleic acid.

Many viruses when present in high concentration form characteristic crystals. The crystals consist of aggregates of virus particles which are released again when the crystal is dissolved. Crystal formation is a consequence of the regular geometry or symmetry of the virus particle. It occurs most readily with purified preparations of virus but in some cases—tobacco mosaic virus and the adenoviruses—virus crystals may be observed in infected cells.

Capsid Symmetry

Three types of capsid symmetry are described—*complex*, *helical* and *icosahedral*.

Complex Symmetry

This describes the structure of complex viruses, e.g. the poxviruses and the bacteriophages, in which a number of major structural components may be identified. In these the geometry of the total particle cannot be treated directly as a function of the geometry of the repeating subunits. Such a treatment, is, however, possible in respect of the helical and icosahedral viruses.

Helical Symmetry

In this the protein subunits are packed in helical array around the viral nucleic acid. The helical virus whose structure was first determined in detail was the tobacco mosaic virus. This was achieved entirely by X-ray diffraction studies which can be attempted only for viruses that can be crystallized. The completely assembled virus consists of rigid rods; the helically disposed structure

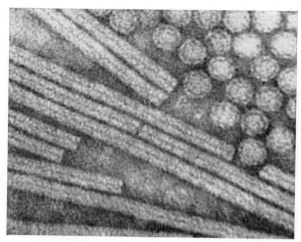

FIG. 42. TOBACCO MOSAIC RODS AND SPHERICAL TURNIP YELLOW MOSAIC VIRUS MIXED IN ONE PREPARATION (*Dr R. W. Horne*)

units—except for those at the ends of the particle—are completely equivalent, i.e. each subunit has identical relations with its neighbours. There is a central, apparently empty core, and the nucleic acid which runs in helical fashion along the length of the particle rests in a groove formed by indentations in the subunits. The complete equivalence of the subunits of the tobacco mosaic virus makes self-assembly a straightforward process, and this has been achieved with the virus under in vitro conditions. It is possible, under appropriate conditions, to disaggregate the protein subunits of the capsid and the nucleic acid and, by reversing these conditions, to reaggregate the complete virus. The protein subunits will also spontaneously reaggregate in the absence of the nucleic acid, to form either the normal helical capsid or a stacked disc structure. The occurrence of the latter in the absence of nucleic acid, and the finding that nucleic acid-free helical capsids are more readily disaggregated than native or reconstituted virus, indicate that some degree of bonding between the nucleic acid and the protein subunits can act as a check on the self-assembly process, and can also contribute materially to the stability of the finished product.

Of the animal viruses, the myxoviruses have clearly been demonstrated by negative staining to possess a helical symmetry but as these viruses cannot be examined by X-ray diffraction little progress has been made in resolving the details of their structure. Recent evidence suggests that the arboviruses may also possess helical symmetry. It is significant that, so far, the viruses possessing helical symmetry have all been RNA viruses. It is possible that this type of capsid would be quite unsuitable for the more rigid DNA double helix. Considered simply as containers, helical capsids are less efficient than icosahedral capsids. On the other hand being capable of exhibiting complete equivalence of subunits they are more readily assembled. Moreover, it is possible that the larger area of contact of the capsid with the environment, and the more intimate association of the capsid subunits with the nucleic acid, may, under certain circumstances, have a specific biological value.

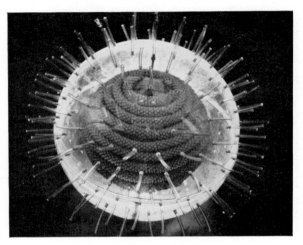

Fig 43. Model of Myxovirus
Note nucleocapsid with helically disposed subunits, envelopes and spikes (*Horne* et al., Virology)

Icosahedral Symmetry

In early electron micrographs many viruses appeared to have a spherical shape. Further studies by X-ray diffraction and, later, by electron microscopy, using the phosphotungstate negative-staining procedure showed, however, that many apparently spherical viruses were in fact icosahedral. Since all the apparently spherical viruses, whether of plant or animal origin, appeared to have icosahedral symmetry it is apparent that icosahedral symmetry fulfils some essential biological structural requirements. An icosahedron is a polygon with 12 vertices, 20 faces and 30 sides, providing axes of fivefold, threefold and twofold symmetry respectively. The biological choice of such a structure for viral capsids was examined by Caspar and Klug, who demonstrated that it was in fact the preferred arrangement for the construction of capsids consisting of a large number of asymmetric subunits, the subunits being arranged in such a way that they possessed a maximum degree of equivalence in their relationships with each other—an essential requirement for self-assembly.

The geometry of icosahedral capsids is complex. The simplest capsid is one in which subunits are located at the apices of the icosahedron. Such a structure, with 12 apical subunits, is found in the bacteriophage φX 174. This structure is in fact the simplest member of a class in which the subunits are located on the edges of the icosahedron, each of the 20 faces of the latter being subdivided into a further series of equilateral triangles, subunits being located at the apices of each triangle. The total number of units required in such a structure is given by the formula $10T + 2$, or $10(N - 1)^2 + 2$, where T is the number of triangles into which each face of the icosahedron is subdivided, and N is the number of subunits arranged on each of the 30 edges of the icosahedron. This type of structure is realized in the adenoviruses, which possess 252 subunits, and in the herpes virus, which possesses 162 subunits.

X-ray diffraction studies, where feasible, have in general indicated that the number of subunits of viral capsids should be 60 or some multiple of 60. This paradox has been resolved by distinguishing between the morphological sub-units, or *capsomeres*, which are demonstrable by electron microscopy, and the fundamental structure units required by X-ray diffraction. The latter would be components of the capsomere and would be located at the apices of each of the small equilateral triangles into which the capsid surface is subdivided. In this way capsomeres at the vertices of the icosahedron would each consist of 5 structural units and capsomeres on the sides or faces of the icosahedron would consist of 6 structure units; because of this is it proposed that they should be designated as *pentons* and *hexons* respectively.

This rationalization fits the observed electron microscopic data well for the herpes virus, the vertical capsomeres of which are clearly pentagonal in outline, and those on the sides and faces hexagonal in outline. If in such a case the structure units which make up the capsomeres are all identical, the 6-component capsomeres should be the most stable arrangement and the 5-component cap-someres should involve some distortion in the normal bonding arrangements, and therefore involve more free energy and possess less stability. They must nevertheless have sufficient stability to function as integral capsid components even if they cannot exist in the free state. It is possible that in the capsid they may be rendered more stable by association with some underlying unit which is not normally revealed by electron microscopy. Units which might possibly fulfil this role have been identified in disrupted preparations of adenoviruses.

Virus Envelopes

As has been indicated some viruses, notably the myxoviruses and the herpes virus, possess an outer layer or envelope surrounding the nucleocapsid. Both the herpes- and myxoviruses possess a high concentration of lipid, the lipid occurring mainly, if not exclusively, in the envelope. In the case of the influenza virus the lipid has been shown to resemble in composition that of the host cell in which the virus is grown, and to be derived mainly from lipid present in the cell before infection. Influenza virus also contains polysaccharide which resembles that of the host tissue. It seems likely therefore that the envelope of the influenza virus is derived directly from the host cell membrane. However, in addition to host cell material the envelope also contains virus specific material, notably the haemagglutinin which appears to be associated with the spikes seen projecting from the surface of the virus, and which are identical with the surface strain-specific antigens involved in haemagglutination inhibition and infectivity neutralization tests (p. 440).

Morphologic evidence on its acquisition indicates clearly that the envelope of the herpes virus is derived from the host cell nuclear membrane, and this is supported by the finding that enveloped herpesviruses are agglutinated by anti-host cell serum, whereas non-enveloped viruses are not agglutinated. That the arboviruses also possess envelopes is suggested by electron microscopic data but the viruses are so small that resolution of their detailed structure has been extremely difficult. The infectivity of all three viruses is destroyed by treatment

STRUCTURAL PROPERTIES OF PRINCIPAL ANIMAL VIRUSES

	Group	Capsid Symmetry	Envelope	Size of Particle mμ	Number of Capsomeres (C) or Helix Width (A°)
RNA viruses	Picornavirus	Cubic	—	18–28	32 C
	Reovirus	Cubic	—	70	92 C
	Arbovirus	?Helical	?+ *	20–100	
	Myxovirus	Helical	+	I 80–120	90 A°
				II 100–300	180 A°
DNA viruses	Papovavirus	Cubic	—	50–55	72 C
	Adenovirus	Cubic	—	60–90	252 C
	Herpesvirus	Cubic	+	150–200 (naked form 100)	162 C
	Poxvirus	Complex	+	200–250 × 250–300†	

* Indirect evidence from ether and desoxycholate sensitivity.
† Envelope of vaccinia about 25 mμ thick.

with ether, and in the case of the herpes and myxoviruses, this has been shown to be associated with disintegration of the viral envelope—a finding clearly consistent with the prominent role of lipid in the composition of the envelope.

RESISTANCE

Heat is the most reliable method of virus disinfection. With the exception of the serum hepatitis virus the human pathogenic viruses are, in general, inactivated by exposure to 60° C for 30 minutes. As in the case of bacteria the inactivating effect of heat depends on the environmental conditions, the presence of organic material affording the virus considerable protection. Viruses, like bacteria, are much less susceptible to dry than to moist heat. Viruses are inactivated by exposure to ultra-violet irradiation and this method is sometimes used in the preparation of viral vaccines. The most active wave-lengths appear to be in the region of 2600 Å. Ionizing radiations on the other hand appear to be much less active against viruses than against bacteria.

As a general rule viruses are more resistant than bacteria to chemical disinfection, presumably because of their deficiency in metabolic enzymes. Of the disinfectants commonly used against bacteria, phenol, the lower alcohols and the quaternary ammonium compounds have very low virucidal activity. On the whole the most generally active agents are chlorine, the hypochlorites, iodine and formaldehyde. Other compounds with appreciable activity against one or more viruses are mercuric chloride, silver nitrate, ethylene oxide and the nitrogen mustards. Ether and sodium desoxycholate have a highly selective action. They have a marked activity against viruses with a high content of lipid, e.g. the arbo- and influenza viruses. The selective action of these compounds is of occasional value in virus identification.

INFECTIOUS NUCLEIC ACID

As we have seen, viruses are completely devoid of metabolic enzymes and are therefore dependent on the metabolic machinery of the host cell. They must, however, carry all the genetic information required for the synthesis of viral material, and this information is contained in the nucleotide sequence of the viral nucleic acid. The nucleic acid can therefore be regarded as the essential virus, the function of the capsid and the envelope being primarily, and in some cases exclusively, that of protecting the nucleic acid. The first clear indication of the essential role of the viral nucleic acid was in the demonstration by Hershey and Chase that, on infection of *E. coli* with T2 bacteriophage, the phage protein coat remained attached to the outside of the cell, only the nucleic acid gaining access to the interior. This finding was soon followed by the extraction—by Girer, Schramm and Fränkel-Conrat—of an infectious protein-free nucleic acid from tobacco mosaic virus and, later, by the extraction of infectious nucleic acid from a number of animal viruses. RNA viruses have been particularly potent in yielding infectious nucleic acids. These have now been obtained from a considerable number of the picorna and arbo groups. Infectious DNA has been obtained from the papovaviruses.

So far, infectious nucleic acid has not been obtained from the larger DNA or RNA viruses. The isolation of infectious RNA from influenza virus has been reported but not confirmed. The failure to extract infectious RNA from these viruses might be due to the fact that their larger nucleic acid threads may be broken down on extraction, or it may be that the capsid and/or envelope may be necessary for the initiation of infection.

The methods most used for nucleic acid extraction have involved as a first stage the rupture of the capsid by treatment with phenol or with a combination of phenol and a detergent, e.g. sodium dodecylsulphate. The nucleic acid is then obtained as the sodium salt, by addition of sodium acetate, and finally precipitated by ethanol. During extraction the nucleic acid must be protected from the action of contaminating nucleases. This can be achieved by the addition of bentonite, which adsorbs these enzymes, and of the chelating agent Versene, which fixes ions necessary for their activity. The recovery of nucleic acid with these procedures is high but the infectivity of the extracted nucleic acid is low, usually less than 1 per cent of that of the original virus, even under optimal conditions. This low infectivity may be due to a low intrinsic capacity of the naked nucleic acid to penetrate susceptible cells. Infectivity of such preparations must be due to nucleic acid since this is lost after treatment of the preparation with the appropriate nuclease and is insusceptible to antiviral antibody.

Although it possesses a low infectivity, infectious nucleic acid usually exhibits a wider host range than does the intact virus. Thus poliovirus RNA will infect a variety of cells which are not infectible by intact poliovirus. This is presumably because, for the cells to be infected with intact virus, they must possess the appropriate receptor capable of combining with the viral capsid. This limitation on infectivity is removed when the capsid-free nucleic acid is used. With the latter, however, only one cycle of virus replication is possible since the product of growth is a complete virus to which the cells are, of course, not susceptible.

VIRUS MULTIPLICATION

Being completely parasitic, viruses can multiply only within susceptible host cells. The mechanism of viral multiplication appears to be fundamentally similar for bacterial, plant and animal viruses. That involved in the multiplication of bacterial viruses, especially of the T series of bacteriophages, which infect *E. coli B*, has been studied particularly intensively (p. 553), and has been the experimental model for attempts to elucidate, at a biochemical level, the stages involved in the multiplication of the animal viruses. Bacteriophage multiplication, as exhibited by phage T2, involves first a highly specific adsorption of the phage to the bacterium, after which the phage proceeds to inject its nucleic acid into the bacterial cell. This initiates the 'eclipse phase' during which no intact bacteriophage can be recovered from mechanically disintegrated cells but during which the synthesis of phage components under the direction of the phage genome is nevertheless proceeding. Eventually, complete fully infective phage is produced and is released from the cell.

Adsorption and Penetration

Similarly in infection with many of the animal viruses we can distinguish first an adsorption phase in which the virus becomes associated with the susceptible cell. The animal viruses, however, do not possess an injection mechanism. It would appear that, for the bacteriophages, the possession of such a mechanism is determined by the necessity for the phage DNA to traverse the rigid bacterial cell wall. With the bacterial viruses, only the nucleic acid gains access to the cell. With the animal viruses, however, the entire nucleocapsid appears to enter the cell, accompanied in the case of enveloped particles by a good deal of the envelope as well. Within the cell the viral capsid disintegrates and the nucleic acid is liberated. Consequently, with animal viruses, as with bacterial viruses, penetration of the cell is followed by an eclipse phase during which virus synthesis is proceeding, and no intact virus is recoverable on disruption of the cell. The sequence of events in the early stages of infection has been examined in most detail for the influenza and polioviruses, and, for both of these, unequivocal evidence for initial adsorption of virus to specific cell receptors has been obtained.

Influenza

The influenza virus is an enveloped RNA virus, the RNA being present in a nucleocapsid possessing helical symmetry. A conspicuous feature of the surface of this virus are the spike-like projections which have been identified as the viral haemaglutinins through which the virus adsorbs to mucoprotein receptors on susceptible red cells. The receptors are susceptible to breakdown by a viral enzyme—neuraminidase or receptor-destroying enzyme—also present on the surface of the virus envelope, and by the neuraminidases of a variety of bacteria. Similar receptors are present on susceptible tissue cells. Thus the susceptibility of the chick chorioallantoic membrane and of mouse respiratory epithelium to infection is lost after treatment with the receptor-destroying enzyme of the cholera vibrio. The subsequent stages in penetration are not clear. There is, however, no evidence of an injection process, as a result of which the viral envelope would be left on the outside of the cell. On the contrary, penetration appears to involve the active participation of the cell, as shown by the fact that it does not occur in the case of non-viable cells. There is some evidence that the first stage is an invagination of the cell membrane around the invading virus, a process which appears to be a strict analogue of the process of pinocytosis, by which tissue cells engulf fluid droplets. The invaginated epithelium is nipped off to form a vesicle round the virus. The breakdown of the viral envelope appears to be initiated by a fusion of the envelope with the cell membrane. It seems likely that the envelope and the capsid are completely broken down within the cytoplasmic vesicles, since virus has not so far been demonstrated microscopically in the cytoplasm.

Poliovirus

In contrast to the influenza virus the poliovirus possesses a non-enveloped capsid with icosahedral symmetry. Receptors which contain a protein component and are probably a lipoprotein mosaic have been demonstrated in the membranes of susceptible cells. They appear to determine the tropism (p. 437) of the virus, being present in tissues susceptible to infection and absent from tissues insusceptible to infection. There is some evidence that the poliovirus receptors of the cells of the central nervous system may differ from those of the alimentary tract, since the latter but not the former were found capable of binding an attenuated strain of virus. A variety of tissues which do not appear to be susceptible to infection in the intact animal are susceptible in tissue culture. This has been shown, by Holland, to be due to the acquisition, under the conditions of in vitro culture, of the specific receptor and only occurs if the tissues are broken down, e.g. by trypsin, so that normal cell contact relationships are destroyed.

Following fixation to the membrane of susceptible cells the virus particles undergo a profound change. The capsids become susceptible to proteolytic enzymes, and lose their capacity to adsorb to susceptible cells. It would therefore appear that the first stages in the disintegration of the poliocapsid is effected by enzymes associated with the cell membrane. These changes are also accompanied by a loss of susceptibility to antibody, but whether this is due to physical inaccessibility of the virus or to a change in the capsid protein has not been determined. The changes produced in the virus by the membrane do not, however, result in the liberation of the nucleic acid. This final stage presumably occurs only when the particle enters the cytoplasm.

Other Viruses

The early stages of viral cell interaction have been less closely studied for other viruses. Nevertheless it is reasonable to assume that they involve an initial adsorption phase, particularly in the case of those viruses which have been demonstrated to possess haemagglutinating activity as an intrinsic function of the virus particle, e.g. the entero, arbo and adeno groups. It must not be assumed, however, that a specific adsorption phase is an essential preliminary to infection. Virus particles could, probably, also be taken up by cells, in the absence of adsorption, by a process of phagocytosis or pinocytosis, as has been shown to occur in addition to adsorption in the case of influenza virus.

In general the breakdown of viral envelopes would appear to be initiated by fusion with the membrane of the host cell. There is evidence that this occurs with the herpesvirus just as it does with the influenza virus. The breakdown of the capsid appears to be essentially an intracellular event carried out by host cell proteolytic enzymes. The enzymic nature of capsid breakdown has been clearly demonstrated for the vaccinia virus. After infection most of the phospholipid of the virus is released in an acid-soluble form, and a considerable amount of protein is dissociated from the virus, possibly in the form of subunits. Both these processes occur close to the membrane, and are due to cellular activity. The final liberation of the viral nucleic acid, however, depends on the activity of an enzyme induced, apparently, by the capsid protein. Heating the virus to 56° C for one hour destroys its capacity to induce this enzyme, and virus heated in this way is therefore incapable of establishing infection. However, heated virus will establish infection if the cell is at the same time infected with another poxvirus which is capable of inducing the uncoating enzyme.

Intracellular Multiplication of Virus

As we have seen, following penetration of the cell there is an interval before infective virus is recoverable. Under the conditions of tissue culture, the length of this interval depends on the particular virus, being about 3 hours for poliovirus, 6 hours for herpes- and vaccinia- and about 15 hours for the adenoviruses. Before the appearance of infective virus, however, it is possible to demonstrate the presence of components which are ultimately destined for assembly into the mature virus. The first component which is directly demonstrable is the nucleic acid. This is not surprising since the nucleic acid carries the genetic code for the synthesis of the viral capsid. The nucleic acid is not detectable, however, for some time after infection. The interval before its appearance allows for the uncoating of the virus particle, for the transport of the viral nucleic acid to the appropriate sites of synthesis in the cell, and, in some cases at least, for the synthesis of the various enzymes necessary for nucleic acid replication.

The final stage in replication is the assembly of the various components into the complete virus. This assembly is known as *maturation*. The primary event in maturation is the coating of the nucleic acid of the virus with the protein capsid. This is envisaged, as previously discussed, as a process of self-assembly, by virtue of which the capsid components arrange themselves around the nucleic acid in a form predetermined by their intrinsic geometry. In the case of enveloped viruses the final stage in maturation is the acquisition of the envelope.

In certain circumstances a defective viral synthesis occurs resulting in the production of an incomplete form of virus of low infectivity. This phenomenon has been most studied in the influenza virus, incomplete forms of which have been found to develop in eggs inoculated with a very large dose of virus and in mouse brain inoculated with a non-mouse-adapted virus; in these circumstances the virus yield has been found to have a very low infectivity titre in relation to its haemagglutination titre. This low infectivity can be related to the fact that the virus has an RNA content very much lower than that of the normal virus. It is possible, although so far no experimental evidence has been obtained for this, that during the synthesis of all viruses a certain amount of the virus produced is of incomplete type. This supposition is supported by the finding that for many viruses the number of infective particles in virus containing fluids as determined by infectivity tests is appreciably less than the number demonstrable by electron microscopy.

On a priori grounds it might be anticipated either that all viruses would be found to multiply in the same compartment of the cell, either in the cytoplasm or the nucleus, or that DNA viruses should multiply in the nucleus, and RNA viruses in the cytoplasm. Neither of these expectations is fulfilled. Some viruses multiply in the nucleus and some in the cytoplasm, the site of multiplication being quite unrelated to the nature of the viral nucleic acid. Viruses multiplying in the nucleus include the DNA-containing adeno- and herpesviruses and the RNA group 1 myxoviruses. With these, the problem of the site of synthesis of the viral protein has not been resolved. The RNA poliovirus, the group 2 myxoviruses and the DNA vaccinia virus multiply in the cytoplasm, and presumably use host cell ribosomes for the synthesis of viral protein.

Much of our present information on the intracellular multiplication of virus has been derived from a study of three viruses, polio, influenza and vaccinia.

Poliovirus

This is a small RNA virus exhibiting icosahedral symmetry. The first effect, appearing almost immediately after infection, is an inhibition of the synthesis of cellular RNA and protein. Whether this is due to the action of some substance synthesized under the influence of the viral genome is not known. About 2 hours after infection, synthesis of viral RNA and of viral protein can be detected. The synthesis of viral RNA is not inhibited by actinomycin D which inhibits DNA-dependent RNA synthesis. It must therefore occur on a template provided by the infecting RNA. This synthesis requires the activity of an RNA polymerase present in the host cell and synthesized under the influence of the viral genome. This polymerase has been identified, and has been found to be insensitive to actinomycin. The first role of the viral RNA must therefore be to code for the synthesis of the RNA polymerase. Synthesis of new RNA proceeds by the formation of a complementary chain which in turn acts as a template for the synthesis of the new viral RNA. This new viral RNA then acts as a messenger for the synthesis of the capsid proteins. This role has been confirmed by the demonstration of the capacity of poliovirus RNA to act as messenger for the synthesis of virus-specific protein on *E. coli* ribosomes, and by the demonstration of its association with polysomes synthesizing poliovirus in infected HeLa cells (p. 435).

The final maturation of the particle occurs about half an hour after the synthesis of its protein and nucleic acid. Evidence from the incorporation of labels into the completed particle supports the view that the nucleic acid, on formation, is coated with prefabricated capsid subunits, a finding which is entirely consistent with the principle of self-assembly. Virus synthesis appears

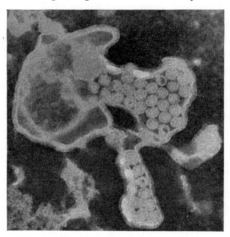

FIG. 44. POLIOVIRUSES IN CYTOPLASMIC
FRAGMENT

Probably the vesicle in which the virus particles are synthesized. Negative staining with phosphotungstate (*Horne and Nagington*, J. molec. Biol.)

to occur in cytoplasmic vesicles which are demonstrable in electron micrographs. The localization of synthesis to these structures is presumably important in preventing the wide dissemination of the viral components through the cytoplasm—a dissemination which might be expected to minimize their chances of assembly into infectious particles.

Influenza and Fowl Plague Myxoviruses

These are enveloped RNA viruses possessing capsids with helical symmetry. The first viral component to appear is the helical nucleocapsid or soluble antigen (p. 440). By the use of the fluorescent antibody technique the protein of the nucleocapsid is first seen in the nucleus. The dominant envelope antigen or haemagglutinin appears later and, as demonstrated by the fluorescent antibody technique, appears to be synthesized in the cytoplasm. The separate synthesis of nucleocapsid and envelope antigens has been confirmed in the case of the fowl plague virus by the finding that exposure of tissue cultures at a critical time after infection to *p*-fluorophenylalanine (FPA) inhibits the production of the haemagglutinin but permits the synthesis of the soluble antigen. If exposed at a somewhat later stage, the production of neither antigen is inhibited, but the soluble antigen is prevented from migrating into the cytoplasm. These findings establish not only the sequence in which these components are produced but also the fact that transfer of soluble antigen from the nucleus to cytoplasm appears to depend on a protein synthesis which is inhibited by FPA. It is by no means certain from these results that the viral nucleic acid is produced in the nucleus, but the fact that the production of both viruses is inhibited by actinomycin suggests that they may be synthesized by the normal cellular DNA-dependent RNA polymerase. By contrast the soluble antigens of the group 2 myxoviruses are first demonstrable in the cytoplasm, and it is of interest that the growth of these viruses is not affected by actinomycin.

Vaccinia Virus

Fluorescent antibody and autoradiographic studies have shown that vaccinia virus is synthesized in areas in the cytoplasm now described as virus 'factories'. These areas have long been recognized by conventional microscopic techniques as inclusion bodies. They are the sites of DNA synthesis and of virus maturation but they do not contain RNA. Consequently, the viral proteins must be synthesized on ribosomes in other areas of the cytoplasm and transported to the 'factories' for final assembly. In HeLa cells vaccinia DNA begins to appear about $1\frac{1}{2}$ hours after infection, and protein synthesis, as determined by inhibition studies, 3 hours after infection. Infectious virus does not begin to appear in the cell until some 5 to 6 hours after infection. The protein coat of the virus appears to be built up piecemeal with the sequential production of various immature virus forms—the final stage in maturation being the acquisition of a surface antigen which can be demonstrated by the fluorescent antibody procedure. About an hour after infection the cells show a considerable increase in three enzymes normally present in the cell: thymidine kinase, DNA polymerase and desoxyribonuclease. It is possible that one or more of these enzymes is coded for by the viral DNA but the evidence so far obtained is not completely conclusive. The production of these enzymes is switched off about 4 hours after infection. This appears to be determined by a protein repressor which is coded for by the viral DNA.

Release of Virus

The final phase in infection is the release of infectious virus from the infected cell into its environment. The extent to which viruses are released from infected cells is variable. With the RNA viruses, most of the virus produced in the cell appears to be released. With the vaccinia- and adenoviruses, on the other hand, only a small part—less than 10 per cent—is released. By analogy with bacteriophage, it might be expected that virus is released by a degeneration of the cell surface analogous to phage bacteriolysis. With respect to the myxoviruses this is patently not the case, the viruses being released as they are formed. In this instance, however, release, involving as it does the envelopment of the viral nucleocapsid with modified host cell membrane, might reasonably be regarded as the final stage in synthesis. It is possible that viral receptor-destroying enzyme plays a part in the final detachment of the virus particle from the membrane surface. Arboviruses also appear to be released from cells which show no significant signs of degeneration. At the other extreme, release of the adenoviruses is preceded by gross disorganization of the nucleus and consequent degeneration of the cell. Cells infected with polioviruses show marked cytopathogenic effects but these are also found in cells in which virus multiplication is inhibited by exposure to p-fluorophenylalanine. In a closely related virus—Coxsackie A10—a cytopathogenic effect has been observed, but only after the virus has been released. These findings suggest that the production of a cytopathogenic effect and virus release should be regarded as two quite distinct events. That the event involved in the release of poliovirus may be an enzymatic one is suggested by its occurrence at 37° C but not at 30° C. Such a process might be the result of an alteration in membrane permeability unassociated with gross cellular degeneration. Such an alteration in permeability has been shown to occur in chick chorio-allantoic membrane cells infected with the PR8 strain of influenza virus, the cells following infection showing a loss of lactic dehydrogenase.

When virus is released from cells into the surrounding medium it will normally readsorb to uninfected cells, and thus initiate a further wave of infection. There is, however, evidence that in certain cases virus can pass directly from one infected cell to an adjacent cell. Thus, tissue cultures infected with herpesvirus will give rise to plaques when covered with an overlay containing immune serum which would neutralize any virus directly extruded from the cell. With viruses which produce a syncytium, e.g. the para-influenza viruses, this would appear to be formed by a fusion of infected cells with normal cells. Spread in this way would explain the persistent carrier state that is not abolished by exposure to immune serum which has been demonstrated with para-influenza 3 virus. For one virus, at least, the varicella zoster virus, direct cell to cell transfer appears to be the main way in which the virus is spread, little virus being found in the surrounding medium.

Inhibitors of Viral Growth

Viruses, being obligatory intracellular parasites, require for the synthesis of their proteins and nucleic acids building blocks—amino acids and nucleotides—fabricated by the host cell. Any attack on the synthesis of these compounds must therefore constitute an attack on the synthesizing functions of the host. The later stages of viral growth, involving the synthesis of viral proteins and of nucleic acids and their assembly into mature virus, are to a considerable extent virus specific, being mediated by the genetic information contained in the viral nucleic acid. These stages are therefore the ones most likely to be vulnerable to specific antiviral agents.

Viral growth will also be specifically inhibited, or more correctly prevented, by any substance which interferes with absorption of virus onto or its penetration into susceptible cells. This is the type of action exerted by antibody (p. 444) and by the non-specific serum inhibitors active against influenza and other myxoviruses (p. 497). An effect on viral penetration is believed to be the basis of the action of *amantadine* (1-adamantanamine)—a substance which has been found to have an inhibitory effect on the multiplication of certain myxoviruses in tissue cultures and in mice. To be effective the drug must be used before or very shortly after exposure to virus. It is of no value in the treatment of established infections but a limited trial appears to indicate that it might have some prophylactic value against Asian influenza in man.

Inhibition of Nucleic Acid Synthesis

Two halogenated deoxyuridines—fluoro- and iodo-deoxyuridine (IUDR)—both of which have marked capacity to inhibit the production of DNA viruses, have been studied extensively. Fluoro-deoxyuridine is an analogue of deoxyuridine. It combines irreversibly with the enzyme thymidilic acid synthetase and as a result blocks the synthesis of thymidilic acid. Its action is, however, quite non-specific. IUDR appears, on the other hand, to have appreciable specificity. It is an analogue of thymidine and its inhibitory action on viral growth may be due either to the production of faulty DNA in which it is incorporated instead of thymidine, or to an inhibition of DNA synthesis. IUDR has been found to have a significant therapeutic effect on herpetic and vaccinial infections in animals. Its apparent specificity has been attributed to the fact that it is converted in significant amounts into a phosphorylated derivative, which is the active inhibitor, only in cells infected with virus.

Inhibition of Protein Synthesis

The production of infective virus can be inhibited by exposure of infected cells at a sufficiently early stage of growth to puromycin (p. 194), which is an analogue of amino-acyl RNA and to *p*-fluorophenylalanine, which is an analogue of the amino acid alanine. Both of these compounds are quite non-specific in action, and are therefore not suitable for chemotherapy.

Two compounds, 2-hydroxy benzimidazole and guanidine, which have been found to inhibit the multiplication of certain picornaviruses appear to act by interfering with the production of viral RNA polymerase. They have not been found to be of value in the treatment or prophylaxis of viral infections in the intact animal. This appears to be primarily due to the rapid emergence of drug resistant viral mutants.

Interferon which may possibly act by interfering with viral protein synthesis is more fully considered on p. 441.

Inhibition of Virus Maturation

The maturation of the poxviruses can be inhibited by isatin β-thiosemi-carbazone and its N-methyl derivative, methisazone. Even in cells which have been exposed to the drug at an early stage the synthesis of viral DNA and of a number of viral antigens is not affected. Because of this the cells develop degenerative changes even though they fail to yield infective virus. Spread of virus to other cells therefore does not occur. This compound appears to have a highly specific effect on the maturation of the poxviruses, no other viruses being susceptible.

CULTIVATION OF VIRUSES

The human pathogenic viruses may be propagated in the laboratory in the chick embryo, in tissue cultures or in the tissues of some laboratory animal.

The Chick Embryo

Inoculation may be into the allantoic or amniotic cavities, into the yolk sac or onto the chorioallantoic membrane, the precise route used depending on the

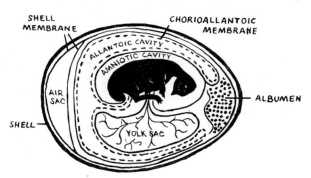

FIG. 45. SECTION OF AN EGG CONTAINING A CHICK EMBRYO.
10TH TO 12TH DAY OF INCUBATION

particular virus being cultivated. The amniotic route is the method of choice for the isolation of the influenza and mumps viruses. The allantoic route, which is technically the simplest, is used mainly for the passage of influenza viruses that have already been established in the embryo. Yolk sac inoculation is of value for the propagation of certain of the rickettsiae and of the chlamydiae. Inoculation on to the chorioallantoic membrane is used for the isolation of the pox- and herpes simplex viruses.

Tissue Cultures

Many of the human pathogenic viruses may be propagated in tissue cultures derived from a variety of animal species. Since, however, a number of common viruses, e.g. the enteroviruses and the adenoviruses, will grow only in the cells of primate tissues the tissue cultures used in diagnostic virology are generally derived from monkey or human sources.

Tissue culture techniques may be divided broadly into three groups— *fragment cultures*, *cell cultures* and *organ cultures*.

(a) Fragment Cultures

The simplest form of fragment culture is the Maitland type culture which consists of fragments of tissue suspended in a fluid nutrient medium. The cells remain viable for several days—sufficiently long to permit virus growth—but do not multiply. In plasma clot cultures the tissue fragments are fixed via a plasma clot to the sides of tubes or bottles; new cells, mostly fibroblasts, then grow out from the tissue fragments. Fragment cultures have no application in diagnostic virology.

(b) Cell Cultures

These are prepared from cell suspensions obtained from intact tissue or from a prior tissue culture. Dispersal of cells is usually achieved by digestion of the tissue or tissue culture with trypsin; this results in the release of single cells and/ or of small aggregates of cells capable of initiating growth. Cell cultures may be prepared as *suspended* cultures or as *monolayer cultures*.

Suspended cell cultures resemble Maitland type cultures in that the cells are simply suspended in nutrient medium. They are extensively used for metabolic inhibition tests which may, in diagnostic work, be applied to the estimation of antiviral antibody. Uninfected cells metabolize and actively produce acid; this causes a colour change in an appropriate pH indicator incorporated in the nutrient medium. If the cells are infected by virus their metabolism is interfered with and the indicator change does not occur. If however the virus is neutralized by antibody the indicator change occurs as in a normal uninfected culture.

In *monolayer cell cultures* the cells are allowed to settle on the sides of a tube or flat bottle and are covered with nutrient medium. Antibiotics are incorporated in the latter in order to control bacterial and fungal contamination. After 5 to 10 days' incubation at 37° C the growing cells will have formed into a continuous sheet or monolayer—so called because it is one cell thick—adherent to the glass of the tube or bottle. The growth medium is then removed and replaced with a maintenance medium which is nutritionally less rich than the initial growth medium but adequate to maintain the viability of the tissue cells. Then the virus inoculum is introduced and the culture again incubated. During incubation tubes are maintained in a slightly sloped, and bottles in a horizontal, position; as a result the cells are continuously bathed by the nutrient medium. Alternatively they may be rolled in a special drum or mechanically shaken. Many viruses when propagated in monolayer cultures produce degenerative changes in the tissue cells readily visible under the lower power objective or, if the area involved is sufficiently large, to the naked eye; this is known as a *cytopathogenic effect*. The type of cellular change produced differs with different viruses. It may consist simply of a loss of normal staining properties. In some cases there is the formation of giant cells and syncytia. In others there may be extensive destruction of the tissue culture sheet. When a virus producing a cytopathogenic effect has been isolated its identity is finally confirmed by neutralization tests with specific immune serum—its cytopathogenic effect being neutralized by homologous serum.

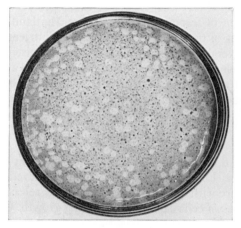

FIG. 46. PLAQUES PRODUCED BY FOWL PLAGUE
VIRUS ON A CHICK EMBRYO MONOLAYER
TISSUE CULTURE (*Dr H. G. Pereira*)

A modification of the monolayer technique, which has been introduced by Dulbecco, will permit the isolation of pure lines of virus. In this, a sheet of cells, which has been grown as a monolayer culture in a flat bottle or Petri dish, is seeded with virus and covered with a layer of agar incorporating the nutrient medium employed. Many viruses produce cytopathogenic effects readily visible to the naked eye as degenerated areas in these plate cultures. If the number of virus particles inoculated into the culture is small, the degenerated areas will appear as discrete plaques analogous to the plaques of bacteriophage (Chapter 41). By subculture from one of these plaques a pure culture of the virus can be obtained which is derived from a single virus particle. The plaques produced in this type of culture frequently have a distinctive appearance which is valuable in identification.

Cell cultures may be divided into three types according to the passage history of the cells used for their preparation:

Primary and Secondary Cell Cultures

Primary cell cultures are prepared from cells obtained directly from the tissues.

A secondary cell culture is the first subculture of a primary cell culture, the cells of which are dispersed by treatment with trypsin or versene for the preparation of the secondary culture. This procedure is particularly convenient for the preparation of monkey kidney cell cultures since the primary cultures can be prepared in a central laboratory, which alone needs to maintain a stock of monkeys, and these cultures are then distributed to satellite laboratories for the production of secondary cultures. Secondary monkey kidney cultures are more likely to show the growth of latent simian viruses (p. 438) than are primary cultures.

Continuous Cell Lines

As a rule when tissue cultures are prepared directly from an animal tissue the cultures cannot be serially propagated, the cells dying out after a few subcultures. A number of lines of mammalian cells are, however, available—mainly derived from foetal and malignant tissues—which can be serially propagated more or less indefinitely. These established cell lines have the advantage of obviating the necessity for procuring fresh animal tissue for each set of cultures. They have the disadvantage, on the other hand, that on prolonged subculture the tissue is liable to undergo spontaneous changes in its susceptibility to infection. Moreover many cell lines which have been directly propagated for long periods have been found to be contaminated with mycoplasmas.

The cells of continuous cell lines differ from the cells of primary and secondary cultures in the following respects. They all present, regardless of source tissue, a similar epithelial morphology, and they are genetically aneuploid, i.e. they possess a variable number of chromosomes. Cells with these characteristics are said to be *transformed*. The established cell line most frequently employed is the HeLa cell culture which was derived originally from a human cervical carcinoma.

Diploid Cell Cultures

The cells of certain tissues notably human embryo cells can, as first shown by Hayflick, be serially propagated for about 50 subcultures without transformation. Genetically they differ from continuous cell lines and resemble normal cells in being diploid, not aneuploid. Diploid cell cultures are highly susceptible to infection by viruses such as the H rhinoviruses and the cytomegaloviruses which may be difficult to propagate in other systems.

(c) Organ Cultures

In this procedure, recently introduced by Hoorn, and adapted by Tyrrell and Hoorn to the cultivation of viruses from the respiratory tract, small pieces of human embryonic nasal and tracheal epithelium in the intact state are grown in Petri dishes containing a thin layer of nutrient medium. Virus growth may lead to impairment of ciliary function, which may be detected by microscopy in situ, and to cellular degeneration, which may be demonstrated in stained sections. The growth of certain respiratory viruses which fail to produce these effects convincingly, may be demonstrable by the interference phenomenon. Organ culture has been recommended for the isolation of cold viruses which cannot be propagated by other procedures. The technique will almost certainly be extended, using tissue from the appropriate organ for the isolation of viruses other than those affecting the respiratory tract.

Animal Inoculation

Of the ordinary laboratory animals the mouse is the most generally useful and, depending on the virus, can be infected by nasal instillation or by intra-peritoneal or intracerebral inoculation. The presence of virus in the inoculated material is shown by the development of appropriate symptoms in the infected animal.

HAEMAGGLUTINATION

A number of viruses possess, or are associated with the production of, haemagglutinins which agglutinate the red blood cells of a variety of animal

VIRAL HAEMAGGLUTININS

Virus	Most Susceptible Species	Notes on Haemagglutinin (HA)
Adeno-	Rat and/or rhesus monkey (a)	Both capsomeres and fibres have HA activity. Maximal at 37° C (b)
Arbo-	Chick (24 hours) and goose	Very sensitive to pH and non-specific serum inhibitors (c)
Coxsackie and ECHO- (certain serotypes) (d)	Human group O	Many elute at 37° C without receptor destruction. Receptors probably protein
Reo-	Human group O (e)	Receptors are polysaccharides insusceptible to receptor-destroying enzyme (RDE)
Vaccinia. Variola Coxsackie A7	Fowl (f)	Soluble lipoproteins
Myxo- (except RSV and measles)	Human group O. Fowl, Guinea-pig	Component of envelope spikes. Virus elutes at 37° C through destruction of red cell receptors by viral neuraminidase (RDE). Highly susceptible to non-specific serum inhibitors (g)
Measles	Rhesus monkey	Maximal at 37° C. No elution (h)

(a) Susceptible cells vary with virus serotype.

(b) HAs associated with fibres and some apical capsomeres agglutinate only with heterotypic serum. They act as red cell sensitizing antigens.

(c) Removed by treatment with lipid solvents or kaolin.

(d) Considerable strain variation in HA capacity.

(e) Bovine cells agglutinated by type 3. Bovine receptors susceptible to RDE.

(f) Red cells of certain fowl only susceptible. Susceptible cells agglutinable also by cardiolipin and certain other lipids.

(g) Mucoproteins susceptible to RDE, KIO_4 and trypsin.

(h) HA preparations highly heterogeneous in size—varying from intact virus to membrane fragments. HA therefore not a satisfactory measure of virus content.

species. In certain cases notably in the myxovirus group the detection of viral haemagglutinins is of considerable value as a method of demonstrating the presence of the virus. Haemagglutination is also used as a basis for antibody estimation since antibody specific for the viral haemagglutinin neutralizes its capacity to agglutinate red cells. Such tests are known as haemagglutination inhibition tests. They are used both for the serological identification of an unknown virus and for estimating the antibody content of a patient's serum.

Viral haemagglutinins are of two types: (a) Haemagglutinins occurring as integral components of the virus particle. Haemagglutinins of this type are found in the myxoviruses, arboviruses, adenoviruses and certain of the ECHO and Coxsackie viruses. (b) Lipid haemagglutinins distinct from the virus particle. This type of haemagglutinin occurs in tissues infected with the vaccinia and variola viruses, the psittacosis virus and Coxsackie A7. The mechanisms involved in the production of lipid haemagglutinins are at present unknown.

PATHOGENICITY

The animal viruses show considerable variability in their host range. Some are highly specific and are capable of infecting only one or a few animal species. Others will infect a wide range of species. Under the conditions of natural infection viruses exhibit a considerable degree of tissue *tropism*, i.e. an affinity for the cells of a particular tissue. In some cases inability of a virus to grow in the cells of a particular tissue may be due to the absence of specific receptors (p. 425); in other cases it is probably due to environmental factors governing the route of access of the virus to that organ, rather than to the fact that it is the only organ in which the virus can multiply.

In general it can be said that viruses damage cells by interfering, during the course of intracellular growth, with their metabolism. In some cases, for example in infection with the papovaviruses (p. 527), this interference leads to cellular hyperplasia. The more usual observable effect of infection however is a progressive degeneration of the cell and it is this degeneration which results in clinical disease.

The extent to which viruses possess an intrinsic toxicity distinct from the effects of virus multiplication is not clear. It has not been established that any virus produces a substance separable from the virus particle analogous to the exotoxins produced by certain bacteria. But some viruses, notably the myxoviruses, appear to be inherently toxic in that they may be rapidly lethal to experimental animals if injected in very large amounts or by a route which does not clearly lead to virus multiplication. Nevertheless it has not been possible to establish in such instances that some restricted virus multiplication has not occurred. In the intact animal overt virus infections are normally associated with pyrexia and general constitutional disturbance—symptoms which in bacterial infections are attributed to the action of bacterial endotoxins. These symptoms are however, not necessarily due to an inherent virus toxicity. Pyrexia may be due to endogenous pyrogens liberated by leucocytes in response to the stimulus of phagocytosed virus. Other constitutional symptoms might be due to the action of breakdown products of tissue cells infected with virus. It has been suggested that severe shock-like systemic reactions, such as are found in small-pox, may be due to some multiplication of virus in vascular endothelium.

A number of viruses are capable of persisting in the animal body for long periods in a latent form which, in normal circumstances, does not produce any obvious lesion. The best documented example of latency amongst the human pathogenic viruses is that of the herpes simplex virus. After initial infection the herpesvirus remains latent, but can, from time to time, be stimulated into activity by a number of environmental factors. Herpes is the only human in-fection which has so far been found to show any resemblance to infection of bacteria with bacteriophage in the prophage state (p. 557). Other viruses which can produce persistent latent infection in man are the adenoviruses, the virus of homologous serum jaundice and the cytomegalovirus.

A number of latent viruses, of which Theiler's mouse encephalomyelitis is an example, have been recognized in laboratory animals. This virus was initially recognized as a latent virus present in the brain of mice and was detected only when the brain tissue of a mouse harbouring the virus was inoculated intra-cerebrally into other mice. Viruses latent in experimental animals may cause considerable confusion in the interpretation of inoculation experiments since, if activated by inoculation, they may be falsely regarded as causative agents of disease in the individuals from whom the inoculated material was obtained.

Latent viruses which give rise to spontaneously occurring cytopathogenic effects have also been recognized in tissue cultures prepared from a variety of apparently normal animal tissues. To date about fifty different types of such latent viruses have been isolated from monkey kidney tissue cultures—the most important of which are the so-called 'foamy' viruses and the adenoviruses. They may cause considerable confusion in diagnosis when monkey kidney cultures are used for virus isolation.

There are now a number of reports of the establishment of persistent carrier infections in tissue cultures with various human pathogenic viruses. In these cases the virus is apparently maintained in cells which have an increased resistance to its pathogenic effects. The study of the carrier state in tissue culture is obviously of considerable importance in the investigation of the mechanisms of latent virus infections in man.

Since viruses do not multiply in tissue fluids, acute inflammatory reactions are not a normal feature of virus infection; pus formation is observed only in infections with the large viruses of the variola-vaccinia group. Chronic in-flammatory cells are, however, frequently observed. These are probably not the direct result of the presence of the virus but are secondary reactions stimulated by degenerative changes occurring in the infected cells.

In many virus diseases, structures known as *inclusion bodies* are present in the cells of infected tissues. Inclusion bodies are homogeneous masses of varying size, usually showing a high affinity with acid dyes. They may be present either in the cytoplasm or the nucleus and frequently have a very characteristic appearance. Some cytoplasmic inclusions have been removed from infected cells by dissection and have been shown to be infective and by special staining procedures to contain large numbers of virus particles. They therefore appear to be intracellular colonies of virus. In some cases intranuclear inclusions also represent colonies of virus. In others, however, e.g. the late intranuclear inclusions of herpes simplex, they are found in nuclei which contain no demonstrable active virus.

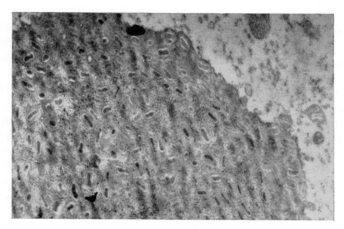

FIG. 47. FOWL POX INCLUSION BODY IN CHORIOALLANTOIC MEMBRANE. ELECTRON MICROGRAPH OF ULTRA-THIN SECTION. × 17,500
The virus particles appear to be embedded in a homogeneous matrix material. (*Dr T. H. Flewett*)

Types of Infection

In some diseases—influenza, the common cold, adenoviruses—the virus appears to remain localized during the entire course of the infection to its initial site of entry. The lesions characteristic of these diseases are the result of local growth of the viruses in the area or organ initially infected. Spread by the blood stream from the initial site of infection with secondary multiplication in some organ remote from the primary site is, however, a feature of many virus diseases —the major symptoms of infection being the result of this secondary multiplication. The frequency with which in this latter group viraemic spread and secondary multiplication supervene on initial infection differs with different viruses. In smallpox, measles, chickenpox and mumps, viraemic spread with secondary multiplication is almost invariable. With other viruses which exhibit this pattern of infection, however, the frequency of secondary multiplication is very low, the virus in most cases remaining localized and causing only mild or inapparent infection. Thus it has been estimated that involvement of the central nervous system occurs in only a small proportion of individuals infected with the poliomyelitis virus, while in the remainder the virus remains localized to the intestinal or pharyngeal mucosa. In certain of the arthropod-borne encephalitides it has been estimated that the frequency of secondary multiplication is even less than in poliomyelitis.

IMMUNOLOGY

Like bacteria, viruses are antigenic and each virus particle possesses, as a rule, a number of serologically distinct antigens. Some viral antigens are characteristic of a particular group or 'species' of virus and these are of considerable importance in viral identification. In many cases e.g. amongst the enteroviruses and myxoviruses it may be possible, within a particular virus species to distinguish a number of different serological types. In certain instances there may be some sharing of antigens by viruses of quite distinct pathogenic properties. Thus the measles virus shows some serological relationship to the rinderpest and canine distemper viruses.

In so far as they have been chemically characterized viral antigens appear to be protein; viral analogues of bacterial polysaccharide and lipid antigens have not so far been identified. Some viruses of which the myxoviruses and adenoviruses are of particular importance produce or are associated with so-called 'soluble' antigens. These are antigens distinct from the virus particle which may be demonstrable in infected tissue cultures, eggs or animals. In general, soluble antigens appear to be serologically identical with protein components of the viral nucleocapsid. Their origin is not clear. They may represent excess material which has not been incorporated into mature virus particles or they may be products of virus breakdown.

Antibody to viral antigens may be demonstrated by the conventional in vitro techniques of complement fixation and precipitation (Chapter 7). Because of the small size of virus particles, however, precipitation techniques are relatively insensitive, since large numbers of particles and correspondingly large amounts of antibody are required to give visible precipitation. Complement fixation tests are more useful since they give positive results with much smaller amounts of antigen. In respect of viruses that possess haemagglutinins as intrinsic components of the virus particle or which produce soluble haemagglutinins, haemagglutination inhibition tests may be used for the demonstration of antiviral antibody. In these the serum under examination or an appropriate dilution thereof is mixed with a standard amount of virus or of soluble haemagglutinin and, after a suitable period to permit combination of antibody with haemagglutinin, susceptible red cells are added. If the serum contains antibody to the viral haemagglutinin haemagglutination will be inhibited.

Neutralization tests are undoubtedly the most sensitive of the methods available for the detection of antiviral antibody. They determine or measure the capacity of antibody to prevent the infection of susceptible cells. The possible mechanisms involved are discussed on p. 444. Neutralization tests may be carried out in experimental animals, in chick embryos if the virus is capable of growing in the chick embryo, but most conveniently in tissue cultures. They can be carried out with quantities of virus which though sufficient to initiate an infection are insufficient to produce any demonstrable in vitro reaction. They will only detect antibody to virus particle antigens. Antibodies to soluble antigens are not demonstrable. Tissue culture neutralization tests may be performed either by demonstrating the capacity of the antibody to prevent the production of a cytopathogenic effect (p. 434) or by *metabolic inhibition tests*. The latter are based on the fact that the metabolism of cells infected by virus is inhibited, whereas if cell infection is prevented by the presence of antibody the cells metabolize normally. The occurrence of cell metabolism is detected by the incorporation of a pH indicator in the nutrient medium. Actively metabolizing uninfected cells produce acid which causes a colour change in the indicator. Non-metabolizing infected cells do not produce acid and therefore fail to produce the colour change.

Interferon

It has been known for many years that infection of cells with one virus may prevent infection of the cells with a second, serologically unrelated virus. The phenomenon, referred to as interference, has been demonstrated in intact animals, in chick embryos and in tissue cultures. Interference differs from acquired immunity (p. 443) in being of very short duration, lasting at most for a few weeks, and in being serologically non-specific. In many cases it can be produced not only by live virus but also by virus which has been rendered incapable of multiplication by heat treatment or by ultra-violet irradiation. The mechanisms involved in interference by inactivated influenza virus have been extensively investigated by Isaacs and his co-workers. They found it to be due to the production by the exposed cell of a substance which they call *interferon* with which the interference phenomenon could be reproduced.

Chemically, interferon is a trypsin-sensitive protein with a molecular weight of approximately 25,000. It possesses considerable species specificity. Thus interferon produced in calf kidney is more active in calf cells than in chick embryo cells; some interferons are in fact only active in the species in which they were produced. Highly purified preparations of chick interferon have been obtained by a combination of ammonium sulphate precipitation, chromatography and electrophoresis. Interferon can be assayed by determining the extent to which it can reduce the capacity of treated cells to produce virus after infection. The most widely used assay procedure is that in which the concentration required to achieve a 50 per cent reduction in the plaque count in a cell monolayer culture is determined.

Although interferon production is most readily studied in cells which have been exposed to inactivated virus it is also produced as a response to live virus. In general, however, live virus is a much less effective stimulus to interferon production than is inactivated virus. When occurring in response to live virus, interferon production is delayed until after virus production has passed its peak. Different strains of virus vary considerably in their capacity to stimulate interferon production. These differences appear to depend primarily on the degree of virulence for the particular host cell system studied. When virulence is high interferon production is minimal. Thus Newcastle disease virus, which is highly virulent for chick cells, produces very little interferon in them. On the other hand, it multiplies poorly in human thyroid cells in which, however, it produces large amounts of interferon. Interferon production is in fact possible in cells that do not support viral growth, e.g. mumps virus does not grow in HeLa cells but nevertheless stimulates them to produce interferon.

The production of interferon in tissue cultures in response to live virus depends also on environmental factors. In general it would appear to be optimal under conditions which limit viral multiplication, e.g. by growth at supra-optimal temperatures, under reduced oxygen tension, after treatment of the cells with interferon or, in the case of poliovirus at least, at an acid pH.

Interferon has no direct action on virus. Its action is entirely on the cell, which it prevents from synthesizing virus and which, instead, on exposure to virus produces more interferon. Tissue cells differ considerably in their response to interferon, embryonic cells and tumour cells being less sensitive than normal cells. Viruses differ from each other in their susceptibility to suppression by interferon, good producers of interferon as a rule being highly sensitive, and poor producers having a low sensitivity.

Interferon production has also been shown to follow exposure of cells to non-viral nucleic acid. Thus exposure of chick cells to mouse RNA has been found to result in the production of a chick interferon. Chick interferon production has been reported following the inoculation of *Br. abortus*—an intracellular parasite. Interferon production is also stimulated by treatment of cells with homologous nucleic acid treated with nitrous acid. More recently it has been found that the production of interferon-like substances may be stimulated by exposure of cells to non-nucleic acid-containing materials, namely, *statolon*—an anionic polysaccharide produced by a *Penicillium* mould, phytohaemagglutinin and *E. coli* endotoxin.

Production of interferon following virus infection is nevertheless probably a response of the cell to the viral nucleic acid. It would appear likely that the response is primarily to nucleic acid which is not replicating; consequently it is favoured by conditions which delay or impede replication. Isaacs suggested that it might act by uncoupling oxidative phosphorylation, and showed a correlation between sensitivity of viruses to interferon and to uncoupling agents. More recently, evidence has been presented by Marcus and Salb that it acts by inducing or derepressing the synthesis of a translation inhibitory protein which inhibits the translation of viral-specific messenger RNA into protein. This is consistent with the findings of a number of workers that interferon prevents the synthesis of viral nucleic acid but has no effect on virus adsorption, uncoating or assembly, and that its action is blocked by inhibitors of protein synthesis. In addition it visualizes interferon triggering a normal cellular control mechanism —the translation inhibitory protein being presumed to have a role in controlling the translation of cellular messenger RNA which must, however, be much less sensitive to interferon than viral messenger RNA.

Evidence has been obtained by Isaacs, Rotem and Fantes of the production in cells infected with some strains of influenza virus of a substance with the capacity to inhibit interferon synthesis. The substance which was resistant to digestion by proteolytic enzymes was demonstrable in crude preparations of interferon. They suggested that the capacity to induce the production of this substance, which they designated 'blocker', might play a role in virus virulence.

There is considerable reason to believe that interferon is the agent primarily responsible for recovery from virus infection. In general, recovery seems not to be due to an immunological mechanism nor does it appear to be due to humoral antibody since antibody may not appear in significant amount until after recovery, and the low concentrations which may be present during the acute stage of infection are regarded as insufficient to prevent the spread of a virus which has already established itself in the tissues. The demonstration, for a number of virus infections, that the administration of gamma globulin has no effect on the course of the infection is further evidence in support of this view. It is also unlikely to be due to delayed-type hypersensitivity since viral infections may regress spontaneously in chick embryos and in tissue cultures in which the development of a delayed-type hypersensitivity is not possible.

The timing of interferon production during the course of infection—peak levels appearing shortly after the peak of virus concentration, but a considerable time before the development of antibody—render its implication as the main agent of recovery extremely plausible. Recent evidence indicates that shortly after the development of viraemia a considerable amount of interferon appears in the blood stream. Circulating interferon is clearly in a favourable position to spread to target organs and protect them from virus attack. In addition experimental evidence suggests that it plays a part in controlling viraemia. Thus mice in which interferon production was suppressed by actinomycin D showed a higher level of viraemia and a greater mortality rate than untreated controls, following infection with Sindbis virus. Protection of sites remote from the initial invasion might be achieved not only by circulating interferon but also by the migration of interferon producing leucocytes.

Since interferon is non-toxic and active against a wide range of viruses it would appear to have considerable potential for the prophylaxis and/or treatment of viral infections in the intact animal. Under laboratory conditions it is most effective if given or exhibited before, or at most shortly after, exposure of cells to virus. It would therefore appear to have more potential as a prophylactic than as a therapeutic agent. That its administration is of prophylactic value has been clearly established under experimental conditions. Thus, in rabbits, rabbit interferon when applied locally will protect against vaccinial infections of the skin and cornea, and in man also intradermal injection of monkey interferon will protect against vaccinia. In animals protection against a number of systemic infections can be produced by parenteral administration of interferon but the doses required are so large as to have excluded, so far, any similar trial in man. As an alternative to the direct administration of interferon the possibility of prophylaxis by stimulating interferon production with agents such as statolon (see above) are currently under consideration.

Acquired Immunity

Humoral antibodies are produced as a result of virus infection and, since their administration both to animals and man will protect against infection, they are presumed to play an important part in specific actively acquired immunity. Further evidence that antibodies can per se protect against natural infection is shown by the fact that in many diseases such protection can be obtained by immunization with killed vaccines of a type unlikely to produce delayed hypersensitivity.

The precise role of antibody in antiviral immunity is not clear. There is no evidence that a virucidal effect mediated by complement is of any immunological importance. Similarly, antibody does not appear to sensitize to phagocytosis by polymorphonuclear leucocytes. Since virus diseases are not associated with a polymorphonuclear leucocytosis—not infrequently they are accompanied by a leucopenia—it is presumed that the polymorphonuclear leucocyte plays no significant part in antiviral immunity. In a number of conditions virus has undoubtedly been demonstrated in leucocytes but has been present in these in a fully infective form. Recent work has tended, however, to attribute an antiviral role to the macrophages of the reticulo-endothelial system. The cells which appear to be of greatest importance in this connexion are the fixed macrophages or Kupffer cells of the liver. The capacity of macrophages to remove virus from the blood stream appears to be considerably enhanced in the presence of antibody, and in the case of the poxviruses there is evidence that the opsonized virus is digested by the macrophage.

Under laboratory conditions antiviral antibody can be shown to have a marked virus-neutralizing effect. It will prevent the infection of susceptible cells by virus—an effect which, in neutralization tests, is the basis of an important method of measuring antibody concentration. Work reported by Mandel, on poliovirus, indicates that two phenomena are involved in virus neutralization: (1) Certain antibodies prevent the adsorption of the virus to susceptible cells, and ipso facto prevent infection. The prevention of adsorption appears to be particularly a function of 19S antibodies. (2) 7S antibodies, on the other hand, permit adsorption of the virus, but interfere with the normal release of the viral nucleic acid. They appear in fact to trigger a reaction in the cell by which the latter is degraded instead of replicated.

That there may also be a cellular component in acquired antiviral immunity appears to be indicated by the finding that persons with hypogammaglobulinaemia not only recover normally from virus infection but appear in most cases to possess a normal resistance to reinfection. Similar evidence has been obtained from the finding that the vaccination of guinea-pigs whose capacity to produce humoral antibody had been destroyed by X-irradiation produced a specific immunity of considerable duration. Such an immunity could clearly not have been due to interferon production since the protection afforded by the latter is of short duration and is non-specific. On the other hand hypogammaglobulinaemics do produce a small amount of gamma globulin and this, if it were highly avid, might serve to protect against virus infection. In this case it would not, of course, be necessary to invoke the participation of delayed hypersensitivity or another type of cellular immunity. The possibility that delayed hypersensitivity may contribute substantially to antiviral immunity, and may be the type of immunity demonstrable in cases of hypogammaglobulinaemia, has received considerable support from the observation of Kempe, that a child who had failed to produce antibody after vaccination, and who had, as a result, developed progressive vaccinia (p. 488), was cured by the injection of leucocytes from a previously vaccinated subject. The possibility is also borne out by the demonstration of parallelism in hypogammaglobulinaemic children between immunity to live vaccinia virus and hypersensitivity to dead vaccinia virus.

The precise way in which delayed hypersensitivity might be responsible for antiviral immunity is entirely a matter for speculation. It is possible that the resultant inflammatory reaction—by lowering pH, increasing local temperature and diminishing oxygen tension—may have a significant antiviral effect, possibly by increasing interferon production. Alternatively, the reaction might be mediated either through sensitized lymphocytes, as has been suggested for homograft rejection (p. 117), or through sensitized macrophages, as is possible in antituberculous immunity (p. 361). A recent suggestion of considerable interest is that sensitized macrophages may respond to virus infection by enhanced interferon production.

Many virus diseases are followed by a long-lasting immunity, one attack of the disease being apparently sufficient to protect the patient for life. In communities in which a particular virus is endemic, and in which, after the first attack, the patient will frequently encounter the virus, such encounters will serve to boost the immunity which he has derived from the clinical attack. There is, however, evidence that antiviral immunity can persist without further contact with the virus, and therefore without further antigenic stimulation. Thus epidemiological evidence has been obtained for the persistence of immunity against measles on the Faroes for at least 65 years, and demonstrable antibodies have been shown to persist for 70 years after an attack of yellow fever in a patient who could not possibly have been exposed to the virus after the initial attack. Antibody to polioviruses has been found to persist amongst Eskimos without any identifiable contact with the virus for 40 years. This long persistence of immunity in the absence of external antigenic stimulation raises the possibility that the virus may continue to be present, though in a latent form, in the tissues. If this were the case one would expect to find, particularly in the poliomyelitis and measles episodes referred to above, cases of contact infection; no such cases have, however, been identified.

The virus infections in which there is a persisting solid immunity are characteristically systemic infections with long incubation periods, and in which the virus has spread through the body via the blood. Under these conditions the invading virus would have considerable opportunity to evoke a secondary immune response in a person possessing some degree of potential immunity. In the case of surface infections with short incubation periods, e.g. influenza, the common cold and adenovirus infections, the virus can establish itself and produce overt infection a considerable time before it succeeds in stimulating a secondary response.

A further factor operating in the case of surface infections is that the virus is much less accessible to antibody than is virus which must first be disseminated by the blood stream. Surface infections of this type are almost entirely due to viruses which exhibit considerable antigenic heterogeneity, e.g. influenza, the common cold and adenoviruses. Because of this, an individual may have a number of attacks of the same disease, each attack being produced by a different antigenic type of virus. For such conditions, therefore, immunity to the homologous antigenic type is much more long-lived than immunity to the disease.

Immunization

Passive immunity can be produced against certain virus diseases by the injection of the gamma globulin fraction prepared from pooled adult plasma. This is the preparation issued commercially as gamma globulin. Its prophylactic value is due to the fact that since adults have been exposed to a number of virus infections their plasma contains a variety of antiviral antibodies. The main use of commercial gamma globulin is for the prevention of measles in very young and debilitated children. It is also of value for passive immunization against rubella, poliomyelitis and infective hepatitis. For the prophylaxis of mumps and smallpox, for which commercial gamma globulin is of little or no value, gamma globulin prepared from convalescent serum, or, in the case of smallpox, from the serum of persons who have been recently vaccinated, is sometimes employed.

Active immunity to a number of virus diseases may be produced by the inoculation of virus vaccines. Of the vaccines currently available the most important are those used for immunization against smallpox, yellow fever and poliomyelitis. The smallpox and yellow fever vaccines are living vaccines. From neither of these viruses is it possible to produce a satisfactory non-living immunizing antigen. This is possibly due to the high lability of the viral antigens responsible for the stimulation of protective antibody to the various inactivation procedures used in vaccine preparation. Alternative possibilities are that the live virus, as a result of multiplication in the body, provides a greater antigenic stimulus than killed virus or that it acts by producing a delayed-type hypersensitivity. Both living and dead poliovaccines are available, and both are highly effective in producing immunity.

Viral vaccines are variously obtained by growth of the virus in the chick embryo, in tissue cultures or in infected animals. It should be noted that when vaccines prepared in the chick embryo are employed they must be administered with caution to individuals showing hypersensitivity to eggs.

THE SPREAD OF VIRUS DISEASES

The majority of the human pathogenic viruses are essentially human parasites, but some are primarily animal pathogens. Thus rabies occurs as a result of the bite of a rabid animal—usually the dog. The arthropod-borne encephalitis viruses appear to be normally parasitic on a variety of bird and animal hosts. The lymphocytic choriomeningitis virus causes a natural infection in mice. The main reservoir of yellow fever infection is in monkeys, although in epidemics the virus is spread by case to case transfer through the intermediary of a mosquito.

In most of the common virus diseases infection occurs through the respiratory tract. The common virus diseases spread by the respiratory route—influenza, the common cold, measles, rubella, mumps—are highly infectious; this is probably because of the large numbers of virus particles in the respiratory secretions. Faeces appear to be a less common source of infection than the respiratory secretions—the enteroviruses and the virus of infective hepatitis being apparently the only viruses which are excreted to any extent by this route. The common wart is the result of direct inoculation of virus into the skin. Rabies occurs as a result of wound infection, and yellow fever, dengue, sandfly fever and the arthropod-borne encephalitides are transmitted by arthropod vectors. In most cases of arthropod-borne disease, transmission is biological —i.e. the virus undergoes a stage of multiplication in the body of the vector. Rabbit myxomatosis provides a clearly established case of mechanical transmission, the virus being mechanically transferred from rabbit to rabbit, without multiplication, by the arthropod—mosquitoes in Australia, rabbit fleas in the British Isles. Some viruses, the most important of which is the virus of rubella, can be transmitted across the placenta from the maternal to the foetal circulation. The homologous serum jaundice virus is unusual in that infection is transmitted artificially, mainly by injection or transfusion.

Most virus diseases occur in epidemic form, the epidemics usually exhibiting a seasonal incidence, and with an interval of one or more years between each major episode. The tendency of respiratory diseases such as influenza to occur during the winter months can probably, in part, be attributed to the fact that it is during these months that people are in closest contact with each other, thereby providing optimum opportunity for spread of virus from one person to another. In general, however, the factors determining the seasonal incidence of different virus diseases are not fully understood. We do not know, for example, why poliomyelitis shows a maximum incidence in the late summer and autumn. It is possible that seasonal alterations in basic host resistance may be involved. The periodic recurrence of many virus diseases—the classic example is measles, which in urban communities recurs at 2- or 3-year intervals—can be explained on the basis of alterations in susceptibility of the individuals comprising the population. Immediately after an epidemic the immunity of the population is high; with the passage of time it gradually wanes to reach ultimately a critical level when a further epidemic can occur.

A great deal has still to be learnt as to what happens to the virus in interepidemic periods. In some, e.g. influenza, it appears to migrate from one susceptible population to another. In others, it persists in the community, and causes subclinical infection or, possibly, remains in a completely latent form. In the case of infections which are exotic for a particular community, e.g. smallpox in the British Isles and United States, the outbreak of an epidemic depends on the adventitious introduction of the disease from outside.

DIAGNOSIS

Although the identification of the aetiological agent of a virus infection is of no value in indicating the use of a particular chemotherapeutic agent, viral diagnosis is of practical importance for a number of reasons: (*a*) The identification of a particular infection as a viral rather than a bacterial infection eliminates the necessity for chemotherapy. (*b*) In certain cases, notably smallpox, rabies and rubella, the information obtained may be of prophylactic value in respect of individuals exposed to the infection. (*c*) When used on a large scale, diagnostic procedures provide a valuable epidemiological record of the infection experience of the community—a record which is of considerable value for the planning of preventive measures on a community scale.

1. Microscopy. Microscopy is of limited but definite value in the diagnosis of viral infections. In smallpox, virus may be demonstrable in cutaneous lesions by special staining procedures as well as by electron microscopy. Electron microscopy has also been used to establish the diagnosis in herpes simplex. Fluorescent antibody techniques are of considerable potential value but so far their most successful application has been in the post-mortem diagnosis of rabies (p. 475) in infected animals. In the live subject they have been used for the diagnosis of herpes simplex and smallpox but in these contexts their sensitivity and specificity requires further evaluation. In general, microscopy is unlikely to be of value in systemic infections in which there are no localized accessible virus-containing lesions. Cytological examination for the presence of characteristic giant cells and/or inclusion bodies is of value in the diagnosis of herpes simplex, varicella-zoster and cytomegalovirus infections and the post-mortem diagnosis of rabies.

2. Detection of viral antigen in lesions by serological methods. In smallpox the virus may be demonstrated in material derived from the skin lesions by serological methods. Virus-containing material may give positive flocculation tests, or positive complement fixation tests with immune anti-vaccinial serum (p. 484).

3. Isolation. An attempt may be made to isolate the virus by inoculation of suitable material, derived from the patient, into the chick embryo, into an experimental animal or into an appropriate tissue culture. Since viruses are very susceptible to drying, swabs should be transmitted to the laboratory in an appropriate transport medium. If the material cannot be examined immediately it should be refrigerated, preferably at $-70°$ C. Most of the human pathogenic viruses can now be isolated by tissue culture. The prospect of isolation is considerably enhanced if a number of different types of tissue culture are inoculated, the particular tissues chosen depending on the identity of the suspected virus. At a minimum the material should be inoculated into primary cultures of monkey or human kidney, and into a human cell line such as HeLa cells. When primary cultures are employed the possibility of activating a latent virus present in the tissue is a considerable diagnostic hazard. The risk appears to be maximal with monkey kidney cultures, from which about 50 latent viruses have so far been isolated. Except for the isolation of the influenza viruses and poxviruses, chick embryo inoculation has been largely superseded by the use of tissue culture methods.

Following inoculation the presence of virus may be inferred from the development of cytopathogenic effects in tissue culture, opacities on the chorioallantoic membrane, or typical symptoms or death in an infected animal or the detection of viral haemagglutinins or complement fixing antigens in infected egg or tissue culture fluids, or the demonstration of haemadsorption in tissue culture. As a final stage in the identification of an animal virus its effects on an experimental animal, tissue culture, or chick embryo or its haemagglutinating capacity should be shown to be neutralized by a specific antiserum.

ISOLATION OF VIRUSES

Tissue Culture or animal	Virus
HeLa cells (C)	Polio. Coxsackie B. Adeno-RSV (a). Herpes simplex
Monkey kidney (P or S)	Polio. ECHO. Coxsackie B. Myxo (b). Reo. M rhino
Human amnion (P)	Polio. Coxsackie B. ECHO. Zoster-varicella. Rubella. Measles
Human diploid cells (lung)	Zoster-varicella. H rhino. Cytomegalo
Chick embryo	AMN: Influenza. Mumps
	CAM: Herpes simplex. Variola. Vaccinia
Mouse	Arbo. Coxsackie A (c). Rabies. Herpes simplex. EMC

C—Continuous cell line   AMN—Amnion
P—Primary culture   CAM—Chorioallantoic membrane
S—Secondary culture   RSV—Respiratory syncytial virus
     EMC—Encephalomyocarditis
(a) Will grow only in sensitive cell line
(b) Para-influenza and mumps grow best in rolled cultures at 33° C
(c) Only suckling mice susceptible

It should be noted that the isolation of a virus from a patient does not necessarily mean that the patient's symptoms are being caused by that virus. This difficulty arises particularly in the case of patients from whom viruses of the ECHO, Coxsackie (Chapter 32) and adenovirus groups (Chapter 38) are isolated. In such cases proof of infection may require a demonstration that the patient has developed antibody against the virus.

4. Serological methods. Where possible two specimens of serum should be examined, one taken during the acute phase of the infection and the second about two weeks later—usually during convalescence. As a rule a diagnosis can be made only if there is a significant rise in antibody titre between the two examinations.

Complement fixation is on the whole the most useful technique for the estimation of antiviral antibody. Since, however, complement fixing antibodies are directed against soluble antigens as well as against constituent antigens of the virus, complement fixation tests are usually less type specific than neutralization tests. Complement fixing antibodies tend to persist for a shorter time after infection than neutralizing antibodies; as a rule, therefore, they are of more value as an index of current or recent infection than neutralization tests. In some cases, notably in poliomyelitis, the maximum titre may have been reached by the time the acute phase specimen of blood has been taken. Under these circumstances a serological diagnosis may have to be made on a single serum examination.

TREATMENT

The treatment of viral infections presents quite different problems from those involved in the treatment of bacterial infections.

1. The integration of the virus with the host cell is so close that most substances which interfere with the multiplication of the virus also interfere with the metabolism of the host cell. Certain substances have been identified, however, which under experimental conditions have a specific antiviral action (p. 431). So far only two of these—IUDR and methisazone—have had any significant application as antiviral agents in man. IUDR has proved to be too toxic for systemic administration but has been used, by topical application, in the treatment of progressive vaccinia and of herpetic and vaccinial keratitis. Its value in these conditions is still to be fully assessed. Methisazone is active only against the poxviruses. It has been used with considerable success in the prophylaxis of smallpox but is of no value in the treatment of this condition. It may possibly have some value in the treatment of eczema vaccinatum and of progressive vaccinia (p. 488). The status of interferon, which is not at the moment a practicable chemotherapeutic agent, is considered on p. 441.

2. In most systemic virus diseases recognizable symptoms only appear after the peak of virus multiplication has passed. In such conditions, therefore, chemotherapy, even if an agent suitable for systemic administration were available, would not appear to be practicable. Conditions which might respond to a specific antiviral agent are those in which there is a prodomal period of non-specific symptoms before viral localization, e.g. smallpox, poliomyelitis and measles or those showing a prolonged slow development e.g. herpetic keratitis, progressive vaccinia and virus-induced tumours.

Although viruses are not susceptible to antibacterial chemotherapeutic agents, such agents are nevertheless of considerable value in controlling the secondary bacterial infection which is liable to complicate certain viral diseases, particularly those, such as influenza, which involve the respiratory tract.

CHAPTER 32

THE PICORNAVIRUSES

These are small icosahedral non-enveloped RNA ether-resistant viruses, with diameters in the range of 15 to 30 mμ.

ENTEROVIRUSES

As their name implies enteroviruses are viruses which are to be found in the alimentary tract, in some cells of which they are able to multiply. Three groups are distinguished: polioviruses, Coxsackie viruses and ECHO viruses.

Enteroviruses are occasionally disseminated through the body, almost certainly by the blood stream, to specific target areas. The most important of these target areas is the central nervous system, which can be invaded by viruses of all three groups but particularly by the poliovirus. Children are more frequently infected than adults, and infection, particularly in younger children, is often asymptomatic. Except for the Coxsackie A group, enteroviruses grow readily in tissue cultures of monkey and human cells. In infected cells they produce a characteristic cytopathic effect, the cells becoming round in shape, smaller and with highly pyknotic nuclei. In agar overlay monolayer cultures each produces distinctive plaques. They are amongst the most stable of the human pathogenic viruses outside the animal body. Since they are resistant to many of the commonly used disinfectants, material which has been contaminated with the more highly pathogenic enteroviruses should be sterilized by heat. Susceptibility to heat inactivation is considerably reduced in the presence of high concentrations of certain cations, particularly Mg^{++}.

The Poliomyelitis Virus

Properties of the Virus

Three antigenically distinct types of poliovirus—types 1, 2 and 3—are known. Although immunologically distinct the types appear to show some minor antigenic overlap. This antigenic overlap is most readily demonstrable in complement fixation tests with virus which has been inactivated by heat or by ultraviolet irradiation. In general the type 1 virus is that most frequently responsible for clinical infection and is the cause of most epidemics. By the use of hyperimmune strain-specific antisera it is possible to demonstrate minor antigenic differences between different strains of the same type. These differences are of value as marker characteristics. They do not appear to affect the response to immunization since vaccine prepared from any one strain will immunize against all other strains of the same type.

In addition to infective virus, infected tissue culture fluids contain a considerable amount of non-infectious, nucleic acid-free, 'incomplete' virus, which can be separated from infectious virus by centrifugation in a sucrose density gradient. This non-infectious or 'incomplete' virus possesses type-specific antigens whose distribution runs parallel with, but which are antigenically distinct from, the type antigens of infectious virus. This non-infectious antigen, known as the C antigen, can be obtained from the D antigen and the antigen of infectious virus by heating. Unlike the C antigen, the D antigen stimulates the production of protective antibody.

Freshly isolated polioviruses will produce infection only in primates; these may be infected by the intracerebral and intranasal routes. Chimpanzees and cynomolgus monkeys may be infected also by the oral route. Certain strains of all three types, but particularly of type 2 have been adapted to mice; these animals are, however, of no value for isolation. Apart from some specially adapted strains the poliomyelitis viruses will not grow in the chick embryo.

The discovery in 1949, by Enders, Weller and Robbins, that polioviruses could be cultivated in tissue cultures of a variety of primate extraneural cells initiated a revolution in the study and control of poliomyelitis. For purposes of isolation, monkey kidney cells and the cells of the HeLa carcinoma have been most used. In the cells of infected tissue cultures all the types produce a well marked cytopathogenic effect.

By passage in rodents or in tissue cultures, strains of attenuated virulence have been derived, some of which, notably those developed by Sabin, are suitable for vaccine production. These strains possess identifiable marker characteristics by which they can be differentiated from virulent strains: (1) They possess neurovirulence for monkeys, but only when inoculated instraspinally— the most sensitive route of inoculation. (2) They grow poorly at 40° C as compared with 34 to 36° C. Virulent strains grow well at 40° C, a property known as the RC/t/40 or temperature marker. (3) Their capacity to produce plaques in agar overlay monolayer cultures is depressed by a reduction in bicarbonate composition of the nutrient medium. (4) They show minor antigenic differences which may be demonstrated by intratypic neutralization tests.

Poliomyelitis

It was at one time thought that poliomyelitis was exclusively an infection of the central nervous system. It is now realized, however, that this is not so and that paralytic symptoms are in fact of infrequent occurrence. According to one widely accepted estimate they appear in only one out of every hundred persons infected with the virus. At least 90 per cent of infections are completely asymptomatic. In others, the only evidence of infection is the occurrence of a mild illness clinically resembling influenza. These symptoms, which are more marked in children than in adults, usually disappear after a few days and the patient makes an uneventful recovery. This form is usually known as *abortive poliomyelitis*. It is due to multiplication of the virus in the alimentary tract and possibly also in other extraneural foci. In only a few cases is this first phase of infection followed by signs of involvement of the central nervous system. These usually appear some 6 to 7 days after the onset of symptoms, and are often preceded by an interval during which the patient feels quite well. In most cases they are simply meningitic in character and the condition progresses no further. In this type of infection, which is known as *non-paralytic poliomyelitis*, the cerebrospinal fluid shows an increase in protein and in leucocytes. In the early stages the cellular reaction is predominantly polymorphonuclear in type, the cell count usually being in the range of 50 to 150 cells per mm³, but after a few days becomes predominantly lymphocytic. Non-paralytic poliomyelitis is clinically indistinguishable from aseptic meningitis caused by a number of other viruses and by leptospirae. In a minority of cases—about 1 to 2 per cent— meningitic symptoms are followed by the development of the typical flaccid paralyses which are the classical signs of the disease.

The characteristic lesions of paralytic poliomyelitis are degenerative change occurring in the anterior horn cells of the spinal cord and in the motor nuclei of the cranial nerves. In fatal cases there is usually extensive involvement of the central nervous system with widespread lesions in the cord, medulla, cere-bellum and motor and premotor areas of the cerebral cortex. By the time the first paralytic symptoms appear, extensive degenerative changes have already occurred in the central nervous system. Since the degenerative process is usually arrested within a few days of the appearance of symptoms, paralysis reaches its maximum extent early in the disease, being complete usually within 3 days of onset of the paralytic phase.

The most widely accepted view on the pathogenesis of poliomyelitis is that proposed initially by Bodian, on the basis of experimental oral infection in chimpanzees. This suggests that the virus multiplies first in the tonsils and/or the Peyer's patches of the small intestine. Coincident with this multiplication there may be, particularly in young children, a short pyrexial phase of a few days' duration, beginning about 3 days after initial infection. During this pyrexial phase the virus gains access to the lymphatics by which it is transported to the local lymph nodes, cervical and/or mesenteric. Further multiplication of virus in lymph nodes is followed by a viraemia by which the virus is carried to the central nervous system. In the spinal cord it probably spreads, like tetanus toxin, in the fluid between the nerve fibres, its spread being facilitated by pressure waves from the aorta. Although difficult to demonstrate, the evidence for a viraemia in man—occurring about the time of the initial general symptoms of infection—is considerable. Some workers consider, however, that it only represents an overflow of virus from extraneural sites of multiplication and is not an essential preliminary to invasion of the central nervous system. On this view the virus is believed to gain access to the nervous system by neuronal routes.

The distribution of lesions in the central nervous system is suggestive of neuronal spread but the fact that gamma globulin and active immunization protect against paralytic infection is more readily explained by the viraemic theory. As yet, however, there is no decisive evidence in favour of either the viraemic or neuronal theories.

In all types of poliomyelitis infection virus is demonstrable in the pharynx and in the faeces. It is present in both these situations immediately prior to and during the acute stages of infection and in the faeces for a variable period—on occasion for some months—after the appearance of paralytic symptoms. It is therefore presumed that the disease is spread both by droplet infection and by infected faecal material. The relative importance of these two routes, however, has still to be determined. Since epidemics of poliomyelitis occur mainly in the summer and autumn, times when gastro-intestinal infections are most frequent, it has generally been assumed that of the two the gastro-intestinal route is the more important. In countries, particularly tropical countries, with relatively low standards of hygiene it is probable that considerable dissemination of the virus occurs, as in the enteric fevers, through large-scale excretal contamination of food and water. In more advanced communities, however, it is unlikely that this mechanism of spread occurs to any significant extent. Under these conditions poliomyelitis appears rather to be a disease of close personal contact— the virus presumably being spread both by casual faecal contamination of the environment and by droplet transfer. Personal contact is maximal within the family group and as a result an individual excreting virus rapidly infects other members of the family. In this case droplet transfer could well be the more important route of spread. In support of this is the fact that the maximum infectivity of the patient occurs at the time that virus is demonstrable in the pharynx. As sources of infection symptomless carriers, because of their numbers, are of great importance. Individually, however, they are less dangerous than overt cases who excrete larger amounts of virus and who usually succeed in infecting most people in their immediate environment.

Poliomyelitis is a disease of world-wide prevalence occurring in both endemic and epidemic forms. Since its first recognition in the first half of the nineteenth century it has shown considerable changes in epidemiological behaviour. Thus whereas prior to 1900 paralytic infection was mainly sporadic, nowadays, in many countries—and this is particularly the case in Europe and North America —it shows a markedly epidemic character. Associated with the increased epidemicity of the disease there has also been a substantial change in the age incidence of overt infection. Formerly paralytic infections were found almost exclusively in children of less than five years of age—hence the name 'infantile paralysis'. Nowadays, however, paralytic infection takes a heavy toll of older children and adults. Thus it has been estimated that the incidence of paralytic cases in young children is about one in 1000 infected, while in adults it may be as high as 1 in 75. These changes in epidemiological behaviour can be attributed to social and hygienic improvements which have diminished the opportunity for infection in early life. Under conditions of overcrowding and poor sanitation the virus can spread readily and as a result, most individuals come into contact with it in infancy. This type of widespread endemic infection is still observed in many parts of the world, particularly in tropical countries with relatively low standards of hygiene. With improvements in hygiene and in social conditions infection in infancy becomes less frequent. As a result there is a larger population of susceptibles with in consequence an increased opportunity for epidemic spread. Furthermore, since many older persons now lack any naturally acquired immunity, there is an increase in the age incidence of infection.

It appears to be a general rule that in communities in which poliomyelitis assumes an epidemic form paralytic cases are more frequent than in communities in which the disease is mainly endemic. This is in part due to a greater physiological susceptibility of the older age groups to paralytic infection. This, however, may not be the only factor involved. It is also possible, as suggested by Sabin, that strains of virus circulating in communities in which early infection is prevalent may be of relatively low virulence for the central nervous system and are therefore less liable to give rise to paralysis.

There is now clear evidence that various extrinsic factors—in particular, fatigue, trauma, pregnancy, tonsillectomy and the intramuscular administration of prophylactics containing alum (Chapter 8)—may favour the development of paralytic poliomyelitis in individuals exposed to infection. These factors are presumed to act by transforming asymptomatic and abortive infections into paralytic ones, rather than by increasing the overall susceptibility to infection but precisely how they do so has not been satisfactorily explained.

Diagnosis

Usually, a diagnosis of paralytic poliomyelitis can be readily made on clinical grounds. It should be remembered, however, particularly with the declining incidence of poliomyelitis, due to vaccination, that a paralytic syndrome can be produced by certain ECHO and Coxsackie serotypes, particularly Coxsackie A7. This distinction can only be made by using laboratory procedures, which are particularly important in the diagnosis of non-paralytic poliomyelitis. This condition, presenting as an aseptic meningitis, may be caused not only by other enteroviruses but also by a number of non-neurotropic viruses, particularly the mumps virus, and also by *L. canicola*. Sporadic cases of aseptic meningitis, occurring during the winter and spring, are usually due to agents other than the enteroviruses.

Where possible an attempt should be made to isolate the virus by culture. Antibodies to the poliovirus may be demonstrated by neutralization tests in tissue culture, and by complement fixation tests. Neutralizing antibody appears early during the course of infection and may be maximal at the time of onset of paralysis. It is therefore frequently impossible to demonstrate a significant, that is a fourfold, rise in antibody titre between the acute and convalescent phase sera. Neutralizing antibody persists for a long time and, sometimes, apparently for life; this reduces the diagnostic significance of such antibody detected by a single examination. Complement fixing antibody appears somewhat later in infection than neutralizing antibody and, in the majority of cases, it is possible to demonstrate a rise in antibody titre. For its demonstration live virus is preferable as an antigen, since the C antigen of heated virus may react strongly with acute phase serum and shows less type specificity. Since complement fixing antibody is of short duration, examination of a single specimen may yield a diagnostic titre. Overall, the complement fixation test permits a serological diagnosis in from 80 to 90 per cent of cases.

Prophylaxis

In the control of poliomyelitis at the community level, isolation of cases for 2 to 3 weeks, covering the period of maximum infectivity, quarantining of contacts of less than 10 years of age for 21 days, and a general restriction of assembly are believed to be of some value. Effective control by such measures is, however, difficult because of the high incidence of asymptomatic infections.

Gamma globulin prepared from pooled adult plasma has some protective value if given early in the incubation period; the protection obtained is, however, of short duration, lasting at most for some 4 to 5 weeks. Its occasional use has, however, been recommended for susceptible persons introduced into an environment in which the disease is prevalent, but it is only effective if given very soon after exposure.

Two types of vaccine are currently available for active immunization: (1) Salk killed vaccine and (2) live vaccine, prepared from attenuated strains of virus.

Salk Vaccine

This consists of virus of all three antigenic types grown in monkey kidney tissue culture and inactivated by exposure to a low concentration of formalin. Three injections of the vaccine are usually given with an interval of 3 to 6 weeks between the first and second injections and an interval of 6 to 7 months between the second and the third. This long interval is required in order to ensure a satisfactory secondary antibody response.

In short-term follow-up a full course of three injections with a satisfactory vaccine appears to give about 90 per cent protection against paralytic infection. Vaccination also protects against pharyngeal infection but not against intestinal infection, the latter requiring considerably higher levels of protective antibody. Because of this the killed vaccine has a greater efficacy in more advanced communities, in which infection is to a large extent by the pharyngeal route, than in less developed communities in which infection appears to be mainly by the alimentary route. Of the three polio types, inactivated type 2 virus is the most effective antigen, and inactivated type 1 virus the least effective. In the preparation of the early killed vaccines, these differences were not realized and the vaccines were therefore relatively deficient in the type 1 component. This deficiency has been corrected in the killed vaccines currently available which, in addition, are more highly purified and contain more concentrated virus. Killed vaccine may be combined with diphtheria, tetanus and pertussis antigens without any diminution in antigenic potency.

Live Vaccine

The feasibility of using live attenuated polioviruses for human immunization was first established by Koprowski who showed that children could be immunized, apparently without risk, by the oral administration of virus attenuated by passage in rodents. Subsequently strains suitable for oral administration were developed by Cox and by Sabin. Sabin's strains derived by plaque selection in tissue culture are the basis of most of the live vaccines currently in use. Live vaccine is now accepted as the antigen of choice for immunization against poliomyelitis. It is easier to administer, cheaper to produce, stimulates an immunity which, resembling that produced by natural infection, develops more rapidly, and is at least as effective in protecting against paralytic infection. Its effectiveness can be gauged by the fact that where it has been used on a community-wide scale wild-type polioviruses have been virtually eliminated. In addition to protecting against paralytic infection live vaccine produces a local immunity of the intestinal tract. To some extent this local immunity may be due to viral interference (p. 441) but it has been suggested that local antibody production, or a local cellular immunity, may also be involved. Whatever its basis, it develops sufficiently rapidly to permit the use of live vaccine as a prophylactic during the course of an epidemic.

There are, however, certain potential disadvantages inherent in the use of live vaccine: (1) Live attenuated virus is not completely avirulent. It multiplies in the intestinal tract. This multiplication is in fact essential to provide an antigenic mass sufficient for the production of a solid immunity. The type 2 component, at least, can produce a viraemia. In addition some residual neurovirulence is demonstrable by intraspinal inoculation of monkeys. It is therefore possible that, on occasion, the vaccine strains might invade the central nervous system and produce paralytic disease, though their diminished neurovirulence would be expected to make this an extremely rare event. From careful scrutiny of data in vaccine associated cases of poliomyelitis occurring in the United States shortly after vaccine administration, it seemed probable that the type 3 component was in fact responsible for some of the cases. These infections occurred only in adults, and with an estimated incidence of 1 in 1,000,000 vaccinations. Because of this it is generally considered preferable not to give live type 3 vaccine to adults. Under present conditions, however, the risk is not such as to modify the use of live attenuated vaccines for childhood immunization. (2) The possibility that the vaccine strains, which are transmissible from the individuals to whom they are administered to others, might, as a result of serial passage through the human intestinal tract regain some of their human pathogenicity. The reality of this danger has been shown particularly by Dick and his associates who found that intestinal passage led to an increase in the neurovirulence of the vaccine strains for monkeys. From the evidence available, however, it seems unlikely that the slight increases demonstrated in this way are associated with increased virulence for man. Any danger to the community of an increase in the virulence of the vaccine strains would presumably be largely eliminated if the vaccine were given to all or most of the susceptible members of the community simultaneously. This procedure has not been adopted in the British Isles, however, although the vaccine is included in routine immunization schedules. There is no evidence that failure to do so has had any untoward effect. (3) The possibility that other enteroviruses prevalent in the community might interfere with the establishment of the vaccine strains in the intestinal tracts of a proportion of the population. This risk would be minimized if the vaccine were given only at times of low enterovirus prevalence. (4) The danger of disseminating other viruses, pathogenic to man, which might be present in the tissue cultures used for vaccine preparation. This danger could probably only be totally eliminated by the propagation of the vaccine in established cell lines proved to be free from contaminating viruses. So far the only virus known to have been transmitted in this way, the so-called vacuolating agent SV 40, is, as far as is known, non-pathogenic for man.

The vaccine may be administered as a trivalent vaccine containing all three antigenic types of virus—this is the vaccine normally used in the British Isles—or as a monovalent vaccine containing only one antigenic type. The trivalent vaccine is given in three doses in syrup or on a lump of sugar with an interval of one month between each feeding. The administration of three doses is essential since the type 2 component frequently establishes itself as the sole inhabitant following the first feeding. If, however, sufficient interval is allowed to permit the elimination of this strain by an immune response, the other strains have a better chance of establishing themselves.

Coxsackie Viruses

The name of this group of viruses is derived from the village of Coxsackie in New York State from which the first member of the group was isolated by Dalldorf and Sickles in 1948 from the faeces of children believed to be suffering from poliomoyelitis. Some 30 serological groups have been distinguished.

On the basis of their pathogenicity for mice they are divided into two groups—A and B. Of the serological types indicated above 25 belong to group A and 5 to group B. Cross reactivity between the different types, due to shared group antigens, is readily demonstrable with human sera. Different strains within each type frequently show considerable antigenic differences.

On inoculation into mice group A viruses produce generalized inflammation and degeneration of the voluntary musculature, the animals eventually dying of respiratory paralysis. On inoculation into mice group B viruses produce localized areas of myositis, degenerative changes in the brown intercaspular fat pads and necrotic lesions in various organs, particularly in the pancreas and, following intracerebral inoculation, in the brain.

The only laboratory animals uniformly susceptible are suckling mice and hamsters; these may be infected by the intracerebral, intraperitoneal or subcutaneous routes. Some strains have been adapted to the chick embryo but will not grow in the embryo on primary isolation. All group B strains grow readily in monkey kidney tissue cultures with the production of cytopathogenic effects, and also, but as a rule less readily, in HeLa cells. Only a few group A strains can be propagated in tissue cultures. A9 will grow in monkey kidney and A-11, 13, 15, 18, 20 and 21 will grow in HeLa cells but not in monkey kidney.

The Coxsackie A7 virus produces a haemagglutinin for fowl red cells which possesses properties similar to those of the vaccinia haemagglutinin. Strains of certain other serotypes are capable of agglutinating human group O red cells, haemagglutination being inhibited by type-specific antiserum.

So far all the Coxsackie group B viruses and about half the group A viruses have been shown to be capable of producing clinical disease. Viruses of both groups can cause aseptic meningitis and mild febrile illnesses. Herpangina, a

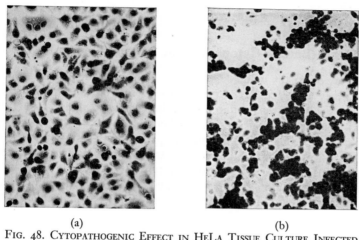

(a)   (b)

FIG. 48. CYTOPATHOGENIC EFFECT IN HELA TISSUE CULTURE INFECTED
WITH A COXSACKIE B3 VIRUS

(a) Uninfected culture   (b) Infected culture

condition occurring in children and characterized by fever and the presence of small ulcers on the tonsils, uvula and soft palate, is caused exclusively by group A viruses. On occasion group A strains have been found to be associated with a paralytic syndrome indistinguishable from paralytic poliomyelitis. This is particularly true of Coxsackie A7, because of which this serotype has been classified by Russian workers as a poliovirus. An unusual syndrome characterized by the occurrence of vesicles in the mouth, and a rash, at first papular and later becoming vesicular, on the hands and feet—hand, foot and mouth disease—and apparently caused by Coxsackie A16 has been reported from Canada and South Africa. Bornholm disease or epidemic myalgia—a febrile condition which is associated with severe attacks of pain in various voluntary muscles, particularly those of the thorax and abdomen, is caused exclusively by group B viruses. Group B viruses can also cause an acute myocarditis in infants occurring mainly in those of less than ten days of age. It is possible that in certain of these cases the foetus may be infected in utero. The disease has a high fatality rate and at post mortem there is usually evidence of involvement of the liver and brain.

Diagnosis

An attempt may be made to isolate virus from the throat or from the faeces, or in cases of aseptic meningitis from the cerebrospinal fluid. The material is usually inoculated first into monkey kidney and HeLa tissue cultures—specimens which are negative in these then being inoculated into suckling mice.

Neutralizing and complement fixing antibodies appear early during the course of infection. The serological heterogeneity of the group is, however, a considerable obstacle to the use of serologic tests as routine diagnostic methods. In addition they are only practicable with strains which can be propagated in tissue cultures. When a Coxsackie virus has been isolated serological tests may be used to demonstrate an antibody rise in the patient's serum against it, thereby confirming its aetiological role.

ECHO (Enteric Cytopathogenic Human Orphan) Viruses

These were originally defined as a group of viruses which could be isolated in monkey kidney tissue cultures in which they produced an enterovirus type of cytopathogenic effect; they differed from the Coxsackie viruses in not infecting mice, and from the polioviruses in not being pathogenic for monkeys. Some viruses, however, which differ in some respects from this original pattern, are now included in the group. Thus many strains of type 9 can produce lesions resembling those produced by Coxsackie type A in suckling mice. Following intracerebral inoculation of monkeys, some types have been found to produce neuronal lesions when large inocula are used. Monkey kidney cells are the cells of choice for isolation but ECHO viruses also grow well in primary cultures of a variety of human cells. They grow poorly in HeLa cells and in most continuous cell lines.

At least thirty serotypes have been differentiated by neutralization and complement fixation tests. As has also been demonstrated for the Coxsackie viruses, some strains—the so-called prime strains—possess an inherently low susceptibility to antibody in neutralization tests. These strains, however, readily stimulate the production of antibody, with a high neutralization titre against normal strains of the same serological type. There is evidence that prime strains consist of a mixture of poorly neutralizable and normally neutralizable particles. In some cases it has been shown that such strains may be transformed, on passage in tissue culture, into normally reacting strains.

Many ECHO viruses are capable of agglutinating human red cells. The red cell receptor is susceptible to trypsin and to reagents reacting with sulphydryl groups. It must therefore be protein, the sulphydryl groups of which are important in the binding of virus to the cell. Virus elutes from the cell with increase in temperature but elution is not associated with breakdown of the receptor. The receptor is quite distinct from that for the myxoviruses.

Most types have now been found to be associated with clinical syndromes, particularly with aseptic meningitis both of sporadic and epidemic type. ECHO viruses appear to be responsible for some cases of summer diarrhoea occurring both in infants and in older children. In this condition they are not infrequently associated with enteropathogenic *E. coli*; it is believed that they may in fact enhance the pathogenicity of the latter organisms. Some types have been incriminated as the causes of indefinite summer febrile illnesses in children. These infections are not infrequently associated with a maculopapular rash. ECHO viruses may cause mild upper respiratory tract infections, and appear to be occasional causes of the common cold syndrome. Very exceptionally they may cause a paralytic syndrome resembling poliomyelitis.

RHINOVIRUSES

It has been known for many years that the common cold can be transmitted to human volunteers by nasal instillation of infected nasal secretions. Colds are also transmissible to chimpanzees, but no laboratory animal is susceptible nor has it been possible to isolate the causative agent in the chick embryo. The first major step in the isolation of a common cold virus was taken by Andrewes and his associates of the Medical Research Council Unit at Salisbury in 1953 when they succeeded in isolating a cold virus in human embryo lung tissue culture. The virus did not have a cytopathogenic effect and its presence could be recognized only by its capacity to produce colds in volunteers. The next advance was the discovery in 1960 by the same group of workers, that viruses capable of producing colds in volunteers could be readily isolated in human embryo tissue cultures maintained at 33° C rather than at the customary temperature of 36° C and with a low biocarbonate concentration and therefore a low pH. Under these conditions a recognizable cytopathogenic effect was produced. For this group of viruses the name *rhinovirus* has been proposed.

The rhinoviruses so far isolated have been subdivided into two groups: the H rhinoviruses, which will grow only in cultures of human tissues, and the M rhinoviruses, which are also capable of growing in monkey kidney tissue cultures. Some 50 serologically distinct types have so far been recognized amongst the H viruses, and 7 distinct serotypes amongst the M viruses. These are specifically human pathogens but similar viruses have been isolated from cattle and horses. Unlike the enteroviruses which they closely resemble, the rhinoviruses are rapidly inactivated at pH 3, and are not stabilized to heat inactivation by high concentrations of divalent cations.

Although the rhinoviruses are almost certainly the main cause of the common cold syndrome, the H rhinoviruses being more frequently involved than the M viruses, colds may also be caused by viruses of other groups. There is clear evidence that parainfluenza viruses, adenoviruses, respiratory syncytial virus and Coxsackie viruses, particularly A21 and B5, are occasionally involved. In addition, some cases of the common cold are due to viruses which can be transmitted to volunteers but which cannot be propagated in the conventional type of tissue culture. From some such cases, Tyrrell and Bynoe have isolated viruses in organ cultures of human embryonic respiratory epithelium in which the presence of virus appears to be most readily detected by electron microscopy. Two such strains, examined by Almeida and Tyrrell, appeared morphologically identical with the virus of infectious avian bronchitis, which they resembled in size, measuring from 80 to 120 mμ in diameter, and in being sensitive to ether. A third strain showed a myxovirus morphology.

The immunity produced by an attack of the common cold appears to be of very short duration and an individual may experience several attacks in a single year. In the experimentally transmitted disease immunity is also of short duration, immunity to the homologous virus appearing to last at most a few weeks. It is nevertheless possible that under natural conditions the duration of immunity may be somewhat longer since in isolated communities the disease dies out rapidly. Repeated attacks may therefore be due to antigenically distinct viruses.

The agents responsible for the common cold are spread by infected respiratory secretions. They appear to be viable for a considerable time on infected clothing, and this therefore could be a source of infection. Children are much more susceptible to infection than adults and are of particular importance in spreading the disease.

THE ENCEPHALOMYOCARDITIS OR EMC GROUP

This comprises the encephalomyocarditis virus, the Mengovirus, the Columbia-SK virus, and the MM virus. They are small RNA viruses measuring about 30 mμ in diameter. They are antigenically indistinguishable and, though isolated in various parts of the world and from different hosts, are probably all strains of a single species. The name of the group derives from the fact that inoculation into mice produces encephalitis and an acute interstitial myocarditis. Only few human infections have been reported; these have varied from a mild febrile disorder to severe encephalitis. EMC viruses are probably maintained in nature as parasites of rodents.

CHAPTER 33

ARBOVIRUSES

The arboviruses are a group of small viruses which are transmitted under natural conditions by arthropod vectors. Some 200 different species are known, each with a characteristic geographical distribution. Only about 50 of these have been identified as causes of overt human infection. The remainder have been isolated from mosquitoes or animals, particularly in equatorial Africa and America. Twenty-one serological groups, each consisting of 2 or more members, have been distinguished while about 50 viruses are serologically ungrouped. The majority of the human pathogens belong to group A, containing 17 viruses, or group B, containing 33 viruses. It is possible that the arboviruses, as at present defined, are in fact heterogeneous, and that with the development of more incisive methods of differentiation some subdivision of the group will be necessary.

1. They are small viruses, those of group A being approximately spherical particles of from 40 to 50 mμ in diameter, and those of group B from 20 to 35 mμ in diameter. The precise structure of these viruses has not yet been determined. The unusually high lipid content which has been demonstrated for certain members of the group—that of the Western equine encephalomyelitis virus amounting to 54 per cent—and their sensitivity to ether suggest the presence of a lipid-containing envelope. Electron micrographs of some group A viruses have indicated the presence of surface projections resembling the spikes of the influenza virus, and which might possibly be the viral haemagglutinin. The symmetry of the viral nucleocapsids is in doubt but recent evidence suggests that in the case of WEE virus it may be helical.

2. All arboviruses which have been examined chemically have been found to be RNA viruses, and some have yielded an infectious nucleic acid. In general, infectious nucleic acid is easier to obtain from infected cells than from purified virus. This may be related to the acquisition of a lipid envelope on release of the virus from the cell.

3. Most possess haemagglutinins which are best demonstrated against the cells of day-old chicks. The haemagglutinin appears to be a component of the virus particle. The optimum conditions for the demonstration of haemagglutination differ considerably with different strains; pH is of particular importance, affecting both the demonstration and stability of the haemagglutinin.

4. Arboviruses are classified serologically by the use of haemagglutination inhibition, complement fixation and neutralization tests. Amongst the viruses

of groups A and B, group relationships are more apparent in haemagglutination inhibition than in complement fixation or neutralization tests. Individual members of the groups are most clearly differentiated by neutralization tests.

The specific geographical location of many arboviruses is probably due to the fact that the presence of established endemic or enzootic infection with a particular virus will tend, by stimulating group antibody, to exclude other viruses of the same serological group.

5. They are pathogenic for mice, in which they produce an encephalitis following intracerebral or intraperitoneal inoculation. As a general rule the susceptibility of mice to infection decreases with increasing age of the animal. Many will grow in the chick embryo—on the chorioallantoic membrane and in the yolk sac and in a variety of tissue cultures in which they produce recognizable cytopathogenic effects.

6. Arboviruses are maintained in nature in insect–vertebrate cycles and except in rare instances direct transmission from one animal to another without the intervention of an insect vector does not occur. With the exception of sandfly fever for which the only known vertebrate host is man the natural vertebrate hosts of the arboviruses are various wild animals and birds. Man is usually only incidentally infected and except for dengue and yellow fever is epidemiologically a 'dead end'. The main arthropod vectors are mosquitoes, ticks and sandflies. Transmission of the virus normally occurs only after its multiplication in the vector, the final stages of multiplication being in the salivary glands. Prior to this the vector is not infective; this period is known as the extrinsic incubation period and its length varies inversely with the ambient temperature. Arboviruses do not produce disease either in the insect vectors or in their natural animal reservoir. In many cases the route by which man is infected from the animal reservoir is not known. It is possible that arbovirus infections which, in temperate climates, are maintained during the summer in mosquito–bird cycles, may be maintained through the winter in a cycle involving small rodents and their parasitic arthropods.

7. In infected animals and man the viruses are present in the blood during the early stages of infection; viraemia is in fact a necessary condition for insect transfer. Following the bite of an infected arthropod it is probable that the virus multiplies first in the lymphatic glands draining the inoculation site. From the glands the virus gains access to the blood stream. As a general rule viraemia is maximal from 1 to 5 days after infection, and it is only during this period that the patient is infective.

8. Asymptomatic subclinical infection is as a rule more frequent than overt symptomatic infection. It has been estimated for example that only one in every thousand persons infected with the Japanese B encephalitis virus shows clinical signs of infection. The type of overt infection which the arboviruses produce is varied. Some give rise to systemic illnesses without localizing signs. These illnesses may be of relatively mild type as in dengue and sandfly fever or severe as in infection with the tick-borne encephalitis group which occasionally produce systemic infections with severe haemorrhagic manifestations. The majority produce overt infections with marked localizing signs. In most cases localization

is in the brain with the production of an encephalitis or in less severe cases an aseptic meningitis but in yellow fever the virus localizes in the liver. In conditions showing localization of virus the illness is frequently diphasic with a saddle-back temperature chart, the first rise in temperature coinciding with the initial multiplication of the virus and the second rise being associated with its localization.

9. Isolation of virus from human cases is frequently difficult. In some cases this can be achieved with blood taken early in the infection. In the encephalitides virus can only rarely be isolated from the cerebrospinal fluid, in general most successes being obtained by inoculation of brain tissue obtained at post-mortem examination.

A serological diagnosis is achieved most readily by the use of haemagglutination inhibition and complement fixation tests. Complement fixing antibody usually persists for only a short time after clinical infection. Haemagglutination inhibiting antibody is more persistent and neutralizing antibody may be detectable for very long periods. In individuals infected for the first time with an arbovirus the reactions in complement fixation and haemagglutination inhibition tests are usually highly specific and may permit a precise serological diagnosis. In those who have suffered from a prior arbovirus infection due to a virus of the same serological group the antibody response shows a much broader pattern, reactions occurring with other viruses of the same group. For groups A and B this overlap is most marked with the haemagglutination inhibition test and least with the neutralization test.

GROUP A VIRUSES

Equine Encephalomyelitis Viruses

These are most frequently encountered, and were originally recognized, as the causes of encephalomyelitis in horses and mules, but they may give rise to both sporadic and epidemic human infections. The Western and Eastern viruses, WEE and EEE, are prevalent in the Western and Eastern parts of North and South America. The Venezuelan viruses are confined to Central and South America. The Eastern equine virus is the most invasive of the three, giving rise to much fewer latent infections and, not infrequently, producing a severe, and often fatal disease. The Venezuelan virus is the least invasive; it frequently causes latent infections and rarely produces a frank encephalitis.

The epidemiology of Western equine encephalomyelitis has been most studied. The main vector of this virus appears to be the mosquito *Culex tarsalis*, and birds, from which the virus has frequently been isolated, probably constitute the main reservoir of infection. Birds are probably also the main reservoir of the Eastern virus, and mosquitoes may be the main vectors as well. Little precise information is available on the natural history of the Venezuelan virus but it seems likely that wild mammals are the main reservoir of infection. Both the Eastern and Venezuelan viruses appear to be capable of being directly transmitted from one animal to another without the intervention of an insect vector.

Though belonging to the same serological group, the equine encephalo-myelitis viruses are relatively easily differentiated by neutralization tests. Formalin inactivated vaccines of all these viruses have been used for the immunization of horses. Vaccines are not available for human immunization.

Chikungunya and Onyongnyong Viruses

The Chikungunya virus was first recognized as the cause of an outbreak of a dengue-like disease in Tanganyika in 1952. A serologically similar virus has also been identified as the cause of dengue-like disease and of severe haemorrhagic fever in Thailand. The virus is probably maintained in a primate–mosquito cycle. The Onyongnyong virus was first isolated as the cause of a febrile disease characterized by joint pains, rash and lymphadenitis which appeared in Uganda in 1959. Over the next few years infection with this virus became widespread in East Africa. The Onyongnyong virus is closely related serologically to the Chikungunya virus and may well be a mutant of the latter. The virus is thought to be spread by Anopheles mosquitoes.

GROUP B VIRUSES

A number of subgroups are distinguished, the individual members of which have a closer serological relationship to one another than to other viruses of the group.

St. Louis Subgroup

This group includes the St. Louis, Japanese B, Murray Valley fever and West Nile viruses. These viruses are closely related to each other serologically and fall into a serological subgroup of group B. Culicine mosquitoes appear to be the main vectors and wild birds the main reservoirs. The St. Louis, Japanese B and Murray Valley are encephalitogenic in man. The West Nile virus produces a mild systemic infection characterized by a general lymphadenopathy and rash. It rarely produces encephalitis, and then, only in older people.

Infection with the St. Louis virus is widespread throughout the United States and in the Caribbean. Infection with the Japanese B virus is found in China, Japan and Far Eastern Russia. The West Nile virus is found in Egypt, India and Palestine. The Murray Valley virus has been found as a cause of an epidemic infection only in South Eastern Australia. The main reservoir of infection, however, is believed to be in Northern Australia and New Guinea, where it is maintained in a bird–mosquito cycle. From these areas it is introduced into South Eastern Australia by migratory birds, from which it is believed to be transmitted to domestic fowl and water fowl. In these areas epidemics have been noted particularly at times of flooding, when water fowl, which carry the virus, are brought into close contact with the human population.

Tick-borne Subgroup

This group comprises a number of tick-borne viruses which have been isolated in various parts of the world, viz. the louping ill virus, the Far Eastern or Russian spring summer and Czechoslovakian or Central European encephalitis viruses and the viruses of Kyasanur Forest disease (India) and of Omsk haemorrhagic fever (Siberia). The louping ill, Russian spring summer and Central European viruses are very similar serologically, but can be distinguished by neutralization tests. The Kyasanur and Omsk viruses closely resemble one another antigenically.

These viruses are apparently capable of being transmitted transovarially in ticks but the extent to which this transmission is responsible for their persistence in nature is speculative. In the case of the Central European virus it has been suggested that the primary reservoir is in a cycle involving wild rodents and tick larvae. It is thought that this cycle may generate a secondary cycle involving adult ticks and larger vertebrates. On occasion, infection with tick-borne viruses may occur in the absence of a tick bite. Thus the Central European and Far Eastern encephalitis viruses can be transmitted by improperly pasteurized goat's milk, and there is reason to believe that the development of louping ill in butchers may be the result of respiratory or alimentary infection.

The pathogenicity of the Kyasanur Forest disease virus is unusual. Like other arboviruses it may produce meningo-encephalitis. In some cases, however, there are severe haemorrhagic manifestations. The disease appears to occur only in the State of Mysore in India. There is believed to be a reservoir in wild rodents from which cattle, monkeys and man may be infected. Transmission to monkeys and man is believed to have occurred on a significant scale only during the last decade.

The louping ill virus is the only arthropod-borne encephalitis virus which occurs in the British Isles. It is enzootic in sheep in Scotland, Northern England, Wales and Ireland. In sheep it gives rise to a condition showing marked cerebellar ataxia—from the symptoms of which the disease derives its name. There have been a few isolated human cases of infection with this virus—in a farmer and a veterinary surgeon working with infected sheep, in some abattoir workers in Glasgow, and in laboratory workers. Serological evidence of infection with the louping ill virus or with an antigenically closely related virus has been obtained by Likar and Dane in Northern Ireland.

Yellow Fever

Yellow fever is a disease of Equatorial Africa and America, occurring in a belt extending from roughly 10° north to 10° south latitude. Its aetiology and epidemiology were first elucidated by Walter Reed and his associates in Cuba in 1911, when Reed succeeded in substantiating the theory of Carlos Finlay that the disease was spread by the mosquito *Aedes aegypti*. The virus was not isolated, however, until 1927 when Stokes, Bauer and Hudson showed that rhesus monkeys were susceptible to infection.

Properties of the Virus

The yellow fever virus is a very small virus measuring from 15 to 28 mμ in diameter. It has not yet been demonstrated by the electron microscope. On primary isolation the virus can be propagated in monkeys by subcutaneous or intraperitoneal inoculation, when it produces necrotic lesions in the liver. This property is referred to as viscerotropism. As first shown by Theiler in 1930, the virus will also infect adult white mice to produce an encephalitis, following intracerebral inoculation. The combination of neurotropism for mice with viscerotropism for monkeys is referred to as pantropism. In serial passage intracerebrally in mice its neurotropism is increased while its viscerotropism diminishes. Chick embryos are not susceptible on primary isolation but can be infected by virus which has been passaged intracerebrally in mice.

Although all yellow fever viruses are of essentially the same immunogenic type slight differences between American and African strains have been shown by haemagglutination inhibition tests. These differences are not, however, sufficient to interfere with the efficacy of current vaccines against both types of infection.

Pathogenesis and Epidemiology

Yellow fever occurs in two epidemiological varieties: urban yellow fever and jungle yellow fever. Urban yellow fever, which is the classical form, is an epidemic disease. It assumed major proportions in Central America at the end of the nineteenth and the beginning of the twentieth centuries. Recent epidemics have occurred mainly in West Africa. The disease is transmitted by the mosquito *Aedes aegypti*. Infection is only possible if the insect has fed from a patient in the first 3 days of the disease, but the insect does not become infective to another person for at least 4 days, and not for a much longer time if the air temperature is low. Thereafter it remains infective for life. Transovarian passage of the virus in the mosquito has not been demonstrated. Infection may also be conveyed directly from man to man by contact with the blood or serum of a patient.

The virus is present in the blood of infected persons and multiplies in the vascular endothelium and in the liver cells. It is believed that following introduction into the tissues the initial multiplication of the virus occurs in the lymph nodes and that it is from these that the blood is invaded. In fatal cases the liver cells show marked necrosis. The necrotic cells, which have a characteristic hyaline appearance, are known as Councilman bodies. Occasionally infected cells show the presence of irregular acidophilic intranuclear inclusions. These are commoner in monkeys than in man; the inclusions do not contain nucleic acid and are apparently not colonies of virus.

When, following the work of Reed, it was found that epidemics of yellow fever could be prevented by measures directed against *Aedes aegypti* it was thought that the problem of the control of the disease had been finally solved. This was, however, found to be far from the case. The source of this continuing infection remained a problem until it was shown by Stokes that the virus is maintained in a reservoir of monkeys and possibly other jungle animals, amongst which it is spread by various mosquitoes. Sporadic human infections occur by direct transmission from this animal reservoir; this epidemiological variety of the disease is known as jungle yellow fever. In Africa the disease is transmitted within the animal reservoir by the mosquito *Aedes africanus*. This mosquito lives in the tree tops and does not normally bite man, the disease being transmitted from monkeys to man by the link vector *Aedes simpsonii*. This mosquito, like *Aedes aegypti*, has a preference for human communities. It usually becomes infected from monkeys raiding villages. Like *Aedes aegypti*, it is capable of maintaining a man-to-man cycle of infection but clearly has not the same devastating epidemic potential. This variety of jungle yellow fever may affect all ages and sexes. In the forests of South America, jungle yellow fever presents a somewhat different picture. It is usually contracted by adult males who work in forests inhabited by an infected monkey reservoir. The main vector appears to be *Haemagogus spegazzinii*.

There is evidence of some degree of cross-immunity between yellow fever and the other group B arbovirus infections, to such an extent as to diminish the spread of yellow fever in areas in which such infections are enzootic or endemic, and in which an animal reservoir of yellow fever and a suitable insect vector are both present. Thus in Trinidad and Ethiopia, in recent years, there has been reason to believe that the spread of yellow fever was restrained by the presence of endemic infection with the dengue virus.

The outstanding features of a typical case of severe yellow fever are high temperature, great prostration, vomiting, haemorrhages and jaundice, the disease in most cases being of a biphasic type with a remission of a few days' duration between the major episodes. Sometimes the infection is fulminating. The disease may also occur as a mild 'flu-like infection, or in a latent asymptomatic form which can be detected only by serological means. In Brazil and in Colombia serological evidence indicates the occurrence of latent asymptomatic infection in as much as 30 to 40 per cent of the population of enzootic areas. Such areas in which the only evidence of the disease is serological but in which the infection is nevertheless widespread are known as 'silent areas'.

Diagnosis

The virus may be isolated by intracerebral inoculation of mice with blood taken in the first few days of the disease. Since a considerable amount of antibody appears at an early stage of infection it is customary to inoculate a number of dilutions of blood so as to dilute out the antibody present.

A serological diagnosis may be made by the use of neutralization, complement fixation or haemagglutination inhibition tests. These tests give highly specific results in individuals who have not previously suffered from a group B arbovirus infection. In people who have had a prior group B infection the antibodies have a broad specificity reacting to a greater or lesser extent with other viruses of the B group. In this type of case antibodies are usually present in much higher titre than in those who have not had a prior group B infection. For the detection of antibody in epidemiological surveys mouse neutralization tests have been mainly used.

A diagnosis of yellow fever can often be made from the histological examination of liver tissue obtained by punch biopsy in fatal cases.

Prophylaxis

As in other mosquito-borne diseases the use of DDT and anti-mosquito measures are of the greatest value in controlling epidemic yellow fever. In America *Aedes aegypti* is mainly domestic in its habits, breeding primarily in household collections of water. These breeding sites are comparatively easy to eliminate. As compared with the American varieties of *Aedes aegypti*, however, the African varieties are less domestic in habit and are therefore more difficult to control. Control of *Aedes aegypti* is in itself sufficient to prevent the development of urban epidemics of yellow fever but will not of course affect the jungle type of the disease.

Active immunity can be induced by the use of a living attenuated vaccine. The vaccine in most use is that prepared by growth of the attenuated 17D variant in the chick embryo. This variant was derived by Lloyd, Theiler and Ricci by passage from the initially fully virulent Asibi strain, which had been isolated from a patient on the Gold Coast. The virus was first propagated in mouse embryo tissue culture and then in chick embryo tissue culture from which the head and spinal cord had been removed. After a total of 176 passages the 17D variant, which was devoid of viscerotropic properties and of diminished neurotropism, appeared. That the virus retains some pathogenic potential is shown by the fact that it can regain full neurovirulence following intracerebral passage in mice, and that it has, though very rarely, produced encephalitis in vaccinated infants. Nevertheless it is probably as safe as any live vaccine can be.

The vaccine is inoculated subcutaneously, one injection being adequate for immunization. It does not normally produce any untoward reactions, although it may do so very rarely in the young infant. Following vaccination, immunity develops rapidly and is sufficient to give complete protection after about 10 days. The immunity produced is of long duration and can be fully relied on to protect against infection for at least 10 years. Immigration authorities of countries in which the insect vector is present, and in which therefore the disease if introduced could be easily spread, require that all immigrants from or who have recently visited yellow fever endemic areas should be vaccinated at least 10 days prior to entry. Yellow fever vaccination should not be carried out within 21 days after a primary smallpox vaccination. If smallpox vaccination is required, yellow fever immunization should be carried out first; smallpox vaccination can then be given after an interval of 4 days, except in the case of children of less than 9 months of age, when the interval should be 21 days. It is generally considered unnecessary, however, to immunize children in this age group.

A neurotropic variant obtained by intracerebral passage in mice has been used extensively by the French in West Africa. It is inoculated by a scratch technique which has considerable advantages for mass immunization. The immunity produced appears to be at least as good as that produced by the 17D variant but in the past it has shown a much greater tendency than the 17D virus to produce encephalitis. There is some evidence that this complication is much less frequent with the vaccine currently used.

Dengue Fever

The dengue viruses are probably the most widely distributed of all the arboviruses. They are, however, extremely difficult to isolate, success having been achieved only by intracerebral inoculation of suckling mice. Four serotypes are recognized, types 1 and 2 being world wide in distribution; types 3 and 4 have so far been recognized only in the Philippines. The viruses produce two distinct clinical syndroms: (1) A febrile disease of several days' duration characterized by severe pains in the back and limbs, because of which it is known as breakbone fever. A similar syndrome is produced by infection with certain other arboviruses, notably West Nile fever, Chikungunya and Onyong-nyong. (2) A much more severe disease with marked haemorrhagic manifestations. This is the main form of the disease in the Philippines and Thailand.

The chief vector is *Aedes aegypti*, which is the sole vector in the Western Hemisphere. In the East, however, other *Stegomyia* mosquitoes, notably *Aedes albopictus*, are of importance and, being less domestic in habit than *Aedes aegypti*, render the disease more difficult to control.

Immunization with attenuated vaccine is still in the experimental stage. The epidemiology of dengue closely resembles that of yellow fever. Dengue is, however, much more readily spread than yellow fever and may be maintained on an epidemic scale by a much smaller population of *Aedes aegypti*.

OTHER GROUPS

Amongst other arboviruses causing disease in man may be mentioned the viruses of Colorado tick fever, Rift Valley fever, vesicular stomatitis and sandfly or phlebotomus fever. The vesicular stomatitis virus is of interest because of its unusual morphology. It is a bullet-shaped particle measuring 200 mμ long by 60 mμ wide. The virus is enzootic in livestock in North and South America. Human infection, though it may occur, is rare.

Sandfly Fever

Sandfly or phlebotomus fever is a mild febrile condition usually of from 2 to 4 days' duration. The virus is spread by the sandfly—*Phlebotomus papatasii*. Only the female of this species bites—usually during the night or in the early hours of the morning. Insects do not become infective for some 7 to 10 days after biting.

Sandfly fever occurs in Europe, Africa and Asia in a belt, corresponding to the distribution of the insect vector, from 20 to 45° north latitude. It has not been recognized in America. The disease does not cause death, and the pathological changes produced are therefore unknown.

The viruses so far isolated fall into two antigenic groups—the Neapolitan and Sicilian—the prototypes of which were first isolated by Sabin. A number of sandfly fever viruses isolated in South America belong to the Neapolitan group. The viruses can be isolated only by intracerebral inoculation of suckling mice but, when established, strains have been propagated in a variety of tissue cultures. Isolation is usually only possible from blood taken during the first or second day of the disease.

CHAPTER 34

RABIES AND MISCELLANEOUS CNS VIRUSES

RABIES

Properties of the Virus

Morphologically the rabies virus resembles the myxoviruses. It is a spherical particle measuring from 100 to 150 mμ in diameter but filamentous forms are occasionally seen. The virus possesses an envelope, the surface of which is studded by spike-like projections. The internal component of the nucleocapsid appears to resemble that of the myxoviruses in having helical symmetry. From the evidence available it appears to be an RNA virus.

All the ordinary laboratory animals are susceptible but mice, particularly, have been used for isolation. They are normally infected by intracerebral inoculation. Strains of rabies virus from different sources show appreciable differences in mouse virulence, the most virulent being those derived from canines. The virus does not infect the chick embryo on primary isolation but rabbit- or mouse-adapted strains will do so.

Strains of rabies virus, irrespective of source, are closely similar antigenically although minor differences are demonstrable by the use of neutralization, complement fixation and agar gel diffusion tests. In addition to the virus particle a soluble complement fixing antigen of about 12 mμ in diameter is demonstrable in infected tissues.

Pathogenesis and Epidemiology

Rabies is primarily a disease of carnivorous animals. Except for certain island countries, e.g. the British Isles, Australia and New Zealand, it is widely prevalent in wild carnivores throughout the world. Notably, it occurs in wolves, which were at one time the main source of human infection in Europe and are now a common source of infection in Iran, foxes, jackals in India and Israel, the mongoose in India and the Caribbean, in North America various species of insectivorous and frugivorous bats, and in Trinidad and Brazil the vampire bat. It has been suggested that the main reservoir of infection are the mustelidae and viveridae in which the disease is maintained as a latent infection, with only sporadic overt cases, which protects them from their natural canine enemies. From this reservoir, the disease is transmitted first to wild canines which in turn infect domestic animals—dogs, cats and cattle, and occasionally, man. In

Trinidad and Brazil the vampire bat, which suffers an asymptomatic infection, can directly infect cattle and man.

In canines rabies is characteristically encephalitogenic. The virus invades the central nervous system and the main symptoms produced are those of an encephalitis. In infected cells characteristic inclusion bodies known as Negri bodies may be found. These are particularly numerous in the pyramidal cells of Ammon's horn of the hippocampus. In addition to the central nervous system the mucus-secreting glands may contain the virus. Of these the salivary glands, from which the virus gains access to the saliva, are the most important for the transmission of the disease. In mustelidae the central nervous system is only infrequently involved. Involvement of the salivary glands, however, ensures that the infection may be spread, via the saliva, from one animal to another.

Human infection usually occurs as a result of the bite of a rabid or pre-rabid animal—the virus present in the animal's saliva coming into contact with exposed nerve endings. Not all persons who are bitten by rabid animals, however, develop rabies. The risk is greatest in cases with severe and multiple wounds and particularly with wounds involving the head, neck and face. Infection may also occur from a lick of a rabid or pre-rabid animal—the virus present in the

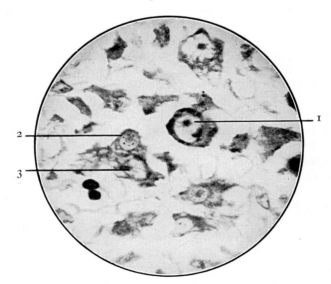

FIG. 49. NEGRI BODY IN A NERVE CELL (× 850)

1. Nucleus of nerve cell.
2. Negri body showing a rosette-like arrangement of its
   granules around a central structure.
3. Degenerated nucleus of nerve cell.

animal's saliva gaining access to nerve endings through scratches and abrasions of the skin. The incubation period of rabies in man is highly variable; it may be anything from 10 days up to 2 years but is usually less than 2 months.

The route by which the virus gains access to the central nervous system is not known with certainty but as viraemia has not been demonstrated, either in experimental animals or in man, it seems likely that it travels by the peripheral nerves. Positive evidence in favour of this view is the finding that, in mice, section of the nerves prior to inoculation prevents infection with virus injected into the foot pad. Similarly, division of efferent nerves interferes with spread of virus centrifugally from the central nervous system to the salivary glands. Thus the centrifugal, as well as the centripetal, movement of the virus probably occurs by neuronal routes. In carnivorous animals infection may also result from eating the flesh of an infected animal. In this case the virus presumably gains entry either through the nasopharynx or the intestinal tract. It is not known whether any local multiplication of the virus occurs at the site of inoculation. In experimental animals there is clear evidence that stress and the administration of ACTH can transform a latent into an overt infection.

In man infection with the rabies virus is invariably fatal. The earliest symptoms are fever, headache and general malaise with, in the majority of cases, pain at the site of the bite. Difficulty in swallowing is the most characteristic symptom of the established disease. When water reaches the fauces it is violently expelled as a result of forcible contraction of the pharyngeal muscles. Because of this the patient develops the fear of water which gives the condition its common name—hydrophobia. This symptom is associated with a progressively increasing excitability of the musculature which gives rise to generalized convulsions in response to minimal stimuli, together with signs of increased stimulation of the sympathetic nervous system, e.g. salivation, perspiration and dilatation of the pupils. Death usually occurs during this phase of the disease but occasionally follows a terminal phase of paralysis and coma.

Diagnosis

The diagnosis of rabies in dogs is of considerable importance as a means of deciding whether a human being, bitten by a suspected animal, should receive prophylactic treatment. As in man, the incubation period in the dog may be very long, extending on occasion up to about 7 months. The dog may show one or other of two contrasting clinical syndromes—the furious, characterized by symptoms of excitation, and the dumb, by the early appearance of paralytic symptoms. If the dog is dead, an attempt should be made to demonstrate the presence of Negri bodies in the hippocampal cells. In addition, the brain should be examined for rabies antigen by the fluorescent antibody technique. If microscopy is negative it may be possible to isolate the virus by intracerebral inoculation of mice. If the dog is alive and has not developed paralysis, it should be kept alive for 10 days, by which time, if it is infected, paralysis should have developed. If it develops rabies the diagnosis should be confirmed as indicated above.

The diagnosis of rabies in man is mainly a clinical problem and usually gives little difficulty. If the case comes to post-mortem examination, the procedure is the same as in the diagnosis of rabies in the dog. In a considerable number of human cases, however, Negri bodies are not demonstrable. During life an attempt may be made to isolate the virus from the saliva, throat swabs or urine by intracerebral inoculation of mice.

There is no treatment for rabies once symptoms have developed.

Prophylaxis

As a general measure the most important step is to abolish rabies in dogs. This can be done by the killing of stray dogs, enforced muzzling, annual vaccination and canine registration. When, as in Britain, the disease has been eliminated, it can be kept out by strict quarantining, for 6 months, of all imported dogs. In countries where there is much wild-life rabies attempts should be made by trapping and other means to reduce the wild animal reservoir. It is doubtful, however, whether it will ever be possible by these measures to eliminate the disease completely.

The feasibility of preventing rabies in persons who have been bitten by rabid animals by active immunization during the incubation period was first shown by Pasteur. The original Pasteur vaccine, known as *virus fixe*, was derived by serial intracerebral passage in rabbits, the preparations used being obtained from infected spinal cords which had been dried for various periods over sodium hydroxide. Pasteur believed that the drying process reduced the virulence of the virus. In fact it appears to cause the death of the virus, very little, if any, remaining alive after 10 days' drying.

Pasteur's method of vaccine preparation is now seldom employed. Most of the vaccines now in use are prepared by Semple's method and consist of a 4 per cent suspension of sheep or rabbit brain inactivated by exposure to 0·5 per cent phenol saline. The virus strains used in these vaccines, however, are all derived from Pasteur's virus fixe. The immunization course consists of from 14 to 21 injections each of 2 ml of vaccine given by the subcutaneous route at daily or twice daily intervals. In the current standard prophylactic procedure rabies hyperimmune horse serum is given immediately after exposure, followed 24 hours later by the first injection of vaccine. There is decisive evidence that such combined active and passive immunization is more effective than active immunization alone. Prophylaxis is however undertaken only if there is clear evidence, or a strong suspicion, that the person has been bitten by a rabid animal.

Anti-rabies vaccination is not without risk—a small proportion of individuals inoculated developing a condition known as a neuroparalytic incident with symptoms referable to damage of the brain, spinal cord or peripheral nerves. This complication usually appears about 2 weeks after the initiation of treatment. Its reported frequency varies from 1 in 800 to 1 in 8000 inoculations. In general it has been less frequent with phenolized vaccine than with the Pasteur type of rabbit cord vaccine. The pathogenesis of the condition is discussed below.

Because of the risk of neuroparalytic incidents after immunization with nervous tissue vaccines considerable work has been carried out in recent years on the feasibility of using living attenuated vaccines propagated in the chick embryo. The most successful of these have been vaccines prepared from the attenuated Flury strain. Two types of vaccine have been prepared from this strain: (1) A low egg passage (LEP) vaccine consisting of virus that has received less than 50 passages in the embryo. LEP vaccine is non-pathogenic for dogs by the intramuscular route but is still pathogenic for mice. It has been used extensively for the immunization of dogs, in which it stimulates a better antibody response than nervous tissue vaccines. Because of this it is now generally accepted as the vaccine of choice for dog immunization. (2) A high egg passage (HEP) vaccine consisting of virus that has been maintained for from 117 to 210 passages in the chick embryo. The vaccine is non-pathogenic for both dogs and mice by the intramuscular route. The HEP vaccine has been used on a limited scale for human immunization. It does not stimulate as good an antibody response in man as nervous tissue vaccines but has the enormous advantage for human immunization that it does not apparently produce neuroparalytic incidents. It is generally considered to be the vaccine of choice for the selective immunization of individuals whose work brings them into contact with rabid animals and for whom frequent inoculation with nervous tissue vaccines would carry considerable risk of allergic sensitization. The vaccine, however, cannot replace nervous tissue vaccine for individuals who have been bitten by rabid animals.

In the prophylaxis of rabies energetic local treatment of the wound is of the greatest importance. The wound should be thoroughly cleaned with soap or a detergent solution and where feasible should be cauterized with concentrated nitric acid. It should be noted that the application of ordinary antiseptics has no effect on the rabies virus. There is evidence that injection of hyperimmune serum around the wound is of considerable value.

LYMPHOCYTIC CHORIOMENINGITIS

The lymphocytic choriomeningitis virus is a natural parasite of mice in which it produces a latent infection and from whom man is almost certainly infected. When enzootic in a stock of mice the virus is transmitted from the mother to the foetus across the placenta. Mice infected in this way continue to maintain a high concentration of virus in the brain and other tissues. In spite of this they exhibit no clinical symptoms of infection. On the other hand, if adult mice are inoculated intracerebrally they develop an encephalitis. Mice infected transplacentally are found to be immunologically tolerant, and develop neither humoral antibody nor delayed-type hypersensitivity. It therefore seems possible that the disease produced in adult mice is the result of an immunological response, either to the virus itself or to some brain antigen liberated as a result of the infection.

In man the virus can produce aseptic meningitis but appears to be a very uncommon cause of this condition. Human infection probably occurs by the respiratory route. It is most readily diagnosed by the demonstration of complement fixing antibody in the patient's serum. The virus measures about 50 mμ in diameter. It can be propagated in mice and in guinea-pigs and will grow in a variety of tissue cultures, in some of which it produces a cytopathogenic effect.

NON-NEUROTROPIC VIRUSES WHICH MAY INVADE THE CENTRAL NERVOUS SYSTEM

The central nervous system may also be invaded by a number of viruses which do not normally infect it, viz. the viruses of mumps, herpes simplex, infectious mononucleosis, zoster, varicella, measles and infectious hepatitis. Infection with these viruses usually gives rise to the syndrome of aseptic meningitis; in some infections the symptoms are those of a definite meningo-encephalitis. In contrast to post-infection encephalitis, meningoencephalitis develops during the course of the primary infection.

ENCEPHALITIS LETHARGICA

This condition occurred extensively in epidemic form in Europe in the early 1920s, but since 1928 no epidemics have appeared. The condition is believed to have been almost certainly of virus origin. The virus of herpes simplex was isolated on a number of occasions from rabbits inoculated with material from fatal cases, but is not believed to have been the causative agent.

POST-INFECTION ENCEPHALITIS

This type of encephalitis may follow infection with a number of viruses but occurs particularly after measles and after vaccination against smallpox (p. 487). A similar condition may also occur following anti-rabies treatment and rarely after other prophylactic inoculations. The pathological changes in post-infection encephalitis consist in a demyelination in the white matter of the central nervous system. These changes are quite different from those occurring in the viral encephalitides, in which the fundamental lesion is a degeneration of nerve cells. This difference renders it unlikely that post-infection encephalitis is the direct consequence of viral infection. More likely alternatives are that it is due to an allergic reaction or to auto-immunization. A possible auto-immune aetiology is suggested by the finding that a similar pathological picture can be produced in animals by inoculation of brain tissue combined with Freund adjuvant. This type of experimental encephalomyelitis would appear to have its strictest analogue in the encephalitis following rabies vaccination with nervous tissue vaccine (p. 476). It nevertheless raises the possibility that when encephalitis follows any viral infection it develops in response to antigens liberated from the brain tissue by the virus infection.

CHAPTER 35

THE POXVIRUSES

This is a group of viruses with a marked affinity for the skin, in which they produce the characteristic lesions or pocks which gives the group its name. They are the largest and, both structurally and chemically, by far the most complex of the animal pathogenic viruses. Nevertheless, they are true viruses, containing only one type of nucleic acid—DNA—and exhibiting an eclipse phase after infection. In electron micrographs they appear as brick-shaped particles measuring from 200 to 300 mμ in length.

They may be divided into five groups: (1) The variola-like viruses, the most important of which, in relation to man, are the vaccinia, variola and cow-pox viruses. The group also includes the rabbit-pox virus, which is possibly a rabbit-adapted vaccinia virus, and the monkey-pox and mouse ectromelia viruses. The viruses of this group resemble one another closely antigenically. A particularly close antigenic relationship exists between the variola, vaccinia and cowpox viruses. (2) The avian poxviruses. (3) Rabbit myxoma and fibroma viruses. (4) The contagious pustular dermatitis (Orf) virus and other poxviruses of ungulates. (5) Miscellaneous viruses including the molluscum contagiosum and milkers' nodule or paravaccinia virus.

VACCINIA VIRUS

Vaccinia is the name given to the strains of virus used for vaccination against smallpox, all of which have had a long history of passage in calves and/or sheep. The origin of many of these strains is obscure but it is believed that most have been derived originally from naturally occurring cowpox virus. Since it has not however so far been possible to transform a wild-type variola virus into a vaccinia virus this proposed lineage cannot be regarded as fully established. The strain in current use in Britain seems likely to have been derived from a smallpox virus isolated from a German soldier during the Franco-Prussian war. Another possibility that has been recently suggested is that vaccinia viruses may have arisen by hybridization between variola and cowpox viruses. Hybrids of this sort have been produced in the laboratory and have been found to possess considerable genetic stability. It is therefore distinctly possible that at least some vaccinia viruses have arisen in this way. Such an origin, followed possibly by the formation of further hybrids would provide a neat explanation for the differences encountered between different strains of vaccinia.

The main component of the vaccinia virus is protein but it has a lipid content of approximately 5 per cent. Highly purified preparations of the virus in addition contain copper, flavinadenine dinucleotide and biotin. There is still considerable doubt as to whether these should or should not be regarded as integral components of the virus particle. On the whole the evidence suggests that they should, but their function is, in this case, unknown. They may have a role in relation to some, so far unidentified, viral enzymes or they may simply be the vestiges of an evolutionary past. No carbohydrate has been detected in the virus other than the deoxyribose of the viral DNA.

Structurally the vaccinia virus is highly complex but the details of the structure have still not been fully resolved. There is evidence for an outer envelope, possibly of lipid, surrounding an indefinite layer containing soluble protein antigens. These superficial layers can apparently be lost without loss of infectivity. The surface of the virus proper has a coarsely granular mulberry-like appearance, due apparently to loops of thread-like protein double helices.

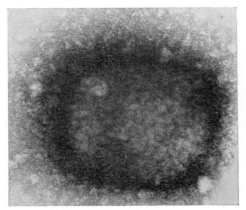

FIG. 50. VACCINIA VIRUS FROM VACCINE LYMPH
Shows mulberry appearance of surface. Electron micrograph. Negative stain. (*Dr T. H. Flewett*)

The centre of the virus is occupied by a nucleoid or core which contains the viral DNA. This is bounded by a coat bearing a characteristically palisaded surface. On cross-section the nucleoid and its coat appear as a biconcave disc, the space between the concavity of the disc and the mulberry surface being occupied by an amorphous structure known as a lateral body.

By the use of the Ouchterlony technique a number of vaccinial antigens have been demonstrated; a maximum of eight have been found in preparations from purified virus, and up to seventeen in preparations from infected cells. It is possible that some of the latter may be enzymes involved in the synthesis of virus rather than integral components of its structure. One of the structural viral antigens—the LS antigen of the literature—is a complex protein consisting of heat-labile and heat-stable components. A nucleoprotein antigen common to all the poxviruses has been described but it has not clearly been demonstrated that this contains only a single component, or that a single component is common to all members of the pox group. The partial purification of an antigen responsible for stimulating neutralizing antibody has been reported but this report still requires full evaluation. If such an antigen can be obtained it could well be of considerable importance in smallpox vaccination.

In infected tissues the virus produces a haemagglutinin which is distinct from the virus particle. The haemagglutinin measures about 15 mμ in diameter, is without regular structure and contains about 75 per cent of lipid. The haemagglutinin is active against fowl red cells but the cells of only about 50 per cent of fowl are susceptible.

The vaccinia virus grows in a variety of tissue cultures in which it produces a well-marked cytopathogenic effect. It also grows readily on the chorioallantoic membrane of the chick embryo, producing large, irregular and frequently haemorrhagic opacities known as pocks. It will infect a variety of animals, particularly calves and rabbits, on intradermal inoculation. By intracerebral passage in rabbits strains of increased neurovirulence, known as neurovaccinia, may be produced. The virulence of the virus for rabbits and calves is considerably diminished by serial passage on the chorioallantoic membrane.

VARIOLA VIRUS

The variola virus has been examined in much less detail than the vaccinia virus but is very similar in its properties. Like the vaccinia virus it will grow in a variety of tissue cultures, though the cytopathogenic effect is slower to appear and less extensive. Inclusion bodies can also be demonstrated in infected cells. Haemadsorption of fowl red cells to the tissue culture can be demonstrated, apparently before the appearance of a significant cytopathogenic effect. Haemadsorption is presumably due to viral haemagglutinin.

The variola virus has a much narrower host range than the vaccinia virus. It will infect monkeys, producing symptoms resembling those of smallpox in man, and most strains will infect rabbits when inoculated onto the cornea. Occasional strains will cause skin lesions in rabbits on intradermal inoculation but serial passage of these strains has not been found possible. Dumbell and Bedson, however, have reported the serial intradermal passage, in rabbits, of virus which had been previously passaged in rabbit kidney tissue culture. Serial passage is also possible in suckling mice by the intracerebral route. Variola virus produces pocks on the chorioallantoic membrane of the chick embryo but these are smaller than those produced by vaccinia, have a smoother surface, are less necrotic and have a uniformly greyish white appearance.

Smallpox virus from cases of variola minor or alastrim are in general less pathogenic for the chick embryo but more readily infect rabbits than strains from variola major. They can be more precisely differentiated, on the basis of growth temperature, on the chorioallantoic membrane variola major strains being capable of producing pocks at both 35 and 38·25° C while alastrim strains will produce pocks at 35° C, but not at 38·25° C. This is consistent with the general principle that virulent viruses will grow at higher temperatures than viruses of low virulence, a difference due, possibly, to their diminished capacity to produce interferon at the higher temperatures.

Smallpox

Smallpox occurs in two clinical forms: variola major which is a serious disease with a high fatality rate, and variola minor or alastrim, which is a relatively mild

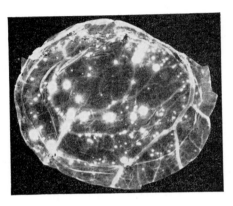

FIG. 51. POCKS PRODUCED BY VARIOLA AND VACCINIA VIRUSES ON THE CHORIO-ALLANTOIC MEMBRANE. THE LARGER POCKS ARE THOSE OF VACCINIA, THE SMALLER THOSE OF VARIOLA. (*A. W. Downie*)

disease with a low fatality rate. Each type breeds true, and there must therefore be some intrinsic differences in the viruses responsible. This is consistent with the differences in pathogenicity that have been demonstrated in the laboratory.

In both types of smallpox, infection usually occurs through the respiratory route by the inhalation of infective material. This material may be droplets from the respiratory tract of a patient, dust containing dried droplets, or material derived from the skin lesions. The danger of infection from such material is considerable since the virus has been shown to be capable of surviving in dried crusts for longer than a year. Epidemiological evidence indicates that cases of smallpox are not infective until the appearance of the skin lesions. These are numerous, and each contains a large amount of virus. On the other hand, the virus present in them does not readily gain access to the exterior, and it is more likely that the main sources of dissemination are the lesions of the mouth and upper respiratory tract.

The disease appears after an incubation period of from 10 to 16 days. It has an acute onset with the development of a high temperature—the characteristic rash appearing on the third or fourth day; when the rash appears the temperature falls. The rash goes through papular, vesicular and pustular stages, its evolution to the pustular stage taking about 10 days. When the pustular stage develops, the patient's temperature again rises; this stage is usually associated with secondary pyogenic infection of the skin lesions. Finally the pustules dry up giving rise to scabs which fall off in 2 to 4 weeks. Since the lesions involve the skin to a considerable depth they leave a permanent scarring which causes considerable disfigurement.

The severity of smallpox varies directly with the extent of the rash. In the classical type of smallpox, with a discrete rash, the mortality is about 10 per cent. Variola major occurring in persons who have been previously vaccinated but who have lost much of their immunity may be indistinguishable from alastrim. If their immunity is of a high order but not sufficient to protect against infection there may be no rash—the so-called variola *sine eruptione*; this type of disease has a very low mortality. Cases in which the rash is confluent are of considerable clinical severity—the mortality in this type usually being about 40 per cent. Occasionally fulminant infections with the early appearance of a generalized purpuric eruption occurs. The majority of these severe infections are fatal. In alastrim the rash is much less profuse than in variola major, there is frequently no secondary fever and the mortality is much lower, being usually less than 1 per cent.

The site of initial viral multiplication is not known with certainty but it is presumably some part of the upper respiratory tract. Since the virus ultimately reaches the skin from the respiratory tract a viraemic stage must occur. Viraemia is readily demonstrable in very severe cases but in others has been found only in the early stages of the disease. From analogy with results obtained by Fenner with mouse ectromelia it is believed that there are in fact two viraemic phases in smallpox. In the first, occurring shortly after infection, reticulo–endothelial cells throughout the body may be invaded, multiplication of the virus in these leading to a second and more intense viraemic stage associated with the development of clinical symptoms.

In fatal cases of smallpox widespread focal lesions are found in the respiratory tract, kidney, liver, spleen and intestines. Infected skin cells show marked degenerative changes. The vesicles have a multilocular character due to the fact that they are traversed by strands of degenerating cells. In the pustular stage large numbers of polymorphonuclear cells are present; these probably accumulate initially as a result of the stimulus of dead or dying epithelial cells, but their presence is also associated with a secondary pyogenic infection. Characteristic acidophilic cytoplasmic inclusion bodies—Guarnieri bodies—are present in infected epithelial cells. In the early stages of the disease the inclusion bodies are usually oval homogeneous masses, lying close to the nucleus and surrounded by a clear unstained area. In older lesions the inclusions are usually granular with an irregular outline, and may occupy most of the cytoplasm. The inclusions are identical with the 'virus factories' demonstrable by electron microscopy (p. 429).

Though it had been endemic in parts of Asia and Africa for centuries, smallpox was only introduced into Europe in the Middle Ages, probably by the Saracens. From the sixteenth to the eighteenth centuries it was a common disease in the British Isles. From the early nineteenth century onwards, however, as a result of the adoption of vaccination as a general prophylactic measure, it showed a marked decrease in incidence until during the course of the nine-teenth century it ceased to exist as an endemic infection. Nowadays, cases occur only when the disease has been introduced from other countries, as in the extensive 1962 epidemic of variola major, when it was introduced by immigrants from Pakistan. Due to the efficacy of control measures, however, this remained largely an institutional outbreak. Smallpox is still endemic in India, Burma, China, the Middle East, Africa and to a lesser extent in South America and Mexico.

Diagnosis

The clinical diagnosis of smallpox in a typical case is relatively easy. Most difficulty is encountered in cases of variola minor, of mild smallpox in vaccinated persons and in cases of the severe haemorrhagic types which do not show the typical rash. Mild cases may be confused clinically with chickenpox, which is therefore usually made notifiable when a smallpox outbreak occurs. Important features differentiating mild smallpox from chickenpox are that in smallpox the lesions have a predominant impact on the extremities, are all at the same stage of development and involve the skin more deeply than do chickenpox lesions.

In the initial febrile stage, prior to the development of the rash, it may be possible to demonstrate the virus in the blood by inoculation onto the chorio-allantoic membrane of the chick embryo. Persistence of the virus in the blood after the second day of the disease is found only in severe haemorrhagic cases. The complement fixation test has been used to demonstrate the presence of virus antigen in the blood but is only likely to give a positive result in very severe cases.

When the rash appears the following methods of diagnosis are available.

1. Virus particles may be demonstrable microscopically in scrapings from papular or vesicular skin lesions. This is best achieved by electron microscopy, using the negative-staining procedure in which the characteristic morphology of the virus is readily demonstrable. Alternatively the material may be examined by ordinary light microscopy, using preparations stained, for example, by Gutstein's method. Stained preparations have little value during the pustular stage when it is virtually impossible to distinguish the virus from the particles of debris present in pustular lesions. The fluorescent antibody technique has also been used but so far has appeared less sensitive than conventional micro-scopic procedures. In addition it has not shown sufficient specificity to consti-tute the sole basis for a positive diagnosis. This situation may however be remedied by improvement in the specificity of the available test antisera.

2. The virus may be isolated by inoculation of scrapings from skin lesions, taken at any stage, onto the chorioallantoic membrane, or into an appropriate tissue culture.

3. Virus may be demonstrable in scrapings from vesicular and pustular skin lesions and in crusts by the complement fixation test. This method is highly reliable and will give a more rapid result than egg inoculation, but will not distinguish between variolous and vaccinial lesions. Virus antigen may also be

demonstrated by the Ouchterlony technique for which the microtest procedure of Dumbell and Nizamuddin has been recommended. This procedure is reported to be highly sensitive for the detection of antigen in vesicle fluid and pus and to permit a specific identification in from 4 to 5 hours.

4. Antibody may be demonstrated in the blood of smallpox patients by the use of haemagglutination inhibition, complement fixation or neutralization tests. The antigens used in these tests may be prepared from vaccinial skin lesions in the rabbit or from chorioallantoic membrane infected with vaccinia. Haemagglutination inhibition and neutralization tests are more sensitive than complement fixation tests and may detect antibody as early as the fifth or sixth day in patients who have not been vaccinated; the complement fixation test is not usually positive before the tenth day. In those who have not been vaccinated a diagnosis may be made on the basis of a single serum examination. For patients who have been previously vaccinated the demonstration of a rising titre of antibody in paired sera is essential. Serological examination is of limited value in the diagnosis of smallpox because of the delay in establishing the diagnosis. Its main value is in the diagnosis of mild atypical cases particularly those presenting without a rash.

Prophylaxis

As has been mentioned smallpox is not now an endemic disease in the British Isles, the cases occurring being the result of the introduction of the disease from abroad. This state of affairs can be attributed in the first place to the adoption of universal vaccination. Vaccination is, however, not now compulsory and immunity from epidemics of the disease is more dependent than formerly on the vigilance of Port Health Authorities, whose duty it is to prevent its reintroduction. When a case of infection is detected it is immediately isolated in an infectious disease hospital. All contacts are vaccinated and are kept under surveillance for a period of 16 days.

Vaccination consists in the intradermal inoculation of vaccinia virus. This results in a local vaccinial lesion which protects against smallpox because of the very close antigenic relationship between the smallpox and vaccinia viruses. Originally vaccination was carried out by arm-to-arm transfer. Nowadays the virus is used in the form of lymph; this is obtained from the lesions produced by inoculation of the virus onto the skin of calves or sheep. The seed virus is maintained by alternate passage in calves and rabbits. For the preparation of lymph the vesicular lesions are curetted, ground up to form a pulpy mass and suspended in 1 per cent phenol. The material is stored for 48 hours at 22° C during which time there is a considerable fall in its bacterial content. Glycerol is then added to give a final concentration of 40 per cent. The glycerinated lymph is stored at $-10°$ C for a further period when there is a further fall in its bacterial content. Before issue it is tested for potency by inoculation into the skin of rabbits or onto the chorioallantoic membrane, and for the absence of pathogenic organisms. If stored at 0° C, lymph retains its potency for months, but if kept at room temperature must not be used after 1 week from the date of issue. Dried calf lymph is now available and is being used on an increasing scale.

It has the advantage of having a much longer 'life'—up to 2 years at 4° C—than ordinary vaccine lymph.

Vaccines prepared from virus grown on the chorioallantoic membrane of the developing chick embryo have been in use in certain areas of the United States for some years. They appear, however, to be less efficient antigens than calf lymph vaccine and have not therefore been adopted for general use in Europe. Vaccines prepared in tissue cultures of bovine skin have also been employed and have given promising results. Chick embryo and tissue culture vaccines have the advantage that they can be prepared under sterile conditions. It has not yet been shown, however, whether they are less likely to give rise to post-vaccinal encephalitis than does the calf lymph vaccine.

It was thought at one time that the hazard of post-infection encephalitis increased progressively with increasing age. It is now generally accepted, however, that the risk is less at 2 years of age than in early infancy. Two years is therefore the age recommended for primary vaccination of children in the British Isles. Children who are debilitated or who have been exposed to an infectious disease or who are suffering from infantile eczema should not be vaccinated. Primary vaccination should not be carried out during the early stages of pregnancy or within 21 days before or less than 4 days after yellow fever inoculation.

A substantial degree of immunity is present by about the eighth or ninth day after vaccination. Since the average incubation period of smallpox is 12 days, individuals who have been in contact with a case are therefore usually protected if vaccination is carried out within the first 2 or 3 days of the incubation period. It can usually be assumed that vaccinated individuals are completely immune to infection for at least 3 years, and a useful degree of immunity persists for life. In countries where smallpox is prevalent it is, however, advisable to carry out re-vaccination at least every 2 years. Immunity to natural smallpox infection in vaccinated individuals appears to be much more persistent than immunity to revaccination.

Vaccination is usually carried out by the multiple-pressure method. In this procedure a Hagedorn needle is pressed through a drop of lymph placed on the skin—the pressure being applied with the needle parallel to the skin surface. The virus gains entry to the skin through the minute pricks produced by the needle in the epidermis. This method has largely outmoded the scratch method formerly in use. Some authorities consider, however, that the latter may give more effective immunity and advise its use in the face of an epidemic. Evidence has been presented that the multiple pressure technique may be more successful than the scratch method for the revaccination of male subjects. After vaccination the vaccination site should be covered with a light dressing to prevent dissemination of the virus.

Following a successful primary vaccination a papule appears within 3 to 4 days at the site of inoculation. The lesion then goes through the stages of vesiculation, pustulation and scabbing, taking approximately 3 days for each stage. The peak of the reaction which, in some subjects, may be associated with considerable swelling of the arm and high fever, occurs at about the ninth or tenth day. The scab falls off finally after about 20 days. This type of reaction to vaccination, which is that occurring in subjects with no previous immunity, is known as a 'primary take'. In those who have previously been vaccinated the reaction appears sooner, evolves more rapidly, and is milder in character than the typical primary reaction. Some show an immediate reaction to vaccination, a small papule appearing within 24 hours; in such cases there is usually no vesicle formation and the reaction fades within about 3 days. This type of reaction has often been referred to in the past as the reaction of immunity. This designation is, however, incorrect; the reaction may be due to immunity but may occur following vaccination with an inactive lymph either as a result of trauma or as an allergic response to the virus or to some other component of the lymph. In some cases no reaction follows vaccination. It should be emphasized that unless there is evidence of a successful recent vaccination the complete absence of a reaction or the development of an immediate-type reaction should be regarded as due to a faulty technique or to the use of inactive vaccine lymph and the vaccination should be repeated.

Vaccination not only protects against infection but also tremendously lowers the fatality rate in patients who in spite of vaccination contract the disease. Thus in cases of smallpox occurring in Britain between 1942 and 1953 the mortality in unvaccinated patients was 48·4 per cent while in vaccinated ones the mortality was only 13·5 per cent. All deaths in the latter group occurred in patients who had been vaccinated at least 13 years previously.

Gamma globulin prepared from the sera of recently vaccinated individuals has definite protective value and is recommended for household smallpox contacts and for persons who cannot be vaccinated within 3 days of contact. There is some evidence that its administration may be valuable in preventing the development of encephalitis in adults who are being vaccinated for the first time, and for the protection of eczematous children who have been in contact with recently vaccinated persons. It has also been recommended for the treatment of complications of vaccination, e.g. corneal vaccinia, but its value for this purpose has still to be determined.

Complications of Vaccination

Post-vaccinal Encephalitis

This is a very rare but grave complication with an overall mortality of about 10 per cent. The frequency with which it occurs has shown considerable variability in different parts of the world. In Scotland in 1942 it occurred once in 8000 vaccinations, whereas in Durban in 1944 no cases were observed in 450,000 vaccinations. Most cases have occurred after primary vaccination of adults, and the hazard is clearly related to age (p. 486).

There is some evidence that the risk of post-vaccinal encephalitis following late primary vaccinations may be considerably reduced if gamma globulin, prepared from the sera of recently vaccinated persons, is given at the same time. Thus in Holland, where all army recruits are vaccinated, the incidence of encephalitis was found to be reduced by 75 per cent by concomitant administration of immune globulin. It has also been suggested that the risk may be reduced by the administration of ultra-violet or formalin-inactivated vaccine and of attenuated live vaccine, prior to immunization with calf lymph. These procedures are still under examination. There is, however, some evidence from work in experimental animals that the administration of inactivated vaccine may induce a state of hypersensitivity which might result in an unduly severe reaction to the live vaccine.

Generalized Vaccinia

In this condition, which usually appears from 9 to 14 days after vaccination, there is a widespread dissemination of the vaccinia virus through the body by the blood with the production of a generalized vaccinial eruption. The condition is rare, occurring about once in 50,000 vaccinations. Recovery is usually rapid.

Eczema Vaccinatum

This is the development of secondary vaccinial lesions on eczematous or burnt skin areas. Because of the risk of such infections children with eczematous lesions or burns should not be vaccinated unless they have been in contact with a case of smallpox. Most cases appear to be the result of contact infection from an individual who has been recently vaccinated.

Progressive Vaccinia

In very exceptional cases the vaccinial lesion fails to heal. In such cases there is a progressive necrosis of the skin at the vaccination site and the development of metastatic lesions in other areas of the skin and in the viscera. Some of the individuals in whom this condition has been described were agammaglobulinaemic. A recent report suggests that methisazone may be of value in treatment.

Chemoprophylaxis

As an alternative to vaccination for the protection of smallpox contacts, the administration of methisazone (p. 432) has been favourably reported on—the degree of protection obtained being of the same order as that following vaccination. When methisazone was combined with vaccination the degree of protection, as shown in data reported by Bauer, was much greater than that following vaccination alone. Thus of 1987 treated vaccinated contacts only 2 developed smallpox whereas of 2380 contacts who were not given methisazone 62 developed smallpox. The protective effect of methisazone is of short duration and administration of this drug cannot therefore be substituted for vaccination as a long-term phophylactic procedure.

MOLLUSCUM CONTAGIOSUM

This condition is characterized by the occurrence of painless pearly white nodules in the skin of various parts of the body. Only man appears to be susceptible.

In infected epithelial cells typical inclusion bodies are seen. These are large acidophilic structures frequently almost completely filling the cell. In electron micrographs the virus appears as a brick-shaped particle, morphologically similar to the other poxviruses. The viruses possess a soluble complement fixing antigen serologically distinct from those of variola and vaccinia. In some cases of molluscum contagiosum antibody to this antigen is demonstrable in the serum but not sufficiently frequently to make its demonstration of diagnostic value. The virus has not been propagated in the laboratory.

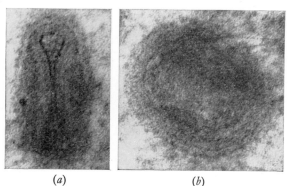

(a)   (b)

Fig. 52. Molluscum Contagiosum

Section (a) across and (b) along length of particle. Note dumb-bell shaped nucleoid in (a) (Dr T. H. Flewett)
Electron micrograph. Negative stain

CONTAGIOUS PUSTULAR DERMATITIS (ORF)

This is a disease of sheep and goats of world-wide distribution. Human infection which occasionally occurs in people in contact with infected animals takes the form of a solitary papulovesicular lesion, with a central ulcer, on the arm, hand or, less frequently, the face.

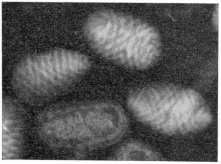

Fig. 53. Orf Virus

Note surface criss-crossed structures. Internal structure of some particles may be seen.
(Horne, Nagington and Newton, Virology)
Electron micrograph. Negative stain

The Orf virus is somewhat smaller than the vaccinia and variola viruses, and in electron micrographs, in contrast to the mulberry appearance of the latter, shows a criss-cross pattern formed by two sets of parallel threads. The virus shows no immunological relationship to the viruses of the variola group. It has not been propagated in the chick embryo or in any of the ordinary laboratory animals but lesions can be produced in the skin of sheep by the inoculation of material obtained from a human lesion. It has been grown in fibroblast mono-layer cultures prepared from sheep skin.

COWPOX

The virus of cowpox closely resembles those of variola and vaccinia but exhibits minor antigenic differences. Man is occasionally infected from cattle, with the production of localized skin lesions.

MILKERS' NODES (PARAVACCINIA)

These are red, papular lesions which occasionally develop on the hands of individuals milking infected cows. The lesions differ from those of vaccinia in not having a vesicular stage and in not being associated with systemic symptoms. A generalized rash is occasionally present. The disease occurs in many countries but appears to be particularly common in Norway. In infected cows the lesions occur on the teats and udder.

Morphologically the virus resembles the Orf virus. It will not grow in the chick embryo or in ordinary laboratory animals but will infect cows on inocu-lation into the skin. It has recently been propagated in tissue cultures of bovine kidney. It shows no antigenic relationship to the vaccinia or cowpox viruses.

CHAPTER 36

THE MYXOVIRUSES

The myxoviruses were originally defined as a group of viruses capable of agglutinating the red blood cells of a variety of animal species through combination with mucoprotein receptors present on the red cell surface, and possessing at the same time an enzyme capable of breaking down the receptors. Subsequently it was found that all viruses possessing these properties were essentially similar in structure, and that the same structure was shown by certain viruses without demonstrable haemagglutinating properties. As a result the group is now defined by structural criteria. As defined in this way, myxoviruses are RNA viruses possessing an internal component or nucleocapsid of helical symmetry. The nucleocapsid is surrounded by an envelope with radially disposed spike-like projections. These projections are the viral haemagglutinins. The myxoviruses have a high content of lipid which constitutes from 20 to 40 per cent of the virus particle. The lipid appears to be confined mainly, or exclusively, to the envelope which, as a result, is disrupted when the viruses are treated with ether. This causes liberation of the internal component or nucleocapsid and a concomitant loss of infectivity. The internal component released by ether treatment shows an appearance in negatively stained preparations consistent with a helical arrangement of protein subunits surrounding a coiled strand of RNA—an arrangement essentially similar to that found in the tobacco mosaic virus. The reported isolation of an infectious RNA from influenza viruses has not been confirmed.

Two subgroups of myxoviruses are distinguished.

Subgroup I

This includes the influenza viruses and virus of fowl plague. These measure from 80 to 120 mμ in diameter, the envelope spikes measuring 90 by 15 to 20 Å. The internal component is a helix 90 Å wide by 6000 to 10,000 Å in length. Its RNA content is about 5 per cent. Filamentous forms, which may be up to 1μ in length, are frequently found, particularly in recently isolated strains. The filamentous forms which appear to be fully infective contain much more RNA per particle than the spherical forms; some of this excess RNA may be of host cell origin.

Subgroup II

This comprises the para-influenza viruses, mumps, measles, respiratory syncytial virus, Newcastle disease virus and the viruses of canine distemper and rinderpest. The viruses of this subgroup are distinctly larger than those of subgroup I, measuring from 100 to 300 mμ in diameter; the spikes are more delicate, measuring 80 by 10 to 15 Å and the internal component is larger— 180 Å wide and 35,000 to 50,000 Å in length. These viruses also have a higher concentration of RNA—around 10 per cent—suggesting that the latter may occur as a double helix. The membranes of the subgroup II viruses undergoes spontaneous rupture, releasing the internal component, much more frequently than the membranes of subgroup I viruses.

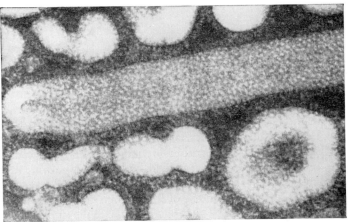

FIG. 54. INFLUENZA VIRUS SHOWING FILAMENT AND PARTICLES
Electron micrograph. Negative stain (Dr T. H. Flewett)

SUBGROUP I MYXOVIRUSES

THE INFLUENZA VIRUS

Two distinct types of influenza virus antigen may be distinguished.

1. Soluble antigens (S antigens). These can be readily extracted from infected tissues and are present also in infected fluids, e.g. allantoic fluid. Although designated as soluble they occur as small particles of 10 to 15 mμ in diameter. Chemically they are ribonucleoproteins, owing their antigenic specificity to the protein component. Antigens of identical chemical and serological specificity can be obtained by rupture of intact virus particles by ether treatment or by ultrasonic disintegration. There is little doubt that the soluble antigens found in infected tissues are in fact fragments of the internal component or nucleocapsid of the virus, their presence in free form in infected tissues and in tissue fluids representing either excess material which has not been incorporated into the completed virus particle or material which has been released by spontaneous rupture of the virus envelope. They are non-infective and non-haemagglutinating and are demonstrable only by complement fixation tests. On the basis of the soluble antigens they possess influenza viruses are subdivided into three completely distinct antigenic types: A, B and C.

2. Strain-specific surface antigens (V antigens). These have been identified with the spikes on the surface of the virus envelope, which are also responsible for haemagglutinating activity. Because of this, antibody to V antigens will inhibit haemagglutination and, since the virus makes contact with the susceptible cell through the spikes, will neutralize infectivity. Hence, this is the antibody responsible for immunity against influenza. The reaction between V antigens and antibody can also be demonstrated by complement fixation tests. Specific reactions, however, are only obtained if purified preparations of virus, freed of soluble antigens, are used. Such preparations can be readily obtained by adsorbing the virus onto red cells and allowing it to elute at 37° C. The supernatants of fully absorbed preparations will contain the soluble antigen.

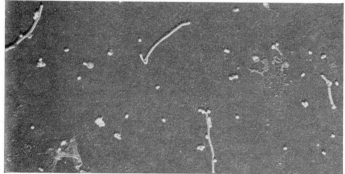

FIG. 55. FILAMENTS AND SPHERES OF INFLUENZA VIRUS TYPE A,
MELBOURNE STRAIN
Platinum shadowed × 10,000
(*Dr A. Isaacs and Dr R. C. Valentine*)

When influenza viruses of types A and B are examined by haemagglutination inhibition and neutralization tests they exhibit considerable antigenic heterogeneity. This heterogeneity is due to differences in strain-specific antigen composition and is most marked in type A strains. Its precise serological basis is not known. Francis and Davenport, however, have brought forward evidence for the presence in various type A strains of at least 18 distinct antigenic components and have suggested that the antigenic differences between the various strains are due to an arrangement of the antigens on the virus surface in which antigens inaccessible in some strains are prominently sited on the surface of other strains, and vice versa. Evidence in favour of this view is provided by Davenport and his associates in their finding that the viral haemagglutinins obtained by disruption of the virus by ether show a broader antigenic reactivity and a capacity to stimulate a broader immune response than does the intact virus. They suggest that in the intact virus the dominant strain-specific antigens are those located at the tip of the spike. This is consistent with the results obtained from electron microscopy of virus particles exposed to ferritin-labelled antibody. Davenport has proposed that, in addition to these antigens, other antigens are located along the sides and at the bases of the spikes; these are normally inaccessible to antibody but become accessible when the virus particle is inactivated by ether treatment. This is also consistent with the evidence obtained from electron microscopy, which in disrupted preparations shows fragments of membrane with attached spikes occurring in the form of rolled-up hedgehog-like balls, or rosettes in which the spikes are considerably more splayed out and separated than in the intact virus. A second possibility is that the antigenic differences depend on variations in the antigenic specificity of one or a limited number of components.

Whatever the basis of these differences may be, an apparently progressive antigenic variation has been observed in the type A strains that have been so far isolated since the discovery of the influenza virus by Smith, Andrewes and Laidlaw in 1933. It has in fact been possible to demonstrate antigenic differences between the strains responsible for every major type A outbreak; as a result, recently isolated type A strains differ sharply from those first isolated. In this progressive antigenic variation there have been two sharp changes in antigenic type—the first occurring in 1947 and exhibited particularly in the FM1 strain, the second occurring in 1957 with the appearance of the Asian strains. These sharp breaks in antigenic behaviour permit the classification of type A strains into three antigenic families: (1) Strains occurring before 1947 and antigenically resembling the prototype PR8 strain; these are known without qualification as type A strains. (2) Strains appearing in the period between 1947 and 1957 and antigenically resembling the FM1 strain; these are known as type A1 strains. (3) Strains antigenically resembling the Asian strains which appeared in 1957; these are known as type A2 strains. Like A1 strains, these have, clearly, been undergoing antigenic variation. Up to 1964 the differences from the earlier strains were insufficient to frustrate the immunity produced by vaccine prepared from the latter. Type A2 strains isolated from 1964 onwards have, however, differed sharply from earlier strains. A similar antigenic variation has been encountered in type B strains but to a lesser extent and with less dramatic breaks in continuity. A strain isolated in Taiwan in 1962, however, showed considerable antigenic difference from previous strains. Nevertheless, further dissemination of this strain has not been observed.

The emergence of new antigenic variants of the influenza virus can be readily explained on the basis of selection in immune populations. When immunity has developed to a current antigenic variety the antibodies responsible tend to suppress this variety; if, however, a new antigenic variant appears which is not inhibited by the prevalent antibodies it will be able to spread until it in turn is replaced by yet another antigenic variant. As a corollary of this view it has been suggested that the type A virus is that most frequently responsible for epidemics of influenza because it possesses an inherently high antigenic lability.

Evidence has been presented by Francis and Davenport that the dominant antibodies in an individual's serum are specific for the antigenic components of the particular virus to which he or she was first exposed. Thus children who were first exposed to influenza during the period of prevalence of the FM1 or A1 types, i.e. from 1947 to 1957, possess antibodies reacting particularly with these varieties. Older people who were first exposed to the pre-1947 or PR8 type virus possess antibodies reacting particularly with PR8 components. Since the sera of individuals over forty were distinguished by the presence of antibodies reacting particularly with the swine influenza virus these workers believe that the virus of the 1918 epidemic was antigenically related to the swine virus. Similarly a high titre of antibodies to the Asian virus has been found by Mulder in the sera of persons old enough to have experienced the influenza pandemic of 1890. This suggests that there may be some antigenic relationship between the Asian virus and the virus responsible for the 1890 pandemic and supports Francis's theory of multiple antigenic components which vary quantitatively in different strains. In addition to differing antigenically, strains of influenza virus of precisely the same antigenic composition may differ in the avidity with which they combine with antibody. This type of heterogeneity was first observed by Mulder in A1 strains. Mulder distinguished three phases—P, Q and R—differing in their behaviour in haemagglutination inhibition tests. P phase strains are normal strains which are inhibited to high titre by homologous antiserum. Q phase strains are poorly inhibited by homologous serum. R phase strains are inhibited by homologous serum and by certain heterologous sera. It is suggested that Q phase strains may be of importance in permitting the virus to persist in immune populations, since they are relatively insusceptible to specific antibody. P→Q variation can be induced under laboratory conditions by growing the virus in the presence of immune serum. Similar differences have been demonstrated for A2 strains, which have been found by Choppin and Tamm to consist of varying proportions of two types of particle—avid particles with a high combining power for antibody, and non-avid particles with a low combining power. The relative proportions of the types of particle present determines the overall behaviour of the strain. Avid particles also appear to have a higher affinity than non-avid particles for red cell receptors and mucoprotein inhibitors.

Growth of the Virus

The influenza virus grows readily in the chick embryo. On primary isolation most strains grow only in the amniotic cavity. When it has been established by amniotic inoculation it may then be propagated by the allantoic route. Allantoic inoculation is usually carried out using 10- or 11-day-old embryos—the infected allantoic fluid being harvested 2 days later. The concentration of virus in the allantoic fluid of infected eggs is high—infectivity titres for 0·1 ml of fluid being of the order of 10^{-9}. The virus will also grow in chick embryo tissue culture, in fragments of chorioallantoic membrane suspended in nutrient medium and in cultures of human amnion and monkey kidney cells. In tissue cultures the cytopathogenic action of the virus is normally slight though it may be appreciable with some strains. Infection of tissue cultures with influenza virus is most readily detected by the *haemadsorption* technique in which a suspension of red cells is added to the culture; if virus is present the red cells adhere to the infected tissue cells. This technique is more sensitive for the detection of virus than the demonstration of haemagglutinin in the culture fluid.

If allantoic cells are simultaneously infected with two strains of influenza virus which differ in properties that can be readily distinguished, the progeny of infection may contain hybrid or recombination forms. The formation of these hybrids is analogous to the recombination phenomenon in bacteria (p. 26) and in bacteriophages. It is not known whether or to what extent recombination can occur under natural conditions but it is potentially a mechanism which might result in the emergence of variants of enhanced virulence or of altered antigenic composition.

If influenza virus is passed serially in eggs, using a concentrated inoculum, e.g. undiluted allantoic fluid, the progeny shows a progressively increasing number of incomplete virus particles. These are particles which, although fully effective in haemagglutination, have a low RNA content and are non-infective. It has been shown, however, that cells producing such virus have a normal content of viral RNA. It is clear therefore that the defect involved occurs in virus maturation. A similar defect in maturation is observed when virus propagation is attempted in mouse brain (except with adapted strains), in certain types of tissue culture, notably HeLa cells, or in the chick chorion as distinct from the allantois. In all these cases virus nucleic acid and protein are formed but are not assembled into mature virus.

Haemagglutination

The influenza virus has the property of agglutinating the red cells of a variety of animal species. The cells which have been most used in the study of virus haemagglutination are those of fowl, man and guinea-pig. Haemagglutination is a function of the envelope spikes which adsorb to the appropriate receptor on the red cell surface, the virus particle then forming a bridge joining one cell to another.

When they are first isolated type A1 viruses are frequently in the phase called by Burnet the O or original phase; in this phase the virus has a low haemag-glutinin titre for fowl red cells relative to its titre for human and guinea-pig cells. On further propagation by the allantoic route it assumes the D or derived phase which has a high haemagglutinin titre against fowl cells. The O phase is presumed to be the form of the virus as it exists in nature and to be the only form which is naturally infective for man.

If red cells which have adsorbed virus are allowed to stand for some time, the virus is released or eluted from the cell. Elution takes place more rapidly at $37°$ C than at lower temperatures. It is due to the action of a virus enzyme which breaks down the receptor substances on the red cell with which the virus combines. Red cells whose receptors have been broken down to the extent that they are no longer agglutinable by the homologous virus may nevertheless be agglutinated by another strain of influenza virus. It is in fact possible to arrange different strains of virus in a series or 'receptor gradient', each strain of which is capable of removing receptors for the viruses below it in the series, but not for the viruses above it. The precise basis of the phenomenon is not understood but, presumably, depends on differences in the extent to which different strains of virus can bind to the receptors.

For many years it was assumed that the viral haemagglutinin and receptor-destroying enzyme (see below) were identical, the virus combining with the cell through specific groups on the surface of the enzyme. Recent evidence, however, suggests that this is not the case. Thus active preparations of the enzyme can be obtained by digestion of the virus particle with trypsin, without any significant disintegration of the envelope spikes. In addition it has been possible to separate the enzyme from the haemagglutinin by electrophoresis of preparations obtained by disrupting the virus with sodium dodecylsulphate. The distinct character of the haemagglutinin and the enzyme is also supported by the finding that anti-body to the haemagglutinin blocks the enzymatic activity of the virus particle against large molecular weight mucoproteins but not against low molecular weight neuraminic-acid containing substrates, e.g. neuraminyl lactose.

In addition to destroying the red cell virus receptors the virus enzyme effects a number of other changes in the cell. (1) Virus-treated cells are agglutinable by the so-called 'incomplete' Rh antibodies; this change is also produced by treat-ment of the cells with trypsin and various proteolytic enzymes. It has not been shown, however, that influenza virus possesses any protease activity. (2) Treated cells differ from normal cells in electrophoretic mobility. (3) Treated cells possess an antigenic specificity different from that possessed by untreated cells. It is not known whether this change is due to chemical modification of the receptor or to the unmasking, by removal of the receptor, of some antigen normally present in the cell.

Because of the capacity of the virus enzyme to break down the virus receptors on the red cell surface it is known as the receptor-destroying enzyme (RDE). The enzyme has been shown by Gottschalk to have the properties of a neura-minidase or sialidase—splitting off N-acetyl neuraminic acid from various mucopolysaccharides. Enzymes with properties similar to those of the virus RDE have been detected in a number of bacterial species, particularly potent preparations being obtained from the cholera vibrio.

The role of the enzyme in infection has not been determined. The initial stage of infection is undoubtedly the adsorption of the virus on to the receptor substances of susceptible cells; these receptors have been shown to have very similar properties to those of red cells. It would therefore seem likely that break-down of the receptors by the virus enzyme permits penetration of the virus into the cell. There is some evidence, however, that the virus can infect cells whose receptors have been modified in such a way that though they can combine with virus they are not broken down by it. It is therefore possible that the virus RDE is more important in securing the release of virus from infected cells than in facilitating its entry.

The virus receptor substance appears to be a mucoprotein. Mucoproteins from many sources—saliva, various types of mucus, serum and urine are capable of inhibiting haemagglutination; this they do by combining with the virus and thereby preventing its adsorption to the cells. Inhibitory mucoprotein has a much more marked effect on virus which has been heated sufficiently to in-activate the receptor destroying enzyme than on unheated active virus. This is presumably due to the fact that inactivated virus enzyme can combine with the mucoprotein but is unable to elute from it.

The inhibitory mucoprotein present in normal mammalian sera is usually known as α inhibitor. It is readily broken down by RDE, by trypsin and by periodate. A second inhibitor known as β inhibitor and distinguished from α inhibitor by its relative insusceptibility to RDE and to periodate and by its heat lability is also present in normal human serum. β inhibitor is readily broken down by trypsin and by proteases present in crude *V. cholerae* filtrates. Serum inhibitors are of considerable practical importance since they cause difficulty in the interpretation of haemagglutination inhibition tests (p. 437).

Influenza

Influenza is a disease of acute onset and of short duration—usually lasting, in the absence of complications, for about 3 days. The essential lesions are degenerative changes in the epithelium of the bronchi and bronchioles, the lesions found being very similar to those encountered in experimental infections of the ferret. There is now clear evidence that influenza virus can, in severe cases, cause a specific type of pneumonia associated with degenerative changes in the alveolar wall, though, for some time, this was doubted. It is not clear, however, that this syndrome is due to invasion of the alveolar cells by virus. It may be due to the toxic effect of a large number of virus particles on the alveolar epithelium, an effect which has been observed in experimental infections of mice. The most serious effect of influenza is, however, the fact that it predisposes, especially in older people, to secondary pulmonary infection by pyogenic organisms, particularly by pneumococci and *Staph. aureus*: a high proportion of staphylococcal pneumonias occur in fact as complications of influenza. Staphylococcal pneumonia complicating influenza is particularly serious and has a high fatality rate. It usually develops during the acute phase of the disease. Pneumonia due to the pneumococcus, on the other hand, usually occurs after the acute phase of the infection has subsided. Influenza is a particular hazard to patients suffering from cardiovascular or renal disease, and epidemics are always associated with an excess mortality in patients with these diseases.

Influenza is a disease that affects all age groups but the decades 5 to 14 years and 25 to 34 years show maximum susceptibility. Following the introduction of a new antigenic variant, as occurred with the spread of the A2 virus in 1957, the main brunt of the disease is borne by the younger age groups. With each successive appearance of the virus, however, the peak incidence moves to an older age group.

Influenza is mainly an epidemic disease but occurs also as a sporadic infection. Serological evidence indicates that during the course of an epidemic, in addition to overt infections, a considerable number of associated subclinical infections also occur. Of the three antigenic types, type A is epidemiologically the most important having a particularly marked capacity for epidemic spread. Epidemics of type A infection tend to occur with a periodicity of 2 to 3 years. Epidemics of type A infection are explosive in onset and tend to spread rapidly by contiguity from the initial focus of infection. Occasionally the disease assumes a pandemic form spreading rapidly from one country to another until the entire world is involved, as in the great pandemics of 1918 and 1957. The type B virus is more frequently responsible for sporadic cases and small localized outbreaks—large epidemics occurring much less frequently than with type A. Type B epidemics tend to occur with a periodicity of 3 to 6 years. The type C virus has not so far been shown to be of any great epidemiological importance and is not known to have given rise to large-scale epidemics. Antibody to the virus is, however, present in the sera of a high number of normal persons. It is consequently believed that subclinical infection is frequent and is the normal result of infection with this type.

There has been considerable speculation as to the way in which the influenza virus persists in interepidemic periods when no virus is recognizable. It is possible that it assumes a dormant or masked form which, though capable of causing sporadic cases, would be incapable of large-scale epidemic spread. It has been suggested that this dormant form might be the Q form referred to above, since this form seems particularly adapted to survival in immune populations. The observation that some large type A epidemics appearing in the autumn were preceded by a summer 'flurry' of infection involving a relatively small number of cases is in support of the masked virus theory. This sequence of events was observed in Sicily in 1948 and in Scandinavia in 1950. Following the minor summer outbreak the virus apparently went 'underground' and became dormant only to be lighted into activity in the following autumn. A somewhat analogous process has been observed by Shope in the epidemiology of swine influenza. The swine virus can apparently persist for long periods in lung-worms. The larvae of the lung-worms are ingested by earthworms which are in turn swallowed by pigs. The lung-worms with their contained virus become parasitic in the pig's lung in which the virus remains latent; if, however, the pig develops a respiratory infection with *H. influenzae*, the latent virus is activated and causes an attack of influenza. There is, however, no evidence that *H. influenzae* plays the role of a precipitating factor in the pathogenesis of influenza in man, but it may give rise to secondary pulmonary infection during the course of the disease.

In recent years the isolation from various animal sources of viruses possessing the type A soluble antigen has suggested the possibility of an animal reservoir for human influenza viruses. Apart, however, from the possible relationship of the swine influenza virus to the virus responsible for the 1918 pandemic—a relationship which can, of course, never be confirmed—the type A viruses isolated from animal sources have shown no relationship in strain-specific antigen composition to human type A strains. The reported isolation of type A2 viruses from horses has not been confirmed.

The capacity of the virus to undergo antigenic variation plays an important part in the epidemiology of influenza. As has been mentioned above the virus appears to be undergoing a progressive antigenic variation, the virus of each epidemic differing detectably from that of the previous epidemic and more markedly from the viruses of still earlier epidemics. Consequently the virus responsible for each major epidemic is to a greater or a lesser extent insusceptible to the immunity persisting from earlier epidemics. Because of this the influenza virus is able to give rise to epidemics which recur at relatively short intervals.

The great severity of the influenza pandemic of 1918–19 is well known. The mortality in this pandemic was very high; it was in fact responsible for more deaths than World War I, killing in all from 10 to 20 million persons. A particularly serious feature of the pandemic was the great severity of the disease in young adults. It has been suggested that the virus responsible differed sharply in antigenic properties from the viruses present before 1918, against which the population possessed appreciable immunity. There is, however, some indirect serological evidence that the 1918 virus antigenically resembled the swine influenza virus and that it was prevalent for some time prior to 1918. If this was the case, the severity of the epidemic could not have been solely due to antigenic variation. An alternative explanation is that the virus, although showing some normal antigenic variation from preceding viruses, was of very much greater virulence. Andrewes suggests that increase in virulence might have resulted from a recombination between two distinct strains of virus producing a vicious new hybrid. In support of this possibility he points out that the virulent form of the disease first appeared around Boston and in Brest—ports of embarkation and disembarkation for American troops going to the European war theatre. At these ports there might well have been a fusion between an American and a French strain of virus. Both these explanations are, however, entirely hypothetical and the great virulence of the 1918 pandemic is likely to remain for ever an unsolved problem.

Diagnosis

The virus may be isolated from the throat during the acute stage of infection. For this purpose chick embryos inoculated by the amniotic route have mainly been used, the presence of virus in the amniotic fluid being detected by haemagglutination tests. Tissue cultures have been favourably reported on for the isolation of type B viruses but do not appear to give satisfactory results with the current type A2 strains.

For clinical purposes serological tests are more valuable than isolation of the virus but have the disadvantage that they only permit a retrospective diagnosis. Two samples of serum are taken—the first, if possible, within the first 3 days of the disease and the second during convalescence about a fortnight later. If the case is one of influenza there should be a rise in antibody titre of at least fourfold between the two examinations. Antibody may be detected either by haemagglutination inhibition or by complement fixation tests. The latter are best carried out with preparations of soluble antigen freed of virus particles by absorption with red cells. Soluble antigens of both type A and type B should be used but need only be obtained from a single strain of each type. Haemagglutination inhibition tests are carried out using allantoic fluid as a source of virus. In this case it is important that the virus strain employed should be of the prevalent antigenic type. Best results are obtained in haemagglutination inhibition tests if the patient's serum is first treated with a preparation of the receptor-destroying enzyme from *V. cholerae* or with trypsin so as to break down the non-specific inhibitors present. Serial dilutions of the serum are made and are mixed with a standard amount, usually four agglutinating doses, of virus. The tubes after addition of red cells are allowed to stand for some time and are then examined for agglutination either by a densitometric or a pattern method. Complement fixing antibody declines more rapidly after infection than haemagglutination inhibiting antibody and is consequently more valuable as an index of recent infection. In addition, it is not produced, as is the latter, by vaccination.

Prophylaxis

A great deal of experimental work has been carried out on the value of killed vaccines in active immunization against influenza. In general the results have been satisfactory; when the virus used for vaccine preparation has been closely related antigenically to the virus responsible for the next epidemic, significant, though by no means complete, protection has been obtained. Thus in the MRC trials of A2 vaccine in England in 1957, protection rates of from 52 to 75 per cent were achieved. A significant degree of protection was demonstrable 8 days after the administration of a single dose of vaccine.

The antibody response to a given amount of antigen can be greatly increased by incorporating the antigen in an adjuvant consisting of mineral oil and an emulsifying agent (p. 110). Limited trials with such mineral oil vaccines have been highly satisfactory, high levels of antibody being found in a considerable proportion of vaccinees for up to 2 years after vaccination. Adjuvant vaccines have the additional advantage of permitting the employment of a much smaller amount of antigen than with the conventional saline vaccines. Because of this they clearly provide a more practicable basis than saline vaccines for a programme of immunization on a community scale.

There are, however, considerable limitations to the practicability of active immunization against influenza. Because of the capacity of the virus to undergo antigenic variation the preparation of an effective vaccine requires anticipation of the antigenic type likely to be responsible for the next epidemic. It is hoped that it may be possible to get over this difficulty by early isolation and antigenic typing of the virus responsible for a major epidemic, so that vaccine can be prepared from it and used for immunization in communities to which the epidemic has not yet spread. If, as Francis believes, the number of possible antigenic components is limited, there is some possibility that an antigenically comprehensive vaccine which would give a wide degree of protection might be produced. Because of this the commercial vaccines available in the United States are usually polyvalent vaccines containing A, A1, A2 and B components.

Though the organization of vaccination programmes on a community scale is not at the moment practicable it is advised that vaccination should be offered to persons suffering from certain chronic diseases—chronic pulmonary disease, chronic heart disease, chronic renal disease, diabetes—in which an attack of influenza might aggravate disability or prove fatal.

For many years Russian workers have experimented with live attenuated vaccines administered by intranasal instillation. The Iksha strain of A2 virus, attenuated by passage in chick embryos, has been particularly used. Small-scale trials have been carried out by British workers, and results sufficiently encouraging to justify further study have been obtained. So far, however, the procedure cannot be accepted as an alternative to immunization with killed virus.

SUBGROUP II MYXOVIRUSES

The morphological features distinguishing these from subgroup I have already been considered. Haemagglutination is not as prominent a feature of these viruses as of the subgroup I viruses. Some, notably the respiratory syncytial virus and the viruses of rinderpest and distemper, are devoid of haemagglutinating and receptor-destroying activity. Subgroup II viruses are more difficult to propagate than those of subgroup I. Only two members of the group—the mumps virus and the Newcastle disease virus—can be isolated in chick embryos. In tissue cultures they have considerable tendency to induce the formation of giant cells and syncytia, and infected cells frequently show the presence of cytoplasmic acidophilic inclusions. The viruses appear to be synthesized exclusively in the cytoplasm and, possibly because of this, incomplete virus is rarely produced. Genetic recombination has not so far been demonstrated amongst any of the subgroup II viruses.

THE PARA-INFLUENZA VIRUSES

Four serotypes are distinguished on the basis of soluble antigen composition. The types show some sharing of envelope antigens. No single envelope antigen is, however, common to all four types. The haemagglutinins are best demonstrated with guinea-pig cells incubated at 37° C. For primary isolation, monkey kidney tissue cultures have given best results. Only type 2 produces a well-marked cytopathogenic effect in monkey kidney but a para-influenza virus is readily recognized by the use of the haemadsorption technique.

The para-influenza viruses have been isolated mainly from mild upper respiratory tract infections in children. Not infrequently, however, they invade the lower respiratory tract where they produce a laryngotracheobronchitis (croup) and very occasionally a bronchopneumonia. Types 1 and 3 have been found to produce cold-like illnesses in human volunteers but whether, and to what extent, they contribute to the total incidence of colds has still to be determined. Similar but antigenically distinct viruses have been isolated from animal sources. The Sendai virus which antigenically resembles type 1, was isolated in Japan from pigs and mice, and viruses resembling type 3 have been isolated from a respiratory infection—shipping fever—in cattle assembled for transport. Viruses similar to type 2 have been isolated from monkeys.

THE MUMPS VIRUS

The mumps virus is serologically homogeneous but shares minor surface antigens with some of the para-influenza viruses. It is completely distinct from the influenza viruses in both V and S antigen content. Like the para-influenza viruses, it possesses a haemolysin which appears to act on the same cell receptors as the receptor-destroying enzyme from which, however, the haemolysin appears to be distinct. The enzymic activity of the mumps virus is appreciably less than that of the influenza virus. After elution at 37° C there still remains a considerable amount of irreversibly bound virus, which is insufficient to cause significant agglutination of the red cells but whose presence can be detected by the occurrence of haemagglutination when the cells are exposed to antiviral serum.

Mumps

Parotitis or inflammation of the parotid gland is the most frequent manifestation of infection with the mumps virus; in addition to the parotid, the sublingual and submaxillary glands are also occasionally involved. In about 20 per cent of infections in males of over 13 years there is an associated orchitis developing from about 4 to 7 days after the appearance of the parotitis. This may result in a pressure atrophy of the affected testis but leads to sterility only if, as only occasionally happens, the condition is bilateral. In the female an oophoritis may develop but this is a very much less frequent complication than is orchitis in the male. It is thought that these conditions may be the result of an auto-immune process triggered by the infection. Aseptic meningitis or meningoencephalitis may also occur as complications of mumps; occasionally they may be the only evidence of infection. In the United States and Britain the mumps virus appears to rank next to the enteroviruses as the most important single cause of aseptic meningitis. Serological evidence shows that the mumps virus frequently gives rise to latent infection. It has been estimated from such data that during the course of an epidemic about 40 per cent of infected persons are without obvious symptoms.

Mumps occurs mainly as an infection of the 5- to 15-year age group. The disease is followed by a high degree of immunity and second attacks are uncommon.

In mumps the virus is present in the saliva, from which it may be isolated just before and for a few days after the onset of parotitis. The virus has also been demonstrated in the saliva of persons who are latently infected and who are therefore of considerable importance in spreading the disease. The virus has been detected in the blood during the first few days of infection, and it is generally believed that involvement of the parotid gland as well as of the central nervous system, testis and ovary are the result of viraemic spread. This would be consistent with the long incubation period of 18 to 21 days.

Diagnosis

The laboratory is not usually called on for assistance in the diagnosis of mumps since the condition is usually quite obvious clinically. When laboratory assistance is required the virus may be isolated from the saliva by amniotic inoculation or in tissue culture. A convenient method of collecting saliva is by the insertion of cotton wool pledgets into the mouth. In cases of aseptic meningitis it may be possible to isolate the virus from the cerebrospinal fluid. Antibodies may be demonstrated by complement fixation or haemagglutination inhibition tests. Of these the complement fixation test is on the whole the more satisfactory. The antibody titre to both V and S antigens should be estimated. Antibody to the V antigen does not usually appear until some 8 or 9 days after infection but persists for a long time after recovery. Antibody to the S antigen is usually demonstrable in the first 2 or 3 days of the disease and declines rapidly after recovery. Where possible an attempt should be made to demonstrate a rising antibody titre, but the demonstration in the early stages of infection of a high S titre in the presence of a low V titre is virtually diagnostic. Serum amylase regularly increases during the course of mumps and its estimation may be of value in differential diagnosis.

In the course of mumps a delayed type of skin hypersensitivity develops which may be detected by the intracutaneous injection of an antigen prepared from infected allantoic fluid. The skin test has no value as a diagnostic test, as it usually does not become positive until some 3 to 4 weeks after the onset of the disease. It may, however, be used for the detection of immunity. The antigen involved has not been identified.

Prophylaxis

The administration of gamma globulin prepared from the serum of convalescents to contacts gives some degree of protection; it is claimed that if given early in the disease gamma globulin considerably diminishes the risk of the development of orchitis.

Immunization with an inactivated chick embryo vaccine appears to give considerable protection but has not been generally adopted as a prophylactic procedure. Some degree of immunity can also apparently be produced by the use of an attenuated vaccine sprayed intra-orally or, as practised by Russian workers, injected intradermally.

RESPIRATORY SYNCYTIAL VIRUS

Although it lacks haemagglutinating properties the respiratory syncytial virus (RSV) shows, on electron microscopy, the general morphology of the myxovirus group. Three distinct antigens are demonstrable in infected tissue culture fluids: (1) An antigen which stimulates the production of neutralizing antibody and which appears to be analogous to the envelope antigens of the influenza virus. (2) A soluble complement fixing antigen which does not stimulate the production of protective antibody, and which is presumed to be an internal component or nucleocapsid. (3) An antigen which appears to be lipoprotein in nature but which has not so far been identified as any particular component of the virus particle. Two serotypes differing in surface antigenic composition have been recognized. RSV shows no antigenic relationship to other myxoviruses.

The virus does not grow in the chick embryo but can be propagated in cultures of various human tissues and in monkey and bovine kidney. The cultures most used have been those of HeLa cells—particularly the Bristol line —and Hep 2 cells. In infected tissue cultures a characteristic cytopathogenic effect with marked syncytium formation is produced but the yield of virus is very poor. The virus is very unstable outside the body, and clinical material should be cultured as soon as possible.

RSV is particularly pathogenic for children, and has emerged as the single most important cause of serious respiratory infection in children of under 1 year of age. In Newcastle it was isolated by Gardiner et al. from approximately 60 per cent of serious respiratory infections of infants, and in a Bristol study 18 out of 21 viruses isolated from children of less than 5 months of age with respiratory infection were RSV. These findings confirm and extend the original observations of Chanock in the United States on the seriousness of RSV as a respiratory pathogen of childhood.

Prophylaxis by vaccination is still in an experimental stage. A vaccine producing appreciable antibody response has been prepared by formalin inactivation but its value has still to be assessed. Vaccination would be required most for very young children in whom, however, the immunological response to infection is poor due to the presence of maternal antibody. This may be expected to interfere seriously with the efficacy of vaccination at such an early age.

NEWCASTLE DISEASE VIRUS

This virus which possesses the influenza type A soluble antigen is responsible for a serious and widespread disease of fowl of considerable economic importance. It is occasionally a cause of infection in laboratory workers and in workers with poultry. In man the virus gains entry through the conjunctiva with the production of a conjunctivitis which in some cases is associated with signs of a systemic infection. The condition is a mild one and no fatalities have been reported.

THE MEASLES VIRUS

The measles virus is an RNA virus with the typical electron micrographic structure of the myxoviruses. It has haemagglutinating properties but only for monkey red cells. Unlike influenza virus, the virus does not elute from the agglutinated cells nor are the red cell receptors destroyed by RDE. Like most of the subgroup 2 myxoviruses it has haemolytic properties. Haemolysis appears to be due to spontaneously released fragments of the membrane of high lipid content. Although these fragments also haemagglutinate, the haemolysin and haemagglutinin appear to be distinct. Only one serological type of the virus is known. There is, however, some sharing of antigens with the rinderpest virus and with the virus of canine distemper.

The virus will grow, though rather slowly, in a variety of tissue cultures but isolation is usually difficult and has been most successful in primary cultures of human and monkey kidney. In infected cultures a cytopathogenic effect characterized by multinucleated giant cells and by syncytium formation is produced.

Measles

Measles is primarily an epidemic disease, the period of maximal incidence being from November to March. Major epidemics show a marked periodicity recurring regularly in urban communities at 2 to 3 yearly intervals, although in Nigeria, where the disease shows a high prevalence, annual epidemics are the rule. Epidemic periodicity appears to be due to the accumulation of susceptibles in the population since the last epidemic. This in turn is due to the combined effect of a natural waning of immunity and to the addition of susceptibles by

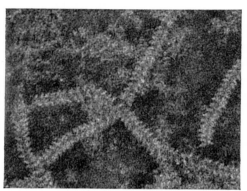

FIG. 56. INTERNAL COMPONENT OF MEASLES
VIRUS SHOWING HELICAL STRUCTURE
Electron micrograph. Negative stain (*Dr June D.
Almeida*)

births in the intervening period. When the proportion of susceptibles reaches a critical level conditions are suitable for epidemic spread. The virus is present in the respiratory secretions and in the urine prior to the development of the rash. It is during this period that infectivity is at a maximum. The main route of infection is almost certainly via the respiratory tract but there is some suggestion that the virus may also gain entry through the conjunctiva.

The disease has a long incubation period of 12 to 14 days. During this period the virus probably multiplies in some part of the respiratory tract from which it gains access to the blood stream. During this phase lymphatic glands through-out the body are invaded. Multiplication of virus in these could then be respon-sible for a secondary viraemia during the prodromal phase by which the virus eventually reaches the skin. The pathogenesis of the skin lesions is not fully understood. They are probably not due to multiplication of the virus but may be the result of damage inflicted by virus antibody complexes.

Children between the ages of 1 and 5 years are mainly affected. In the more severe cases there is evidence of extensive involvement of the respiratory tract with symptoms of laryngotracheitis, bronchitis or interstitial pneumonia. On rare occasions the disease assumes a severe haemorrhagic form with a high mortality rate. Secondary bacterial invasion, the most important manifestations of which are bronchopneumonia and otitis media, is found in about 5 per cent of cases. There is now convincing evidence that most, if not all cases of a rare, but invariably fatal disease of children—giant cell pneumonia—are caused by the measles virus. This condition has been found only in children who have been unable to develop antibodies to the virus; most reported cases having been in children with leukaemia. The absence of a rash in these cases supports the hypothesis that the measles rash is due to an antigen–antibody reaction.

In more highly developed countries mortality from measles has declined dramatically over the last 50 years. Hence, in Glasgow the mortality in children aged 1 to 5 years was, in 1908, approximately 5 per cent, but fell, in 1960, to about 0·2 per cent. In England and Wales, in general, mortality has been maximal in children of under 1 year. In West Africa, however, the disease showed, in the period 1958–61, a case mortality for all age groups of over 20 per cent—the highest mortality being in children of over 1 year. There is some epidemiological evidence that high mortality rates are associated with low nutritional status.

One attack of measles produces lifelong immunity. Consequently, in isolated communities, the disease tends to die out. When reintroduced into such populations it has been found to assume a very severe form with a high incidence and a high mortality in the adult population. The disastrous effect of measles on a virgin population was clearly shown in the 1875 epidemic in the Fiji Islands (Chapter 8), and more recently in a somewhat similar epidemic in Greenland.

The simplest diagnostic test for measles is the demonstration of multinucleated giant cells, known as Warthin-Finkeldey cells, in sputum and nasal secretions taken during the prodromal period. These cells, which may measure 100μ in diameter and contain up to 100 nuclei, are very similar to the multinucleated giant cells seen in infected tissue cultures; they appear to be derived from lymphoid tissues. Their demonstration may be of some diagnostic value. Isolation of the virus in tissue culture is not a practicable diagnostic procedure.

Prophylaxis

Measles can be partly or completely prevented by the administration of commercial gamma globulin prepared from pooled adult plasma. Children who have been fully protected will again become susceptible when their passive immunity wears off. On the other hand children who are partly protected and who develop a mild attack acquire an active immunity and will therefore be insusceptible to future infection. Complete protection is considered desirable only for the very young—under 1 year—or for debilitated children. It can be achieved only if gamma globulin is given within 5 days of contact, the amount required depending on the weight of the child. After the fifth day only attenuation is possible and little if any protection can be achieved by passive immunization after the ninth day.

The first attempts at active immunization against measles were with the attenuated Edmonston strain of virus developed, by Enders and his colleagues, by passage in tissue culture. Although this strain proved to be a highly efficient immunizing agent it was by itself unacceptable for general immunization because of the severity of the reactions it produced. Since then further attenuated variants have been developed but in general the greater the degree of attenuation the less effective is the virus as an immunizing agent. Some further attenuated variants have been derived, however, which appear to produce an acceptable degree of immunity. Thus the Schwarz variant of the Enders–Edmonston strain was found in a recent Medical Research Council trial to give a protection rate of approximately 85 per cent over a follow-up period of 6 months. Children who, in spite of vaccination, developed measles experienced only a mild form of the disease. The duration of the immunity produced by this vaccine has, however, still to be determined. If this were only for a short period immunization might simply defer an attack to an age at which it could be less readily withstood by the patient. Immunization with live attenuated vaccine is nevertheless now recommended by the British Ministry of Health for all children not previously protected, and ultimately when the majority of children have been protected it is envisaged that routine immunization should be carried out in the second year of life.

Killed vaccines have also been tried. They give rise to negligible immediate reactions but have proved to be poor immunizing agents, the antibody levels produced being low and transient. It has been suggested that killed vaccine might be inoculated as a preliminary to live vaccine in order to reduce the number and severity of the reactions produced by the latter, thereby permitting the use of a less attenuated, more highly immunogenic live strain. It has recently been reported from the U.S.A., however, that children who had been given repeated injections of killed vaccine developed severe local and systemic reactions on subsequent exposure to measles or following the injection of live vaccine. Under these circumstances combined immunization with killed and live vaccines cannot at the moment be recommended.

CHAPTER 37

THE HERPESVIRUSES

This is a group of moderately large ether-sensitive DNA viruses of apparently identical morphology. The important human pathogens are the herpes simplex virus, varicella-zoster virus and the cytomegalovirus.

HERPES SIMPLEX

In infected tissues and fluids the herpes simplex virus is found in two morphological forms, an enveloped form and a naked non-enveloped form, both of which appear to be infective. Enveloped forms are roughly spherical, measuring from 130 to 180 mμ in diameter. The envelope has a high content of lipid and has been shown to possess host cell antigens. Like the myxovirus envelope it is probably derived from the membrane of the host cell. The non-enveloped forms represent the naked viral nucleocapsid. The nucleocapsid possesses icosahedral symmetry and contains 162 capsomeres. The twelve apical capsomeres are pentagonal in outline, and the remainder, on the edges and faces of the icosahedron, are hexagonal. Many virus particles, both of enveloped and naked types, appear in electron micrographs to be empty. They are presumably incomplete or non-infective particles lacking DNA.

Although all strains of herpes simplex virus closely resemble one another antigenically and may therefore be regarded as belonging to a single antigenic type, minor antigenic differences are demonstrable between strains. In addition to antigens associated with the virus particle, a number of soluble antigens have been demonstrated in infected fluids by complement fixation and agar gel diffusion.

The herpesvirus is highly unstable and is rapidly inactivated on standing. It is susceptible to ether. This would be readily understandable if only the enveloped forms were infective. Since, however, the naked forms are also infective their ether sensitivity suggests that they contain some lipid as an integral component of the nucleocapsid.

The virus can be readily propagated on the chorioallantoic membrane of the chick embryo on which it produces small discrete pocks visible to the naked eye (Fig. 57). The rabbit is highly susceptible to the herpesvirus and can be infected by intradermal or by corneal inoculation. Suckling mice may be infected by both intracerebral and intraperitoneal inoculation but adult mice, as a rule, only by intracerebral inoculation. The virus grows in a variety of tissue cultures with the production of a cytopathogenic effect, the most characteristic feature of which are multinucleated giant cells which may form a syncytium.

Infected cells show characteristic intranuclear inclusions the development of which can be followed in preparations stained with haematoxylin and eosin. The inclusions are at first basophilic, rich in virus and have a high concentration of DNA; later they become acidophilic and at this stage are devoid both of DNA and of virus. The latter, which are known as Cowdray type A inclusions, fill most of the nucleus and appear to compress the nuclear chromatin into a peripheral ring. A clear area or halo is usually demonstrable between the inclusion body and the compressed chromatin; this appears to be a fixation artefact. Inclusions are also demonstrable in the cytoplasm after degeneration of the nucleus. Infected epidermal cells show in addition a characteristic ballooning degeneration.

By the time they reach adult life the majority of people have been infected with the herpesvirus. Antibody surveys show that infection is most frequent in

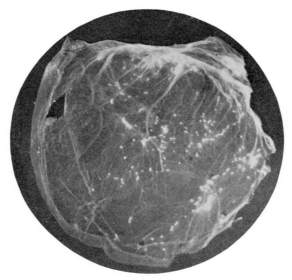

FIG 57. POCKS OF HERPES SIMPLEX VIRUS ON THE CHORIO-
ALLANTOIC MEMBRANE

the lower social groups. Primary infection usually occurs before the age of 5 years, and almost certainly through contact, e.g. in kissing, with virus present in the saliva of an infected person. It is probable that in most cases children are infected in this way by their mothers. Primary infection of adults who have escaped childhood infection is uncommon, possibly because of a greater resistance of adult epithelium to invasion by the virus. When primary infection occurs in the adult it appears to be quite often through a wound, e.g. of the fingers, with the formation of a herpetic whitlow or, in the female, through the genital tract, with the development of vesicles on the external genitalia.

The majority of primary infections are asymptomatic but in some cases primary infection may be quite severe. The commonest type of symptomatic primary infection is aphthous stomatitis, a condition in which there is an extensive eruption of vesicles in the buccal mucosa; the regional lymph glands are usually enlarged and fever is generally present. Kerato-conjunctivitis, vulvo-vaginitis and aseptic meningitis may also occur as primary herpetic infections. It seems probable that in most cases with involvement of the central nervous system the virus gains access by neuronal routes. Some cases of an uncommon but severe generalized skin disease known as Kaposi's varicelliform eruption are also caused by the herpes simplex virus. This condition occurs most frequently as a primary herpetic infection in children with eczema but involving the normal, as well as the eczematous, skin. In premature infants and in neo-nates born of mothers without circulating antibody the virus may, though rarely, produce a generalized infection with lesions in the viscera, particularly in the liver and the brain.

Following the primary infection the virus in many cases, possibly in all, assumes a latent form in which it persists in the tissues without the production of obvious lesions. In this state it is liable to be aroused into activity by a variety of debilitating factors. Persons latently infected are therefore liable to recurrent herpetic lesions. The commonest manifestation of recurrent herpes is the appearance of small vesicles at various mucocutaneous junctions particularly around the lips and nostrils. Vesicles may also appear on the genital mucosa, on the conjunctiva and cornea and in the mouth. One of the most effective precipitating factors in stimulating an attack of recurrent herpes is fever, hence the name 'fever blisters' formerly applied to herpetic vesicles occurring in the course of such bacterial infections as lobar pneumonia. Attacks are also commonly precipitated by exposure to sunlight.

The nature of the immunity in herpes is of some interest. Individuals who are subject to recurrent attacks nevertheless possess a considerable amount of antibody in their blood; they can also be experimentally infected by their own strain of virus. Under these circumstances the development of overt lesions is probably due to the fact that the virus can pass directly from one cell to another (p. 430), and thereby escape contact with antibody in the extracellular fluid.

Herpes provides the best example in man of a persistent latent viral infection. The precise relationship between the persisting virus and the infected cells is not understood. It is possible that the virus becomes integrated into the host cell genome in a manner analogous to prophage in lysogenic bacteria (p. 557), but no definite evidence has been obtained that this is the case. If it were so, environmental factors might interfere with the control exerted by the cell over virus multiplication, in a manner analogous to prophage induction.

The multiplication of the herpesvirus in tissue cultures can be inhibited by exposure of the culture to 5-iodo-2-deoxyuridine (p. 431). This compound has been found to have a considerable ameliorative effect on superficial herpetic infections, e.g. of the cornea, in experimental animals. In general, however, withdrawal of the drug results in renewed proliferation of the virus. The drug has been used in the treatment of human herpetic infections but initial reports of its value have not been adequately confirmed. A recent report of the effectiveness of an ultra-violet irradiated vaccine in cases of recurrent herpetic infection still requires evaluation.

Diagnosis

The diagnosis of recurrent herpes is mainly a clinical problem. Laboratory assistance is usually only required in the diagnosis of primary infections. The procedures principally used are: (1) The demonstration of giant cells and inclusion bodies in scrapings obtained from the base of the vesicles. (2) The direct demonstration of virus by electron microscopy. (3) The demonstration of viral antigen by the fluorescent antibody technique. An attempt may also be made to isolate the virus either from the lesions or from the throat, saliva or faeces. Antibodies are best demonstrated by the neutralization test. Because of the wide prevalence of herpetic infection the demonstration of a rising antibody titre is of particular importance.

'B' VIRUS

In morphology, growth characteristics and in antigenic structure, this virus closely resembles the herpes simplex virus. The most important distinguishing features are the failure of B virus to infect adult mice, and the fact that, though it stimulates antibodies against herpes simplex virus, it is not neutralized by herpes simplex antiserum. The virus is a natural parasite of monkeys in which it is the analogue of the herpes simplex virus. Human infection usually occurs as a result of a monkey bite but it has also been recorded after contamination of a wound from an infected monkey kidney tissue culture.

ZOSTER AND VARICELLA

Although presenting quite distinct clinical syndromes there is now conclusive evidence that zoster and varicella are caused by the same virus, the differences in the clinical and epidemiological features of the two conditions depending on host factors. The virus, which is known as the varicella-zoster virus, has been found to be morphologically identical with the virus of herpes simplex from which, however, it differs considerably in growth characteristics and in antigenic structure. The virus will grow on primary isolation in a variety of human and monkey tissue cultures. Its cytopathic effect consists of focal lesions much less marked than those of herpes simplex; these are characterized by cell rounding, formation of multinucleated giant cells and the occurrence in infected cells of intranuclear inclusions resembling those produced by the herpes simplex virus. In tissue cultures the virus appears to spread directly from cell to cell, and infective virus is not found free in the tissue culture fluid. The latter, however, contains large numbers of non-infective particles with a ragged appearance on electron microscopy. By contrast, large numbers of infective non-ragged particles are present in the vesicle fluid of human lesions.

So far, it has not been possible to prepare immune animal sera against any varicella-zoster viruses. Serological examination using human immune sera has, however, failed to reveal any difference between strains of virus from cases of zoster and those from cases of varicella. Although a number of antigens have been demonstrated in agar gel diffusion tests, all strains so far isolated have belonged to a single antigenic type.

Varicella or chickenpox is a mild febrile disease of childhood characterized by the presence of a generalized rash. Adults are occasionally infected, the disease being much more severe than in childhood. The rash is at first papular, later vesicular, the lesions finally drying up with the formation of crusts. The lesions, which are most marked on the trunk and face, tend to appear in successive crops; these features are of value in distinguishing varicella from mild smallpox. The histology of the skin lesions is very similar to that of herpes simplex, infected cells showing a ballooning degeneration and intranuclear inclusions which are at first basophilic later becoming acidophilic with accumulation at the base of the lesion of multinucleated giant cells. The mortality of the condition is extremely low except in the case of neonatal infections contracted from the mother in which it may be as high as 20 per cent. Varicella has a well marked seasonal incidence, epidemics occurring mainly in the winter and spring. It is a disease of very high infectivity. Infection is via the respiratory tract where initial multiplication of the virus probably occurs, and from which the virus is disseminated by the blood stream.

In contrast to varicella, zoster is a disease mainly of adults in which after a few days of fever a vesicular eruption appears in the area of distribution of one or more sensory nerves. The thoracic nerves and the ophthalmic division of the fifth cranial nerve are those most frequently involved. The condition is usually unilateral. The virus appears to multiply mainly in the posterior root ganglia from which it spreads centrally to the cord and peripherally along the nerve trunks to the skin. Occasionally the anterior horn cells of the cord are involved with the development of paralysis in the corresponding muscles. The disease shows no seasonal incidence and its frequency is not increased during varicella epidemics. No evidence has been obtained of direct transmission of zoster from one person to another.

The epidemiological evidence supporting the identity of the varicella and zoster viruses is considerable. Children experimentally infected with zoster fluid have been found to develop varicella; contacts of these children have also developed varicella, contacts of zoster cases frequently develop varicella. The incidence of varicella in contacts of zoster cases is, however, lower than it is in the contacts of varicella cases presumably because of the absence of virus from the respiratory and salivary secretions in zoster.

The differences in the clinical and epidemiological manifestations of varicella and zoster are believed to be due to differences in the immune status of the host. In non-immune persons the virus produces a generalized disease—varicella—because, in the absence of humoral antibody, it is able to spread widely throughout the body. In the immune on the other hand the virus is not able to spread widely and because of this produces zoster—a localized disease. It is possible that zoster resembles recurrent herpes in being due to the activation of a latent virus possibly maintained since primary childhood infection in the posterior root ganglia. Although there is no decisive evidence in support of this hypothesis the fact that a history of having had varicella in childhood can be elicited from most adults with zoster and the finding that in zoster antibody generally rises more rapidly and attains a higher level than in varicella—suggesting a secondary antibody response—make it plausible.

Microscopic examination of smears from the skin lesions in both zoster and varicella is of considerable diagnostic value. These show the presence of characteristic giant cells—Tzanck cells—with intranuclear inclusions. Similar cells are found in cases of herpes simplex but not in material from cases of smallpox or vaccinia. The identification of viral antigen in vesicle fluid by the complement fixation test, isolation of the virus by tissue culture and the demonstration of complement fixing antibodies in the patient's serum have also been used on a limited scale as diagnostic procedures.

CYTOMEGALOVIRUSES

Cytomegaloviruses are a group of viruses which, both in the intact animal and in tissue culture, give rise to infections, the characteristic feature of which is the presence of greatly enlarged cells with large nuclei containing prominent acidophilic inclusions. The inclusion fills most of the nucleus but is separated from the nuclear membrane by a clear well-defined halo. Acidophilic juxtanuclear cytoplasmic inclusions may also be present. Cytomegaloviruses have been isolated from a variety of animals, in all of which they have a particular predilection for the salivary glands. The strains isolated from different animal species possess a high degree of species specificity and grow, in culture, only in cells of the species which they naturally infect.

Cytomegaloviruses are classified in the herpesgroup on the basis of particle morphology, and the fact that, in the case of human strains, the nucleic acid has been identified as DNA. Electron micrographs show the nucleocapsid of the human virus to measure about 100 mµ in diameter and to contain 162 hollow capsomeres, many of the particles surrounded by a loose irregular envelope similar to that of the herpesvirus.

Cytomegaloviruses of human origin can be cultivated in tissue cultures of human fibroblasts and human muscle cells; they grow poorly in epithelial cell cultures. On primary isolation growth is slow, with the production of focal cytopathic lesions in which the virus, like that of zoster, is transmitted directly from cell to cell. Also like in zoster, the extracellular fluid contains mainly noninfective virus with a ragged appearance on electron microscopy. So far, antigenic analysis has been possible only with human sera, the results obtained indicating considerable sharing of antigens, with at the same time appreciable strain differences.

There is a fair amount of evidence indicating that in man infection with cytomegaloviruses is widespread: (1) The frequent recognition of enlarged cells with inclusions, resembling those known to be produced by cytomegaloviruses, at routine post-mortem examination, in the salivary glands of children who have died from a variety of causes. (2) The presence of complement fixing antibodies in a high proportion of adult human sera. In a recent study in the London area the proportion of positive sera ranged from 4 per cent, in the 6-month to 5-year age group, to 54 per cent in the 35- to 75-year age group. The precise nature of the latent infections responsible for these findings is not known but many are presumably infections of salivary glands. (3) Isolation studies indicate that from 1 to 2 per cent of children actively excrete the virus in the saliva and/or urine.

The results of infection depend on age. In new-born infants it gives rise to a severe and usually fatal generalized disease with symptoms referable particularly to involvement of the haemopoietic tissues. This type of infection clinically

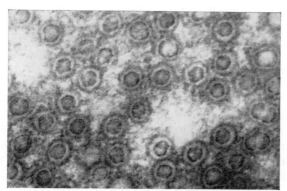

FIG. 58. CYTOMEGALOVIRUS, INTRANUCLEAR FORM (*Dr T. H. Flewett*)

resembles erythroblastosis foetalis and presents like the latter, at post mortem, evidence of extensive extramedullary erythropoiesis. Since in these cases virus has been isolated from the placenta and from the urine of the mother it seems likely that the infection is contracted in utero. In older children and adults generalized infection is infrequent and appears to occur only in the presence of some debilitating factor. Under these conditions the symptoms depend on the organ primarily involved—usually the intestine, liver, kidney, lungs or brain. Recent evidence suggests that cytomegaloviruses may be significant causes of hepatomegaly in older children and of infectious mononucleosis not associated with a positive Paul–Bunnell reaction in adults.

A diagnosis of cytomegalic inclusion body disease is most simply made by the demonstration, in urine and saliva, of the characteristic enlarged cells with intranuclear inclusion bodies. Where possible, the virus should, however, be isolated by tissue culture. The development of antibody may be demonstrated by the complement fixation test.

CHAPTER 38

HEPATITIS

Two types of viral hepatitis—infective hepatitis and serum hepatitis—are distinguished, each with different modes of infection and apparently due to different viruses. In both conditions recovery is usual, but in a small proportion of cases the process develops into an acute yellow atrophy which is almost invariably fatal. In a few cases hepatitis results in permanent damage to the liver which leads ultimately to cirrhosis.

There have been a number of reports of the isolation of hepatitis viruses from the blood of infected persons, in tissue cultures and in experimental animals. The most suggestive of these has been of the isolation of some strains of infective hepatitis virus in tissue cultures of the Detroit 6 line of cells, in which it is claimed that, under appropriate conditions, a characteristic cytopathogenic effect is produced. The significance of these observations remains to be determined. It is, however, evident that both infective and serum hepatitis are caused by infective agents presumed to be viruses since they can be transmitted experimentally to human volunteers. From the limited experimental data, it has been estimated, on the basis of ultra-filtration studies, that the serum hepatitis virus is a small virus measuring not more than 25 mμ in diameter. The size of the infective hepatitis virus has not been determined.

Both viruses appear to be highly resistant to both physical and chemical disinfection, the serum hepatitis virus being capable of withstanding exposure to 60° C for several hours.

Because of the lack of a laboratory method for propagating hepatitis viruses, there are no specific diagnostic tests. A variety of biochemical liver function tests are employed clinically, however, to indicate the extent of liver involvement. Of these the most sensitive is the estimation of serum glutamic oxaloacetic transaminase (SGOT) activity; the levels of this enzyme have been found to be elevated in the pre-icteric phase of the infection.

Evidence supporting the antigenic distinctness of the two viruses has been obtained from cross-infection experiments in human volunteers. Patients who have recovered from infective hepatitis appear to have acquired substantial immunity to infective hepatitis but to be fully susceptible to serum jaundice. Conversely, though in this case the evidence is less clear-cut, patients recovered from serum jaundice appear to have developed a homologous immunity, yet remain fully susceptible to infectious hepatitis. The nature of the immunity which follows serum jaundice, however, requires further assessment.

A number of viruses capable of causing hepatitis in animals have been described; these appear to have no relationship to those infecting man.

INFECTIVE HEPATITIS

(Catarrhal Jaundice)

This condition is endemic in most countries, occurring mainly in sporadic and occasionally in epidemic form. Epidemics were particularly numerous in service personnel during World War II. Normally the maximal incidence is between the ages of 5 and 15 years. During epidemics many non-icteric infections occur—particularly in the very young. The incubation period is from 15 to 40 days. In icteric cases jaundice usually appears after a febrile period of 5 to 7 days, but occasionally this pre-icteric phase may be as long as three weeks. Infective hepatitis is usually much more severe in the adult than in the child.

The virus is present in the blood and faeces of cases in which it has been demonstrated during both the incubation period and the acute phase of the disease. A carrier state may persist for some months after infection, and the disease can be transmitted to volunteers by inoculation or by oral administration of serum or stool ultra-filtrates. The virus has not been recognized in the nasopharynx or in throat washings. Epidemiological evidence on the whole supports the view that the disease is spread mainly by the intestinal route but the possibility of droplet transmission cannot be ruled out, particularly in view of the fact that, in temperate climates, the disease is most prevalent in the winter and autumn.

Epidemiologically, infective hepatitis shows considerable resemblance to poliomyelitis: (1) Its primary impact is in childhood. (2) Subclinical infection is frequent. (3) It shows a predominant incidence in the summer and autumn. (4) Transmission of the disease is mainly a result of close contact. Extensive involvement of children in the same institution or of the same family is usual.

Large-scale epidemics initiated by contaminated water and food have been described, e.g. the water-borne epidemic in Delhi of 1955–56, but these are uncommon. In this context the considerable resistance of the virus to chlorine disinfection is of importance.

A high proportion of sera from cases of infective hepatitis contain agglutinins for the red cells of day-old chicks and of rhesus monkeys. Since, however, agglutinins for chick and rhesus red cells are occasionally present in the sera of normal individuals the diagnostic value of these reactions is limited.

Pooled normal gamma globulin has considerable value as a prophylactic. As in the case of poliomyelitis it apparently does not prevent alimentary infection but does prevent the development of jaundice. Complete resistance to infection has been found up to 3 months after the administration of gamma globulin, and in some cases for considerably longer, possibly because it has permitted the development of latent immunizing infections.

SERUM HEPATITIS

(Homologous Serum Jaundice)

This type of hepatitis is an entirely artificial disease. The virus is present in the plasma of a small number of healthy persons and the disease may occur following the injection of whole blood, serum or plasma from such subjects. The condition rarely occurs after the administration of gamma globulin. The incidence of hepatitis following the transfusion of whole blood appears to be somewhat less than 1 per cent; this figure indicates that probably at least 1 per cent of people carry the virus. The concentration of virus in icterogenic plasma is extremely high and one estimate has supplied a figure of 10^6 infective doses per ml.

At one time hepatitis was of frequent occurrence in patients attending venereal disease and other injection clinics, as a result of the use of the same syringe, although with a different needle, for the injection of a number of patients. In these circumstances, a small amount of tissue fluid inevitably finds its way into the syringe from one individual and is then inadvertently introduced into the next individual to be injected. In the era of disposable syringes such infections should no longer occur. An unusual, though important, mode of infection is in tattooing.

Serum jaundice may occur at any age, but there is evidence that adults are more susceptible than children. In contrast to infective hepatitis, serum jaundice has an insidious onset and is usually afebrile. The incubation period is much longer than that of infective hepatitis, generally being from 40 to 150 days. Incubation periods of more than 40 days have however been observed following the experimental transmission of infective hepatitis by inoculation. Consequently, the difference in the incubation periods of the two types of hepatitis may be due to the different routes of infection rather than to any intrinsic differences in the properties of the viruses.

The virus of serum jaundice is present in the blood of patients, but has not so far been identified in faeces. Oral administration of blood known to contain the virus has failed to produce the disease and contacts of serum jaundice cases do not become overtly infected. These findings provide further grounds for believing that the virus of serum jaundice is distinct from that of infective hepatitis.

Although serum jaundice is an artificially produced condition the virus must nevertheless be transmitted from one person to another by some natural route. This has been suggested by a number of reported incidents of the development of hepatitis in contacts of serum jaundice cases. Contact infection of this sort is not, however, a normal occurrence. Another possible route of natural infection is through the placenta, and a case has been described in which this appeared to have occurred. Following placental transmission the patient might develop a state of immunological tolerance and might, because of this, carry the virus for life. Some such explanation is clearly required for the persistence of the virus in the blood of carriers. Alternatively, it is possible that the virus may persist in a form which cannot be neutralized by antibody. Thus it might be present as an infectious nucleic acid.

Prophylaxis

The incidence of hepatitis following transfusion of plasma or serum can be reduced by using plasma or serum pools derived from a small number of donors —the smaller the pool the less is the chance that one of the donors is a carrier of the virus. In one investigation it was found that 11·9 per cent of individuals receiving plasma pooled from a large number of donors developed hepatitis, whereas only 1·26 per cent of those receiving plasma from pools derived from not more than ten donors became infected. It is of particular importance that subjects with a history of jaundice should not be accepted as blood donors.

There is evidence that the virus can be inactivated by ultra-violet irradiation and by exposure to β-propiolactone and sulphur mustard and that it dies out on storage at 27 to 29° C for some months. So far, however, a reliable method of treating plasma and serum to ensure inactivation of the virus has not been devised. Consequently in passive immunization against virus infections, gamma globulin preparations, which have not so far been observed to produce serum jaundice, should be used in preference to serum. Normal gamma globulin is of no value in the prophylaxis of serum jaundice. It has recently been suggested, however, that some protection may be afforded by immune globulin obtained from the sera of recently recovered cases. The value of this procedure has still to be determined. It would, however, because of the scarcity of convalescent immune serum, be clearly impossible of wide application.

CHAPTER 39

MISCELLANEOUS VIRUSES

THE ADENOVIRUSES

Adenoviruses are a group of ether-resistant, non-enveloped viruses possessing classical icosahedral symmetry. They were first recognized by Rowe et al. in 1953 in tissue cultures of human adenoids and tonsils undergoing spontaneous degeneration and in which they were producing latent infection. They were subsequently independently isolated by Hilleman and Werner from cases of upper respiratory tract infection. Similar viruses have since been isolated from monkeys, cattle, dogs, mice and birds. Twenty-eight serotypes distinguishable by neutralization tests have been recognized amongst strains derived from human sources. All the types possess a common complement fixing antigen. The group antigen is also present in adenoviruses derived from simian, bovine and canine sources.

In purified preparations the adenoviruses appear as regular icosahedra measuring from 70 to 80 mμ in diameter. The capsid is made up of 252 capsomeres. On disruption of the virus the capsomeres appear as tubular structures with a central hole. The apical capsomeres of types 3 and 5 show, in electron micrographs, attached knob-like (type 3) or thread-like (type 5) structures. Since purified viral haemagglutinin contains only capsomeres of this apical type, the haemagglutinin is presumed to be identical with the thread-like or knob-like structure. Purified preparations of tubular capsomeres, and of fibres, have been prepared from type 5 virus by column chromatography. Group complement reactivity has been found to be associated with the tubular capsomeres, and type specificity with the fibres. Although showing a high degree of cross reactivity, group antigens from different adenoviruses nevertheless show individual antigenic characteristics.

Except for types 12 and 18, all adenovirus serotypes possess haemagglutinins for rat and/or rhesus monkey red cells. Some types, in addition, agglutinate human group O red cells. The viruses do not elute from red cells, and the nature of the virus receptor is not known. Attachment of virus to red cells is prevented by type-specific antibody. Haemagglutination inhibition techniques therefore can be used for the estimation of type-specific antibody and for the determination of the antigenic type of an unknown strain.

Adenoviruses will grow in a variety of tissue cultures, but growth is best in continuous cell lines, e.g. HeLa, of human epithelial origin. They multiply in the nuclei of infected cells in which basophilic inclusion bodies can be demonstrated by conventional staining procedures. With certain serotypes—3, 4, 7 and 8—the intranuclear virus aggregates in the form of a crystal. The evolution of the nuclear changes in cells infected with these serotypes has been found to be recognizably different from those occurring in cells infected with types 1, 2, 5 and 6, which do not produce crystals and which, in HeLa cells, exhibit a longer eclipse phase before the appearance of virus. Except for the oncogenic serotypes, adenoviruses are not pathogenic for laboratory animals, though they may give rise under certain conditions to latent infection. In suckling rats and hamsters a number of serotypes of which types 12, 18 and 21 are the most active are oncogenic and can induce the production of sarcomata (p. 529).

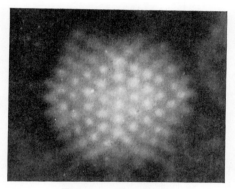

FIG. 59. ADENOVIRUS
Negative staining with phosphotungstate.
Arrangement of capsomeres in triangles is
clearly seen (*Horne* et. al., J. molec. Biol.)

There have been a number of reports of the occurrence in tissues infected with adenoviruses of virus-like DNA-containing particles, of about 20 mμ in diameter. The particles are defective in that they cannot replicate by themselves, but multiplication occurs when the cells are also infected with a 'helper' adenovirus. In this respect they resemble the small tobacco necrosis virus (p. 417) and the Rous sarcoma virus (p. 529). So far no role in pathogenicity has been identified for these particles to which the name adenosatellite virus has been applied.

Antibodies to many adenovirus types are widely prevalent in adult human sera. Adenovirus infection must therefore be of frequent occurrence. Some of the types are capable of causing latent infections, particularly of children; others tend to be associated with specific disease syndromes of which the most frequent is some type of mild upper respiratory tract infection. This may be a simple pharyngitis or a febrile influenza-like illness usually lasting 3 to 4 days and, often, with well-marked constitutional symptoms. Respiratory infection may be associated with conjunctivitis, as in pharyngoconjunctival fever, or conjunctivitis may on occasion be the only symptom of infection. In rare cases, the virus produces a pneumonia resembling PAP but without cold agglutinins. The sero-types particularly involved in these infections are 3, 4, 7 and 14. Latent in-fection of tonsils and adenoids in children are mainly caused by types 1, 2 and 5. Type 8 is uniquely involved in the production of epidemic kerato-conjunctivitis. There is evidence suggesting that adenoviruses of a variety of serotypes can cause mesenteric lymphadenitis, and that this condition may in turn be the precipitating cause of an intussusception. The pathogenicity for man of a number of adenovirus types, notably types 11, 12, 13, 15, 16, 17, 18 is still in doubt.

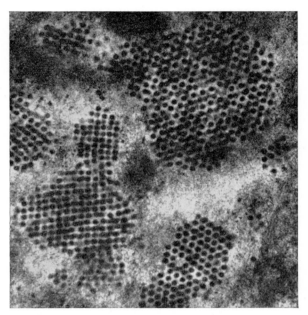

FIG. 60. INTRANUCLEAR CRYSTALS OF ADENOVIRUS TYPE 8
(*Dr T. H. Flewett*)

Inactivated vaccines have been prepared from some of the antigenic types—3, 4 and 7—but are still in the experimental stage.

Diagnosis may be achieved by isolation of the virus from throat swabs, conjunctival swabs or faeces or by the demonstration of a rising titre of anti-body in the complement fixation test against the group antigen. If a strain of adenovirus is isolated from a case its aetiological role can be confirmed by demonstrating a rise in neutralizing antibody titre against it.

REOVIRUSES

Reoviruses were first classified as ECHO virus type 10 but have now been assigned to a distinct group. They are considerably larger than picornaviruses—with a diameter of 60 to 75 mμ. They are non-enveloped RNA viruses possessing icosahedral symmetry; the capsid contains 92 capsomeres. The nucleic acid of the viruses is unusual in being a double-stranded RNA.

Three serotypes are demonstrable by neutralization tests, the types sharing a common complement fixing antigen. Reoviruses have the property of agglutinating human red cells, the red cell receptors being destroyed by periodate but not by RDE. In addition, type 3 strains are capable of agglutinating bovine cells.

Reoviruses will grow in tissue cultures of a variety of human and animal cells. They produce a cytopathogenic effect which is recognizably distinct from that of the enteroviruses. Suckling mice and a variety of laboratory animals can be infected, but infection is often asymptomatic. Reoviruses have a wide host range, and have been isolated not only from man but also from a variety of animal hosts. Most human isolations have been from the faeces but the viruses have also been recovered from the throat. In man they have been found in association with both respiratory disease and gastro-intestinal disease—hence their name. They can, however, be isolated from apparently normal individuals. Their precise pathogenic role is still far from clear.

RUBELLA

The virus of rubella was first isolated by Weller and Neva, in 1962, by the inoculation of blood and urine of rubella patients into tissue cultures of primary human amnion. On passage of the virus, though not on primary isolation, a cytopathogenic effect characterized by the development of focal areas of degeneration, and involving only a limited number of cells in the culture, was observed after 17 to 21 days' incubation. Affected cells showed nuclear disruption and acidophilic cytoplasmic inclusions. A similar cytopathogenic effect, but without the development of inclusion bodies, was found by McCarthy et al. in rabbit kidney and human thyroid tissue cultures. The virus will grow in grivet, patas and rhesus monkey kidney but without the production of a demonstrable cytopathogenic effect. Under these conditions its presence may however be demonstrated by showing the culture is protected from infection with another potentially cytopathogenic virus. The demonstration of interference in an appropriate tissue culture has proved to be a much more satisfactory method for isolating the virus than by the demonstration of a cytopathogenic effect. For this purpose, grivet monkey kidney—for isolation, with challenge by ECHO type 11 have been most used. The rubella virus cannot be propagated in the chick embryo or in suckling mice.

Filtration data indicate a diameter in the range of 50 to 150 mμ but the precise size of the virus has still to be determined. It is ether sensitive, and as its growth in tissue culture is not inhibited by bromo- or fluoro-deoxyuridine, it is presumed to be an RNA virus—probably enveloped. Its resemblance to the myxoviruses is further supported by its reported susceptibility in tissue culture to inhibition by amantadine (p. 431). The virus has not so far been shown to possess a haemagglutinin and satisfactory electron micrographs have still to be produced. Because of the long-lasting and solid immunity which follows infection there is probably only one serological type.

In contrast to measles, rubella is characteristically a disease of the older child and young adult. When it occurs in postnatal life the disease is a mild one. If, however, a mother is infected during the first 4 months of pregnancy the foetus may develop a severe systemic infection resulting in death or, if it survives, in congenital defect. The most important defects observed are deaf mutism, congenital heart disease, cataract, mental retardation and microcephaly. The association between maternal rubella and congenital defect in the foetus was first observed by Gregg in Australia in 1941. Gregg's survey was a retrospective one, and estimated the hazard for the birth of a child with a congenital defect to a mother contracting rubella in the first 4 months of pregnancy at 70 per cent. Prospective surveys in which the diagnosis can be much more accurately determined, however, have given somewhat lower figures. In a survey carried out by the British Ministry of Health, covering the period 1950–52, of 279 pregnancies in women who had contracted rubella in the first 16 weeks of pregnancy, 11 aborted, 11 gave birth to stillborn children and 16 of the children born alive died before the age of 2 years. These figures represent a total foetal loss of 7·3 per cent. Of the remainder, 37 showed major congenital anomaly and 37 a minor anomaly, giving an overall figure for death or some degree of congenital defect of 40 per cent.

In general, the more severe congenital defects have been found in women infected in the first 6 weeks of pregnancy. A high incidence of congenital defect was found by Coffey and Jessop in women who had been in contact with cases of rubella but who had not actually developed the disease, indicating that the foetus may be exposed as a result of asymptomatic infection of the mother. In the severe epidemic of rubella that affected the United States in 1964 many cases were described in which congenital rubella infection resulted in a severe systemic disease which showed, in addition to previously recognized defects, splenomegaly, pneumonitis, hepatitis and bone involvement.

Virus can be isolated from throat swabs or nasopharyngeal washings of the great majority of children showing the congenital rubella syndrome. In some cases of congenital infection, excretion of the virus has been found to continue up to the age of 6 months. Such children are therefore an important community source of infection. Excretion of virus has also been found in normal children born of mothers who had contracted rubella in early pregnancy. In the development of foetal rubella there is evidence that infection of the foetus is associated with infection of the placenta, which may therefore be the primary site of multiplication of the virus in the foetus.

Immunological tolerance does not develop as a result of foetal rubella infection. There is in fact considerable evidence that infected children can produce antibodies against the virus in utero. This is shown by the fact that (a) they frequently have a serum antibody titre which is higher than that of the mother, and (b) a considerable amount of the antibody is mercapto-ethanol sensitive, and is therefore of the IgM type, which is not transmitted across the placenta from the maternal to the foetal circulation. Why there should be a persistent excretion of virus in the presence of a high antibody titre is not known nor why some infected children escape with minimal damage while in others the damage is severe, nor why foetal damage is restricted to infection in the first four months of pregnancy.

Rubella infection in postnatal life is believed to occur via the respiratory secretions. The virus can be isolated from nasopharyngeal washings and throat swabs from about a week before to a week after the appearance of the rash. The virus can also be demonstrated in the urine and faeces; these may be important sources of infection in infants with the congenital rubella syndrome. The primary site of multiplication is presumed to be in the respiratory tract. Dissemination is clearly by the blood stream, a viraemia being demonstrable before the development of the rash. The incubation period under the conditions of natural infection is from 12 to 23 days, but epidemiological, virological and immunological studies suggest that latent infection occurs with about the same frequency as overt infection.

Laboratory diagnosis is not normally required for the individual case of postnatal rubella. Nevertheless the identification of an outbreak of rubella is desirable so that adequate prophylactic measures to protect pregnant women exposed to infection can be undertaken. For the isolation of the virus most success has been achieved in tissue cultures of grivet monkey kidney. Antibody is usually demonstrated by neutralization tests. Complement fixation tests, utilizing a soluble complement fixing antigen which is demonstrable in infected tissue cultures, have also been employed but, so far, only on a limited scale. The precise relationship of the complement fixing antigen, which appears to be a protein, to the virus particle has not been determined. Immunofluorescence, using infected tissue culture cells as antigen, has also been used for antibody detection.

In view of the association of congenital defect with rubella in pregnancy it is generally considered advisable to ensure that all girls should have been exposed to rubella before they reach the child-bearing age. To achieve this some workers have deliberately infected girls by instillation of infective nasopharyngeal washings. Gamma globulin is reported to be of value in preventing the development of rubella in contacts. Whether a suppressive effect on the development of clinical rubella in pregnant women who have been in contact with the disease is sufficient to prevent transmission to the foetus is not yet known. So far, however, it is the only prophylaxis available but experimental work on a live attenuated vaccine is currently in progress.

GLANDULAR FEVER

(Infectious Mononucleosis)

This is a relatively mild febrile disease which occurs mainly in childhood—usually in sporadic form. The characteristic features of the disease are glandular enlargement and large numbers of abnormal mononuclear-type cells in the peripheral blood. In exceptional cases the infection may involve the central nervous system, producing the symptoms of aseptic meningitis or, in severe cases, encephalitis.

There is suggestive but by no means conclusive evidence that glandular fever is due to a virus in the reported transmission of the condition to human volunteers and in the production of symptoms, resembling those found in man, in monkeys inoculated with blood and throat washings from patients. A possible relationship with group II myxoviruses is suggested by the observation that the sera of patients may possess agglutinins for red cells to which Newcastle disease virus has adsorbed. Recent work suggests the possibility that some cases of infectious mononucleosis in adults may be due to a cytomegalovirus (p. 515).

The sera of most patients suffering from infectious mononucleosis show a high titre of agglutinins for sheep red cells, and the demonstration of this antibody in the Paul–Bunnell test is of considerable diagnostic value. This antibody must be distinguished from the species antibody for sheep cells present in normal human serum. The latter is rarely present in a titre as high as 1 in 80 (using 2 per cent red cells), which can be accepted as the diagnostic level for infectious mononucleosis. A high titre of antibody for sheep red cells may also be found following the injection of horse serum. The three antibodies are heterophile antibodies (Chapter 6), but have distinct serological specificities and may be distinguished by absorption tests. The normal serum antibody is removed by absorption with guinea-pig kidney, the antibody produced following the injection of horse serum is removed both by guinea-pig kidney and ox red cells, while the infectious mononucleosis antibody is removed only by ox red cells.

VIRUSES AND TUMOURS

A number of viruses are capable of producing tumours in experimental animals and, in certain cases, of inducing a malignant transformation of primary or secondary tissue culture cells in vitro. The RNA tumour-producing (oncogenic) viruses include the avian leucosis group—to which the Rous sarcoma virus belongs, the murine leucosis group and, probably, the mouse mammary cancer (Bittner) agent. The DNA viruses include the polyoma, SV 40 and papilloma viruses (including the rabbit papilloma and human wart viruses)—these are known collectively as papovaviruses—and various oncogenic adenovirus serotypes.

In many cases virus-induced tumours carry new antigens not present in the corresponding normal tissue cells. Two types of such antigen are described. *1*. Intracellular antigens—in the case of the papovaviruses these antigens are formed in the nuclei—demonstrable by complement fixation tests. These antigens are virus-specific in that they are present in all cells transformed by the same virus and the antigens produced in response to any one oncogenic virus are distinct from the antigens of cells transformed by other such viruses. The new antigens, which are known as T antigens, are distinct from any antigens which have been identified as components of the virus particle and they persist in transformed cells which no longer produce infectious virus. *2*. Antigens which occur as components of the surfaces of transformed cells. These were demonstrated in the first place by transplantation tests as histocompatibility antigens, but in some cases have been visualized by the fluorescent antibody technique.

The nature of the change which occurs in cells transformed by oncogenic viruses is not known but it is probably some alteration in the surface character of the cell which results in the loss of normal contact inhibition. The change may be related to the presence of the new surface antigens referred to above.

PAPOVAVIRUSES

This name is applied to a group of small, non-enveloped DNA viruses, 45 to 55 mµ in diameter, possessing icosahedral symmetry. The capsids of the more intensively studied members of the group have been shown to contain 42 capsomeres. They multiply in the nuclei of infected cells, and crystal formation is frequent. The group comprises the polyoma virus, the papilloma viruses of rabbits and of man and simian virus (SV) 40. These viruses differ antigenically and in growth properties but share the capacity of inducing tumours in susceptible animals. They are exceptional amongst the animal viruses in possessing a circular chromosome, resembling in this respect the bacteria and bacterophages.

The Polyoma Virus

This virus, which, of the group, has received most attention, was isolated from the tissues of leukaemic mice. It is apparently a natural parasite of wild mice which excrete it in the saliva and urine, but without showing any evidence of clinical disease. The disease is imported into laboratory stocks of mice by contaminated grain. The virus can be propagated in mouse embryo tissue culture in which it produces a cytopathogenic effect. It possesses a haemagglutinin as an integral component of the virus particle. The haemagglutinin appears to combine with the same red cell receptors as the myxovirus haemagglutinins. Unlike the myxoviruses, however, the polyoma virus does not possess a receptor-destroying enzyme.

Tumours are most readily produced in young animals. In mice the commonest tumours are cancer of the parotids and of the breast. In rats, hamsters and ferrets the virus produces sarcomata. Malignant transformation can also be demonstrated in cells that have survived the cytopathogenic effect of the virus in tissue culture. The transformed cells appear triangular in form, assume a random arrangement in irregular masses—instead of forming cell sheets—as a result of loss of normal contact relationships, and show a high rate of glycolysis. Infective virus cannot be isolated from transformed cells, and since the cells can be reinfected with fresh virus, the virus initially present appears to have been lost. The persistence of virus is therefore not necessary for the perpetuation of the malignant change. In tissue culture only about 3 per cent of cells are transformable by polyoma virus and these can be transformed not only by intact virus but also by viral DNA. The transformation, clearly, is not due to the selection of spontaneous mutants since these have not been demonstrated by cloning experiments. The polyoma virus has been of great interest by providing a possible model for the development of malignancy in man. The mechanism by which it induces malignant transformation is, however, not known.

Recently evidence has been obtained that some portion of the viral genome persists in transformed cells from which no infectious virus can be isolated. Thus Benjamin has found that some of the RNA of polyoma transformed cells will hybridize with viral DNA and is therefore presumably virus specific and transcribed from persisting viral genome in the transformed cell. The persistence of some of the viral genome would explain the continued production of viral antigen in transformed but non-virus producing cells. It is possible in fact that the new antigens are enzymes coded for by the viral genome and required by the virus in the early stages of virus synthesis.

Papilloma Viruses

The rabbit papilloma virus has been extensively studied, particularly by Shope, who was responsible for its isolation in 1933. The virus is readily recoverable from the papillomata of wild rabbits but only infrequently from the papillomata of domestic rabbits. Infectious nucleic acid, however, can be recovered from the latter, and the infected cells continue to synthesize a viral antigen. The papillomata readily undergo malignant change. This change may, as in the case of polyoma induced tumours, be associated with the disappearance of infective virus.

SV 40

Simian virus 40 was first isolated as a contaminant of rhesus and cynomolgus monkey kidney tissue cultures in which it produces a latent infection. In vervet monkey kidney tissue cultures it causes a destructive lesion with marked vacuolization of the cytoplasm, to which it owes its name of simian vacuolating virus. On inoculation into suckling hamsters it produces sarcomata, and, as in the case of polyoma virus, the persistence of virus is not necessary for continued malignancy.

SV 40 has considerable practical importance because of its presence in monkey kidney tissue cultures used for the preparation of poliomyelitis vaccine. It has been found as a contaminant of live polio vaccine and, since it may resist formaldehyde inactivation, has been found also in inactivated polio vaccine. It is capable of multiplying in the human subject and of stimulating the production of antibodies. So far, however, there is no evidence that it can produce neoplastic proliferation in man, but it is conceivable that it might do so after a prolonged incubation period. Because of this hazard it is essential that monkey kidney tissue cultures used for the preparation of poliovirus vaccine should be completely free of SV 40.

Human Warts

That the common wart—*verruca vulgaris*—is due to a virus is rendered very probable by the occurrence of intranuclear inclusions and virus crystals in infected cells, and by the fact that warts can be transmitted experimentally to human volunteers. The virus is provisionally classified with the papovaviruses. It has a high degree of host specificity and the reported isolation of a common wart virus in monkey kidney tissue cultures has still to be confirmed. The condition appears to have a very long incubation period, and susceptibility to infection appears to depend to some extent on psychological factors.

OTHER ONCOGENIC VIRUSES

A number of RNA-containing viruses are known which have the capacity of inducing tumours in a variety of experimental animals. They include the Rous sarcoma virus and the viruses of avian and mouse leukaemias. The Rous sarcoma virus has been particularly studied. In contrast to the papovaviruses infectious virus continues to be produced by most transformed cells. The Bryan strain of Rous sarcoma virus is unusual in that, although capable of initiating malignant transformation, it cannot by itself produce infective progeny. This it can only do in association with a helper virus known as Rous associated virus (RAV).

Adenoviruses

As a result of routine screening tests for oncogenic potentiality certain adeno-virus serotypes were found capable of producing malignant tumours in rats and hamsters. As with papovaviruses infective virus disappears from the trans-formed cells but virus-specific antigen continues to be produced. Hybridization of adenovirus type 7 with SV 40 has been described, the hybrids possessing adenovirus type 7 capsids, but inducing the production in transformed cells of SV 40 type tumour antigen.

Burkitt Lymphoma

This condition, which is a malignant lymphoma, primarily of the jaw and, secondarily, of other tissues, is of wide distribution in Africa. Principally, it affects children, 87 per cent of the cases being aged from 3 to 12 years. Its geographical distribution closely parallels that of *Glossina* mosquitoes. Because of this it has been proposed by Burkitt that the condition may be due to infection with an arthropod-borne virus. That there may be an infective factor in its causation is suggested epidemiologically by the finding of tumour-free areas within the susceptible belt. Laboratory evidence suggesting a viral origin has been obtained by a number of workers who have found that cultured lympho-blasts from Burkitt lymphomas contained virus particles with a morphology very similar to those of a herpesvirus. Immunofluorescent studies, however, have failed to reveal any antigenic relationship between these particles and the herpes simplex or varicella-zoster viruses. Further evidence of a viral aetiology is provided by the finding of Henle that infected cells possess a high resistance to vesicular stomatitis virus, which would point to the production of interferon. Henle has also demonstrated the presence, in lymphoma tissue culture fluids, of material with interferon-associated properties. Whether the virus is the cause of the condition has yet to be determined. It could be a passenger virus with a predilection for Burkitt lymphoma cells.

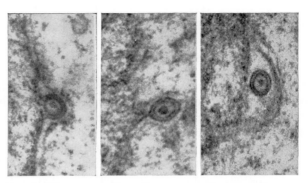

FIG. 61. HERPES-LIKE VIRUS PARTICLES IN CULTURED BURKITT TUMOUR CELLS

Photographs show passage of virus particle through nuclear membrane, acquiring an outer envelope as it goes (*Epstein et al.*, 1967, Brit. med. J.)

Spontaneous Human Cancers

Apart from the Burkitt lymphoma virus, no virus has so far been associated with any spontaneous human malignant state. A suspected virus claimed to be isolated from some cases of leukaemia was subsequently shown to be a *Myco-plasma* (p. 379).

CHAPTER 40

CHLAMYDIAE

Organisms of this group are, like the viruses, obligatory intracellular parasites. Because of this they have in the past been classified as viruses. They show, however, a much closer resemblance to bacteria. Like bacteria, they possess a murein-containing cell wall. They contain both DNA and RNA, do not undergo a genuine eclipse phase and multiply by binary fission. Their obligatory parasitism appears to be due mainly to a deficiency in energy-producing metabolic equipment. Their properties are consistent with an evolution, through a loss of synthetic properties, from highly parasitic bacteria.

There is no general agreement on the nomenclature of the group. It has been widely suggested they should be called *Bedsonia* after Sir Samuel Bedson, the discoverer of the psittacosis agents. The genetic name *Chlamydia* has, however, secured wide acceptance, particularly in the United States. The important human pathogens are the psittacosis, lymphogranuloma, trachoma and inclusion conjunctivitis agents.

All are Gram negative, non-motile spherical organisms of identical morphology, which exhibit a characteristic cycle of intracellular growth, and which possess a common group antigen. As observed in the electron microscope, chlamydiae show considerable heterogeneity in size and structure. At one extreme is a small particle of about 0·3μ in diameter with a dense central body, and presenting the so-called 'wrinkled pea' appearance. At the other extreme is a large particle from 0·5 to 1μ in diameter of granular appearance and without a central body. Between these extremes there is a continuous spectrum of intermediate forms. The dense central body of the small form does not appear to be a nuclear equivalent since, on treatment of small particles with desoxycholate, the DNA is lost, without any alteration in the appearance of the central body. It probably represents some, yet unexplained, condensation of cytoplasmic material within the cell wall. At the end of the growth cycle, in infected cells, small forms predominate. They appear to be forms particularly fit for survival in an extracellular environment, and for the penetration of fresh cells. The large particles, on the other hand, seem specially adapted to multiply in an intracellular environment.

Both types of particle are surrounded by a cell wall which is appreciably thinner than that of a bacterium. The cell walls contain murein, and, like the Gram negative bacteria, a high concentration of lipid. The particles may be stained by Machiavello's, Castaneda's or Giemsa's methods. When stained by

Machiavello's method, which is that most generally used, the small particles are stained red and the large particles blue.

Observations with the electron microscope have given more precision to the concept of an intracellular developmental cycle. The time required for a complete cycle of intracellular multiplication varies from 24 to 48 hours, depending on the type of host cell involved. During the first half of the cycle the small particles increase in size and transform into large particles. During the second half of the cycle, the large particles multiply by binary fission, and, as the cycle proceeds, an increasing number of them undergo transformation into small particles. The population of intracellular particles constitutes an inclusion body demonstrable by light microscopy.

In some cases the particles are embedded in a homogeneous glycogen-containing matrix which can be demonstrated by staining with iodine. The glycogen appears to be produced by the chlamydia itself, rather than by the host cell, since its production is inhibited by penicillin. Glycogen-containing inclusions are much more compact than inclusions lacking glycogen. They are produced by the lymphogranuloma venereum, and trachoma and inclusion conjunctivitis (TRIC) agents, but not by the majority of psittacosis or ornithosis strains or most chlamydiae isolated from animals. Glycogen-producing chlamydiae are in general much more susceptible to sulphadiazine and cycloserine than non-glycogen-producing chlamydiae. Because of these associations it has been suggested that the capacity to produce glycogen may be of phylogenetic significance. In this case, the lymphogranuloma venereum, TRIC agents and chlamydiae isolated from rodents would be closely related and would be distinct from avian chlamydiae and chlamydiae isolated from other animals. This raises the possibility that the characteristically human chlamydiae may have evolved from rodent strains.

Antigenic Structure

The chlamydiae possess both group and specific antigens. The specific antigens are certainly components of the cell wall, and the group antigens probably so. The group antigens, however, are less firmly attached, and can be removed by treatment of the organisms with desoxycholate, which does not remove the specific antigens. Group antigens are heat stable and are inactivated by periodate and lecithinase. They are therefore probably complexes of polysaccharide and lecithin. Chlamydiae possess haemagglutinating activity which appears to be due to the group antigen. The specific antigens are heat labile and are probably protein. The psittacosis, lymphogranuloma venereum and trachoma agents possess different specific antigens.

All the chlamydiae possess heat-labile toxins which are lethal for mice on intravenous inoculation. The toxins have the same serological specificity as the specific antigens. Since, however, the isolated cell walls, though capable of absorbing antitoxic antibody, are not themselves toxic, the specific antigen is probably only a component of the toxin. The specific antigens stimulate the production of protective antibody, while the group antigens do not.

Metabolism

Since chlamydiae only grow intracellularly it has not been possible to define their synthetic capabilities in detail. However, it has been clear from the differential incorporation of labelled phosphorus that they can carry out the terminal stages, at least, of DNA and RNA synthesis. Moreover they have been found to possess ribosomes, and can synthesize their own protein. They must also be able to synthesize murein and its constituent muramic acid, and agents sensitive to the sulphonamides must be able to synthesize folic acid.

The principal metabolic deficiency in the chlamydiae appears to be in energy-yielding metabolism. They are deficient in cytochromes and other components of the electron transport chain, and are therefore incapable of carrying out aerobic oxidations. Anaerobic glycolysis though for many years thought not to occur, has recently been demonstrated. The capacity of the chlamydiae in this respect is only partial, however, since they do not appear to be capable of generating ATP or of reoxidizing reduced NADP. These functions must therefore be supplied by the host cell. The chlamydiae must therefore, unlike bacterial cells, be permeable to ATP and NADP.

Chlamydiae are susceptible to many of the chemotherapeutic drugs active against bacteria, viz. penicillin and cycloserine, which inhibit cell wall synthesis, and erythromycin, chloramphenicol and the tetracyclines all of which appear to act at ribosomal level. Some chlamydiae are also susceptible to the sulphonamides, sulphadiazine being the most effective. As therapeutic agents the tetracyclines are the drugs of choice.

The way in which chlamydiae damage their host cells is not understood. Whether the toxin, which is lethal for mice on intravenous inoculation, has a damaging effect when produced within infected tissue cells is not known. A possible method of damage to the cell is by nutritional deprivation. Thus there is some evidence that the intra-cellular growth of chlamydiae can inhibit host cell DNA synthesis by a diversion from the latter of precursors and energy sources. When released from infected cells in the intact animal, chlamydiae stimulate inflammatory reactions which are frequently of polymorphonuclear type.

Chlamydiae have considerable tendency to establish latent infections. Under experimental conditions latency has been induced by starvation and exposure to a drug to which the chlamydiae are susceptible, or by rapid serial passage. It has been suggested that these various procedures act by interfering in some way with the reorganization of the small particles into the larger multiplying forms.

Outside the body the chlamydiae are highly unstable. They are susceptible to the range of disinfectants active against bacteria. To ensure maximum viability infective material should be stored at $-20°$ C.

The Psittacosis Group

Chlamydiae of this group were first isolated from psittacine birds and these are the most important sources of human infection. Similar chlamydiae are also present in a great variety of non-psittacine birds including pigeons, ducks and domestic fowl. Strains isolated from non-psittacine birds are often referred to as ornithosis agents. Psittacosis-like agents have also been isolated from cat, mouse, calf, sheep and opossum sources. These show significant differences in range of pathogenicity from strains isolated from human and avian sources and are probably of negligible importance in human infections.

The psittacosis chlamydiae grow readily in the chick embryo, particularly in the yolk sac. Mice, guinea-pigs and rabbits are also susceptible. The mouse is the most generally useful animal and may be infected by the intranasal, intraperitoneal or intracerebral routes. Psittacosis chlamydiae isolated from different sources show significant differences in animal pathogenicity. In general, strains from psittacine birds and turkeys exhibit the widest range of pathogenicity and give rise to the most severe lesions. Following intranasal inoculation of mice they produce areas of pulmonary consolidation. Following intraperitoneal inoculation they usually kill the mouse in 3 to 10 days; at post mortem an exudate in which elementary bodies may be demonstrated is found on the surface of the peritoneum, the spleen is enlarged and the liver shows areas of necrosis. Following intracerebral inoculation they produce an encephalitis. The psittacosis chlamydiae can also be propagated in a variety of tissue cultures but the yields obtained are generally low. Tissue cultures have, however, been of particular value for experimental purposes.

By the use of toxin neutralization, infectivity neutralization and complement fixation tests, together with fluorescent antibody studies of cell walls extracted with desoxycholate to remove group antigen, considerable serological heterogeneity has been demonstrated in psittacosis and ornithosis agents and in similar chlamydiae isolated from animal sources. Some of the specific antigens are widely distributed while others are characteristic of strains isolated from particular sources. Thus avian strains have been shown to possess specific antigens absent from mammalian strains, and vice versa, and strains from psittacine birds have been found to possess antigens not present in strains from non-psittacine birds.

A haemagglutinin acting on mouse red cells has been described in some strains. The haemagglutinin which is separable from the virus particle appears to be a complex of lecithin and nucleoprotein. It possess group serological specificity. Dermal hypersensitivity to psittacosis or lymphogranuloma venereum antigen sometimes develops as a result of infection with chlamydiae of the psittacosis group but not as frequently as in lymphogranuloma venereum. The antigen responsible is group specific.

Psittacosis

It should be noted that the term psittacosis is applied to infection by chlamydiae of this group occurring in psittacine birds and in man; the term ornithosis is used for infections occurring in non-psittacine birds.

The disease in birds usually occurs as a latent infection and appears to be transmitted from the mother to the young in the nest. In the case of parrots this latent infection can be transformed into active infection by debilitating factors dependent on capture and transportation. Consequently newly imported birds frequently develop a severe form of the disease in the course of which they excrete large amounts of the agent and are more liable to transmit infection to man.

The great majority of human infections are derived from avian sources and particularly from psittacine birds. They appear to be contracted mainly as a result of the inhalation of infected dust and droppings. Some infections have occurred in individuals who have been bitten by infected birds. Infection by ingestion of infected birds, e.g. of poultry, has not been described. The disease can also be transmitted from one human case to another via the respiratory secretions and a considerable number of infections have occurred in nurses and attendants of psittacosis patients. Many laboratory infections from the handling of infected material have been described.

In man psittacosis may give rise to inapparent infection or to a relatively mild illness clinically resembling influenza. In severe cases the presenting syndrome is that of pneumonia, usually of the lobar type, and on occasion resembling PAP (p. 379) but without the presence of cold agglutinins. Following recovery the agent can apparently persist in the respiratory tract in a latent form for a considerable time; the frequency with which this occurs, however, is not known.

The tetracyclines, especially chlortetracycline, are the drugs of choice in treatment. Chemotherapy, however, though controlling the clinical manifestations of the disease is not always successful in eliminating the chlamydiae from the body. The development of antibiotic resistance has been reported.

An effective vaccine is not available. As a control measure, because of the predominance of psittacine birds as sources of infection, the quarantine of imported psittacine birds is of great importance.

Diagnosis

The organism may be isolated from the blood during the first week of the disease and from the sputum in pneumonic cases. Isolation is usually attempted by yolk-sac inoculation of the chick embryo or by intraperitoneal or intranasal inoculation of mice. The organism may be demonstrated microscopically in the yolk sac of infected eggs and in smears from the liver and spleens of infected mice. Final identification is carried out by the use of complement fixation and toxin and infectivity neutralization tests.

Antibody may be detected in the patient's serum by the complement fixation test using a heat-inactivated and phenolized yolk-sac antigen. Two specimens of serum should be examined: one taken as early as possible in the acute stage; and the other at a later date. If the case is one of psittacosis, a rise in titre should be demonstrable between the two examinations. On account of the sharing of antigens, positive complement fixation reactions with psittacosis antigen are also obtained in cases of lymphogranuloma venereum. Specific complement fixation may be obtained by the use of a living antigen and sera which have been exhausted of group antibody by absorption with heated antigen. This procedure is not, however, suitable for ordinary diagnostic use. The complement fixation test remains positive for long periods after recovery—psittacosis differing in this way from most virus infections.

Lymphogranuloma Venereum

The lymphogranuloma venereum agent is more difficult to propagate than the psittacosis agent but can be isolated in the yolk sac of the chick embryo and by intracerebral inoculation of mice. It can also be grown in HeLa cell tissue cultures.

Lymphogranuloma venereum is a venereal disease affecting only man. It is of world-wide distribution, but commonest in tropical countries. Three stages of the disease are distinguished. In the first stage a primary lesion in the form of a small papule which progresses to ulceration appears on the genital mucosa or in the anterior urethra in from 3 days to 3 weeks after infection. In the secondary stage, which appears about 2 weeks after the development of the primary lesion, the patient becomes febrile and there is enlargement of the local lymphatic glands. In most cases the glands involved become purulent and discharge through the skin. Apart from local lesions, some cases show signs of generalized infection with widespread lymph gland involvement; occasionally arthritis and meningitis are observed. The tertiary stage, which may be highly chronic and which is commoner in the female than in the male, is characterized by the appearance of granulomatous lesions around the genitalia and in the perineal region. Lymphatic involvement in this region may lead to the development of localized elephantiasis. The discharging granulomatous lesions of the tertiary stage are very liable to secondary bacterial infection.

Though usually of venereal origin non-venereal infections may occur; a number of such infections in which the virus has gained entry through the conjunctiva have been described.

Very satisfactory results have been obtained in the treatment of lymphogranuloma venereum with the tetracyclines and these are the drugs of choice. The sulphonamides are also reported to be of value.

Diagnosis

The organism may be demonstrable microscopically in smears of pus from infected glands or in material taken from the glands by biopsy. An attempt may also be made to isolate it by intracerebral inoculation of mice or inoculation into the chick embryo yolk sac but is frequently unsuccessful.

The complement fixation test using inactivated yolk-sac antigen may be used for the demonstration of antibody. Positive reactions with lymphogranuloma venereum antigens are, however, also given by the sera of patients suffering from psittacosis, and on occasion by sera which give a positive Wassermann reaction.

A skin test using antigen prepared from infected yolk sac inactivated by heat is widely used as a diagnostic method. This test, which is known as the Frei test, depends upon a delayed-type allergy. In positive cases, following intradermal injection of the antigen an inflammatory swelling appears within a few days around the site of inoculation. Hypersensitivity is usually sufficiently established to give a positive skin test within 2 to 6 weeks after infection and persists for long periods, possibly for life. Positive reactions in the Frei test may also be obtained from patients who have been infected with the psittacosis and other chlamydiae of the group. The antigen responsible for the skin reactions appears to be distinct from the group complement fixing antigen. It is reported that a skin test antigen specific for lymphogranuloma venereum can be obtained by extraction of crude yolk-sac antigen with 0·02N.HCl.

Trachoma and Inclusion Conjunctivitis

The agents responsible for these diseases have long been known, on morphological grounds, to be chlamydiae. They were not isolated, however, until 1957 when Tang showed that agents from trachoma could be isolated by inoculation

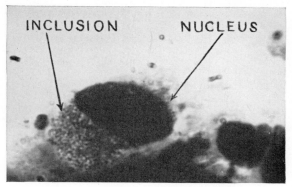

Fig. 62. Inclusion Body of Trachoma Virus in an Infected Conjunctival Cell. Giemsa–May–Grünwald Stain × 1820 (*Dr L. H. Collier and J. Sowa*). The inclusion body fills most of the cytoplasm and has compressed the nucleus

of the yolk sacs of 6- to 8-day chick embryos. Only a few strains appear to be capable of growth in tissue culture. Lesions can be produced in the eyes of monkeys, but no other laboratory animal is susceptible. In their morphology, developmental cycle, common group antigen and toxicity they resemble the psittacosis lymphogranuloma venereum agents. A completely species-specific antigen has not been demonstrated.

It has not so far been possible to differentiate the trachoma and inclusion conjunctivitis agents by laboratory procedures. Since, however, the diseases are epidemiologically clearly distinct it is reasonable to assume that there is some difference between the agents involved. Yet the strains from each condition produce the same type of lesion on inoculation onto the conjunctivae of human volunteers and of monkeys. At present they are therefore grouped together without distinction as TRIC agents. TRIC agents resemble the lymphogranuloma venereum agent and differ from psittacosis chlamydiae in producing glycogen-containing inclusion bodies.

Trachoma is a form of follicular conjunctivitis which is of world-wide distribution. It is particularly prevalent in the Middle East but is rare in the British Isles. The organism is very susceptible to drying, and spread of the

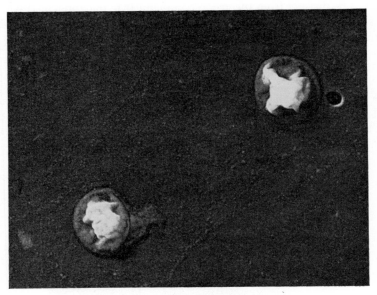

FIG. 63. TRACHOMA ORGANISM × 22,000
Electron micrograph. Shadowed preparation.
(*Dr R. C. Valentine and Dr L. H. Collier*)

disease from one person to another requires close contact and occurs mainly under unhygienic conditions. Trachoma is a serious disease, since after the acute stage has passed it develops into a chronic form with the formation of scar tissue in the eyelids, conjunctiva and cornea leading ultimately to blindness. In communities in which it is prevalent infection usually occurs within the first year of life, the disease as a rule being acquired from the mother. The condition is considerably more severe in the adult than in the child. Secondary bacterial infection, which increases the amount of damage caused by the organism, is usual.

By contrast the lesions of inclusion conjunctivitis are milder than those of trachoma and occur mainly in the lower lid; the cornea is rarely involved and when it is the lesions are transient and show no residual scarring. The disease is of world-wide distribution.

Inclusion conjunctivitis occurs in two clinical forms: (1) As a neonatal infection, the infant's eyes being infected during delivery by organisms present in the mother's genital tract. The condition is an acute one with the accumulation of pus cells in the conjunctival exudate. It must be distinguished clinically from gonococcal ophthalmia from which it differs in that it usually appears between the fifth and fifteenth day after birth. (2) As an infection of adults. This variety is less acute than the neonatal infection and the conjunctival exudate usually shows the presence of lymphocytes as the predominant cell type. The infection appears to be contracted mainly in swimming baths contaminated with infected genito-urinary secretions.

The sera of patients from both conditions may give positive complement fixation tests with chlamydial group antigen but these tests have no diagnostic value. Although isolation of the agent is possible by chick embryo inoculation, diagnosis is more readily achieved by demonstration of the typical cytoplasmic inclusion bodies in infected conjunctival cells. In trachoma these are most numerous in cells from the upper tarsal conjunctiva and in inclusion conjunctivitis from those of the lower tarsal conjunctiva.

Sowa et al. have found, however, that virus isolation is much more sensitive than the demonstration of inclusions for the diagnosis of established trachoma infection. Chlamydiae are not susceptible to streptomycin and this drug can therefore be used for the control of bacterial contamination in the isolation of these agents by yolk-sac inoculation. More recently the examination of smears by the fluorescent antibody technique has been favourably reported on.

Sulphonamides and tetracyclines are effective therapeutic agents in both conditions.

Non-bacterial Regional Lymphadenitis
(Cat Scratch Disease)

This condition, which usually follows the scratch of a cat, after an interval of 1 to 7 weeks, is characterized by a mild degree of fever and a regional lymphadenitis which may progress to pus formation. The syndrome has also resulted from other types of scratch, e.g. from thorns. A possible relationship of the agent to the chlamydiae is suggested by the observation that some patients give positive complement fixation tests with chlamydia group antigen. A skin test using pus or macerated lymph node tissue is claimed to be highly specific.

CHAPTER 41

THE RICKETTSIAE

Properties of the Group

The rickettsiae are a group of small organisms which, because of their apparently obligatory intracellular parasitism, have in the past been regarded as intermediate between viruses and bacteria. There is now, however, little doubt that like the chlamydiae they are in fact very small bacteria. Like bacteria they possess a murein-containing cell wall; they contain both RNA and DNA, multiply by binary fission, and have considerable independent metabolic activity. Under in vitro conditions they have been found to be capable of carrying out certain transamination reactions and of oxidizing some small molecular weight substrates, notably glutamate, which is possibly their main source of energy under natural conditions. Unlike the chlamydiae they can generate high-energy phosphate bonds. However, unlike bacteria they cannot break down glucose. Apart from *Rickettsia quintana*, which has recently been reported to grow on a blood agar medium, rickettsiae have not so far been cultivated in the laboratory on cell-free media.

Rickettsiae may be demonstrated in infected tissues by Macchiavello's, Castaneda's or Giemsa's methods. In Giemsa stained preparations they appear as bluish-purple structures; when stained with Macchiavello's stain they appear bright red showing up in sharp contrast against a blue background. They also stain by Gram's method and are Gram negative. Gram's stain is, however, not a satisfactory routine stain for demonstrating them.

Smears from infected tissues show considerable pleomorphism—coccal, oval and bacillary forms being observed. The average size of the rickettsiae is from $0 \cdot 3$ to $0 \cdot 4\mu$ in width and up to $1 \cdot 5\mu$ in length. In electron micrographs a central structure analogous to a nucleus, a cell wall, and a peripheral layer resembling a bacterial capsule have all been demonstrated. This capsular layer probably contains the group-specific soluble antigens. None of the rickettsiae are motile. In smear preparations they are frequently found as pairs of flame-shaped organisms, somewhat resembling pneumococci, and occasionally in short chains. In infected tissue cells they usually appear in large clumps.

Rickettsiae are heat labile, being destroyed at $50°$ C in half an hour, and are fairly susceptible to the action of chemical disinfectants; they are readily destroyed by low concentrations of phenol and formalin. They undergo inactivation rapidly at room temperature but may be preserved for long periods by freeze drying.

The rickettsiae appear to be primarily parasites of insects, particularly of ticks and mites and to a lesser extent of fleas and lice, and infect animals on which their insect host is parasitic. Ticks and mites are capable of transmitting rickettsiae transovarially to their offspring. In these cases though the animal

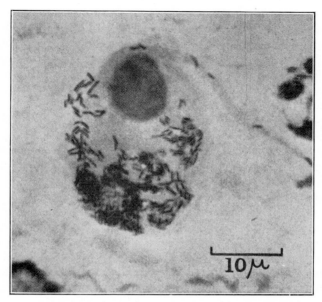

FIG. 64. *Rickettsia typhi* IN AN ENDOTHELIAL CELL OF A GUINEA-
PIG TESTIS
(Electron micrograph)

host of the insect is also infected the insect should probably be regarded as the primary natural reservoir of infection. Epidemic typhus and trench fever are unusual in that the only animal naturally infected is man.

In their insect vectors the rickettsiae multiply in the epithelium of the intestinal tract; they are excreted in the faeces but occasionally gain access to the insect's salivary glands. In their animal host they are found principally in the endothelium of the small blood vessels particularly in those of the skin, brain and heart. In infected endothelial cells they produce proliferative and, in the more severe infections, as in Rocky Mountain spotted fever, necrotic changes. These endothelial changes result in vascular thromboses and in haemorrhages.

The rickettsiae are pathogenic on experimental inoculation for a wide range of animals. For their isolation guinea-pigs and mice have been most used. They will grow in the developing chick embryo, the highest concentrations being obtained on inoculation into the yolk sac. They can also be propagated in cultures of certain rat and mouse tissues. In general, growth of the rickettsiae is maximal when the metabolism of the host cell is proceeding at a low rate as in growth in eggs or tissue cultures at suboptimal temperatures or in the presence of metabolic inhibitors. In infected cells the rickettsiae of the spotted fever group and *Rickettsia akari* are found in the nucleus where they appear to multiply. Other rickettsiae are not found in the nucleus and appear to multiply in the cytoplasm.

Concentrated rickettsial suspensions are lethal for mice on intravenous inoculation. In addition they are haemolytic for the red cells of a variety of animal species. Toxicity and haemolytic activity are both intrinsic properties of the organism and on storage are lost concomitantly with infectivity. There is some evidence that these properties, though not requiring multiplication of the rickettsiae, depend on enzymatic activity since suspensions which have become non-haemolytic and non-toxic on storage regain these capacities, as well as their infectivity, if suspended in NAD.

Three major types of rickettsial antigen have been identified:

1. Group-specific soluble antigens. These are demonstrable in the environment of the organism and appear to be derived from the surface capsular layer. The soluble antigens of the typhus fever group and of the spotted fever group are group-specific, the same, or similar, soluble antigens being present in different members of the group. The soluble antigens of the scrub typhus group, on the other hand, show considerable heterogeneity.

2. Species or, in the case of the scrub typhus rickettsiae, strain-specific antigens associated with the bodies of the rickettsiae. In order to demonstrate these antigens, well-washed suspensions, from which the group antigens present in the capsular layer have been removed, must be employed.

3. Antigens shared with various strains of *Proteus*. Sharing of antigens has been shown between various rickettsiae and *Proteus* strains OX19, OX2 and OXK. These antigens appear to be polysaccharides. The antigens do not react in agglutination tests, and therefore do not appear to occur as surface components.

In the diagnosis of rickettsial infections serological tests are of primary importance. The most generally applicable test is the Weil-Felix reaction which measures the titre of antibody against the *Proteus* strains OX19, OX2 and OXK. The Weil-Felix reaction is specially valuable in the diagnosis of epidemic and murine typhus, in both of which there is a high titre of antibody to OX19. For the differentiation of these two conditions, however, complement fixation or agglutination tests with well-washed rickettsial suspensions are required for the identification of antibody to the specific antigens. Complement fixation tests with soluble antigens have a particular value in the diagnosis of infections with the spotted fever group. Here again, however, species differentiation requires the use of complement fixation or agglutination tests with specific antigens.

A substance capable of sensitizing red cells so that these are agglutinated specifically by rickettsial antibody has also been prepared from *R. prowazeki* and *R. typhi*. The sensitizing antigen can be extracted by heating the rickettsiae under alkaline conditions. It does not fix complement; haemagglutination tests, however, give results which parallel those obtained in complement fixation tests with the group-specific soluble antigen. A similar but serologically distinct red cell sensitizing antigen, also possessing group specificity, has been isolated from certain of the tick-borne spotted fever group. The demonstration of antibody to red cell sensitizing antigens has been used as a diagnostic procedure.

For diagnostic purposes an attempt may be made to isolate rickettsiae by the intraperitoneal inoculation of guinea-pigs or mice with blood taken during the febrile stage of infection. For this purpose defibrinated, heparinized or citrated whole blood or ground-up clot may be used. If sampled later than the first week ground-up clot is preferable because of the presence of antibodies which might otherwise inhibit rickettsial growth. Isolation of rickettsiae is technically difficult and, because of their high infectivity, should be attempted only in specialized laboratories where adequate safety measures can be employed.

In identifying a *Rickettsia*, the clinical response of the animal is of considerable importance. Thus all rickettsiae will give rise to fever in the guinea-pig following intraperitoneal inoculation, but the rickettsiae of spotted fever and murine typhus will produce also inflammation of the testes. It may be possible to demonstrate rickettsiae microscopically in the organs of animals which have been sacrificed or which have died from the infection. When guinea-pigs are used confirmation of the presence of rickettsiae can be obtained by demonstration in their sera of complement fixing antibody. Inoculation into the yolk sacs of developing chick embryos is a feasible but not very satisfactory method for isolation since satisfactory growth can only be obtained after the organism has been adapted to the chick embryo by a number of blind passages.

Like the psittacosis-lymphogranuloma group, rickettsiae are sensitive to chloramphenicol and the tetracyclines, and these agents have proved of great value in the treatment of rickettsial infections. The rickettsiae are not inhibited by penicillin or the sulphonamides. The latter in fact have a definite stimulatory effect and when given to a patient adversely affect the course of the disease. PABA has been found to have an inhibitory effect and prior to the introduction of the wide-spectrum antibiotics was used with some degree of success in the treatment of infections of the typhus group.

Four groups of rickettsiae may be distinguished: (1) The typhus fever group comprising *R. prowazeki*, the cause of epidemic typhus, and *R. typhi*, the cause of murine typhus. These rickettsiae share a common soluble antigen. (2) *R. tsutsugamushi*, the cause of scrub typhus. (3) The spotted fever group. (4). *R. quintana*, the cause of trench fever.

EPIDEMIC TYPHUS

Epidemic typhus was at one time a common disease of world-wide distribution but has now been eliminated from Western Europe, North America and many other parts of the world where it was formerly prevalent. Endemic foci of infection, however, still exist in Eastern Europe and parts of Asia, Africa and South America. These endemic foci may be the site of origin of large-scale epidemics.

Typhus is spread from case to case by lice, and on this account epidemics are particularly associated with war, cold and dirt—conditions which favour louse infestation. During World War II a very large epidemic occurred in Naples. The disease first appeared in air-raid shelters in which many people were closely confined under highly insanitary conditions and in which they rapidly became infested with lice. Lice do not become infective until 4 to 6 days after biting an infected patient. Thereafter they remain infective until they die, which usually occurs within a further 2 weeks. The rickettsiae are present in considerable numbers in the intestinal contents of the louse but do not apparently gain access to its salivary glands. Infection is therefore probably due to the contamination of scratches and abrasions by louse faeces rather than to the bite of the insect. Infection by the respiratory route has been shown to occur in the laboratory and may also occur under epidemic conditions from rickettsiae in dried louse faeces.

Typhus is a severe disease marked clinically by considerable prostration; a characteristic rash which in severe cases is purpuric in character appears about the fifth day. The mortality from typhus has been found to vary considerably in different epidemics and is highest in individuals over forty.

SOME FEATURES OF RICKETTSIAL INFECTIONS

Organism	Disease	Vector	Reservoir	Proteus agglutinins	Isolation (intraperitoneal)
R. prowazeki	Epidemic typhus	Louse	Man	OX19	GP. Fever
R. typhi	Murine typhus	Flea	Rats	OX19	GP. Scrotal swelling
R. tsutsu-gamushi	Scrub typhus	Mites	Wild rodents	OXK	Mice. Ascites
R. rickettsi	Rocky Mountain spotted fever	Tick	Wild rodents and dogs		GP. Scrotal necrosis
R. conori	Fièvre bouton-neuse (and African tick typhus)	Tick		OX19 and/or OX2	GP. Scrotal swelling
R. australis	Queensland tick typhus	Tick	Wild rodents and mar-supials		GP. Scrotal swelling
R. akari	Rickettsial pox	Mite	House mice	—	Mice. Ascites
R. quintana	Trench fever	Louse	Man	—	—
C. burneti	Q fever	Tick	Cattle, sheep, goats, gerbil-les, bandicoots	—	GP. Fever

Brackets at left of figure indicate species sharing group complement fixing antigens.

During the course of an epidemic, as well as cases of the classical type, relatively trivial and asymptomatic latent infections also occur. Latent infection may persist for many years. The epidemiological variety of typhus known as Brill's disease is a well-documented example of such persistence. Brill's disease is a form of typhus observed on the Eastern sea-board of the United States in European immigrants who were almost certainly latently infected before they left Europe. Persistent latent infections of this type may be important as a reservoir of the rickettsiae under natural conditions. Some such reservoir is necessary since *R. prowazeki* has not so far been identified as a natural parasite of any animal host.

Prophylaxis

A formolized egg yolk vaccine is widely used for immunization against typhus and is of value in preventing the disease and in considerably diminishing its severity in inoculated individuals. The immunizing potency of the vaccine appears to depend on soluble antigens as well as on antigens present in the bodies of the rickettsiae. Consequently, in modern methods of vaccine preparation, the techniques used are designed to retain a considerable amount of soluble antigen. Following inoculation of rickettsial vaccine there is an increase in specific rickettsial antibodies, as detected by rickettsial agglutination and complement fixation tests; there is, however, no increase in the antibody demonstrable in the Weil-Felix reaction. Although there is a high degree of cross immunity, under natural conditions of infection, between epidemic typhus and murine typhus, inactivated *R. typhi* vaccines do not protect against epidemic typhus and inactivated *R. prowazeki* vaccines do not protect against murine typhus. Immunization against epidemic typhus has also been carried out on a limited scale with the living attenuated E strain of *R. prowazeki*. For the control of epidemics disinfestation, particularly by the use of DDT, is of primary importance.

MURINE TYPHUS

Like epidemic typhus, murine typhus is a disease of world-wide distribution. The rickettsia responsible—*R. typhi*—is a natural parasite of the rat. *R. typhi* is also parasitic on fleas and lice, and these appear to be mainly responsible for transmitting the organisms from rat to rat. Transmission of the disease to man is almost certainly due to the rat flea. There is some evidence that body lice infected from patients with murine typhus may cause epidemic spread of the disease.

Clinically murine typhus is a much milder disease than epidemic typhus. Involvement of the central nervous system, heart and kidneys is considerably less frequent. Except in individuals over 50 the mortality is negligible.

The control of the disease depends essentially on the use of DDT and on measures designed to control the rodent population. Immunization, though feasible, is not considered necessary.

SCRUB TYPHUS

This disease, which is caused by *R. tsutsugamushi*, occurs in the Far East and Japan—where it is known as Tsutsugamushi—in Malaya and in the Pacific area. The disease is transmitted to man by the bites of the larvae of certain trombiculid mites. The parasite is transmitted from one generation of mites to the next transovarially. Wild rodents, especially rats, on which the mites are parasitic, constitute an animal reservoir of infection. Scrub typhus occurs particularly in areas where the jungle has been cut down and replaced by low scrub—an environment in which rats and mites multiply rapidly. It was very common amongst troops in the Pacific theatre of World War II, where these conditions frequently prevailed.

In its main clinical features scrub typhus resembles epidemic typhus. A distinctive characteristic of the disease is the appearance in most cases, either just before or at the onset of symptoms, of a small, punched-out ulcer covered by a dark scab at the site of the insect bite.

Rickettsia tsutsugamushi is antigenically very heterogeneous. Because of this, in endemic areas, second attacks are common. The antigenic heterogeneity of the group has so far made it impossible to develop an effective vaccine.

The sera of patients suffering from scrub typhus may show a high titre of agglutinins for *Proteus* OXK. No rise in titre is demonstrable against *Proteus* OX19 or OX2. A considerable proportion of cases, however, fail to produce detectable *Proteus* agglutinins. Because of the antigenic heterogeneity of the species rickettsial agglutination and complement fixation tests are of very limited value in diagnosis.

SPOTTED FEVER GROUP

Under this heading are included a number of rickettsial infections caused by rickettsiae possessing a common group or soluble antigen. The infections fall into three groups: (1) Rocky Mountain spotted fever. (2) Tick-borne rickettsioses of the Eastern hemisphere. (3) Rickettsial pox.

Rocky Mountain Spotted Fever

This condition, which is much the most severe of this group of rickettsial infections, is due to *R. rickettsi*, first identified as the cause of Rocky Mountain spotted fever by Ricketts in Montana. *R. rickettsi* is now known to be of wide distribution in North, Central and South America. It occurs as a parasite of various ticks in the Rocky Mountain region. The main vector is *Dermacentor andersoni* which is parasitic on a variety of wild animals. Ticks, e.g. *Dermacentor variabilis* and, in Mexico, *Rhipicephalus sanguineus*, which infest dogs, are probably of considerable importance in spreading the disease, because of their close association with men.

Rickettsia rickettsi produces marked necrotic changes in the endothelium of the small blood vessels and frequently also in the smooth muscle cells of the arterioles. In the skin these vascular changes result in an extensive haemorrhagic rash which in severe cases may progress to necrosis of large areas of skin. There is usually extensive involvement of the blood vessels of the brain; in recovered cases this may lead to permanent neurological sequelae. The sera of the majority of patients show a high titre of agglutinins against one or more *Proteus* strains, the highest titres usually being found against OX19. Complement fixation tests with group antigens will differentiate Rocky Mountain spotted fever from the typhus group. Differentiation from other members of the spotted fever group, by the use of specific rickettsial antigens, is not normally required.

Inactivated vaccines of *R. rickettsi* prepared from infected yolk sacs or from the tissues of infected ticks are available and have been found to give a considerable degree of protection. Effective vaccines have not yet been prepared from the other members of the spotted fever group.

Tick-borne Rickettsial Infections of the Eastern Hemisphere

These are much less severe than Rocky Mountain spotted fever and characteristically show a local lesion at the site of the bite. Three species are involved each with a characteristic geographic distribution: (1) *R. conori* produces infection in Africa—South African tick fever, Kenya tick fever, Indian tick typhus— and, along the Mediterranean littoral, fièvre boutonneuse. (2) *R. australis*, the cause of Queensland tick typhus. (3) *R. siberica*, prevalent in Siberia and Mongolia. These rickettsiae are readily distinguished from one another and from *R. rickettsi* and *R. akari* by complement fixation tests with specific antigens, and by toxin neutralization tests. Agglutinins develop to Proteus OX19 and OX2 but to a lower titre than in Rocky Mountain spotted fever. All these rickettsial species are maintained in nature in wild rodents. Dogs and marsupials appear to be important in the maintenance of *R. conori* and *R. australis*, respectively.

Rickettsial Pox

This is a mild disease—usually lasting less than a week—which was first recognized in New York in 1946. The condition has since been reported from Africa and the U.S.S.R. In the majority of cases a local lesion appears at the site of the bite. A maculopapular rash later becoming vesicular is a characteristic feature. The disease shows a mainly urban distribution.

The causative organism, *R. akari*, is transmitted by mites; house mice appear to be the animal reservoir from which human infection occurs. *R. akari* is closely related to the tick-borne rickettsiae considered above with which it shares a common group-specific soluble antigen. It is consequently usually classified as a member of the spotted fever group.

Agglutinins for *Proteus* are not produced during the course of infection, but specific rickettsial antibodies may be detected by complement fixation tests. *R. akari* is usually isolated by inoculation of mice.

TRENCH FEVER

Trench fever is a febrile influenza-like disease associated with a rash. The disease was first recognized in troops in World War I in whom it occurred in epidemic form. It appeared again in troops on the Eastern Front in World War II. Apparently it is never fatal. There is no known animal reservoir. The disease was spread by lice, and *Rickettsia*-like organisms were demonstrated, by a number of workers, in the intestinal epithelium of infected lice. To these organisms the name *R. quintana* has been given. *R. quintana* cannot be grown in ordinary laboratory animals, in tissue cultures or in the chick embryo, but lice bred in the laboratory have been infected by intrarectal inoculation. Its isolation on a blood agar medium has been recently reported.

Q FEVER

Q fever (Query fever) was first recognized by Derrick of Brisbane in 1935 and the causative organism first isolated by Burnet and Freeman from meat workers in Queensland in 1937. The disease appears to be of world-wide distribution. It is usually a mild febrile illness clinically resembling influenza and with a very low mortality. In contrast to other rickettsial infections there is no rash. In about half the cases there is radiographic evidence of lung involvement. In some of these the consolidation shows the patchy distribution characteristic of primary atypical pneumonia but in the majority it has a more segmental or lobar distribution. Very occasionally the infection assumes a chronic form presenting the picture of subacute bacterial endocarditis, the vegetations being particularly prominent on the aortic valves.

The causative organism was first classified as a *Rickettsia—R. burneti* but since it shows a number of distinctive characteristics it is now assigned to a separate genus *Coxiella* as *C. burneti*. *C. burneti* is appreciably more resistant to heat, desiccation and chemical agents than the rickettsiae proper. It resists heating to 60° C for one hour and will survive for several years in dried tick faeces. It is moreover not toxic for mice on intravenous administration, and soluble complement fixing antigens are not produced in infected tissues.

Two antigenic phases of *C. burneti* can be distinguished on the basis of their reactivity with guinea-pig convalescent sera. On first isolation the organisms are in phase 1 in which they react in complement fixation tests only with late convalescent serum. On passage in the chick embryo they pass into phase 2 which reacts with both late and early convalescent serum. Phase 1 is regained on passage of egg-adapted phase 2 strains in guinea-pigs. Minor antigenic differences have been demonstrated in strains of *C. burneti* isolated from different geographical areas. These differences are not, however, of immunological importance.

Coxiella burneti grows readily in the yolk sac of the developing chick embryo, the infection killing the embryo in 7 to 10 days. Of the ordinary laboratory animals guinea-pigs are the most susceptible, and are readily infected by the peritoneal route. The infection in the guinea-pig is latent, however, and the diagnosis can only be established by the demonstration some 5 to 6 weeks later of antibody production in the infected animal.

Coxiella burneti is widely distributed in nature and is responsible for infection in various wild animals, and in birds, cattle, sheep and goats, as well as in man. Amongst wild animals it is probably maintained by ticks, many species of which have been found to be infected. Human infection appears to be derived almost exclusively from infected domestic animals—cattle, sheep and goats—to which *C. burneti* is probably transmitted from a wild animal reservoir by ticks. In animals other than man it produces latent asymptomatic infection. Infected domestic animals excrete the organism in milk, urine and faeces, but in much larger amounts in the placental and uterine discharges, and the latter therefore appear to constitute the main sources of infection for other domestic animals and for man. Considerable numbers of rickettsiae are also present in the faeces of ticks parasitic on infected domestic animals.

Human infection appears to occur mainly through the respiratory tract. Q fever occurs principally in persons whose occupation brings them into contact with infected animals or with the products of infected animals, e.g. wool, hair, hides and meat. Some human infections may occur as a result of ingestion of rickettsiae in infected milk but in general it would appear that the gastro-intestinal route is of minor importance in the spread of the disease. Case to case infection does not normally occur but some infections have been described in hospital personnel infected during the performance of a post-mortem examination. A number of laboratory infections have been described, as a result of the manipulation of infected materials.

The wide-spectrum antibiotics, of which the tetracyclines are preferred, though valuable in the treatment of Q fever, appear to be appreciably less effective than in the treatment of rickettsial infections.

Vaccination against Q fever is still in the experimental stage.

Diagnosis

Though it may be possible to isolate *C. burneti* from the blood in the early febrile stages of the disease, or from the sputum, urine or cerebrospinal fluid, the diagnosis is usually established by serological methods using either complement fixation or agglutination tests. The complement fixation test, using an egg-adapted phase 2 strain is the more widely used. In acute human infections, only antibodies reacting with phase 2 organisms are produced. In chronic human infections, however, antibody may be present both to phase 2 and phase 1 organisms. The Weil-Felix reaction has no value in diagnosis.

CHAPTER 42

BACTERIOPHAGES

Bacteriophages are viruses that are parasitic on bacteria. As a rule they exhibit a marked specificity of action, each phage being capable of attacking only groups of closely related bacteria. In general, phage specificity follows taxonomic boundaries closely—a particular phage attacking only organisms belonging to a single species. In certain cases phages are not only restricted in action to a particular species but will attack only certain strains of that species. In such cases susceptibility to a particular bacteriophage forms a very convenient basis for species subdivision or typing and one which has been found to be of considerable epidemiological value.

On the basis of the types of relationship they establish with their bacterial hosts, bacteriophages are subdivided into two main groups—the *lytic* or *virulent* and the *symbiotic* or *temperate*. Lytic phages are phages which when they infect and multiply in bacteria always produce lysis of the infected cells. The most closely studied of the lytic phages are the T series of coliphages, T1 to T7, which infect certain strains of *E. coli*. Symbiotic phages are phages which are maintained parasitically in the bacterial host; they are transferred from parental to daughter cells at cell division and do not cause lysis except in a very small proportion of the organisms infected. Cultures which carry symbiotic bacteriophages are described as being *lysogenic*. In lysogenic bacteria the carried bacteriophage is known as *prophage*.

Propagation of Phage

Bacteriophages may be demonstrated in two ways: (1) By inoculation of material containing the phage into a young broth culture of a sensitive strain. In a short time, usually from half an hour to 1 hour after infection, the culture will undergo lysis. When infection is due to a lytic phage the culture will become completely clear. If it is due to temperate phage, a partial clearing will occur and the culture will then become turbid through growth of lysogenic organisms. (2) Plate method. A bacterial lawn is spread on the surface of an agar plate either over the entire surface or in small patches. The lawn is allowed to dry and a loopful of a preparation containing phage is deposited on its surface. After incubation a patch of clearing will be seen in the part of the culture attacked by the phage. If the phage is a lytic one and its concentration has been high, there will be complete clearing or confluent lysis over the inoculated area. If the concentration of phage in the preparation is low, there will instead be a number of very small areas of lysis; each of these areas is the result of growth of a single phage particle and is known as a plaque. The plaques produced by lytic phages are completely clear; areas of confluent lysis are also clear but may occasionally show a few colonies of phage-resistant mutants. The plaques produced by symbiotic phages on the other hand show a central area of growth surrounded by a ring of lysis; most of the organisms in the central area are lysogenic.

In order to isolate a phage in pure culture a small piece of agar is cut from a single plaque; the agar should include some of the area of lysis and some of the growth of the indicator strain at the periphery of this area. The agar is inoculated into broth and after incubation should contain a considerable amount of phage—of the order of 10^8 to 10^9 phage particles per ml. Single plaque isolation is essential if a pure strain of phage is to be obtained; its role in work with phage

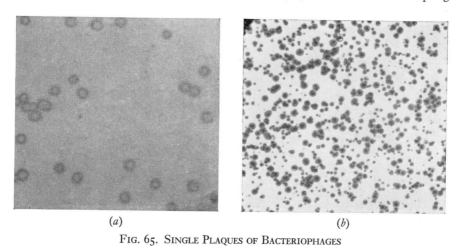

(a)   (b)

FIG. 65. SINGLE PLAQUES OF BACTERIOPHAGES

(a) A symbiotic phage active against *Salm. typhimurium*. Note growth of lysogenic organisms in centre of each plaque. (b) A lytic phage active against *E. coli*.

is precisely comparable to single colony isolation in bacteriology. Most phages are less sensitive to heat than their host organisms. In such cases phage preparations free from residual unlysed bacteria can be obtained by heating. Where heat cannot be used bacteria-free preparations of phage may be obtained by filtration.

Morphology

The majority of phages are tadpole-shaped structures, each of which possesses a head, functioning as a container for the phage nucleic acid, and a tail. The heads are of variable shape but all exhibit some sort of cuboidal symmetry; they may be bipyramidal, hexagonal prisms as in the T-even coliphages, or octahedra or icosahedra. The heads appear to be built up from protein subunits, approximately 1000 of such units comprising the heads of the T-even phages. The phage tails, which are of variable length, are normally surrounded by a sheath; in some cases this is contractile, in others non-contractile. In the T-even coliphages, which possess contractile tail sheaths, there is a collar between the base of the head and the top of the sheath and, in addition, a base plate with projecting spikes at the lower end of the tail. In the normal untriggered state of the phage a network of fibres extends from the base plate to the collar. Like

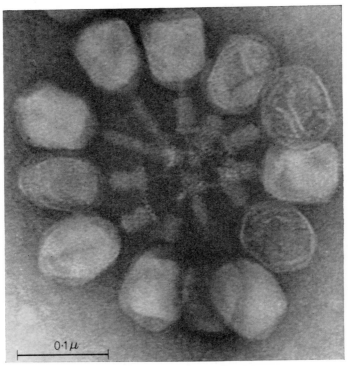

0·1 μ

FIG. 66. T2 COLIPHAGE PARTICLES SHOWING HEADS AND SHEATHS
Electron micrograph. Negative stain.
(*Brenner and Horne*, J. molec. Biol.)

the head, the tail sheath has a subunit structure. The sheaths show a lateral striation due to the arrangement of the component subunits in parallel rings along the length of the sheath. In the sheaths of T2 and T4, in the uncontracted state, each ring appears to consist of six subunits; on contraction of the sheath the number of subunits per ring is increased to 12, thereby allowing a halving of the total length of the sheath. The core of the tail is hollow with a central channel of about 20 Å in diameter. It is through this channel that the phage injects its nucleic acid into the bacterium. Each of the protein subunits of the contractile sheaths of the T-even phages is associated with one molecule of a nucleoside triphosphate, notably ATP, the breakdown of which, by the appropriate phosphatase also present in the sheath, provides the energy for its contraction. The tail structure of the T-even phages also contain a lysozyme-like enzyme which, by causing a local breakdown of the mucopeptide layer, facilitates the penetration of the cell wall in infection. Not all phages, however, possess obvious tails. Some, e.g. T3, have very short tails, while others, e.g. the coliphage ϕX174, appear to possess no tail at all. ϕX174 is a phage with icosa-hedral symmetry, possessing specialized apical subunits which appear to fulfil the function of a tail. An unusual filamentous bacteriophage, which is specific for F+ bacterial cells (p. 553), and morphologically quite distinct from those considered above, has recently been described.

In the majority of phages that have been investigated, including the T phages, the nucleic acid is a double-stranded DNA. In the case of T2 this has a mole-cular weight of circa 10^8, contains about 2 by 10^5 base pairs, and when fully extended, is about 50 mμ in length. Hence its dimensions are from 1 to 2 per cent of the bacterial chromosome. The T-even phages contain an unusual pyrimidine—5-hydroxymethyl cytosine—the demonstration of which has been of considerable value for the detection and estimation of intracellular phage-specific DNA. The pyrimidine is present in a glucosylated form, the extent of glucosylation varying with different phages.

Growth of Bacteriophages

As it occurs within the phage head, T2 phage DNA is in a highly condensed form. It is associated with a small amount of protein—the *internal protein*—whose function appears to be to bind to, and maintain, the DNA in the con-densed state. In addition to the internal protein, the head contains a polypeptide and a small amount of the polyamines spermidine and putrescine. The latter appear to be of importance in neutralizing the high negative charge on the phage DNA. Some very small phages, e.g. ϕX174 contain a single-stranded DNA, and in a few cases the nucleic acid is RNA. The most interesting of the latter are the icosahedral phages specific for F+ cells which adsorb to the sides of the specialized F pili.

The intracellular growth of bacteriophages has been most studied in connec-tion with the T coliphages. The first stage in infection is a random collision between phage and bacteria, as a result of which the phage adsorbs to specific receptors on the surface of the bacterial cell wall. The receptors for each of the T phages are different. This is shown by the fact that bacteria which have mutated to resistance to a particular phage may still retain the power to absorb other T phages. Adsorption, in the case of the T-even phages, appears to occur in the first place through the fibres attached to the tail plate. Some strains of T-even phages adsorb only in the presence of amino acid co-factors, the most effective of which is tryptophane. Adsorption co-factors appear to act by allowing the tail fibres to free themselves from the sheath and collar of the phage. Tailless phages, such as ϕX174, appear to adsorb through the specialized subunits located at the apices of the icosahedron.

Following adsorption the phage proceeds to inject the nucleic acid contained in its head membrane into the bacterium. The whole structure of the phage—head membrane and tail—can in fact be regarded as a micro-syringe developed precisely for this purpose. Neither the protein head nor tail enter the cell; they remain attached to the surface and play no further part in infection.

In the case of phages with contractile sheaths injection is associated with a contraction of the sheath, the energy for which is supplied by the breakdown of the nucleoside triphosphate associated with the tail subunits. Presumably the contraction of the sheath assists in forcing the tip of the tail through the bacterial surface. In some cases the phage tail carries a lysozyme-like enzyme which causes a local breakdown of the cell wall mucopeptide at its point of contact with the tail. Following this local break in the wall the phage DNA is believed to be forced into the bacterium by mechanical pressure resulting from its condensation in the phage head. Active participation of the cell is not required since injection occurs following adsorption of phage to killed bacteria.

If a large number of phages adsorb to a single cell the damage to the wall produced by the phage lysozyme may be sufficient to result in the death of the cell. This is known as *lysis from without*. Under normal conditions of infection with one or a few phage particles, repair of the damaged wall is initiated immediately after infection, and usually results in a considerable increase in the strength of the wall. As a result further phages, which may subsequently adsorb, are unable to inject their DNA into the cell but instead release it into the surrounding medium. This is referred to as *superinfection breakdown*.

Though the tail assembly is necessary for injection of the phage DNA, infection has, in certain cases, been produced by extracted protein-free phage DNA. Thus T2 and ϕX174 DNA will infect protoplasts and lambda (p. 559) phage DNA will infect cells exposed at the same time to intact 'helper' phages. *B. subtilis* is reported to be susceptible to infection with phage DNA when it is in a state of competence in which it is transformable by transforming DNA (p. 29).

The period elapsing between the initial contact of the bacterium with phage and the lysis of the infected cell, with the release of the new phage progeny, is known as the *latent period*. For the T-even phages it lasts about 25 minutes at 37° C. The number of phage particles liberated at the end of the latent period varies with the bacteriophage and the host strain but is usually of the order of 100 phage particles per cell. This is known as the *burst size*. Neither the duration of the latent period nor the burst size is affected by the number of particles initially infecting the cell.

The sequence of events occurring during the latent period can be studied in cells which have been artificially disrupted, e.g. by lysis with another phage, by ultrasonic irradiation or by exposure to chloroform. During approximately the first half of the latent period, no infective intracellular phage is detectable. This period is known as the *eclipse phase*. Around the middle of the latent period the first infective phage particles start to appear, and thereafter increase in number until lysis. During the eclipse phase there is however an active synthesis of phage components and, to an extent depending on the particular phage, of the enzymes necessary for the synthesis of these components. The T-even phages are outstanding in their independence of host cell synthetic enzymes—all the enzymes they require being coded for by the phage DNA. In such cases the first obvious effect of infection is disruption of the nucleus. With many other phages, e.g. T1, T3, T7, the nucleus is not disrupted and the phage utilizes enzymes such as DNA polymerase coded for by the host cell DNA. Because of the disruptive effect of T-even phages on the nucleus these phages block all cellular synthesis. Though highly independent of host synthetic mechanisms they nevertheless depend on the host cell for their energy.

In T-even phage infection the first phage-specific component to appear is an RNA whose phage specificity is shown by the fact that it is capable of hybridizing with phage DNA. The newly synthesized RNA is a messenger RNA which participates in the synthesis of the so-called 'early' enzymes. These are enzymes necessary for the synthesis and replication of the phage DNA. At least twelve such enzymes have been described, including deoxycytidylate hydroxymethylase required for the synthesis of hydroxymethyl cystosine; a DNA polymerase specific for the synthesis of phage DNA, and a glucosyl transferase responsible for the transfer of glucose from UDP-glucose to hydroxymethyl cytosine. In T2 infected cells the next stage is the synthesis and replication of the phage DNA which is distinguishable from the host cell DNA because of its content of hydroxymethyl cytosine. Phage DNA begins to appear in about the sixth or seventh minute after infection, and continues to increase in amount until the end of the latent period. Since mature phage starts to appear at about the middle of the latent period there is, when the cell eventually undergoes lysis, an excess of DNA over that which is incorporated into mature phage.

In the early stages of DNA synthesis the DNA can be seen in electron micrographs as delicate fibrils in the bacterial cytoplasm. Shortly afterwards the fibrils condense into polyhedral structures with the general appearance of phage heads. Condensation appears to be a consequence of binding of the DNA strands with the internal phage protein which is synthesized along with the early enzymes. At about the time of appearance of the condensates the phage head protein, which can be detected serologically, begins to make its appearance. It then proceeds to coat the condensates, presumably by a process of spontaneous aggregation or self-assembly (p. 418). The heads next acquire tails, a process which occurs by the sequential addition of cores, sheaths, tail plates and fibres. The final stage of the maturation process appears to be the setting of some cementing substance which confers stability on the completed structure. Rupture of the cell before this occurs leads to disintegration of the nascent phage. This final stage in maturation is inhibited by proflavine.

The precise way in which the co-ordinated synthesis of the various components and enzymes is controlled has not been determined. It would appear, however, that the messenger RNA involved in the synthesis of the early enzymes and proteins is derived from parental phage DNA and that the messenger RNA required for the synthesis of the structural head and tail proteins and of the 'late' enzymes—lysozyme and ATPase—is derived from the DNA after its replication. How this distinction is made in the cell is not known. The final release of the phage from the cell appears to be achieved as a result of the action of the lysozyme produced in the later stages of growth.

The problems involved in the synthesis of viral capsids such as those of the T phages are considerably more complex than those involved in the synthesis of the helical or simpler icosahedral capsids of the plant or animal viruses (p. 418) since their shape is not solely determined by the geometry of the capsid subunits. The problem of the assembly of the T4 capsid has been examined particularly by Kellenberger. Kellenberger has found that the assembly of the head of this phage is directed by at least two genes in addition to the gene specifying the major structural capsid subunits—namely a gene determining elongation of the developing capsid and a gene controlling completion of the elongation process. The nature and location of the factors controlling these functions is unknown. They are possibly present in an internal scaffolding, distinct from the viral DNA, which appears to be present in electron micrographs. In addition to these two genes the T4 genome contains genes controlling the amount of DNA which is ultimately incorporated into the viral head and a gene determining the production of a solubilizing factor without which the capsid protein subunits precipitate from solution in the form of random aggregates.

In the multiplication of single-stranded DNA phages the first event following infection is the synthesis of a complementary DNA strand. This is achieved through the activity of the bacterial DNA polymerase. The double-stranded DNA thus formed then appears to code for a new phage DNA polymerase. In the synthesis of RNA phages a new enzyme—an RNA polymerase—is required for the synthesis of the phage RNA. The latter then functions as a messenger for the synthesis of phage proteins.

Phage Genetics

The study of the genetics of bacteriophages has been of enormous value in elucidating fundamental genetic mechanisms. That this should be so is not surprising since phages are essentially genes which can be transferred from one organism to another, and whose effect can be precisely evaluated under defined conditions. Bacteriophages differ from one another in a great variety of genetically controlled properties. Those which have been of most value in the study of genetic mechanisms have been: (a) Host range, that is the range of organisms against which the phage is active, and (b) The type of plaque produced. Both of these properties can be readily determined and are therefore particularly suitable for experimental work. Thus by the use of host range mutations in T2 (r II mutants) Benzer and his colleagues have been able to establish the unit of mutation and of recombination, in mixed infections, as being a single nucleotide.

If bacteria are infected with two recognizably different phages or with two different mutants of the same phage, recombination with the formation of hybrids occurs not only between the parent phage DNAs but also between the daughter phage DNAs. The genetic evidence indicates that prior to withdrawal of the DNA for naturation multiple rounds of mating occur in the replicating DNA pool. There is evidence that mating occurs both by breakage and reunion of paired DNA strands and by a copy choice mechanism in which replication of a new DNA begins on one strand and continues on another. When bacteria have undergone mixed infection with two phages the phenomenon of *phenotypic mixing* may also occur. In this process the DNA of one phage is accidentally coated with the head protein of another. The issuing phage has the host specificity of the second phage but on replication in a new host regains its original specificity.

Lysogeny

The elucidation of the precise relationship of a temperate phage with its lysogenic host bacterium first became possible with the discovery that *E. coli* K12, which is capable of undergoing conjugation (p. 26), carried a temperate phage called lambda (λ). Strains of K12 carrying λ are known as K12 (λ). In crosses between a non-lysogenic F$^+$ parent and a lysogenic F$^-$ parent, non-lysogenicity for λ was found to be linked to the *gal* locus. Similarly in crosses between an F$^+$ or Hfr parent—both of which are lysogenic for λ phages carrying different markers—with a non-lysogenic F$^-$ parent, the same linkage with the *gal* locus was found. These findings clearly established the location of the λ prophage on the bacterial chromosome.

The model currently accepted for the association of the prophage with the chromosome is that proposed by Campbell. This envisages recombination between areas of homology on a circular prophage and a circular bacterial chromosome, as a result of which the prophage becomes inserted linearly into the continuity of the bacterial chromosome. When non-lysogenic susceptible bacteria are infected with a temperate phage capable of lysogenizing them, the phage undergoes a lytic cycle of development in the majority of the infected cells but, in a small number of cells, becomes incorporated into the chromosome. The evidence indicates, however, that it is not the infecting phage DNA which is incorporated, but a replica of the infecting DNA. For some prophages more than one chromosomal locus at which the phage can be inserted has been identified. For others, e.g. the P1 coliphages, the chromosomal site is not known. This is believed to be due to the fact that in conjugation experiments—the only means of determining the chromosomal locus—the phage is released on conjugation from its chromosomal location.

When non-lysogenic F$^-$ cells are mated with lysogenic F$^+$ or Hfr cells lysogenic recombinants are never found. Instead the prophage embarks on a lytic cycle of multiplication in the infected F$^-$ cells. The discovery of this phenomenon, known as *zygotic induction*, established that the maintenance of the prophage state depends on the production, under the direction of the prophage genome, of a cytoplasmic repressor which prevents its transcription. When the prophage gains access, on conjugation, to a non-lysogenic cell which does not possess the cytoplasmic repressor, transcription is derepressed, and the lytic cycle of multiplication can occur. Derepression or *induction* (p. 30) of prophage can be achieved in a variety of ways, e.g. by exposure to various chemicals, but particularly by ultra-violet irradiation. In the small proportion of cells in a lysogenic culture which undergo lysis and liberate phage, induction of the prophage is a spontaneous event occurring, possibly, as a result of the action of some inducing substance liberated during bacterial growth. The establishment of the lysogenic state in a small proportion of the infected cells, when non-lysogenic bacteria are exposed to phage, is best interpreted as a race between the production of repressor with its effective control of the phage genome, and the translation of the genome into the synthesis of phage enzymes and phage components. In most cases the latter is dominant, and the phage undergoes a lytic cycle of infection but, in some cells, the repressor wins and the phage is incorporated into the bacterial chromosome.

A symbiotic phage may give rise to mutants which have lost their capacity to lysogenize. This may occur as a result of mutations in different parts of the phage genome: (1) The phage may lose its capacity to synthesize repressor, as a result of mutation in the regulator gene. (2) The phage operator may become insensitive to the repressor. (3) A mutation may occur affecting the area of the phage genome which is homologous with, and pairs with, the bacterial genome; recombination between the bacterial and phage genomes cannot then occur.

Transduction

This is a process in which genetic material is transferred by the agency of bacteriophage from one bacterium to another. Transduction may be effected by both symbiotic or temperate phages. They may acquire host cell genetic material in one of two ways: (1) Through an exchange between homologous areas on the phage and host cell chromosomes; as a result some of the host cell chromosome is incorporated into the phage chromosome. (2) By a process of phenotypic mixing in which the host cell genetic material is incorporated, together with the phage genome, in the phage head. Transduction was first described by Ledeberg and Zinder who found that certain auxotrophic mutants of *Salm. typhimurium* were converted into prototrophs by exposing them to filtrates of other strains possessing the nutritional capacity in which they were deficient. The agent responsible was shown to be a bacteriophage, designated P22. Transduction has also been demonstrated in *E. coli, Shigella, Pseudomonas, Staph. aureus* and *B. subtilis*.

Two types of transduction may be distinguished: (1) Generalized or unrestricted, and (2) Localized or restricted.

1. Generalized Transduction

Transduction in *Salm. typhimurium* with phage P22 is an example of generalized transduction. In this, any gene of the donor cell can be transduced. In respect of any particular marker only 10^{-5} to 10^{-7} P22 particles are capable of transducing. The fragment of host cell genome transferred appears, in the case of P22, to be incorporated into the phage head as a result of phenotypic mixing. On infection of the recipient strain the chromosomal fragment is integrated into the recipient's chromosome but the recipient does not become lysogenic for the transducing phage, possibly because the latter is defective and has lost its region of homology with the recipient chromosome. In some cases the chromosomal fragment is not integrated but is maintained in the cytoplasm and is transmitted to one daughter cell only at each subsequent division. In the cytoplasm it is genetically active and determines the phenotypic expression of the transduced property; this can of course only occur in the single cell in which the fragment is present. This phenomenon, known as *abortive transduction*, was first observed by Stocker, who found flares of growth at various distances from the site of inoculation of a strain of *Salm. typhimurium* which he had attempted to transduce for motility, the flares being due to the movement over the surface of the medium of a single abortively transduced and, consequently, motile cell leaving behind it a trail of non-transduced, non-motile cells.

2. Localized or Restricted Transduction

This type is effected by prophages which have a permanent locus on the bacterial chromosome, and which, on induction, are capable of transducing only those genes which are adjacent to this locus. Thus lambda phage is capable of transducing only the genes for galactose fermentation. When lambda prophage is induced some of the prophage particles incorporate a chromosomal segment carrying the *gal* locus, at the same time leaving behind a segment of their own genome in the bacterial chromosome. On infection of the recipient cell the prophage carrying the donor chromosomal fragment is integrated into the recipient chromosome. Since, however, the prophage is defective, lacking some of its own chromosome, it is incapable of yielding infective phage on induction. On induction it may, however, if the defect in the genome is relatively slight, determine the synthesis of phage components and cause lysis of the cell. If the defect in the phage genome is more severe, lysis does not occur on induction, and phage components are not synthesized. In this case the presence of the prophage on the bacterial chromosome may be demonstrated by the immunity of the cell to superinfection with fully infective phage.

Lambda transductants are diploid for the *gal* locus and segregate out *gal*-positive and *gal*-negative cells. Partial diploids of this type are known as *heterogenotes*, and appear to represent an intermediate phase in which the phages associate with, but are not stably integrated into, the chromosome.

Transducing phages can transfer episomes or plasmids as well as chromosomal genes. C factors (p. 567), F factors (p. 26) and R factors (p. 195) have all been transferred in this way, as have penicillinase plasmids in staphylococci (p. 249). Transduction is in fact the only way in which these plasmids can be transferred.

Phage Conversion

This phenomenon, which closely resembles transduction, consists in the genetic alteration of the cell, either (1) by a temperate phage which can establish the lysogenic state, or (2) by lytic variants of temperate phages which can only undergo a lytic cycle of infection. The best known example of (1) is the control of toxin production in *C. diphtheriae* by β phage (p. 284). In this case, toxin is only produced when the phage is induced. In salmonellae in which conversion has been demonstrated in respect of antigenic composition, induction of the prophage is not necessary for the appearance of the new property.

Sexduction

A process of genetic transfer basically similar to transduction (p. 29) has been shown to be mediated in *E. coli* K12 by substituted or intermediate—F'—sex factors. These are sex factors that have undergone recombination with an area contiguous to the F locus on the bacterial chromosome. Substituted sex factors appear to migrate rapidly to and fro, between the chromosome and the cytoplasm. They resemble F in being transmissible to F⁻ cells, and they resemble Hfr (p. 28) in determining high frequency chromosomal transfer.

Phenotypic or Host-controlled Modification

Bacteriophages may, in addition to genotypic modification or mutation, also undergo a non-genetic form of variation known as host-controlled modification. This is a variation of a temporary nature in the host range of the phage, occurring as the result of a single cycle of growth in a new bacterial host. It appears to be due to a modification produced in the phage DNA by the new host and manifesting itself in an increased capacity of the phage to infect and multiply in the host and/or a decreased capacity to infect and multiply in an alternative host. If one host is designated as A and the second as B the process may be illustrated as follows. When propagated on host A the phage has a high capacity to grow on host A but a low capacity to grow on host B. This is most conveniently represented by the term efficiency of plating (EOP). Taking the EOP on host A to be 1 and assuming that only 1 in 100,000 particles growing on host A propagates on host B then the EOP on host B is 10^{-5}. If propagated on host B, however, the EOP of the issuing phage in host B is equal to that on host A, i.e. 1. From these observations alone it would clearly be impossible to distinguish between an extension of host range produced by phenotypic modification and an extension produced by mutation. The distinction may however be made by examination of the fate of the modified phage when propagated again on host A. Phenotypically modified phage when so propagated regains its original specificity, i.e. it again has a low EOP on strain B. Mutated particles on the other hand retain their mutant host range with a high EOP on strain B.

The most extensively studied example of phenotypic modification is that which occurs in phage λ when propagated in a strain of *E. coli* K12 lysogenized by the symbiotic phage P1, the lysogenic strain being known as K12(P1). If the phage is first grown on non-lysogenic K12 its EOP on *E. coli* K12(P1) is approximately 2×10^{-5}. There is considerable evidence that the majority of the particles fail to grow on K12(P1) because the DNA of the infecting particles is, shortly after infection, degraded to small molecular weight components, presumably as a result of the action of a nuclease synthesized under the influence of the P1 genome. The few particles which succeed in infecting K12(P1) are not mutant particles and differ in no way from the rest of the λ population derived from K12. They multiply in K12(P1) because they have infected a small number of cells in the K12(P1) population which have, for some reason a diminished phage-inactivating capacity. This capacity is markedly influenced by environmental factors and, as recently shown by Schell and Glover, is heat labile. It therefore seems likely that the diminished capacity of a minority of K12(P1) cells to inactivate the phage is due to the influence of physiological conditions within the bacterial cells. The particles issuing from K12(P1), in contrast to those coming from K12, are unrestricted and plate efficiently both on K12(P1) and K12. They have been modified as a result of growth on K12(P1) so that they are insusceptible to inactivation by K12(P1). It is thought that this modification may take the form of a specific alteration in certain base sequences in the phage DNA possibly as a result of methylation. Whatever the basis of the modification, non-lysogenic K12, by reversing it, can be regarded as producing a modification of its own which renders the phage normally unacceptable by K12(P1). In this particular case, as in many others that have been studied, restriction is related to lysogenization which is not however necessary for restriction since Cλ, when propagated on another strain of *E. coli*, is found to be restricted for non-lysogenic K12. From the above it will be seen that the modifying host has two actions, (1) it can break down unmodified phage and (2) it can modify the survivors so that they are resistant to this breakdown.

A particularly important example of host-controlled modification is that observed in the adaptation of *Salmonella typhi* Vi II phage which has been grown on *Salm. typhi*, type A, and which as a result is active only on type A, by growth on certain other non-lysogenic *Salm. typhi* phage types (p. 564). Thus if phage grown on type A and with a low EOP against, for example, non-lyso-genic type C1 is grown on C1, the issuing particles after a single cycle of growth plate efficiently on C1. If however they are again propagated on type A they revert in a single cycle of growth to the wild type Vi II phage. Type adaptation due to phenotypic modification can in practice be distinguished from type adaptation due to mutation by the fact that the phenotypically modified phage when propagated on type A reverts to type A; a host range mutant on the other hand, when propagated on Type A, retains its mutant specificity.

Bacteriophage Typing

Bacteriophages are of considerable practical value to the bacteriologist as epidemiological tools since certain bacterial species can be subdivided on the basis of their susceptibility to various phages into a number of stable phage types. The value of phage typing in epidemiological studies has already been discussed (Chapter 11).

Salmonella typhi

The phages used in the typing of *Salm. typhi* are active only on Vi-containing strains and are consequently known as Vi phages. All are derived from a parent phage—Vi phage II—isolated by Craigie and Yen. These workers found that by propagating this phage on different strains of *Salm. typhi* it could be rendered specific for the strain on which it was propagated; the adapted phages produced in this way are the specific typing phages. The phages and their corresponding bacterial types and subtypes, of which a total of 72 have been described, are designated by letters, A, B, C, D, E etc. and numbers 25 to 46.

In order to determine the phage type of a typhoid bacillus the phages are first propagated on a broth culture of the homologous type so as to yield a high titred preparation of the phage. The culture is then heated to 58° C for half an hour in order to kill any unlysed organisms present. The highest dilution of the resulting preparation which causes confluent lysis of the homologous type—the routine test dilution or RTD—is used in the test. In most cases confluent lysis is produced by a few hundred phage particles. Some of these may however be able to produce isolated plaques on heterologous types. In routine tests such

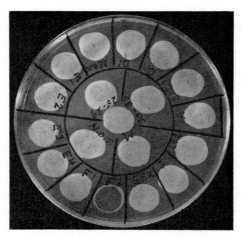

FIG. 67. BACTERIOPHAGE TYPING OF *Salmonella typhi*. The strain tested was of phage type F2 (*Dr E. S. Anderson*)

plaques are more likely to be found with adapted phages which produce very small plaques since with these a much greater number of particles are required to produce confluent lysis on the homologous type. The strain to be typed is spread either as a lawn, or in a number of areas each about the size of a sixpence on the surface of an agar plate. The inoculum is dried and a loopful of each of the test phages is placed on it. After incubation the type of the organism is shown by the presence of an area of confluent lysis with the homologous phage or, in the case of subtypes, by a pattern of lysis with a number of related phages.

The reactions of a representative series of typing phages and of the corresponding phage types are shown in the table below. It will be seen that type A differs from other types in being lysed by all the typing phages. On the other hand the type A phage, which is in fact the wild-type Vi II phage, is the most specific of the typing phages. In contrast to type A many types are lysed by only a single typing phage while others occupy an intermediate position in being lysed by a number of related phages. Such related phages define subgroups, namely C, D, E, F, J, K, L, M the first member of which shows the same relation to the other members of the group as does type A to all other phage types in that it is lysed by all the phages defining the subgroup.

Each of the Vi phage types of *Salm. typhi* is capable of absorbing the full range of typing phages. Type specificity cannot therefore be due to differences in the nature of the phage receptors on the bacterial surface. In fact it would

VI Phage Typing of *Salmonella typhi*

Salm. typhi types	Reactions of representative types*												Structural formula†	Change in phage‡
	Typing phages													
	A	B1	B3	C1	C2	C3	D1	D2	D6	F1	F2	29		
A	CL	CL	CL	CL	CL	CL	CL	CL	CL	CL	CL	CL	A	
B1	+	CL	++	−	−	+	+	−	−	+	+	+	B1	G
B3	−	−	CL	−	−	−	+	+	−	−	−	−	A(b3)	G
C1	+	++	−	CL	CL	CL	+	−	+	+	+	+	C1	P
C2	−	−	−	−	CL	−	−	−	+	−	−	−	C1(d6)	P/G
C3	−	−	−	+	CL	CL	−	−	+	−	−	+	C1(f2)	P/G
D1	−	+	−	+	CL	−	CL	CL	CL	−	+	−	A(d1)	G
D2	−	−	−	−	−	−	−	CL	−	−	−	−	D2	G/P
D6	−	−	−	−	SCL	++	+	−	CL	−	++	+	A(d6)	G
F1	−	−	−	−	−	−	−	−	−	CL	CL	−	F1	P
F2	−	−	−	−	−	−	−	−	−	+	CL	−	F1(f2)	P/G
29	−	+	++	+	CL	CL	+	−	CL	+	CL	CL	A(f2)	G

* CL = confluent lysis, SCL = semi-confluent lysis, + and ++ = increasing numbers of isolated plaques.

† Structural formula is indicated as non-lysogenic precursor, in capitals, followed by designation of type-determining phage, in parentheses. The latter are identified according to phage type of strain from which they were isolated.

‡ Change in phage indicates the change involved in adaptation of the wild-type Vi II phage to yield the specific typing phage. P = phenotypic or host controlled modification, G = genotypic modification, i.e. mutation.

Data from Bernstein, A. and Wilson, E. M. J. (1963). *J. gen. Microbiol.*, **32**, 349.

appear that all the typing phages are adsorbed to the cell through the same receptor, viz. the Vi antigen. In some cases the occurrence of transduction in the absence of multiplication has established not only that the phage is adsorbed but that its DNA gains entry to the cell. Specificity must therefore depend on differences in the capacity of the different phage types to permit the growth of the typing phages. The mechanisms involved have been extensively investigated by Felix and Anderson. These workers have shown that the specificity of several of the types can be related to the presence in them of symbiotic type-determining phages. At least 16 different type-determining phages have so far been isolated. With these it is possible to alter deliberately the phage type of any strain. The type-determining phages would appear to act by preventing in some way the growth of heterologous typing phages, presumably by some sort of interference mechanism. A number of the phage types, however, are not demonstrably lysogenic or not lysogenic with a phage capable of type determination. The non-lysogenic types would appear to be the precursors from which other types are derived by lysogenization with the appropriate type-determining phage. The different non-lysogenic types differ, however, in the way in which their type specificity is modified by infection with a particular type-determining phage. Thus infection of the non-lysogenic type A with the type-determining phage (d6) from type D6 yields type D6 but infection of the non-lysogenic type C with the same phage yields type 33. Consequently a limited number of non-lysogenic precursor types and a limited number of type-determining phages can give rise to a large number of Vi phage types.

Of the various non-lysogenic types type A appears to be in a special position. It is the non-lysogenic precursor of many lysogenic phage types, many of which appear to be capable of spontaneously reverting to it. The fact that it is lysed by all the typing phages suggests that it is the most primitive of all the types and that other non-lysogenic precursor types have also been derived from it. This might conceivably occur as a result of a mutation affecting the capacity of the organism to be infected by, or to support the multiplication of, the wild-type Vi II phage. In some cases it is possible that the apparently non-lysogenic precursor type is in fact lysogenic for a defective prophage (p. 559) or for a phage with a high tendency to lysogenization and which cannot as a result be detected by ordinary lytic indicator tests. This may be the case in respect of types such as B1 (see above table), phage adaptation to which resembles adaptation to types whose specificity is determined by type-determining phages in being purely genotypic in nature.

The nature of the adaptation of wild-type Vi II phage to yield the specific typing phages has been examined extensively by Anderson and his co-workers. The changes involved may be purely genotypic i.e. they may be host range mutations or purely phenotypic, in other words they may be host-controlled modifications achieved by one cycle of growth on the new type, the adapted phage reverting to the wild type when propagated on type A, or they may represent a combination of genotypic and phenotypic modification. When adaptation occurs to types derived from type A by lysogenization with type-determining phages the changes involved are purely genotypic. In most cases of adaptation to non-lysogenic types other than type A, the change is phenotypic while adaptation to types derived by lysogenization of non-lysogenic precursors other than type A involves a combination of genotypic and phenotypic modification.

Other Salmonellae

Phage typing is also applied to the typing, for epidemiological purposes, of *Salm. paratyphi B*, *Salm. typhimurium*, *Salm. enteritidis*, *Salm. dublin* and *Salm.*

paratyphi A. With these organisms, however, the types are defined by the pattern of reactions obtained with a number of phages rather than by specific reactions with type-specific phages. Many of the phages used are symbiotic. Phage typing has been used most for *Salm. paratyphi B*, in which, in the scheme elaborated by Felix and Callow, a total of 30 types, subtypes and variations have been described and for *Salm. typhimurium* in which 24 types have been described. There is some evidence that as in the case of *Salm. typhi* certain of these types are determined by the presence of type-determining symbiotic phages.

A different technique has been described by Boyd for the typing of *Salm. typhimurium*; in this the types are defined not by the susceptibility of the organisms to various typing phages but according to the nature of the symbiotic bacteriophages which they carry. This procedure is technically more difficult and slower than the conventional technique and has had as a result only limited epidemiological application. It has the additional defects that it can be applied only to lysogenic strains and that it will not differentiate strains carrying the same symbiotic phage but which may be derived from different non-lysogenic precursors.

Staphylococcus aureus

The phage typing of *Staph. aureus* is technically considerably more difficult than the typing of the salmonellae. The phages employed are symbiotic phages derived from lysogenic strains of *Staph. aureus*. Twenty-one of these phages constitute the basic set of typing phages in the scheme described by Williams and Rippon. They fall into four groups of antigenically related phages. An individual strain of *Staph. aureus* is usually lysed only by phages of one serological group. Virtually all strains derived from human sources belong to groups I, II and III. In this scheme strains are distinguished by the pattern of results they give with the typing phages and are designated by formulae indicating the individual phages to which they are susceptible; they cannot, as can *Salm. typhi*, be assigned to types on the basis of reactions with type-specific phages. The precise basis for this pattern specificity has not been determined but since many strains of *Staph. aureus* are lysogenic it is probable that in such cases it is determined by symbiotic type-determining phages.

Other Species

Bacteriophage typing has also been found to be of value for the epidemiological typing of *Ps. aeruginosa* and of *V. cholerae*.

BACTERIOCINES

This name is applied to a group of antibiotic proteins produced by strains of a number of bacterial species and which show a highly specific action against other strains of the same or closely related species. Bacteriocine-producing strains are resistant to their own bacteriocine, though they may be sensitive to bacteriocines produced by other strains of the same species. So far bacteriocine production has been demonstrated in the following genera: *Escherichia, Klebsiella, Arizona, Serratia, Pseudomonas, Pasteurella, Bacillus, Listeria* and in *Strep. faecalis* and *Staph. aureus*. In *E. coli* bacteriocinogeny is determined by the presence of cytoplasmic genetic determinants or episomes. Whether this is true of all bacteriocines remains to be seen.

Bacteriocines have not been used, so far, as chemotherapeutic agents, and it is on the whole unlikely that they have any significant therapeutic application: (1) Their molecules are too big for free diffusion in the body and for traversing membrane barriers. (2) They would almost inevitably stimulate antibody production. (3) Their spectrum of action is extremely restricted. (4) Their

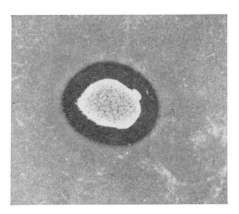

FIG. 68. ACTION OF A BACTERIOCINE PRODUCED BY ONE STRAIN OF *Str. faecalis* ON A SECOND INDICATOR STRAIN OF *Str. faecalis*

Producing strain (in centre) is grown first as a macrocolony on surface of agar plate. After incubation a second layer of agar incorporating the indicator strain is poured over the first

susceptibility to proteolytic enzymes would prevent their being administered orally. Bacteriocine susceptibility is however proving of considerable value as an epidemiological marker, e.g. in the typing of strains of *Sh. sonnei* and of *Ps. aeruginosa*.

Colicines

The production by strains of *E. coli* of bactericidal substances active against other strains of *E. coli* was first demonstrated by Gratia in 1925, and much of our present knowledge has derived from the work of Gratia and of Fredericq.

Approximately 30 to 40 per cent of randomly selected strains of *E. coli* are colicinogenic, and 60 to 70 per cent of *E. coli* strains are sensitive to one or more colicines.

Colicine production is most readily demonstrated by the macrocolony technique. In this, the producing strain is inoculated over an area of about 1 cm in diameter, on the surface of an agar plate. After overnight incubation the organisms present in the macrocolony are killed by exposure to chloroform vapour. This is most readily achieved by pouring some chloroform into the lid of the plate and holding the plate in an inverted position over the lid for half an hour. The plate is then seeded by flooding with a broth culture of the appropriate indicator strain, the excess fluid being pipetted off. After further incubation, colicine activity produces a clear zone of growth inhibition around the macrocolony—the organisms originally seeded in this zone having been killed by the action of colicine. As might be expected from diffusion of colicine through the agar, colicines are also demonstrable in cell-free filtrates.

Colicines appear to be liberated by only a minority of the cells of a colicine-producing culture. In these, colicine liberation is associated with the death of the cell. Because of this, colicine production has been described as a lethal biosynthesis, but the mechanisms involved are not understood. In many cases colicine liberation can be induced in all of the cells of a colicinogenic culture by exposure of the culture to ultra-violet light. This phenomenon shows a marked resemblance to the induction of symbiotic bacteriophage and, like the latter, is associated with lysis of the producer.

Colicines adsorb to specific receptors on the surface of susceptible cells. An organism may acquire resistance to a particular colicine by mutation. This resistance has been shown to be due to loss of the appropriate receptor. On the basis of their spectrum of action and their cross resistance patterns, Fredericq has distinguished a total of seventeen colicines. The differentiation of types of colicines and of different colicine receptors therefore makes possible the use of colicinogeny and colicine sensitivity as strain marker techniques in epidemiological procedures.

In some cases the same receptor is involved in the adsorption of a colicine and of a bacteriophage. Thus bacteriophage T6 has the same receptor as colicine K. In this case there is a complete cross resistance between the bacteriophage and the colicine. There is also evidence that some colicines may adsorb to receptors involved in conjugation.

The genetic determinants of a number of colicines have been shown to be extrachromosomal, and therefore to come within the general category of episome. They are known as C factors. There is however no evidence that C factors can, like prophages and sex factors, become integrated at any stage into the bacterial chromosome. In certain cases C factors can transfer spontaneously from organisms possessing them to organisms lacking them, the latter becoming, as a result, colicinogenic. Spontaneous transfer requires cell contact, and is analogous to F transfer in conjugation. Some C factors are, however, incapable of mediating their own transfer but may be transferred, as in the case of *Col* E1 by the F factor or by other C factors. Self-transfer of C factors is most readily achieved with newly acquired C factors, a phenomenon known as high frequency colicinogeny transfer (HFCT).

C factors create immunity to the corresponding colicine and, as a general rule, to other colicines of the same type. The lack of cross immunity between colicines of similar specificity has provided the basis for a further subdivision of colicines. Thus, type E can be divided into E1 and E2, both combining with the same receptors but differing in that the E1 C factor confers resistance only against E1, and the E2 C factor only against E2. The resistance produced by C factors shows considerable resemblance to the resistance produced by prophage to superinfection with the same or with a closely related phage. It presumably involves a block, probably at an early stage, in the colicine biosynthetic passway.

In cases in which their composition has been investigated, C factors have been found to be composed of DNA, that of colicine E2 having been estimated to contain 3 by 10^4 nucleotide pairs. This would be sufficient DNA to code for about twenty proteins of molecular weight of about 40,000. It seems likely therefore that C factors possess genetic information capable of determining properties other than colicinogeny.

Colicines appear to have a primarily bactericidal action. It the case of colicines K and E2, the colicines whose action has been examined in most detail, adsorption of the colicine is followed very rapidly by a cessation of all macromolecular syntheses. After adsorption there appears to be an appreciable period during which the lethal effect of the colicine can be prevented by treatment of the cells with trypsin, which destroys the adsorbed colicine. It seems likely therefore that the biochemical lesion which results in the death of the cell is produced by the colicine while adsorbed. This lesion has not been identified with any demonstrable alteration in the permeability of the cytoplasmic membrane, though the possibility of the occurrence of a highly specific membrane lesion cannot be excluded. In some cases it would appear that the cell can be killed by the action of a single colicine particle, a finding which suggests an analogy between colicine action and the action of complement. This might, however, require, as in the case of complement lysis, the adsorption of a large number of particles, only one of which has a lethal effect.

Colicinogeny determinants clearly show considerable resemblance, on the one hand, to symbiotic bacteriophages and, on the other, to sex factors. They can occur as cytoplasmic determinants, they can replicate in phase with the nucleus and they are transmissible. Their resemblance to bacteriophage genomes, and the occasional sharing of receptors by bacteriophages and colicines, have prompted Fredericq to speculate that they are defective bacteriophages synthesized by a genome which is incapable of synthesizing the entire bacteriophage. Evidence in support of this view has been obtained by Bradley, who has found, on electron microscopy, bacteriophage-like particles sedimenting with certain colicines at 15,000 g. Other colicines were not sedimented under these conditions, however, and the group would appear to be heterogeneous. The non-sedimentable type might possibly be colicines, like colicine K, which have been found by Goebel to be associated with the somatic antigens of the producing strains into which they appear to be incorporated as additional components. Bradley also found structures resembling bacteriophage tails in preparations from bacteriocinogenic strains of *Ps. aeruginosa*, the central channel of the tail containing what may have been a DNA strand. He has suggested that death of the cell could be due to injection of this DNA which, however, unlike phage DNA is incapable of replication. Structures resembling bacteriophage tails have also been identified in a bacteriocinogenic strain of *V. cholerae*.

Recently a number of C factors (*col* factors) have been found to determine the production of specialized pili (sex pili) morphologically distinguishable from the common (type 1) pili frequently found in Gram negative bacteria (p. 11). The specialized pili so far described fall into two groups: 1. Pili resembling morphologically, and in their capacity to adsorb specific male (F +) bacterioghages, the pili whose production is determined by the sex factor (F) and by fi + R factors. 2. Pili resembling morphologically and in their capacity to adsorb a different specific bacteriophage—I—the pili produced by the majority of fi − R factors. It is proposed that the two types of pili should be designated F and I respectively. From the evidence available it would appear that the types are antigenically distinct but that all pili of the same type are antigenically closely related. F and I pili almost certainly constitute the conjugation tubes through which C factors are transferred from one strain to another. Pili to which neither F nor I bacteriophages adsorb have been identified in some R + bacteria but similar pili have not so far been shown to be determined by C factors. It is clear that a rational classification of colicines requires not only the identification of those whose production is associated with the presence of bacteriophage components but also the recognition of C factors determining the production of specialized pili as well as the identification of the type of pilus produced.

CHAPTER 43

THE PATHOGENIC FUNGI

Although widely distributed in nature and of considerable importance as causes of disease in plants and animals fungi are very much less frequently the cause of disease in man than are bacteria.

Most of the fungi pathogenic for man belong to the large class of fungi known as *fungi imperfecti*. These are fungi which have no demonstrable sexual stage, and reproduce by the formation of various types of asexual spores. On the basis of their microscopic morphology they can be conveniently divided into four morphological groups:

1. *Filamentous fungi.* The most important of these are the dermatophytes or ringworm fungi. The basic morphological elements of the filamentous fungi are long branching filaments or hyphae which intertwine to produce a tangled mass of filaments or *mycelium*. When such fungi are grown on solid media some of the mycelium, known as *vegetative* mycelium, penetrates deeply into the medium while some grows above the surface of the medium as an *aerial* mycelium. The filamentous fungi reproduce by a variety of asexual spores—*arthrospores*, *chlamydospores* and *conidia*. Arthrospores are spores formed by fragmentation of the hyphae into small more or less rectangular segments. Chlamydospores are spores formed by migration of the protoplasm from a number of hyphal segments into a single segment which becomes much enlarged and acquires a thick cell wall. They are in some ways analogous to bacterial spores being produced under conditions unfavourable to the growth of the fungus proper and capable of remaining dormant for long periods. Conidia are spores formed at the tips or sides of the hyphae. They may be directly attached to the hyphae or may be carried on special supporting structures known as conidiophores. Conidia may be small and single—called *microconidia*, or large and multicellular—*macroconidia*. The various types of asexual spores referred to above are seen only when the fungi are grown in the laboratory at room temperature. In the body or when grown at 37° C only arthrospores are produced.

Because of their mycelial character the colonies of the filamentous fungi are strongly adherent to the medium and, unlike most bacterial colonies, cannot be emulsified in water. The surface of the colony may be warty, velvety or powdery or may show a cottony aerial mycelium. Pigmentation of the colony itself and of the underlying medium is frequently present. The macroscopic appearance of the colonies are very susceptible to slight differences in cultural conditions and since their interpretation in species identification requires considerable experience will not be considered in detail.

2. *Yeasts.* These occur in the form of round or oval bodies which reproduce by the formation of buds known as blastospores. Yeast colonies resemble bacterial colonies in appearance and consistency. The only pathogenic yeast is *Cryptococcus neoformans.*

3. *Yeast-like fungi.* These are fungi which occur both in the form of budding yeast-like cells and as chains of elongated unbranched filamentous cells which present the appearance of broad septate hyphae. New buds are formed at the points of constriction of the hyphae. The latter intertwine to form a *pseudo-mycelium* which has some capacity to penetrate into the underlying medium. The yeast-like fungi are grouped together in the genus *Candida.*

4. *Dimorphic fungi.* These are fungi which exhibit a filamentous mycelial morphology—the saprophytic phase—when grown at room temperature, but have a typical yeast morphology—the parasitic phase—in the body and when grown at 37° C in the laboratory.

All the pathogenic fungi grow readily on the ordinary media used for the cultivation of bacteria. They are aerobic in character and grow best under humid conditions. Growth, however, is frequently slow and cultures may require incubation for one or more weeks. As a routine medium for fungal isolation Sabouraud's glucose agar is mainly used. This medium is highly acid in reaction —pH 5·5—because of which it is strongly inhibitory to bacteria. For the isolation of the yeast-like and dimorphic fungi, blood agar, which may be rendered selective for fungi by the incorporation of penicillin and streptomycin or of chloramphenicol, should also be employed. Certain other media are used for special purposes, e.g. corn meal agar to encourage the development of chlamydospores by *Candida albicans.* For the isolation of filamentous fungi, cultures should be incubated at room temperature or in an incubator at 22° C to 26° C at which temperature the characteristic morphology of these fungi is best seen. In other cases incubation should be both at 37° C and at room temperature.

The pathogenic fungi most frequently encountered in medical practice are the dermatophytes which cause the various conditions known colloquially as ringworm. These are entirely superficial infections, the fungus growing in the skin or its appendages and showing no tendency to invade the deeper tissues. In contrast to the dermatophytes the yeast-like and dimorphic fungi are capable of invading the tissues and of giving rise to generalized or systemic infections. Fungal infections of this type are very uncommon in the British Isles. Since fungi do not produce toxins the tissue reactions found in the systemic mycoses are characteristically of a granulomatous type. In general, fungal diseases differ from bacterial diseases in being much more chronic in character and, except in certain types of ringworm in children, in not occurring in epidemic form.

Diagnosis of Fungal Infections

An attempt should be made to demonstrate the fungus by direct microscopic examination of the suspected material. In the identification of the filamentous fungi microscopic examination is usually carried out with unstained wet preparations. Fungi which invade the tissues can usually be demonstrated in sections stained with haematoxylin and eosin or with Gram's stain but better results are obtainable with the periodic acid Schiff technique (p. 38). With this method most fungi are stained a bright red. The method can be used to restain sections already stained with haematoxylin and eosin.

When a fungus has been isolated on culture morphological examination is of paramount importance for its identification. For the examination of filamentous fungi and of dimorphic fungi in the saprophytic phase wet preparations are essential since the organized structure of the fungus is broken up in the preparation of fixed films of the type used for the demonstration of bacteria. For this purpose a small portion of the growth should be gently teased out on a slide in a drop of lactophenol blue and the preparation covered with a coverslip. A permanent preparation can be made, if required, by sealing the edges of the coverslip with nail varnish. The morphology of filamentous fungi is most satisfactorily studied in situ. For this, various types of slide culture, which are inoculated from the primary culture, may be used. For the demonstration of yeast forms satisfactory preparations may be obtained by simply emulsifying a small amount of the growth in a drop of water.

Except for the differentiation of *Candida* and *Cryptococcus* species biochemical tests are of no value in species identification. Pathogenicity tests are rarely used but are sometimes of value in the identification of *C. albicans* and in the differentiation of *Cryptococcus neoformans* from non-pathogenic cryptococci. Serological tests are not of value in fungal identification.

Antibodies detectable by ordinary in vitro tests are not produced during the course of superficial fungal infections but are sometimes demonstrable in the sera of patients suffering from systemic mycoses. Delayed type hypersensitivity, demonstrable by the intradermal injection of an appropriate fungal extract, is, however, frequently present in both superficial and systemic fungal infections. Its demonstration may sometimes be of value in diagnosis.

Chemotherapy

Most fungi are quite insusceptible to the chemotherapeutic agents used in the treatment of bacterial infections. The following substances, which are inactive against bacteria, are however effective in the systemic treatment of certain types of fungal infection. Their action appears to be purely fungistatic.

Iodides. These are reported to be of value in the treatment of sporotrichosis, phycomycosis and pulmonary aspergillosis.

Nystatin (Mycostatin). This antibiotic, derived from *Streptomyces noursei*, possesses considerable in vitro activity against *Candida albicans* and certain of the dimorphic fungi. Administered by the oral route it has been found to be useful in the treatment and prophylaxis of oral and intestinal candidiasis induced by wide-spectrum antibiotic therapy. The drug is, however, poorly absorbed from the alimentary tract and is therefore relatively ineffective in the treatment of systemic *Candida* infections.

Amphotericin B. This antibiotic, which is produced by *Streptomyces nodosus*, is chemically similar to mycostatin and possesses a similar range of action. Of the two, amphotericin B appears to be the more active under in vitro conditions. It is not significantly absorbed from the alimentary tract and, like mycostatin, has been favourably reported on for the prophylaxis of oral and intestinal candidiasis induced by wide-spectrum antibiotic therapy. Administered by the intravenous route it is of established value in the treatment of North American blastomycosis, chromomycosis, coccidioidomycosis, histoplasmosis, crypto-coccosis and sporotrichosis.

Griseofulvin. This antibiotic, which is produced by various species of *Penicillium*, possesses a high degree of activity against all species of dermatophytes. It is well absorbed from the alimentary tract following oral administration and attains a high concentration in newly formed keratin. Since, however, it is not taken up significantly by keratin already formed administration of the drug must be continued until the latter has been allowed to grow out. In general the length of treatment required depends on the thickness of the epidermal structure affected; thus infections of the nails as a rule necessitate administration of the drug for several months. Griseofulvin has no action against *Candida albicans*, a fungus which can cause a variety of superficial infections resembling those produced by the dermatophytes. A precise mycological diagnosis is therefore an essential preliminary to its clinical use. In its action griseofulvin is fungistatic rather than fungicidal and although it has revolutionized the treatment of the dermatomycoses it has not eliminated the necessity for various forms of ancillary local treatment. The mechanism by which it inhibits fungal growth is unknown, but it is presumed to be by some type of specific interference with the synthesis of the fungal cell wall. It is significant that it acts only against fungi whose cell walls contain chitin as the main structural component. In high concentration griseofulvin is a potent inhibitor of mitosis but, apart from the occasional development of a transitory leucopenia which disappears when the drug is withdrawn, no serious toxic reactions following its administration have been described.

Stilbamidine. This compound and its 2-hydroxy derivative appear to be of value in the treatment of North American blastomycosis and sporotrichosis. Both compounds must be administered intravenously.

The Dermatophytes

The fungi of this group attack the keratinized surface of the body—the skin, hair and nails, producing the various conditions known collectively as ringworm. Dermatophytes have marked powers of digesting keratin which they can utilize for growth. They do not invade the tissues or cause systemic infection. They differ from other fungi in being transmissible from one infected animal or person to another. They may be divided into species which only infect man—*anthropophilic* species and species which primarily infect animals—*zoophilic* species.

Three pathogenic genera are distinguished, viz. *Microsporum, Trichophyton* and *Epidermophyton*. In culture all produce a typically filamentous growth.

Recent evidence suggests the identification of dermatophytes as the asexual forms of various ascus bearing fungi or *Ascomycetes* whose natural habitat is the soil.

Microsporum

The microspora attack the skin and hair but not the nails. The principal species are *M. audouini*, *M. canis* and *M. gypseum*. *M. audouini* is the commonest cause of ringworm of the scalp. It does not attack the glabrous skin. It is a specifically human parasite. *M. canis* is the cause of ringworm in cats and dogs and is a fairly frequent cause of human infections of the scalp, beard and glabrous skin. *M. gypseum* is a rare cause of ringworm in the British Isles but is common in South America. It is primarily an animal parasite.

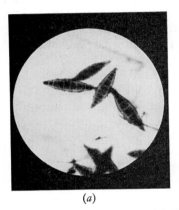 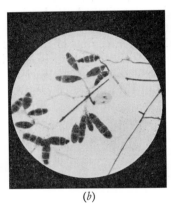

(a)   (b)

FIG. 69. MACROCONIDIA OF (a) *M. canis*, (b) *E. floccosum* (Lactophenol cotton blue)

Macroconidia are numerous in cultures of *M. canis* and *M. gypseum*. They are typically large—40 to 150μ in length by 8 to 30μ in width—thick-walled and spindle-shaped. They are uncommon in cultures of *M. audouini* but when present they are long and rudimentary. As a rule microconidia are few in number in primary cultures of microspora; when present they are borne singly along the sides of the hyphae.

Trichophyton

The trichophyta attack the skin, hair and nails. A great number of trichophyta have been described but these are now reduced to 14, the remainder being regarded as variants. The most important species are *T. mentagrophytes*, *T. verrucosum*, *T. rubrum*, *T. tonsurans* and *T. schoenleini*. *T. verrucosum* is the commonest cause of ringworm in cattle. *T. mentagrophytes* is also primarily an animal parasite producing ringworm in a variety of domestic and farm animals. *T. schoenleini*, *T. tonsurans* and *T. rubrum* are specifically human parasites.

Macroconidia are rare or absent in culture of trichophyta; when present they are typically thin-walled, narrow and pencil-shaped and smaller than those found in *Microsporum* cultures—4 to 6μ in width by 10 to 50μ in length. Microconidia are produced profusely by some species but rarely or not at all by others, e.g. *T. verrucosum* and *T. schoenleini*. They may be borne on the sides of the hyphae (*T. rubrum* and *T. tonsurans*) or in grape-like clusters (*T. mentagrophytes*). Certain special structures, e.g. 'favic chandeliers', i.e. hyphae with antler-like processes, which are seen particularly in cultures of *T. schoenleini*, and coiled hyphae known as 'spiral bodies' which are especially numerous in cultures of *T. mentagrophytes*, are found in *Trichophyton* cultures and are of value in identification.

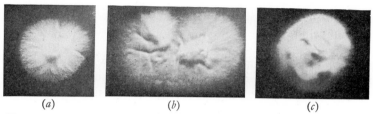

(a)   (b)   (c)

FIG. 70. COLONIES OF VARIOUS DERMATOPHYTES ON SABOURAUD'S MEDIUM
(a) *M. audouini*, (b) *M. canis*, (c) *T. mentagrophytes*

Epidermophyton

Only one species is described: *E. floccosum*. This species attacks the skin and nails but not the hair. Macroconidia are numerous in culture. They are large and club-shaped and are borne either singly or in clusters from the ends or sides of the hyphae. Microconidia are not produced.

Infections Caused by the Dermatophytes

Tinea capitis

This condition is almost entirely restricted to children in whom it is most frequently caused by *Microsporum* species, particularly by *M. audouini*. This is a specifically human pathogen and has a marked tendency to give rise to epidemics of infection.

In ringworm of the scalp the infection starts in the skin and invades the hair from the follicle mouth. As a result of the growth of the fungus in the hair the hair shaft is weakened and breaks off a short distance above the skin surface. In infections due to *M. audouini* the lesions are dry and scaly, the fungus does not stimulate an inflammatory reaction and the condition has little tendency to spontaneous cure. If untreated the infection may persist until puberty when it usually undergoes spontaneous involution. It has been suggested that this is due to the high fatty acid content of the adult hair. In infections due to *M. canis*, *M. gypseum* and the animal trichophyta there is frequently a marked inflammatory reaction with the production in the skin of a boggy, tumour-like mass known as kerion. This may result in damage to the hair bulb resulting in epilation and spontaneous cure. Infection with *T. tonsurans* produces a characteristic 'black dot' appearance of the scalp.

Tinea circinata (Ringworm of the Glabrous Skin)

This variety is usually caused by one of the animal trichophyta; the infection is usually derived from infected animals, although in children it may be secondary to *tinea capitis*. The lesions have a characteristic ring-form, healing in the centre, which has a dry scaly appearance, and spreading peripherally.

Tinea barbae (Ringworm of the Beard)

This is usually caused by one of the animal trichophyta—*T. mentagrophytes* or *T. verrucosum*. Deep infections, with the production of follicular pustules and of kerion-like lesions, are common. The deep type of lesion is known as sycosis.

Favus

This condition at one time not uncommon is now rarely seen; it is most frequently caused by *T. schoenleini*. The infection is usually limited to the scalp but may occasionally involve the glabrous skin and the nails. The disease, which is contracted in childhood but tending to persist into adult life, occurs only under very unhygienic conditions. The fungus tends to invade the skin more deeply than do other dermatophytes. It accumulates in large masses at the mouths of the hair follicles forming a cup or scutulum the apex of which is directed into the follicle. The scutula have a very characteristic mousy odour. Because of the deep nature of the infection scarring is frequent. The hairs are only slightly invaded and consequently do not break; as a result they may be seen standing out prominently from the centre of the scutulum.

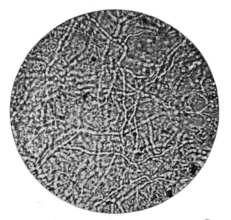

FIG. 71. HYPHAE OF DERMATOPHYTE IN SKIN

Tinea pedis

This condition, commonly known as 'athlete's foot', is nowadays the most frequently encountered of the dermatophyte infections. It is usually caused by *Trichophyton* species, particularly *T. mentagrophytes* and *T. rubrum* and occasionally by *E. floccosum*. The infection is frequently contracted in communal dressing rooms and swimming baths; infected shoes and socks are important sources of reinfection. The condition is uncommon in children.

Tinea cruris (Dhobie Itch)

This condition is characterized by the appearance of bilateral scaly lesions in the inguinal region. Similar lesions may also occur in the axillae and in the sub-mammary folds. *Tinea cruris* is usually caused by *E. floccosum*, less frequently by *Trichophyton* species.

Tinea unguium (Ringworm of the Nails)

This condition is the most intractable of all the dermatomycoses. It is usually caused by *T. rubrum*, *T. mentagrophytes* or *E. floccosum* and is quite frequently secondary to athlete's foot. The most severe infections are those produced by *T. rubrum* which tends to cause a destructive lesion involving the entire thickness of the nail plate. Nail infections similar to those caused by the dermatophytes may also be caused by *C. albicans* (p. 578).

In infections caused by the dermatophytes, particularly those due to *Tricho-phyton* species, a cutaneous hypersensitivity which can be detected by the intradermal injection of a fungal extract—*trichophytin*, which contains both group-specific and species-specific antigens—is frequently present. Hypersensitivity is present in the entire skin and is responsible for the secondary skin lesions or *mycids* which occasionally occur in the course of these infections. These are due to the action of fungal breakdown products, spread through the blood, on the sensitized skin.

Diagnosis of the Dermatomycoses

Three procedures are available:

1. Examination of the lesions under a Wood's lamp. This procedure is of particular value in the diagnosis of ringworm of the scalp and beard. Wood's lamp is a mercury vapour lamp fitted with a special filter which cuts off the visible light rays. Hairs infected with *Microsporum* species or with *T. schoenleini* fluoresce a bright green under the lamp. Hairs infected with other species either do not fluoresce or fluoresce a greyish white.

2. *Microscopy*. Before they are examined microscopically epithelial scrapings, nails and hairs must first be 'cleared'. This is done by suspending them in 10 to 20 per cent potassium hydroxide on a microscope slide when the alkali will dissolve the keratin thereby rendering the mycelium and spores of the fungus more readily visible. If necessary clearing may be accelerated by gently warming the preparation. Epithelial scales and hairs are usually adequately cleared in 10 to 15 minutes at room temperature but nail fragments may require some hours incubation at 37° C.

In infected epithelial cells and nails all the dermatophytes present an identical appearance, appearing as branching filaments which may or may not show fragmentation into arthrospores. From this appearance although a diagnosis of fungal infection can be made, generic or species differentiation is not possible. More precise information may be obtained from the microscopic appearance of the fungus in infected hairs. The microspora and *T. mentagrophytes* produce small spores 2 to 3μ in diameter which are arranged in a tightly packed mosaic on the outer surface of the hair (ectrothrix infections). *T. tonsurans* and *T. schoenleini* produce chains of large spores 4 to 6μ in diameter confined entirely to the interior of the hair (endothrix infections). *T. verrucosum* and *T. rubrum* produce large spores on the outer surface of the hair. A characteristic feature of infection with *T. schoenleini* is the occurrence of bubbles of gas in the infected hairs.

3. For complete identification of the infecting species cultural examination is essential. For this purpose Sabouraud's medium is generally used. Fragments

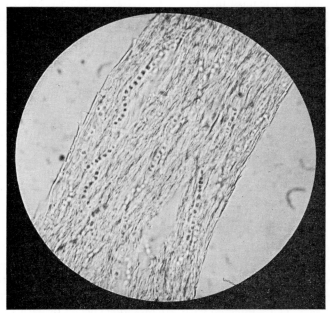

FIG. 72. ENDOTHRIX *Trichophyton* INFECTION OF HAIR (wet alkali preparation)
Note chains of arthrospores within hair shaft

of the hairs, epithelial scales or nail scrapings are planted firmly on the surface of the medium which is incubated at room temperature or in an incubator at 22 to 26° C. The identification of the species present depends on the rate of growth of the fungus and on its macroscopic and microscopic colonial morphology.

Candida albicans

This organism occurs both in the form of oval yeast-like bodies and as thick septate pseudo-hyphae (p. 571). *C. albicans* stains well by Gram's method and is Gram positive.

Candida albicans occurs as a normal inhabitant of the mouth and intestinal tract. It is the cause of thrush, a condition at one time common in children, in which white patches containing the fungus are found on the mucous membrane of the mouth. A similar condition may occur on the vaginal and vulval mucosa giving rise to vaginal irritation and discharge. This type of infection is particularly likely to occur in pregnancy and in diabetic subjects. *C. albicans* occasionally causes infections of the skin, especially intertriginous lesions of the

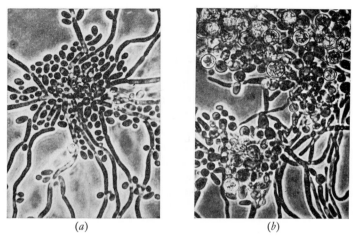

(*a*) (*b*)

FIG. 73. CULTURES OF *Candida* ON CORN MEAL AGAR (Phase contrast)
(*a*) Non-pathogenic species, (*b*) *Candida albicans*
Note chlamydospores in (*b*)

hands in people whose occupation involves frequent immersion of the hands in water. The fungus may also cause an infection of the nails resembling that produced by the dermatophytes but which is less destructive and is usually associated with a considerable degree of paronychia. It is an occasional cause of athlete's foot. During the course of wide-spectrum antibiotic therapy there may be considerable overgrowth of *C. albicans* in the lungs and in the alimentary and urogenital tracts. It is doubtful whether this overgrowth is associated with any significant degree of tissue invasion. Pulmonary invasion may, however, occur in individuals with prior lung disease, e.g. tuberculosis or cancer. Allergic vesicular skin lesions—*monilids*—may occur in any type of *C. albicans* infections.

The diagnosis of mucosal lesions is readily achieved by the examination of Gram stained films—the oval budding bodies being highly characteristic. For the diagnosis of cutaneous infections the methods described for the diagnosis of ringworm are employed.

Candida albicans grows readily on blood agar at 37° C, producing after 24 to 48 hours' incubation small greyish bacteria-like colonies. On Sabouraud's medium the colonies are cream-coloured and pasty and on prolonged incubation develop a honeycombed appearance as a result of glucose fermentation. A number of tests have been described for the differentiation of *C. albicans* from other *Candida* species. The most valuable of these are the demonstration of chlamydospore production on corn meal agar and sugar fermentation reactions. The chlamydospores which are large, round and thick-walled are produced at the tips of the hyphae. *C. albicans* ferments glucose and maltose, producing acid and gas, and sucrose, producing acid but no gas; it does not ferment lactose. In cases of doubt a pathogenicity test may be carried out in the rabbit. Rabbits inoculated intravenously with a suspension of the organism die in 4 to 5 days and show at post mortem multiple small white abscesses in the cortex of the kidney.

Cryptococcus neoformans

This fungus occurs both in the tissues and in cultures in the form of round yeast-like cells surrounded by a large gelatinous capsule. In the tissues the individual cells measure from 5 to 20μ in diameter but in culture they are considerably smaller, usually measuring from 2 to 5μ in diameter. No mycelium is produced either in the tissues or in culture but elongated tube-like cells are occasionally found. On Sabouraud's medium at room temperature *Cryptococcus neoformans* produces a glistening mucoid colony of brownish colour which in course of time flows down the slope to the bottom of the tube. The fungus may

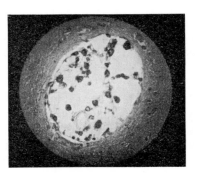

FIG. 74. *Cryptococcus neoformans* IN BRAIN. CRYPTOCOCCI ARE FREE IN CYSTIC CAVITY IN BRAIN SUBSTANCE (Haematoxylin and mucicarmine)

be distinguished from *Candida* species and non-pathogenic yeasts by its positive urease reaction, and from non-pathogenic cryptococci by its capacity to grow well at 37° C and by its lethal effect on mice on intraperitoneal inoculation.

Cryptococcus neoformans has a marked predilection for the central nervous system in which it produces a subacute or chronic meningitis—sometimes known as torula meningitis. In the lungs it may produce low grade inflammatory lesions which may be mistaken for tuberculosis or neoplasm. In addition the fungus may give rise to localized nodular lesions in the skin, or to a generalized infection with lesions in the skin, bones or viscera. The primary habitat of *Cryptococcus neoformans* is not known with certainty but may be the soil which appears to be the usual source of human infections. Infection is not transmitted from man to man.

In cases of meningitis the organism can be demonstrated in the centrifuged deposit from the cerebrospinal fluid and is readily recognized by its conspicuous capsule; the latter is best demonstrated in wet India ink preparations. The diagnosis of cryptococcal meningitis is, however, sometimes missed, the fungi being mistaken for lymphocytes. Immunofluorescence has been used for the demonstration of cryptococcal antigen in tissues. Antibodies may be demonstrated by immunofluorescence, complement fixation and passive haemagglutination.

Histoplasma capsulatum

This is a dimorphic fungus occurring in the tissues as small oval yeast-like bodies of from 3 to 5μ in length. In the body it multiplies mainly within the cells of the reticulo-endothelial system. On Sabouraud's medium, at room temperature, it produces a mould-like colony in which may be seen filaments, conidia, borne singly on short branches or sessile on the sides of the hyphae, and large chlamydospores—up to 15μ in diameter—with characteristic radiating processes. The tissue form is best obtained by growth in sealed tubes on Francis's cystine glucose blood agar. *H. capsulatum* is often difficult to grow and colonies frequently take some weeks to develop.

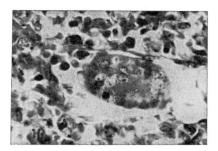

Fig. 75. Tissue Phase of *Histoplasma capsulatum* in Macrophage. Lymph Gland

Histoplasmosis is a common disease in certain parts of the United States and Central America but appears to be uncommon in other parts of the world. The infection primarily involves the lungs and in most cases is asymptomatic. In symptomatic infections the lung lesions are usually multiple and heal slowly by calcification. A generalized progressive infection occurs in a small proportion of cases. In this type of infection the liver, lymph nodes and spleen are particularly involved. In many cases of generalized infection the portal of entry of the fungus appears to be the skin or intestinal tract. The disease is not transmitted from case to case. In endemic areas the fungus is present in the soil, which is probably the main source of human infection. Fowl appear to constitute an important animal reservoir.

Antibodies detectable by complement fixation tests appear within a few weeks of infection. Cutaneous hypersensitivity is also present and may be detected by the intracutaneous injection of a filtrate of a fluid culture of *H. capsulatum* known as *histoplasmin*. The reaction is of delayed type and is indicative of past as well as of current infection. Histoplasmin contains a number of antigens some of which are non-specific. The specific antigen appears to be a polysaccharide.

The diagnosis of histoplasmosis is made by demonstrating the intracellular fungus in Giemsa-stained smears of peripheral blood, sternal bone marrow, sputum or infected lymph nodes—the histological appearance of macrophages filled with capsulated yeasts being highly characteristic. Isolation of the fungus should also be attempted.

Blastomyces

Two species of *Blastomyces* are described—*B. brasiliensis*, prevalent in Brazil and other parts of South America, and *B. dermatitidis*, which is apparently restricted to North America, occurring particularly in the eastern United States. Both are dimorphic fungi.

Blastomyces dermatitidis. In the tissues this fungus appears either free or within phagocytic cells as a round yeast-like body 8 to 15μ in diameter with a thick highly refractile cell wall. The cells, which in the tissues reproduce by the formation of a single bud, are often seen as pairs of cells of unequal size. On Sabouraud's medium at room temperature the growth is at first yeast-like but later assumes a typical mould form showing filaments, arthrospores and conidia resembling those of *H. capsulatum*. The yeast phase may be obtained on blood agar at 37° C when, in addition to the yeast form, characteristic short undeveloped mycelial fragments may also be seen.

Blastomyces dermatitidis causes both cutaneous and systemic granulomatous lesions. The cutaneous type of the disease is usually due to introduction of the organism through a wound in the skin. In the systemic type of infection lesions may occur almost anywhere in the body except the intestinal tract, but the lungs are principally involved and the organism probably gains entry through the respiratory tract. The disease does not spread from man to man but the source of infection is not known.

Delayed type hypersensitivity develops as a result of infection and may be detected by the intradermal injection of an extract of the fungus—*blastomycin*. Positive skin reactions to blastomycin are also given by persons with histoplasmosis and less frequently by those suffering from coccidioidomycosis. The complement fixation test using a suspension of living organisms as antigen has some diagnostic value. It is also of prognostic value, a high titre indicating a poor prognosis.

Blastomyces brasiliensis. The tissue form of this organism is somewhat larger than that of *B. dermatitidis* being usually from 20 to 30μ in diameter and occasionally larger. It reproduces both in the tissues and at 37° C by the simultaneous formation, around the periphery of the cell, of several buds each about 1μ in diameter. Mycelium, conidia similar to those of *B. dermatitidis*, and arthrospores are present in cultures grown at room temperature.

The organism appears to gain access to the body mainly through the mucous membrane of the mouth or alimentary tract. It may produce local lesions on the oral mucosa and adjacent skin, lymph node involvement particularly in the neck region, or a systemic infection in which the initial lesion is usually in the ileocaecal region and in most cases involves the lungs. The source of infection is not known. Sulphonamides appear to be of therapeutic value in early cases.

Coccidioides immitis

Coccidioides immitis is a dimorphic fungus which in the body appears as a large spherule or sporangium of 15 to 70μ in diameter with a thick wall measuring about 2μ in cross section. Characteristically the spherules are filled with endospores measuring from 5 to 8μ in diameter, but some of the spherules may be immature and these do not contain spores. The fungus reproduces by bursting of the spherule thereby releasing the spores which in turn germinate into fresh spherules. In the body the parasite is found mainly within multinucleate giant cells. In culture only a mycelial form which reproduces by the formation of arthrospores is found. Cultures of *C. immitis* are extremely infectious and require very careful manipulation.

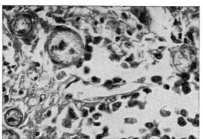

Fig. 76. Tissue Phase of *Coccidioides immitis* in Lymph Gland. Spherules containing Endospores

Coccidioidomycosis occurs as an endemic infection in certain desert areas in the south western United States, particularly in the San Joaquin Valley in California. The fungus vegetates in the soil and human infection appears in most cases to be due to inhalation of contaminated dust. The disease is not transmitted from case to case. In endemic areas it shows a maximal prevalence in the dry months of the year. It occurs in two forms: (1) A primary type usually involving the lungs, less frequently the skin. Primary pulmonary infection is frequently asymptomatic or may appear as a relatively mild upper respiratory tract infection. (2) A disseminated type known as coccidioidal granuloma. This type occurs in about 1 per cent of white individuals infected but in about

10 per cent of infected negroes and has an overall mortality of about 60 per cent. The main lesions, which are in the lungs, are granulomatous in character and are similar to those found in miliary tuberculosis. In addition to the lungs the subcutaneous tissues, skin and central nervous system are also frequently involved.

During the course of coccidioidomycosis a delayed type hypersensitivity which may be detected by the intradermal injection of coccidioidin—obtained from cultures of the fungus in fluid media—develops. The active agent in coccidioidin appears to be a polysaccharide. The skin reaction is positive in individuals with asymptomatic infection. In severe primary infections and in coccidioidal granuloma positive precipitin and complement fixation tests with coccidioidal antigen are also obtained. High titres in the complement fixation test appears to be a bad prognostic sign.

Sporotrichum schenckii

Sporotrichum schenckii is a dimorphic fungus. On Sabouraud's medium at room temperature it produces a filamentous colony with a slender branching mycelium and oval microconidia which in the early stages of growth are arranged in clusters but which later envelop the hyphae in a sheath of spores. On blood agar at 37° C the yeast phase consisting of fusiform to round budding cells is found. The fungus can rarely be seen in infected tissues. When demonstrable it appears as an oval or fusiform, frequently intracellular Gram positive organism.

Sporotrichosis is an uncommon disease of world-wide distribution. It appears first as a granulomatous ulcerated or purulent lesion of the skin. As the lesion progresses the fungus invades the lymphatic vessels which become thickened and develop subcutaneous abscesses along their course. A systemic form of sporotrichosis, frequently without an obvious primary lesion and characterized by the appearance of multiple subcutaneous nodules throughout the body, also occurs but is relatively uncommon. The fungus is present in the soil, on wood and on various plants and the localized type of infection is usually due to the contamination of wounds or abrasions from these sources. Not infrequently patients give a history of having been pricked by a thorn.

For the diagnosis of sporotrichosis, isolation of the fungus is essential. Antibodies demonstrable by the complement fixation, agglutination and precipitation tests develop during the course of the disease. Hypersensitivity to an extract of the fungus—*sporototrichin*—is also demonstrable.

Miscellaneous Fungi

Aspergillus

Aspergillus species are occasionally responsible for otomycosis, a superficial scaly infection of the skin of the external auditory meatus. They also appear to be capable of invading the lungs; this, however, is a very uncommon type of infection occurring as a rule only in patients with established pulmonary disease. Since aspergilli are common contaminants a diagnosis of aspergillosis should be made only when the organisms have been repeatedly isolated and when in addition it has not been possible to demonstrate any other pathogen.

Phialophora and Hormodendrum

Species of these closely-related genera—*H. pedrosoi, H. compactum* and *P. verrucosa*—are responsible for chromomycosis—a chronic localized granulomatous infection of the skin characterized by the appearance of small wart-like nodules which later develop into large fungating papillomatous masses. This condition occurs mainly in labourers, particularly those working with wood, the fungus invading the skin through cuts and abrasions. In the tissues the fungi occur in the form of groups of brown thick-walled spherical to oval bodies measuring about 10μ in diameter.

Piedrai hortai and Trichosporon beigelii

These fungi cause piedra—an infection of the hair characterized by the appearance of hard, black or white nodules on the hair shaft. Unlike the dermatophytes they do not invade the hair nor are they capable of dissolving keratin.

Monosporium apiospermum

This fungus is the asexual stage of an ascomycete—*Allescheria boydii*. It ranks next in importance to *Nocardia* species (Chapter 27) as a cause of mycetoma (Maduromycosis). In the tissues it occurs in the form of white to yellow granules which on microscopic examination are seen to consist of tangled fungal mycelium. A minority of cases of mycetoma are due to various saprophytic fungi.

Rhinosporidium seeberi

This organism is the cause of rhinosporidiosis—an infection of the skin and mucous membranes characterized by the development of friable, pedunculated tumour-like masses. The commonest site of infection is the anterior nares. The disease is endemic in India and Ceylon but occurs also in many other parts of the world. The fungus has not been grown in laboratory culture. In the tissues it occurs in the form of large sporangia measuring up to 300μ in diameter, resembling but considerably larger than those of *C. immitis*. When fully developed the sporangia contain large numbers of small endospores measuring from 5 to 8μ in diameter.

Malassezia furfur

This species, which has not been grown in laboratory culture, is the cause of tinea versicolor—a chronic superficial scaly infection of the skin. In the skin it appears as round budding yeast-like cells surrounded by short hyphal fragments.

Basidiobolus

This phycomycete is the commonest cause of phycomycosis, an unusual infection of the subcutaneous tissues and skin, which has so far been reported only from Indonesia and Africa. The lesions are most numerous on the limbs and consist of circumscribed granulomatous swellings. The condition responds to treatment with iodides.

The fungus consists of large branching septate hyphae which frequently appear empty. It grows well on Sabouraud's medium and on blood agar. It may be identified by its characteristic zygospores, which are demonstrable in culture after about a week.

APPENDIX

SCHEDULE PROPOSED FOR IMMUNIZATION OF CHILDREN
Schedule P (Modified), Ministry of Health, London (1963)

Age	Visit	Vaccine	Injection	Interval
1 to 6 months	1	Diphtheria, tetanus, pertussis	1	4 to 6 weeks
	2	Diphtheria, tetanus, pertussis	2	4 to 6 weeks
	3	Diphtheria, tetanus, pertussis	3	
7 to 11 months	4	Poliomyelitis (oral)	—	4 to 8 weeks
	5	Poliomyelitis (oral)	—	4 to 8 weeks
	6	Poliomyelitis (oral)	—	
18 to 21 months	7	Diphtheria, tetanus, pertussis	4	

Measles immunization recommended during the second year (1968)
Smallpox during the first two years, preferably in the second year

School entry[a]	Diphtheria and tetanus
8 to 12 years	Diphtheria and tetanus
	Smallpox revaccination
Over 12 years	BCG[b]

[a] All immunized children joining school should be offered a reinforcing dose of poliovirus vaccine.
[b] This timing of BCG immunization is acceptable for communities with a low incidence of tuberculosis. In communities with a high tuberculosis incidence BCG should be given in the neo-natal period.

In an alternative schedule (Q) three doses of oral polio vaccine are given between the 6th and 10th months. These are followed by two doses of triple vaccine (diphtheria, tetanus, pertussis) between the 11th and 13th months and a reinforcing dose of triple vaccine between the 18th and 21st months. Thereafter the procedure is as in Schedule P.

SUGGESTIONS FOR FURTHER READING

GENERAL

BULLOCH, W. (1938) *History of Bacteriology.* Oxford University Press

DUBOS, R. J. & HIRSCH, J. G. EDS (1965) *Bacterial and Mycotic Infections of Man.* 4th ed. London: Pitman Medical

HORSFALL, F. L. & TAMM, I. EDS (1965) *Viral and Rickettsial Infections of Man.* 4th ed. Philadelphia: Lippincott

MOSS, E. G. & McQUOWN, A. L. (1960) *Atlas of Medical Mycology.* London: Baillière, Tindall & Cox

WATERSON, A. P. ED. (1967) *Recent Advances in Medical Microbiology.* London: Churchill

WILSON, G. S. & MILES, A. A. (1964) *Topley and Wilson's Principles of Bacteriology and Immunity.* 5th ed. London: Arnold

GENERAL PROPERTIES OF BACTERIA

BRIEGER, E. M. (1963) *Structure and Ultrastructure in Micro-organisms.* London: Academic Press

BRITISH MEDICAL BULLETIN (1965) *Recent Research in Molecular Biology.* Vol. *21*, No. 3

GUNSALUS, I. G. & STANIER, R. Y. (1962) *The Physiology of Growth.* Vol. 4 of *The Bacteria.* London: Academic Press

HAYES, W. (1964) *The Genetics of Bacteria and Their Viruses.* Oxford: Blackwell Scientific Publications

ROSE, A. H. (1965) *Chemical Microbiology.* London: Butterworths

SALTON, M. R. J. (1964) *The Bacterial Cell Wall.* Barking, Essex: Elsevier

15TH SYMPOSIUM OF THE SOCIETY FOR GENERAL MICROBIOLOGY (1965) *Function and Structure in Micro-organisms.* Cambridge University Press

TECHNICAL METHODS

ACKROYD, J. F. ED. (1964) *Immunological Methods.* Oxford: Blackwell Scientific Publications

BUSBY, D. W. G., HOUSE, W. & McDONALD, J. R. (1964) *Virological Technique.* London: Churchill

COLLINS, C. H. ED. (1967) *Progress in Microbiological Techniques.* London: Butterworths

COWAN, S. T. & STEEL, K. J. (1965) *Manual for the Identification of Medical Bacteria.* Cambridge University Press

CRUICKSHANK, R. ED. (1968) *Medical Microbiology.* 11th ed. Edinburgh: Livingstone

MEYNELL, G. G. & MEYNELL, ELINOR (1965) *Theory and Practice in Experimental Bacteriology.* Cambridge University Press

STOKES, JOAN (1960) *Clinical Bacteriology.* 2nd ed. London: Arnold

ANTIMICROBIAL AGENTS

BARBER, MARY & GARROD, L. P. (1963) *Antibiotic and Chemotherapy.* Edinburgh: Livingstone

BARRY, V. C. ED. (1964) *Chemotherapy of Tuberculosis.* London: Butterworths

DATTA, NAOMI (1965) Infectious drug resistance. *Brit. med. Bull.,* Vol. *21*, No. 3

GINOZA, W. (1967) The effects of ionizing radiation on nucleic acids of bacteriophages and bacterial cells. *Ann. Rev. Microbiol.,* Vol. *21*

REEVES, P. (1965) Bacteriocines. *Bacteriol. Rev.,* Vol. *29*, No. 1

STEWART, G. T. (1965) *The Penicillin Group of Drugs.* Barking, Essex: Elsevier

SYKES, G. (1958) *Disinfection and Sterilization*. London: Spon
16TH SYMPOSIUM OF THE SOCIETY FOR GENERAL MICROBIOLOGY (1966) *Biochemical Studies of Antimicrobial Drugs*. Cambridge University Press

INDIVIDUAL BACTERIA

ELEK, S. D. (1959) Staphylococcus pyogenes *and its Relation to Disease*. Edinburgh: Livingstone
HAYFLICK, L. & CHANOCK, R. M. (1965) Mycoplasma species of man. *Bacteriol. Rev.*, Vol. *29*, No. 2
KLIENEBERGER-NOBEL, E. (1962) *Pleuropneumonia-like Organisms. Mycoplasmataceae.* London: Academic Press
MOULDER, J. W. (1964) *The Psittacosis Group as Bacteria* (CIBA Lectures). London: John Wiley
SOWA, S., SOWA, J., COLLIER, L. H. & BLYTH, W. (1965) Trachoma and allied infections in a Gambian village. *Med. Res. Counc. spec. Rep. Ser.*, *308*, H.M.S.O.
TURNER, T. B. & HOLLANDER, D. H. (1957) *The Biology of the Treponematoses*. Geneva: World Health Organization

EPIDEMIOLOGY AND PATHOGENESIS

BURNET, F. M. (1962) *The Natural History of Infectious Disease*. 3rd ed. Cambridge University Press.
14TH SYMPOSIUM OF THE SOCIETY FOR GENERAL MICROBIOLOGY (1964) *Microbial Behaviour in vivo and in vitro*. Cambridge University Press
WILLIAMS, R. E. O. & SHOOTER, R. A. EDS (1963) *Infection in Hospitals*. Symp. Council int. Org. med. Sci. Oxford: Blackwell Scientific Publications

IMMUNOLOGY

BRITISH JOURNAL OF CLINICAL PRACTICE (1963) *Symposium on Immunology*. Vol. *17*, No. 11
BRITISH MEDICAL BULLETIN (1965) *Transplantation of Tissues and Antigens*. Vol. *12*, No. 2
BRITISH MEDICAL BULLETIN (1967) *Delayed Hypersensitivity*. Vol. *23*, No. 1
CHERRY, W. B. & MOODY, M. D. (1965) Fluorescent antibody techniques in bacteriology. *Bacteriol. Rev.*, Vol. *29*, No. 2
CIBA SYMPOSIUM (1965) *Complement*. London: Churchill
CRUICKSHANK, R. ED. (1963) *Modern Trends in Immunology 1*. London: Butterworths
CRUICKSHANK, R. & WEIR, D. M. EDS (1967) *Modern Trends in Immunology 2*. London: Butterworths
GELL, P. G. H. & COOMBS, R. R. A. EDS. (1963) *Clinical Aspects of Immunology*. Oxford: Blackwell Scientific Publications
GLYNN, L. E. (1965) *Auto-Immunity and Disease*. Oxford: Blackwell Scientific Publications
HUMPHREY, J. H. & White, R. G. (1964) *Immunology for Students of Medicine*. 2nd ed. Oxford: Blackwell Scientific Publications
KABAT, E. A. & MAYER, M. M. (1961) *Experimental Immunochemistry*. 2nd ed. Springfield: Thomas
LUDERITZ, O., STAUB, A. M. & WESTPHAL, O. (1966) Immunochemistry of O and R antigens of *Salmonella* and related enterobacteriaceae. *Bacteriol. Rev.*, Vol. *30*, No. 1
PARISH, H. J. & CANNON, D. A. (1962) *Antisera, Toxoids, Vaccines and Tuberculins*. Edinburgh: Livingstone
PIKE, R. M. (1967) Antibody heterogeneity and serological reactions. *Bacteriol. Rev.*, Vol. *31*, No. 2
PORTER, R. R. (1967) Structure of immunoglobulins. In *Essays in Biochemistry*. No. 3. London: Academic Press
STERZL, J., RIHA, J. & JAROŠKOVÁ, L. EDS (1965) *Molecular and Cellular Basis of Antibody Formation*. London: Academic Press
WILSON, G. S. (1967) *The Hazards of Immunization*. London: Athlone Press

VIROLOGY

BRADLEY, D. E. (1967) Ultrastructure of bacteriophages and bacteriocines. *Bacteriol Rev.*, Vol. *31*, No. 4

BRITISH MEDICAL BULLETIN (1967) *Aspects of Medical Virology*. Vol. *23*, No. 2.

CIBA SYMPOSIUM (1964) *Cellular Biology of Myxovirus Infections*. London: Churchill

COLD SPRING HARBOUR SYMPOSIUM ON QUANTITATIVE BIOLOGY (1962) *Basic Mechanisms in Animal Virus Biology*

JOKLIK, W. K. (1966) Pox viruses. *Bacteriol. Rev.*, Vol. *30*, No. 1

STENT, G. S. (1963) *Molecular Biology of Bacterial Viruses*. London: Freeman

18TH SYMPOSIUM OF THE SOCIETY FOR GENERAL MICROBIOLOGY (1968) *Molecular Biology of Viruses*. Cambridge University Press

TYRRELL, D. A. J. (1965) *Common Colds and Related Diseases*. London: Arnold

WILSON-SMITH, W. ED. (1963) *Mechanisms of Virus Infection*. London: Academic Press

INDEX

Abortion, 348, 524
Acetyl choline, 388, 392
Acetyl methyl carbinol, 22, 227
Acid-fast bacilli, 353
Acids, antibacterial action of, 62
Acquired immunity, 153, 443
Acridines, 68, 194
ACTH, 108
Actinobacillus actinomycetemcomitans, 374
  mallei, 375
  lignieresii, 374
Actinomyces israeli, 373
Actinomycetes, 3, 373
Actinomycin D, 109, 194, 428
Actinomycosis, 374
Acute glomerulonephritis, 187, 258
Acute rheumatism, 258
Acute ulcerative gingivitis, 402
Adamantanamine, 431
Adaptation, 196
Adeno-satellite virus, 521
Adenosine triphosphate (ATP), 21, 533
Adenoviruses, 422, 520
Adenylosuccinic acid, 193
Adjuvants, 110, 161, 501
Aedes aegypti, 87, 467
  africanus, 87, 469
  simpsonii, 87, 469
Aerobes, 19
Aerosols, 89
Agammaglobulinanaemia, 123, 444
Agar, 41
Agglutination, 128
  lysis test, 412
  test, 229
Aggressins, 76
Aggressiveness, 75
Agranulocytosis, 151
Air, filtration of, 60
Alastrim, 481
Alcohol, antibacterial action of, 67
Alcoholism, 151

Alkalies, antibacterial action of, 62
Allescheria boydii, 585
Allosteric proteins, 32
Allotypes, 102
Alum, 161
Amantadine, 431
Amoebic dysentery, 321
Amphotericin B, 572
Anaemia, haemolytic, 126, 384
Anaerobic bacteria, 19, 44, 224, 299, 386
  streptococci, 262
Anamnestic reactions, 108
Anaphylactoid reactions, 172
Anaphylaxis, 168, 173
Aniline dyes, antibacterial action of, 68
Animals, as sources of infection, 84
Antagonism between drugs, 202
Anthrax, 278
Antibacterial drugs, 189
Antibiogram, 206
Antibiotics, 189
Antibodies, properties of, 99
Antigens, properties of, 92
  distribution of, 95
Antiglobulin test, 130, 231, 312, 350
Antihistamines, 172, 175, 177
Antilymphocyte serum, 118, 183
Antistreptolysin O, 141, 256
Antitoxin, 106, 141, 154, 165
Apo-repressor, 32
Appendicitis, 295, 336
APT, 110, 288
Arboviruses, 422, 463
Arizona, 317
Arsenicals, organic, 178, 408
Arthritis, 272, 274, 379, 382
Arthropod vectors, 87, 463
Arthrospores, 570, 577
Arthus reaction, 176, 259
Ascoli's test, 280
Asian influenza, 494
Aspartokinase, 32

591